Emergency Drug Therapy

WILLIAM G. BARSAN, M.D.
Associate Professor
Department of Emergency Medicine
University of Cincinnati Medical Center
Cincinnati, Ohio

MICHAEL S. JASTREMSKI, M.D.
Professor and
Director of Program in
Critical Care and Emergency Medicine
SUNY Health Science Center at Syracuse
Syracuse, New York

SCOTT A. SYVERUD, M.D.
Assistant Professor
Department of Emergency Medicine
University of Cincinnati Medical Center
Cincinnati, Ohio

1991
W.B. SAUNDERS COMPANY
Harcourt Brace Jovanovich, Inc.
Philadelphia
London   Toronto   Montreal   Sydney   Tokyo

W. B. SAUNDERS COMPANY
Harcourt Brace Jovanovich, Inc.

The Curtis Center
Independence Square West
Philadelphia, PA 19106-3399

Library of Congress Cataloging-in-Publication Data

Emergency drug therapy / [edited by] William G. Barsan,
    Scott A. Syverud, Michael S. Jastremski.
        p.   cm.
    Includes index.
    ISBN 0-7216-2584-3
    1. Emergency medicine.   2. Chemotherapy.   I. Barsan,
William G.   II. Syverud, Scott A.   III. Jastremski,
Michael S.
    [DNLM: 1. Drug Therapy.   2. Emergencies.   WB 105
E5327]
RC86.7.E5655   1991
616.02′5—dc20
DNLM/DLC   90-8657

Editor: Darlene Pedersen
Developmental Editor: Lawrence J. McGrew
Designer: Dorothy Chattin
Production Manager: Bill Preston
Manuscript Editor: Tina Rebane
Illustration Coordinator: Brett MacNaughton
Indexer: Helene Taylor
Cover Designer: Karen O'Keefe

Emergency Drug Therapy   ISBN 0-7216-2584-3

Last digit is the print number: 9   8   7   6   5   4   3   2   1

To Mary, David, Blake, and Anna for their continued love, support, and understanding during the production of this book.

WGB

To all the students that I've taught over the years.

MSJ

To Janet, Geraldine, and Lauren Syverud for their love and support during my continuing education.

SAS

Contributors

William G. Barsan, M.D.
Associate Professor, Department of Emergency Medicine, University of Cincinnati College of Medicine; Attending Physician, University of Cincinnati Hospital, Cincinnati, Ohio
Respiratory Drugs; Anticoagulants and Thrombolytics

Michelle H. Biros, M.S., M.D.
Senior Associate Staff Physician, Department of Emergency Medicine, Hennepin County Medical Center, Minneapolis, Minnesota
Anticonvulsants

Bryan Blackwelder, Pharm.D.
Clinical Assistant Professor, College of Pharmacy, University of Florida Health Science Center/Jacksonville; Pediatric Practitioner, Department of Pharmacy, University Medical Center, Jacksonville, Florida
Considerations in the Dosing of Pediatric Patients

Steven C. Carleton, M.D., Ph.D.
Chief Resident, Department of Emergency Medicine, University of Cincinnati College of Medicine, Cincinnati, Ohio
Endocrine and Miscellaneous Agents

Lynnette Doan-Wiggins, M.D., FACEP
Assistant Professor of Medicine, Loyola University Stritch School of Medicine; Associate Director, Emergency Department, Loyola University Medical Center, Maywood, Illinois
Drug Therapy During Pregnancy and Lactation; Obstetric and Gynecologic Emergency Drug Therapy

Steven C. Dronen, M.D.
Associate Professor of Emergency Medicine, University of Cincinnati College of Medicine; Staff Physician, University of Cincinnati Hospital, Cincinnati, Ohio
Plasma and Volume Expanders

Susan M. Dunmire, M.D., FACEP
Assistant Professor of Medicine, Division of Emergency Medicine, University of Pittsburgh School of Medicine; Attending Physician and Academic Coordinator, Emergency Department, Presbyterian–University Hospital, Pittsburgh, Pennsylvania
Analgesics

Frederick B. Epstein, M.D., FACEP
Assistant Clinical Professor of Surgery and Emergency Medicine, University of Florida College of Medicine, Gainesville; Director, Department of Emergency Medicine, Bay Medical Center, Panama City, Florida
Endocrine and Miscellaneous Agents

Douglas Evans, M.D.
Assistant Instructor, Department of Ophthalmology, State University of New York Health Science Center at Syracuse, Syracuse, New York; Captain, United States Air Force Ophthalmology Clinic, Lakenheath, Great Britain
Ophthalmic Agents

John I. Gerson, M.D.
Associate Professor, Department of Anesthesiology, State University of New York Health Science Center at Syracuse, Syracuse, New York
Injected Anesthetics

v

W. Brian Gibler, M.D., FACEP
Assistant Professor of Emergency Medicine, Department of Emergency Medicine, University of Cincinnati College of Medicine; Attending Emergency Physician, Department of Emergency Medicine and Center for Emergency Care, University of Cincinnati Hospital, Cincinnati, Ohio
Antiarrhythmics

John Hoepner, M.D.
Chairman, Department of Ophthalmology, State University of New York Health Science Center at Syracuse, Syracuse, New York
Ophthalmic Agents

Michael S. Jastremski, M.D.
Associate Professor, State University of New York Health Science Center at Syracuse; Director of Program in Critical Care and Emergency Medicine, University Hospital, Syracuse, New York
Antihypertensives

Louis J. Ling, M.D.
Medical Director, Hennepin Regional Poison Center; Assistant Director, Emergency Medicine Residency Program, Hennepin County Medical Center, Minneapolis, Minnesota
Antidotes

Mariane McLaughlin, Pharm.D.
Clinical Coordinator, Pharmacy Department, University Hospital, State University of New York Health Science Center at Syracuse, Syracuse, New York
Basic Clinical Pharmacokinetics

Edward J. Otten, M.D.
Associate Professor, University of Cincinnati College of Medicine; Director of Prehospital Care, University of Cincinnati Hospital, Cincinnati, Ohio
Antivenins and Antitoxins

Paul M. Paris, M.D., FACEP
Associate Professor and Chief, Division of Emergency Medicine, University of Pittsburgh School of Medicine; Chief, Division of Emergency Medicine, Presbyterian–University Hospital; Attending, Children's Hospital of Pittsburgh, Western Pennsylvania Hospital, and Mercy Hospital, Pittsburgh, Pennsylvania
Analgesics

Leo C. Rotello, M.D.
Assistant Professor, Program in Critical Care and Emergency Medicine, State University of New York Health Science Center at Syracuse, Syracuse, New York
Osmotic Agents

Charles E. Saunders, M.D., FACP
Associate Professor of Clinical Medicine, University of California, San Francisco; Director, Paramedic Division, Department of Health, City and County of San Francisco; Attending Physician, Emergency Services, San Francisco General Hospital, San Francisco, California
Vasoactive Agents

Daniel L. Savitt, M.D.
Assistant Clinical Professor of Surgery, Brown University; Attending Physician, Department of Emergency Medicine, Rhode Island Hospital, Providence, Rhode Island
Therapeutic Gases

Jay L. Schauben, Pharm.D., FABAT
Clinical Associate Professor, College of Pharmacy and Division of Emergency Medicine, College of Medicine, University of Florida Health Science Center/Jacksonville; Director, Clinical Toxicology Services, University Medical Center, Jacksonville, Florida
Considerations in the Dosing of Pediatric Patients

Clifton A. Sheets, M.D., FACEP
Assistant Clinical Professor, Wright State University; Attending Physician, Miami Valley Hospital, Dayton, Ohio
Emetics and Antiemetics

Bonita Singal, M.D.
Assistant Professor, Department of Emergency Medicine, Wright State University; Attending Physician, Good Samaritan Hospital, Dayton, Ohio
Acidifying and Alkalizing Agents

Mark S. Smith, M.D.
Professor and Chairman, Department of Emergency Medicine, George Washington University Medical Center, Washington, D.C.
Anticoagulants and Thrombolytics

William H. Spivey, M.D.
Associate Professor and Chief, Division of Research, Department of Emergency Medicine, Medical College of Pennsylvania, Philadelphia, Pennsylvania
Routes of Drug Administration

Scott A. Syverud, M.D.
Assistant Professor, Department of Emergency Medicine, University of Cincinnati College of Medicine, Cincinnati, Ohio; Attending Physician, University of Cincinnati Hospital, Cincinnati, Ohio, and St. Luke West Hospital, Florence, Kentucky
Muscle Relaxants

Thomas E. Terndrup, M.D.
Assistant Professor, Critical Care and Emergency Medicine and Pediatrics, State University of New York Health Science Center at Syracuse; Attending Physician, Emergency Department, and Research Director, Emergency Medicine, University Hospital, Syracuse, New York
Sedative-Hypnotics

Alexander Trott, M.D.
Associate Professor, Department of Emergency Medicine, University of Cincinnati College of Medicine; Attending Physician, University of Cincinnati Hospital, Cincinnati, Ohio
Antimicrobials

Peter Van Ligten, M.D.
Assistant Professor, Department of Emergency Medicine, Ohio State University, Columbus, Ohio
Endocrine and Miscellaneous Agents

Jonathan Warren, M.D.
Assistant Professor, Critical Care and Emergency Medicine and Medicine, State University of New York Health Science Center at Syracuse; Attending Physician, University Hospital, Syracuse, New York
Fluid and Electrolyte Therapy

Preface

All physicians involved in the care of acutely ill patients are faced with decisions regarding drug therapy. When treating a common condition with which one has extensive experience, the choice of drug therapy is usually not difficult. Problems can arise (1) when treating uncommonly encountered conditions, (2) when treating commonly encountered conditions in patients who have unusual characteristics (e.g., pregnancy, liver failure), and (3) when standard therapy is not having the desired therapeutic effect and more intensive (and possibly less familiar) therapy is needed. This text is designed to lend guidance and give solid guidelines and dosing information for the tough cases, although it will also be useful when treating the easy cases.

Typically, when one encounters a condition with which one has had little experience, an expert can be consulted for help. There are, however, emergent situations where treatment must be given and expert help is not immediately available. In these cases, one may consult several different texts for information regarding the diagnosis, indications for treatment, and actual dosage and method of drug administration. However, specific indications and end-points for drug treatment are often difficult to find in standard texts. It is also frequently difficult to decide what to do next when your first drug choice does not have the desired effect. We have attempted to address these issues in one text so that the physician does not have to consult several different references and *still* be in doubt as to the next step.

Chapters 1 through 4 discuss the basics of drug therapy and special considerations that affect drug therapy. Chapters 5 to 26 discuss specific drug types. Each of these chapters first lists **Conditions** for which treatment with the type of drug is indicated. The text for each condition is divided into **Diagnosis, Indications for Treatment, a Drug Treatment Outline,** and **Discussion.** The **Diagnosis** section is not meant to be a complete discussion of the condition, but rather an attempt to point out the salient differential features of that condition or to hit the high points in diagnosis. The **Indications** section gives *specific* indications for drug treatment for each condition. When specific indications are unclear, this section will usually present a consensus opinion. Although not all authorities will agree with all the specific indications for treatment given in this book, we anticipate that our recommendations represent a majority view. This text gives very specific criteria for treatment with different drugs.

The **Drug Treatment Outline** provides a quick reference for initial dosage, repeat dosage, end-points, and second- and third-line treatment for each condition discussed. These outlines can be used alone, especially when a fast answer is needed, or with the textual material. Significant cautions are usually listed in the outlines (e.g., pretreat children with atropine prior to succinylcholine use). Although the outlines make more sense when used with the text, they can also stand alone.

The **Discussion** section gives a brief rationale for the preferred use of one drug over another and offers tips and advice based on clinical experience. The discussion section fills in any gaps not covered in the drug treatment outline.

At the end of each chapter, each drug covered in the chapter is outlined separately under the heading **Specific Agents.** Information on distribution, elimination, and dosing is given, as is information on toxicity and treatment of toxicity. Dosing adjustments for organ failure and Food and Drug Administration categories for use in pregnancy are given for each drug.

It is important to understand that this book addresses, for the most part, only *emergency* drug therapy, and, more specifically, parenteral drug therapy. The outpatient treatment of nonemergent conditions is not covered in most instances. Drug treatment that needs to be given within the first 1 to 2 hours, and often within the first 1 to 2 minutes, is under the purview of this text. Hence, this book is written for those physicians who deal with such conditions. Physicians involved in the day-to-day care of critically ill patients will find useful information, as will the clinician who only occasionally deals with critically ill patients. To reflect this wide audience, the contributors to this text range from intensivists to ophthalmologists, anesthesiologists, emergency physicians, and pediatric pharmacologists.

We have attempted to be up to date with our drug selections, but the lag time between writing and final publication always ensures that something will be out of date by the time of publication. This is especially true in a technologically advanced area like drug treatment. We hope, however, that the reader will find this book useful not only when decisions must be made rapidly, but also when time is available to read in more detail. If this book can be used to enhance patient care in critical situations and at the same time be user friendly, our goal for this text will have been reached.

William G. Barsan, M.D.
Michael S. Jastremski, M.D.
Scott A. Syverud, M.D.

Contents

CHAPTER 1

Basic Clinical Pharmacokinetics

MARIANE McLAUGHLIN, PHARM.D.

Over the past 20 years the science of clinical pharmacokinetics has evolved from simple observation of how a drug is handled by the body to complex monitoring of drug concentration on an individual patient basis. The many advances made in this discipline apply to the relatively small number of pharmacologic agents for which a relationship between serum concentration and desired (or adverse) effect has been established. In general, a basic knowledge of pharmacokinetic principles has become a necessity to the clinician in order to effectively initiate and adjust the dosage regimens of patients receiving pharmacologic treatment. This chapter addresses pharmacokinetic principles, individual variability, and drug concentration monitoring. The pharmacokinetic information presented here is introductory, and the reader is referred to the pharmacokinetics texts in the References following this chapter for more detailed information. Specific pharmacologic agents are addressed in subsequent chapters.

Pharmacokinetics is defined as the time course of drug absorption, distribution, metabolism, and excretion. The effect of these functions on drug concentration is of major importance because an alteration in any one of them has the capacity to drastically change the concentration of active drug reaching its receptor site. In addition, the dosage form itself can delay or enhance drug entry into the systemic circulation. A separate discipline known as biopharmaceutics is devoted to the study of product formulation and its effect on the release and absorption of the active drug. Yet another discipline, pharmacodynamics, is concerned with the study of biochemical and physiologic effects of drugs, or, in other words, their mechanism of action. Last, clinical pharmacokinetics is the science that relates the biopharmaceutic, pharmacokinetic, and pharmacodynamic information to patient care (Fig. 1–1).

LADME

The acronym LADME, which stands for *l*iberation, *a*bsorption, *d*istribution, *m*etabolism, and *e*xcretion, is used to represent the pharmacokinetic processes that occur after administration of a medication. *Liberation* refers to the release of the active drug from the dosage form following oral administration. *Absorption* is defined as the transfer of the drug from the site of administration to the general circulation. *Distribution* refers to the movement of the drug from the circulation to various body fluids and tissues. *Metabolism* is defined as the biotransformation of the drug, usually to inactive, excretable forms. *Excretion* is the elimination of the

1

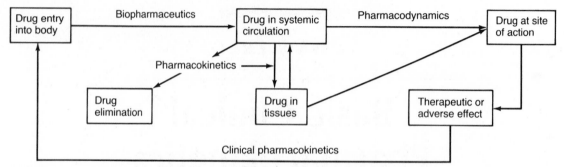

FIGURE 1–1. Interrelationship of biopharmaceutics, pharmacodynamics, pharmacokinetics, and clinical pharmacokinetics.

drug by the kidneys, bile, or lungs, in active or inactive forms.

The effect of these functions on drug concentrations is easily demonstrated using concentration versus time curves. Figure 1–2 represents the changes in serum drug concentration, as effected by LADME, following a single oral dose of a drug.

LIBERATION AND ABSORPTION

Liberation refers to the disintegration of the dosage form of the drug in the gastrointestinal (GI) tract and subsequent dissolution

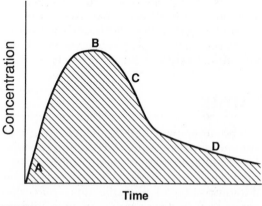

FIGURE 1–2. Graph representing changes in serum drug concentration following a single oral dose of a drug. Section *A* represents the initial absorption of the drug, resulting in increasing serum concentrations. Section *B* reflects the combination of continuing absorption and distribution; thus the serum concentration tends to level off as absorption decreases and distribution commences. Section *C* represents continued distribution and initiation of elimination. Finally, in Section *D*, all other functions are completed, and the concentration versus time curve reflects only elimination. The area under the curve (AUC) represents the total amount of drug reaching the systemic circulation (*shaded area*).

of the active drug in GI fluids. It is generally considered after oral administration of tablets and capsules. Once the drug is released from the dosage form and is in solution, it can be absorbed. Liberation and absorption can be altered by patient factors and/or product formulation factors. Product formulation plays a critical role in these processes, since it can cause changes in the rate and/or extent of absorption and thus ultimately affects the serum concentrations achieved.

Problems with formulation can result in a detrimental decrease in serum concentration due to poor tablet disintegration, binding of the active drug to inert ingredients, and other such factors. However, many benefits are also gained from altered product formulation, such as those provided by the many sustained-release dosage forms developed over the past 10 years. Physiologic factors also have an important role in drug liberation and absorption. Factors such as GI motility, pH of GI fluids, disease states, and food and drug interactions can affect drug liberation and absorption.

RATE AND EXTENT OF ABSORPTION

The rate of absorption of a drug directly affects the peak concentration attained. A drug that is absorbed quickly will attain its peak concentration earlier than a drug that is absorbed more slowly. Figure 1–3 represents the concentration versus time curves of two formulations of the same drug, administered at the same dosage. Formulation *A* is rapidly absorbed and attains a high peak concentration (C_{max}) at 1 hour after administration. Formulation *B* is absorbed more slowly and therefore has a lower C_{max} and a greater time to reach that C_{max}. However, the sys-

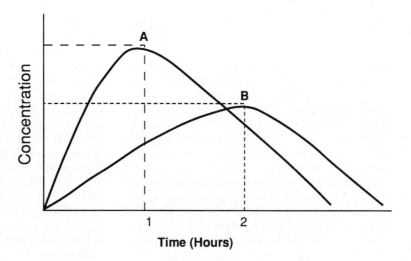

FIGURE 1–3. Effect of the rate of absorption on the concentration versus time curve. Formulation *A* is rapidly absorbed and attains a high peak concentration (or C_{max}) at 1 hour after administration. Formulation *B* is absorbed more slowly and therefore has a lower C_{max} and a greater time to reach that C_{max}. However, the systemic availability of the two formulations, as reflected by the AUC, is identical.

temic availability of the two formulations, as reflected by the AUC, is identical.

Alterations in the rate of absorption can become clinically significant when a minimum concentration must be attained in order for the drug to elicit its desired effect. In such a case, a rapidly absorbed formulation, such as formulation A in Figure 1–3, might be more desirable. In general, changes in the extent of absorption have more clinical significance than do changes in the rate of absorption because they can cause the amount of drug in the body to vary greatly. Figure 1–4 represents the concentration versus time curves of two formulations of the same drug, with equal dosages and equal rates of absorption. However, formulation D is not completely absorbed and therefore may not reach the minimally effective concentration. In addition, the AUCs of the two formulations in Figure 1–4 are quite different.

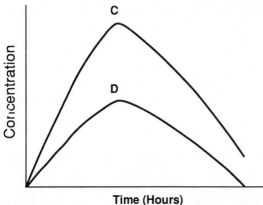

FIGURE 1–4. Effect of the extent of absorption on the concentration versus time curve.

BIOAVAILABILITY

Bioavailability is defined as the rate and extent of drug movement from the site of administration to the systemic circulation. Drugs administered intravascularly are used as a reference point, since 100% of the dose reaches the systemic circulation. The bioavailability of drugs given by other routes of administration is generally less than 100% and reflects the effect of numerous factors on the drug and its dosage form. For example, the bioavailability of medications administered orally reflects the liberation of drug from the dosage form, absorption across the gastrointestinal mucosa, and the effect of hepatic first-pass metabolism (discussed in the following section). In addition, drug solubility, gastric pH, gastric emptying time, intestinal motility, disease states, and interacting substances may all affect a drug's bioavailability. The cumulative effect of all these factors is conveniently reflected numerically as the bioavailable fraction, or f. Drugs administered intravascularly have a bioavailable fraction of one (1), since the entire dose is systemically available, whereas drugs administered extravascularly generally have a bioavailability of less than 100% and a bioavailable fraction of less than one.

HEPATIC FIRST-PASS METABOLISM

Hepatic first-pass metabolism refers to the biotransformation of active drug by the liver prior to the drug's reaching the systemic circulation. Before reaching the systemic circulation, blood from the gastrointestinal tract empties into the portal vein and subsequently into the liver. Any orally administered drug that is subject to hepatic metabolism may have decreased bioavailability as a result of this phenomenon. Medications that exhibit first-pass metabolism generally have a large difference between effective oral and intravenous (IV) doses. Examples of such drugs are propranolol, verapamil, hydralazine, and terbutaline.

Hepatic first-pass metabolism can be expressed numerically by using the hepatic extraction ratio, or E, which is equal to the fraction of the absorbed dose that is metabolized during each pass through the liver. The fraction of drug escaping first-pass metabolism is referred to as $(1 - E)$. The hepatic extraction ratio can also be used to calculate the bioavailable fraction, using the following equation:

$$f = \text{fraction absorbed} \times (1 - E)$$

For example, if 90% of a drug is absorbed after oral administration, and 20% of the absorbed dose is metabolized during first pass, the bioavailable fraction is 0.72. This means that 72% of the dose administered reaches the systemic circulation, or f × the dose.

DISTRIBUTION/VOLUME OF DISTRIBUTION

Once the drug reaches the systemic circulation, it mixes in the plasma, binds to erythrocytes and plasma proteins, and diffuses from the plasma to other body fluids and tissues. The plasma and rapidly equilibrating tissues are referred to as the *central compartment*. Any movement of drug from this central compartment to peripheral or more slowly equilibrating tissues is known as *distribution*. The term *volume of distribution* (Vd) is useful in relating the peak concentration and the dose of drug, as noted in Equation 1.

$$\text{Equation 1: } C_{max} = \frac{\text{dose}}{\text{Vd}}$$

The Vd does *not* represent an anatomic moiety but rather the volume of serum that would be required to accommodate all of the drug present in the body, *if* it were present in all tissues at the same concentration at which it is present in the serum or plasma.

(Vd is expressed in liters/kilogram [l/kg]). Equation 1 is useful for calculating the initial drug dosage for patients if the population average for Vd of the drug is known. For example, if you are giving a loading dose of gentamicin and know that the average Vd is 0.22 l/kg, and your patient weighs 80 kg, then you could calculate the dose required to attain the peak concentration you desire. If you wanted a peak concentration of 8 mg/liter, in this case the loading dose would be 140 mg. This equation, however, is only valid if the dose of drug is administered by IV bolus injection, and if the patient has no pathologic condition that could alter the Vd. Equation 1 can be modified to estimate concentrations of orally administered medications by including the bioavailable fraction (f) as in Equation 2.

$$\text{Equation 2: } C_{max} = f \times \frac{\text{dose}}{\text{Vd}}$$

The two major factors that can alter the Vd of a drug are a change in the medium in which it is distributed and a change in its protein binding. In the case of water-soluble medications, which are primarily distributed in extracellular fluids (ECF), any disease state or condition resulting in a change in the ECF volume alters the Vd. Examples include dehydration, which generally results in a decreased volume of drug distribution, and congestive heart failure, liver disease, ascites, and iatrogenic fluid overload, all of which result in an increased Vd. The Vd of lipid-soluble drugs is not as easily altered, but obesity is one factor that can cause a large increase in their Vd.

Any change in the plasma or tissue protein binding of a drug has the potential to alter the Vd of that drug and subsequently the serum concentration. Drugs that are highly bound to plasma proteins usually have a low Vd, whereas drugs primarily bound to tissue proteins have a high Vd. Displacement of the drug from plasma proteins by other drugs or endogenous substances results in an increased free or unbound concentration that is available for elimination or distribution to other tissues. This elevation in the free concentration is generally transient, since the body will redistribute or eliminate the excess free drug in an effort to reattain the pre-displacement equilibrium. If other distribution sites are available, the drug may be shunted there, resulting in an increased Vd and a decrease in the serum concentration. If no other distribution sites are available, the Vd will be decreased and the serum concentration may increase. In the latter case, the increase in the concentration is followed by an increased elimination of the free or unbound drug, so the elevation in the serum concentration is usually transient. Any change in the Vd, such as those described, affects the serum concentration, as shown by Equations 1 and 2. Drug displacement from protein binding sites is discussed further in the section entitled Drug Interactions.

ELIMINATION

Drugs are eliminated from the body by excretion or metabolism. Excretion involves primarily the kidney, but the biliary tract and the lungs are other possible sites of drug excretion. The major site of drug metabolism is the liver, although drug-metabolizing enzymes are found in other tissues. The metabolites formed during biotransformation in the liver are often excreted renally.

Drug elimination can be expressed numerically in terms of the elimination rate constant, half-life, or body clearance. The elimination rate constant (k_e) equals the fraction of the drug eliminated in a given time period and is most commonly expressed in units of inverse hours (hr^{-1}). For example, if the k_e of a drug is 0.15 hr^{-1}, then 15% of the total amount of that drug in the body is eliminated in 1 hour. The k_e of a drug demonstrating linear or first-order kinetics can be determined in several ways. Graphic determination of the k_e involves plotting serum con-

centration data on a semi-log plot, as shown in Figure 1–5. Two concentrations and time data points from the terminal or elimination phase of the concentration versus time curve are then used to calculate the slope of the line.

With the data from Figure 1–5, the k_e can be calculated using Equations 3 and 4. These equations apply to drugs exhibiting linear or first-order kinetics, in which the rate of drug elimination is proportional to the concentration of drug in the serum and the half-life of the drug is independent of the concentration.

Equation 3: $Slope = \dfrac{(\log C_1 - \log C_2)}{T_1 - T_2}$
Where C_1 and C_2 and T_1 and T_2 are the first and second concentration plus time data points

Equation 4: $k_e = (-slope) \times 2.303$

For example, if $C_1 = 10$ µg/ml, $C_2 = 5$ µg/ml, $T_1 = 2$ hours, and $T_2 = 3$ hours, then the slope equals -0.30 hr^{-1} and thus k_e equals 0.69 hr^{-1}. Therefore, 69% of this drug is eliminated from the body per hour.

The k_e can also be determined from the Vd and clearance (Cl), as demonstrated by Equation 5 for drugs with linear kinetics. (Clearance is discussed in more detail in the following section.)

Equation 5: $k_e = \dfrac{Cl}{Vd}$

The half-life ($T\frac{1}{2}$) can also be used to describe drug elimination. Half-life is defined as the time required for the serum concentration to decrease by one-half. The first-

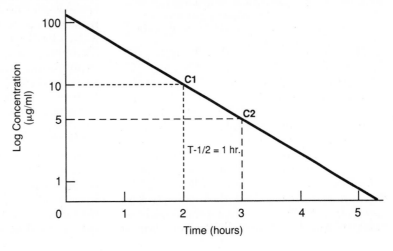

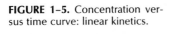

FIGURE 1–5. Concentration versus time curve: linear kinetics.

order elimination rate constant, ke, can be used to calculate the $T_{\frac{1}{2}}$ using Equation 6, or it can be graphically determined as shown in Figure 1–5. Using the data from the previous example, the $T_{\frac{1}{2}}$ is calculated to be 1 hour.

Equation 6: $T_{\frac{1}{2}} = 0.693/ke$

CLEARANCE

Systemic or total body clearance is defined as the rate at which a certain volume of plasma is cleared of a drug and is expressed in units of volume/time (i.e., ml/min). Clearance, therefore, is a measure of the body's efficiency of eliminating the drug in question. Just as elimination is the sum of metabolic and excretory functions, clearance is the sum of the drug's elimination rates, corresponding to each of these functions as shown in Equation 7.

Equation 7: $Cl = Cl_R + Cl_H + Cl_O$

Where Cl is total body clearance, Cl_R is renal clearance, Cl_H is hepatic clearance, and Cl_O is clearance by other routes

Renal Clearance

Renal clearance is the rate at which the plasma is cleared of unchanged drug or metabolite by the kidneys per unit time. Just as systemic clearance is the net result of several rates of clearance, renal clearance is also the net result of several different functions (Equation 8). Renal filtration, secretion, and reabsorption of drugs all affect the final clearance.

Equation 8: $Cl_R =$
(filtration clearance
+ secretion clearance)
$\times$ (1 − fraction reabsorbed)

Each of these functions can be affected by different variables. Filtration can be altered by changing the free or unbound fraction of a drug because only drug not bound to protein is filtered. Secretion can be changed by alterations in plasma flow, changes in the fraction of unbound drug, and also by substances that compete for the same carrier-mediated secretory pathways. Reabsorption can be altered by changes in lipid solubility, fraction of un-ionized drug, and the concentration gradient between the renal tubule and the plasma. Renal clearance (Cl_R) is not only a measure of the efficiency of the kidney at removing drugs from the body, but it can also be used to determine whether the predominant pathway for removal is filtration, secretion, or reabsorption. The Cl_R of a drug is determined by measuring the amount of drug or metabolite excreted in the urine in a given time period and comparing this to the concentration in the serum midway through the time interval. These data are then used as in Equation 9, where Au equals the amount of drug in the urine, t is the time period over which the urine was collected, and C_{mid} is the serum concentration midway through the time interval.

Equation 9: $Cl_R = \dfrac{dAu}{dt} \div C_{mid}$

Once calculated, the Cl_R is compared to the glomerular filtration rate (GFR), which is approximately 130 ml/min in patients with normal renal function. The predominant mechanism by which a drug is excreted is determined using a ratio of the GFR and Cl_R, called the *excretion ratio*. If the Cl_R is greater than 130 ml/min (and the excretion ratio is greater than 1), then the predominant method of excretion is renal tubular secretion. If the Cl_R is approximately equal to 130 ml/min (and the excretion ratio equals 1), the drug is predominantly filtered *or* it is secreted and then reabsorbed. Finally, if the Cl_R is less than 130 ml/min (and the excretion ratio is less than 1), the predominant action is renal tubular reabsorption.

Hepatic Clearance

Hepatic clearance (Cl_H) is defined as the rate at which the plasma supplied to the liver is cleared of drug and the drug is converted to active or inactive metabolites. The two major determinants of Cl_H are the volume of blood flow through the liver and the intrinsic ability of the liver to extract the drug. Cl_H is equal to the product of the volume of blood flow through the liver (Q) and the hepatic extraction ratio (E).

Equation 10: $Cl_H = Q \times E$

Therefore, any change in Q or E directly affects Cl_H. Hepatic extraction is also influenced by such factors as the liver's enzyme activity, the fraction of unbound drug, and the rate of blood flow to the liver. Most drugs can be divided into one of two classes as determined by the degree of hepatic extraction. Drugs that are highly extracted by the liver are subject to a high degree of enzymatic activity, which generally results in the extraction of more than 50% of the drug in the body during each hepatic pass. The Cl_H of these drugs is almost entirely dependent on Q because as the extraction approaches 100%, E in Equation 10 approaches 1, and therefore Cl_H is approximately equal to Q.

Drugs that are poorly extracted by the liver are generally subject to a low level of enzymatic activity; therefore, their extraction (E) is small (generally less than 10%). The two major determinants of the Cl_H of these drugs are the fraction extracted and the fraction of free or unbound drug, since that is the portion available for extraction. In the case of poorly extracted drugs, Q is generally much larger than Cl_H, as demonstrated by Equation 10 when E is <0.1.

STEADY STATE

Steady state is defined as that point during drug therapy when the amount of drug administered during a dosing interval is equivalent to the amount of drug eliminated during that interval. Steady-state concentrations (CSS) are achieved after four to five half-lives of a drug. The time required to reach steady state varies with each drug and each patient, depending on the rate of elimination. Once steady state is achieved, there is little fluctuation in the serum concentrations if the same dosage is maintained and the patient's renal function and hepatic function are constant. In the case of oral or intermittent IV dosing, the same patterns of peak (C_{max}) and trough (C_{min}) concentrations are attained, as demonstrated in Figures 1–6 and 1–7. When monitoring serum concentrations of drugs, steady-state concentrations are

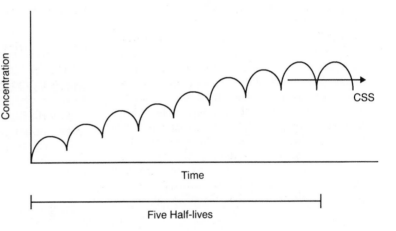

FIGURE 1–6. Steady-state concentration (CSS) achieved after multiple oral doses.

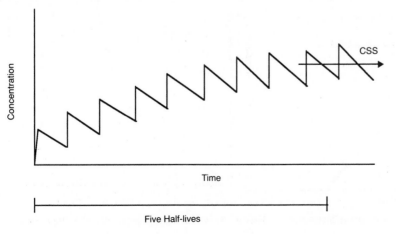

FIGURE 1–7. Steady-state concentration achieved after multiple IV bolus doses.

used to evaluate how the body handles the drug during repetitive dosing. In addition, if serum concentrations are measured prior to reaching steady state, dosage adjustments based on these concentrations may be erroneous because serum concentrations may still be increasing.

FIRST-ORDER KINETICS

The majority of drugs exhibit what is called linear or first-order kinetics. Under first-order conditions, the rate of drug elimination is directly proportional to the concentration of that drug. Other factors such as half-life, total body clearance, and volume of distribution are independent of the serum concentration. Figure 1–8 depicts drug handling by the body under first-order conditions.

ZERO-ORDER KINETICS

Zero-order or nonlinear kinetics is defined as capacity-limited elimination. This means that once a drug's concentration reaches a certain level, its elimination processes become saturated and the drug will be eliminated at a constant rate no matter how high the serum concentration. This saturability is due to the finite number of hepatic enzymes or limited carrier-mediated pathways in the kidney. Capacity-limited processes are also referred to as Michaelis Menten kinetics or dose-dependent kinetics. Two examples of

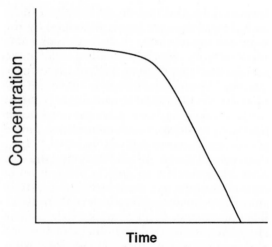

FIGURE 1–9. Zero-order kinetics: concentration versus time—elimination phase.

drugs that exhibit nonlinear kinetics are ethyl alcohol and phenytoin. Figures 1–9 and 1–10 show representative examples of drug handling by zero-order kinetics.

THERAPEUTIC RANGE AND SERUM CONCENTRATION MONITORING

The therapeutic range of a drug is defined as the concentration between the minimum effective concentration (MEC) and the minimum toxic concentration (MTC). Ideally,

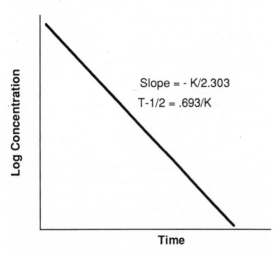

Slope = - K/2.303

T-1/2 = .693/K

FIGURE 1–8. Drug handling by the body under first-order kinetics.

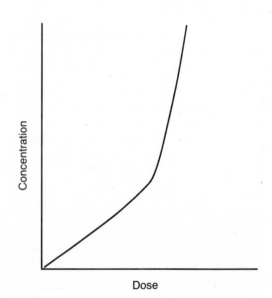

FIGURE 1–10. Zero-order kinetics: concentration versus dose.

serum concentrations should be maintained within this range to obtain maximum therapeutic effect with the least amount of adverse effects. Drugs that have a narrow therapeutic range are monitored most frequently. These same drugs seem to have a high degree of individual variability. In fact, the most common reason for serum concentration monitoring is to document a patient's serum drug concentration relative to the therapeutic range. In addition, serum concentration monitoring can be used to assess patient compliance, evaluate the effect of a change in the dosage regimen, assess the effects of an interacting drug, or document a change in the drug's pharmacokinetics secondary to disease. Thus, serum concentration monitoring can be used in a wide variety of ways, with the same goal—to individualize drug dosage in order to optimize therapeutic effect. Care should be taken to make dosage adjustments based on *both* serum concentration and clinical condition of the patient. There will always be a small number of patients who experience therapeutic or toxic effects outside the normal range.

Serum concentrations can also be used to determine patient-specific pharmacokinetic parameters, which can then be used to further individualize drug dosing. This is generally done by measuring several serum concentrations following a single (or first) dose of the drug and using the obtained data to calculate parameters such as clearance, volume of distribution, and half-life, as described previously.

Individualization of drug dosing initially referred to dosing simply by weight, age, or body surface area, rather than giving each patient the same dose of drug. Today, individualization of drug therapy takes into account not only these three factors, but many more, such as genetics, diet, drug interactions, and disease states, which all have a profound effect on drug pharmacokinetics. For example, diseases affecting the GI mucosa can alter drug absorption; burns, cardiac disease, and neoplastic disease tend to alter drug distribution; malnutrition affects protein binding; and renal and hepatic diseases affect drug elimination. In each of these circumstances serum drug concentrations should be used whenever possible to assess the extent of the disease's effect on drug pharmacokinetics. The reader is referred to the pharmacokinetics texts listed in the References following this chapter and to

the appropriate chapters in this text for specific drug information in these circumstances.

DRUG INTERACTIONS

There are three basic types of drug interactions: physical incompatibilities, pharmacodynamic interactions, and pharmacokinetic interactions. Physical interactions are important to rule out when administering different medications together (e.g., when running medications through the same IV line or mixed in a syringe). Several reference texts are available with this type of information (see Appendix 2). Pharmacodynamic interactions are those that occur at the site of action, for example, agonist–antagonist interactions or interactions causing a potentiation of effect or side effect. Pharmacokinetic interactions are those that alter pharmacokinetic parameters in some way.

The clinical significance of most drug interactions depends on the magnitude of the serum concentration change relative to the therapeutic range. In the majority of cases, drug interactions can be managed by altering administration times or by altering the dosages of the medications. Pharmacokinetics and serum concentration monitoring can aid the clinician in the readjustment of the drug dosage regimens.

Interactions Affecting Absorption

Drug interactions affecting absorption occur most frequently and in a variety of ways. First, drugs can interact with various foods, resulting in decreased absorption. For example, ingestion of tetracycline with calcium-containing foods results in decreased tetracycline absorption. A second type of drug interaction affecting absorption is the formation of drug complexes that are less soluble and therefore not absorbed. Examples of this are binding of digoxin by antacids and of warfarin by cholestyramine. A third type of drug interaction affecting absorption is a change in the gastric pH caused by one drug that alters the solubility, ionization, and subsequently the absorption of another drug. For example, administration of antacids with ketoconazole decreases the absorption of ketoconazole, which requires an acid environment in order to be absorbed. These interactions can all be managed by separating the administration time of the interacting medications by at least 2 to 3 hours.

Drugs that affect gastric emptying time or intestinal motility can also affect the absorption of other medications. Changes in the gastric emptying time alter the rate at which a drug is delivered to intestinal absorption sites and subsequently alter absorption. Changes in intestinal motility alter the amount of time the drug is in contact with absorptive surfaces. Examples of drugs that alter gastric emptying time or intestinal motility are anticholinergics, narcotics, and metoclopramide.

As noted earlier in the discussion on pharmacokinetics, changes in the extent of drug absorption are usually more significant than are changes in the rate of absorption.

Interactions Affecting Distribution

Numerous drug interactions result in changes in the balance of drug bound to serum and tissue proteins. The free or unbound drug is considered to be not only the active fraction but also that fraction available for distribution and elimination. The displacement of even a small percentage of drug can double or quadruple the free concentration. Most of the time the displacement of a drug from proteins results in a transient elevation in the free concentration. This increased free drug is then redistributed to other sites or eliminated, and a new equilibrium is established. The relevance of this type of drug interaction depends on the drug's therapeutic range and the patient's ability to eliminate the drug. If the therapeutic range is wide, an increase in the serum concentration may have little consequence. However, if the therapeutic range is narrow or the patient's elimination of that drug is compromised, a prolonged elevation of the free concentration of the drug may occur.

Interactions Due to Change in Drug Metabolism

Interactions involving drug metabolism generally involve induction or inhibition of the cytochrome P-450 enzymes. The clinical relevance of such interactions is a function of a given drug's therapeutic range. Drugs that tend to induce enzyme activity are barbiturates, ethanol, rifampin, phenytoin, and carbamazine. The onset of enzyme induction is slow, and it may take weeks to see an effect. Also, if the inducer is withdrawn, it takes some time for the enzyme activity to decrease. Drug concentrations (or effect) need to be monitored at initiation of therapy and also when the inducing drug is discontinued.

Some drugs, such as cimetidine, amiodarone, and erythromycin, tend to inhibit cytochrome P-450 enzyme activity. The onset and offset of this interaction tend to be rapid, and the time required to reach maximal effect depends on the new half-life of the drug in question. Dosage adjustments may be necessary in both induction- and inhibition-type interactions, at the onset of therapy with the interacting drug, and again after the drug is discontinued.

Drug Interactions Affecting Drug Excretion

Drug interactions in the kidney are generally of two types: interactions affecting the glomerular filtration rate (GFR) and interactions affecting tubular secretion or reabsorption. Any drug that causes a change in the GFR ultimately has the potential to alter the clearance of other drugs eliminated by that mechanism. The clinical significance of such an interaction depends on the extent of the change in the GFR and on the therapeutic range of the drug in question.

Interactions resulting in inhibition of tubular secretion are more common and generally more clinically significant. The kidney has two nonspecific transport systems, one for organic acids and one for organic bases. Endogenous compounds as well as numerous drugs compete for these carrier systems. Inhibition of tubular secretion of one drug by another can result in significant elevations of serum concentrations; the most common examples of this are penicillin with probenecid and digoxin with quinidine.

Interactions can also occur in the kidney when two compounds compete for tubular reabsorption pathways. One example of this is the increased reabsorption of lithium in place of sodium in dehydrated patients.

TITRATED DRUG THERAPY

The pharmacokinetic principles outlined in this chapter form the basis of emergency drug therapy. However, in most emergency situations, one cannot wait for drug level determinations to guide therapeutic actions, but must use an understanding of these basic principles to adjust therapy based on clinical response. It is important for the physician to understand the concept of titrated drug therapy in which drug dosing is based on objective, measurable physiologic end-points and the pharmacokinetic properties of the administered drug.

The use of intravenous nitroprusside in the treatment of a hypertensive emergency serves as a good example of this concept. Nitroprusside is both rapidly acting and rapidly metabolized, so the physiologic effect (a reduction in blood pressure) of any given dose is fully realized in several minutes and disappears within several minutes of the drug's discontinuation. One sets a therapeutic goal, e.g., a 25% reduction of the patient's starting blood pressure reading, and begins a nitroprusside infusion. Continuous intra-arterial blood pressure monitoring provides real-time knowledge of the physiologic end-point. Since the effect of a given nitroprusside infusion dose is realized in minutes, the clinician can start at a low dose that is not likely to induce complications and advance the infusion dose in gradual increments every 5 minutes until the desired reduction in blood pressure is achieved. If hypotension occurs, the infusion is discontinued. This adverse effect disappears quickly because of the rapid metabolism of the drug, and the nitroprusside infusion is then restarted at a lower dose. A continuous infusion of the drug at the appropriate infusion rate then maintains a constant plasma level and the desired physiologic effect.

As another example, consider the use of intravenous lidocaine for the treatment of premature ventricular contractions. One or several loading doses are given to achieve a therapeutic drug level quickly as evidenced by the disappearance of the premature ventricular contractions. Then a continuous infusion of the drug is instituted to maintain this therapeutic level. If breakthrough premature ventricular contractions occur during a lidocaine infusion, another bolus is given to achieve a higher blood level rapidly, and the infusion rate is simultaneously increased to maintain the higher level.

When selecting drug therapy for the acute management of critically ill patients, the optimal drug should be an intravenous agent with a rapid onset of action, easily monitored physiologic and/or toxic effects, and rapid metabolism. This set of properties facilitates titrated therapy, which will maximize results and minimize toxicity.

REFERENCES

Chernow B: The Pharmacologic Approach to the Critically Ill Patient, 2nd ed. Baltimore, Williams & Wilkins, 1988.

Craviness M, Taylor W: Therapeutic Drug Monitoring. Irving, TX, Abbott Laboratories, 1987.

Evans W, Jusko W, Schentag, J: Applied Pharmacokinetics. San Francisco, Applied Therapeutics, 1980.

Gibaldi M: Biopharmaceutics and Clinical Pharmacokinetics. Philadelphia, Lea & Febiger, 1984.

CHAPTER 2

Routes of Drug Administration

WILLIAM H. SPIVEY, M.D.

Routes of drug delivery may be divided into two general categories: enteral and parenteral. When drugs are administered by the enteral route, absorption occurs in the gastrointestinal tract and may take place in the stomach, intestine, mouth, or rectum. Drugs administered by the parenteral route bypass the gastrointestinal system. Common examples of parenteral routes are the intravenous, intramuscular, subcutaneous, transcutaneous, endotracheal, and pulmonary. In common medical usage, however, the term *parenteral* refers to the intravenous, intramuscular, and subcutaneous routes.

Several factors must be taken into consideration when choosing a route for drug administration. Can the drug be safely and effectively administered by the route under consideration? Some drugs are not absorbed well or their effectiveness may be altered if given by the wrong route. Many drugs cannot be given by the endotracheal route because of potential damage to the pulmonary surfactant and alveoli. Will the drug be adequately absorbed to be of therapeutic value? This takes into consideration absorption characteristics of the route and drug both during normal function of the body and in acute pathologic states. For instance, when treating asthma, drugs such as epinephrine are effectively absorbed after subcutaneous administration. However, during cardiac ar-

rest, the subcutaneous route is of no value. The physician must understand the limitations of each route and how drug dosage and method of administration affect drug absorption. Table 2–1 provides a comparison of the different routes of drug administration.

INTRAVENOUS

The most common route of emergency drug administration is by intravenous injection. It provides almost immediate drug delivery to tissues and allows the drug to be closely titrated. This is especially important when a rapid response to a drug is necessary.

There is no delay in absorption of drugs administered by the intravenous route. As seen in Figure 2–1, the peak serum level for drugs administered by the intravenous route occurs immediately after injection and rapidly tapers off. In contrast, drugs administered by other routes take much longer to reach peak serum levels and have lower peak concentrations.

In order to produce sustained therapeutic levels, an intravenous infusion may be used to supplement the initial bolus of a drug. This offers the advantage of maintaining therapeutic levels while providing the capacity to stop the drug quickly in case of adverse effects. Drugs such as nitroprusside and es-

TABLE 2–1. Comparison of Routes of Drug Administration

Drug	Intravenous Dose	Endotracheal Dose	Intraosseous Dose	Comments
Epinephrine	1 mg/10 ml (1:10,000)	1 mg/10 ml (1:10,000)	1 mg/10 ml (1:10,000)	Dose for cardiac arrest. Animal data strongly suggest that up to 10 times this dose is needed for endotracheal administration.
NaHCO$_3$	1 mEq/kg initially; 0.5 mEq/kg q 10 min	Not applicable	1 mEq/kg initially; 0.5 mEq/kg q 10 min	As demonstrated in Figure 2–3, central venous administration of NaHCO$_3$ increases pH more than does peripheral administration. Blood gases should be closely monitored.
Atropine	0.5–1 mg IV push	1 mg	0.5–1 mg	The endotracheal dose is based on limited clinical data and animal data that suggest a higher dose may be needed than for the intravenous route.
Lidocaine	1 mg/kg initially, followed by 1–4 mg/min infusion	2–3 mg/kg	1 mg/kg initially, followed by 1–4 mg/min infusion	A higher dose of endotracheal lidocaine may be needed in low flow states. No maintenance information is available for the endotracheal route.
Bretylium	5 mg/kg initially, followed by 10 mg/kg q 15 min × 2 if needed	Not applicable	No data available	Bretylium can probably be given by the intraosseous route, but no data regarding potential marrow toxicity are available.
Dopamine	2–30 μg/kg/min	Not applicable	2–30 μg/kg/min	Only short-term infusions have been studied using the intraosseous route.
Diazepam	5–10 mg in adults; 0.2–0.5 mg q 2–5 min in children	5 mg in adults; 0.5–2 mg in children	0.2–0.5 mg q 2–5 min in children	Dosages for seizure control. Endotracheal dosages are based on isolated case reports.
Naloxone	2 mg	2 mg	2 mg	No data currently exist for intraosseous naloxone use, but it should be safe by this route.

molol require a maintenance infusion for therapeutic value but may need to be terminated rapidly in case of an adverse effect.

An advantage of the intravenous route is the relative safety it provides for drugs with a narrow margin between therapeutic and toxic levels. For example, the therapeutic range for lidocaine is 1 to 4 μg/ml. Below this level the patient may be exposed to potentially serious arrhythmias, and if the level is

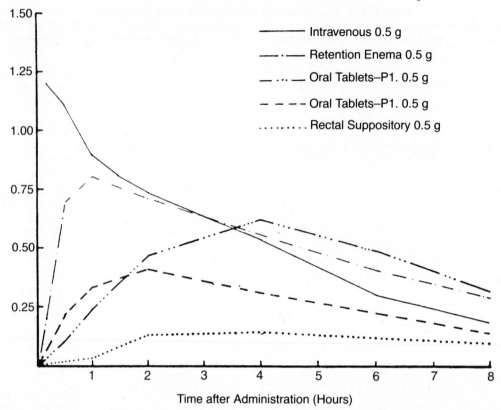

FIGURE 2–1. Comparison of serum levels of theophylline following administration by different routes. (Reproduced with permission from Trvitt EB, McKusick VA, Krantz JC: Theophylline blood levels after oral, rectal, and intravenous administration, and correlation with diuretic action. J Pharmacol Exp Ther 100:309–315, 1950.)

exceeded, the drug may cause respiratory depression, seizures, and cardiac arrest. Maintaining this narrow margin of safety is not possible with other routes of drug administration.

The intravenous route provides a good route of administration for drugs that are not well absorbed from the tissues, such as diazepam. It may also be used for drugs that are tissue irritants when locally concentrated, drugs not absorbed by the gastrointestinal tract, or those destroyed by first-pass metabolism in the liver.

Despite its many advantages, the intravenous route does have drawbacks. Because of the rapidity with which an intravenously administered drug enters the system, side effects may occur that are not commonly seen with other routes. For example, lidocaine may produce cardiac arrest if too rapidly administered, and potassium chloride, while relatively safe if taken orally, is potentially fatal if injected as an intravenous bolus. Allergic reactions are also potentially more se-

vere if a drug is administered intravenously. Once a drug has been administered intravenously, it cannot be removed. Unlike topical drugs, which can be wiped off, or oral drugs, which can be lavaged from the stomach, drugs administered intravenously are dependent on the kidney or liver for elimination.

Other potential complications include precipitation of drug from the vehicle in which it is suspended and subsequent intravenous infusion of the precipitant. Dilantin is well known for precipitating in an intravenous line that contains a dextrose solution. Potential complications of using the intravenous route are embolism due to injected particulate material and bacterial contamination with subsequent infection.

Of the many potential uses for the intravenous route of drug administration, none has been investigated as extensively as its use in cardiopulmonary resuscitation (CPR). The intravenous route is the route of choice for administering drugs during a cardiac arrest. Other routes, such as intramuscular and subcutaneous, are not acceptable, and the intracardiac and endotracheal routes both have limitations. The intravenous route provides an adequate rate of transport, even during CPR, and delivers a high concentration of drugs to tissues. Current guidelines from the American Heart Association's *Standards and Guidelines for Cardiopulmonary Resuscitation and Emergency Care* (1986) recommend that "during CPR, cannulation of peripheral or femoral veins should be the choice of first site since CPR may have to be interrupted if either jugular or subclavian veins are chosen." Peripheral vascular access is recommended because it is simple and does not interfere with CPR. However, data from animal studies suggest that drug delivery by a peripheral intravenous line is not as rapid as by a central intravenous line. Hedges and Barsan (1984) compared peripheral versus central injection of technetium in dogs receiving closed-chest CPR. The mean time to peak counts in the left ventricle after central injection was 118 ± 54 seconds, versus 258 ± 142 seconds for the peripheral route. Although the times to peak activity were significantly different, there were no significant differences in maximum peak activities.

Few flow studies in humans during CPR have been performed. In one recent study, a small but significant difference in time to first appearance and time to peak levels of indocyanine green occurred when the dye was injected through the subclavian or a peripheral intravenous line (Lacy et al, 1987). Another study that compared use of the two routes in 233 patients found no difference in outcome of patients who received drugs by the peripheral versus by the central route.

An antecubital line is acceptable for the initial management of a patient in cardiac arrest. Flow from this site may be improved by elevating the arm and by following drug injection with a saline flush. If circulation is not restored, a subclavian or internal jugular line should be established, if possible, with minimal interruption of CPR.

INTRAMUSCULAR

Absorption from the skeletal muscle is relatively fast and produces predictable serum drug levels. It requires approximately 10 to 30 minutes for absorption to occur, depending on the blood flow through resting mus-

cle, which ranges from 0.02 to 0.07 ml/min/g of tissue. Blood flow and absorption increase during exercise. Most small molecules are absorbed directly into the capillaries, whereas larger molecules, such as proteins, are transported by the lymphatics. Studies in rat muscle have demonstrated that the molecular weight of compounds and the concentration do not significantly affect drug absorption. The rate-limiting factor is blood flow. Other factors that may influence the absorption of a drug from skeletal muscle include the ionization and lipid solubility of the drug, polar versus lipid vehicle, and volume of vehicle. Drugs that are ionized at tissue pH and dissolved in small amounts of aqueous vehicle are more rapidly absorbed than are insoluble drugs or drugs dissolved in an oily vehicle. A common example of this is diazepam, which is poorly soluble in water and has propylene glycol, sodium benzoate, and benzoic acid as its solvents. This leads to slow erratic absorption of diazepam from skeletal muscle and prevents the intramuscular route from being effective for acute seizure control with this drug.

Common uses for the intramuscular route include administration of narcotics, antibiotics, phenobarbital, and tetanus immunization. Drugs used for resuscitation and arrhythmia control are not administered intramuscularly.

Complications of intramuscular injection include pain, inflammation, abscess formation, inadvertent intravenous injection, nerve injury, and injection site lesions. The latter are caused by subcutaneous injection rather than by intramuscular injection. Most complications can be avoided by sterile technique and aspiration of the syringe before injection.

SUBCUTANEOUS

The subcutaneous route is used for drugs that need to be absorbed slowly but that cannot be administered orally. Epinephrine for the treatment of asthma is a common example. Epinephrine is slowly released from the subcutaneous tissue and provides a constant blood level for 20 minutes or longer.

The same factors that affect intramuscular absorption also affect subcutaneous absorption. Blood flow is the predominant factor, with lymphatic drainage assuming a lesser role. Blood flow may be diminished by applying a tourniquet, cooling the extremity, or, as in the case of local anesthetics, adding a vasoconstrictor such as epinephrine. This decreases blood flow at the injection site and prolongs the effect of the drug while minimizing systemic absorption.

Because of the slow absorption and restrictions on the volume that can be injected subcutaneously, this route is somewhat limited. It should not be used in patients who are hypotensive or who have a significant decrease in cardiac output. In these cases, the drugs are poorly absorbed and should be administered intravenously.

The usefulness of the subcutaneous route is further limited by local necrosis, tissue sloughing, and pain that may occur with some drugs. For this reason, many drugs must be given by the intravenous or oral route. Other potential complications include sterile abscesses and injection site lesions.

TOPICAL

One of the primary functions of the skin is to provide a barrier against foreign substances. Given how effective the skin is in preventing transport or diffusion of such substances, it is not surprising that the topical or transdermal route has not been widely used for drug administration. Few drugs that can be administered transdermally have practical use in emergency situations.

The skin is a three-layered structure consisting of the stratum corneum, the epidermis, and the dermis. The stratum corneum is the principal barrier to drug penetration because of its lipid concentration, which permits only slow diffusion of solutes. Furthermore, the lipid content of the stratum corneum is variable and allows variability in absorption. In order for a drug to be used transdermally, it must have the following characteristics. First, it must be potent, requiring a low dose. Second, it should have a short half-life. Third, the drug's partitioning characteristics must favor the stratum corneum over the delivery vehicle and viable tissue over the stratum corneum. Finally, the drug cannot be an irritant or produce allergic reactions.

Most drugs that have been developed for transdermal delivery are prepared in the form of slow-release patches. They include estradiol, nitroglycerin, scopolamine, and clonidine. Nitroglycerin also comes in the form of a paste, which may be applied to the skin to dilate the coronary arteries or decrease blood pressure. Although nitroglycerin paste was often used in the past for decreasing an elevated blood pressure during acute congestive heart failure, it is now rarely used for this purpose because of the variable absorption caused by peripheral vasoconstriction and diaphoresis.

Local anesthetic use in minor surgical procedures has been extensively studied in recent years. Preparations of lidocaine ranging in concentration from 10 to 30% have demonstrated a variable degree of local anesthesia. The gel or cream is covered by an occlusive patch, which improves diffusion into the subcutaneous tissue. In order to produce anesthesia suitable for surgical procedures, however, the gel or cream must be kept in contact with the skin for approximately 30 to 60 minutes.

A combination of tetracaine 0.5%, epinephrine 1:2,000, and cocaine 11.8% (TEC), when placed on a laceration, has been demonstrated to produce local anesthesia in a short period of time. In addition to providing pain relief, this technique produces less tissue destruction and distortion than does a subcutaneous injection. It also produces a local vasoconstriction that decreases bleeding. It does, however, have disadvantages. TEC is absorbed much better in children than in adults and often is of limited value in the latter. It is expensive and has been associated with a high incidence of wound infection in animal studies.

Another form of transdermal delivery of drug that may have benefit is iontophoresis. With this technique, a low-voltage current is used to move ions from a reservoir attached to the skin into the dermis and epidermis. When 2 to 3 ml of lidocaine is placed in a reservoir near a laceration or over a venipuncture site and current is applied for 10 minutes, anesthesia suitable for minor surgical procedures is produced. Disadvantages of iontophoresis include a rash at the site of diffusion that often lasts 1 to 2 days. Little information is available about further damage that may occur to injured tissue in lacerations or about the potential for seizures if the technique is used on scalp or face lacerations.

ENDOTRACHEAL

The endotracheal route was used widely in the late 1930s and 1940s for the administration of epinephrine and antibiotics. However, the route was all but abandoned because of the technical limitations encountered in administering drugs to conscious patients with an intact cough reflex. In 1967, Redding and co-workers, in a comparative study, demonstrated that epinephrine administered by the endotracheal route was as effective as the intravenous and intracardiac routes for resuscitating dogs in experimental cardiac arrest. Later, Roberts and Greenberg (1978, 1979a, 1979b) published a series of papers on endotracheal drug administration and popularized the technique.

Use of the endotracheal route is indicated at present for emergencies in which another acceptable route is not available. The intravenous route is preferred, but the endotracheal route may be used in instances where vascular access cannot be readily obtained.

Several factors affect the delivery and absorption of drugs administered endotracheally. Most importantly, drugs should be aerosolized to ensure maximal transport to the alveoli. In most cases, this is not possible, since it requires special equipment that is not always available. Catheters that spray the solution into the trachea and side ports in endotracheal tubes for instillation of the drug while simultaneously ventilating the patient have been developed, but little data regarding their effectiveness are available.

Various diluents have been demonstrated to affect the absorption of drugs from the lung. Distilled water is more effective than saline in promoting absorption across the alveolar capillary membrane, probably because of the hypo-osmolality of the former (hypo-osmolar solutions are absorbed more rapidly than are iso-osmolar solutions). However, although distilled water may improve absorption, it has been shown to decrease the paO_2 in animals. Greenberg and associates (1982), in an animal model, demonstrated a decrease in paO_2 to 51% of baseline for endotracheally administered distilled water and to 74% of baseline with saline. The dose of diluent used was 2 ml/kg, which would be equivalent to 140 ml in a 70-kg man, far more than is routinely administered to humans. Rusli and co-workers (1987) demonstrated no significant change in arterial pO_2, pCO_2, or pH over 20 minutes in cats that received endotracheal saline, 0.1 ml/kg. This same study demonstrated no significant effect on the same parameters with the administration of diazepam suspended in propylene glycol. Both propylene glycol and

95% ethanol have been used as diluents for diazepam, and both have been shown to be effective in promoting diazepam absorption across the alveolar capillary membrane.

Although little data are available regarding the optimal dose of diluent, most authors empirically recommend 5 to 10 ml. Higher doses may interfere with gas exchange in adults and lower doses do not provide sufficient surface contact with absorptive membranes to maximize absorption. Few data are actually available comparing different volumes.

Once the drug is delivered to the lungs, absorption is determined by the drug's size and structure, ionization, and lipophilic versus polar characteristics, and by the characteristics of the alveolar capillary membrane.

Although areas of the respiratory tree are strongly absorbent, the alveoli have the greatest absorptive capacity. Large pores in the alveoli allow different-size hydrophilic and ionized molecules to diffuse passively into the capillary system. Also, hydrophobic pores allow the absorption of lipophilic molecules. A transport system in the alveoli actively transports the molecules of some drugs across the membrane. Each of these mechanisms may be affected by the underlying state of the membranes. Chronic diseases, such as emphysema, chronic obstructive pulmonary disease (COPD), and acute inflammatory reactions, may affect the transport of molecules across the alveolar capillary membrane.

Of the drugs commonly used in emergency situations, only five, epinephrine, lidocaine, atropine, diazepam, and naloxone, have undergone significant study for use by the endotracheal route. Several other drugs have been studied but are not suitable for use in emergency settings.

Epinephrine

Epinephrine is the drug most commonly administered by the endotracheal route. Roberts and Greenberg (1979a) demonstrated that epinephrine delivered by the endotracheal tube to anesthetized dogs produced peak serum levels in 15 seconds and a maximum blood pressure response within 60 seconds of administration. Furthermore, the serum levels of epinephrine administered endotracheally remained elevated much longer than serum levels following intravenous administration.

More recent experiments by Ralston and

co-workers (1985) have demonstrated that, in an animal model of electromechanical dissociation, epinephrine must be administered in doses approximately 10 times higher by the endotracheal route as compared with doses by the intravenous route (Fig. 2–2). Epinephrine in doses of 30 µg/kg produced the same success rate of resuscitation as did doses of 300 µg/kg when administered by the endotracheal route. When administered by the endotracheal route, 30 µg/kg produced no successful resuscitations.

The current American Heart Association recommended dose for intravenous epinephrine is 7.5 to 15 µg/kg for adults. The same dose is recommended for the endotracheal route. However, based on experimental data, a much higher dose of endotracheal epinephrine may be necessary to produce the same cardiovascular effects.

One potential danger of endotracheal epinephrine administration is the depot effect. Once patients are resuscitated and catecholamines circulated, a large increase may occur in blood pressure and heart rate. Normally, these will again decrease, but, with high doses of endotracheal epinephrine, there may be a release of epinephrine from the lungs for 30 minutes or longer following the return of a heartbeat and blood pressure.

Lidocaine

Lidocaine has been recommended for endotracheal use for over 30 years. However, little information is available about the drug's pharmacokinetics in the hypotensive or cardiac arrest state. To date, most studies have been performed on healthy volunteers or in anesthetized animals. The clinical studies have used a wide variety of lidocaine concentrations and techniques, such as spraying the trachea with lidocaine and transtracheal injection of lidocaine. Translaryngeal injection of 10% lidocaine (5 mg/kg) in humans has produced therapeutic serum levels (over 1.4 µg/ml) in a mean time of 5.1 ± 3.2 minutes, with a peak at 20 minutes.

Data from anesthetized mongrel dogs demonstrate peak serum lidocaine levels at 5 minutes, with a gradual decline over 30 minutes (Mace, 1987). Lidocaine (4 mg/kg) when diluted with saline (3.2 ml) produced a higher mean plasma level (4.7 ± 1.3 µg/ml) at 5 minutes than did the same undiluted concentration (1.94 ± 0.5). There was very little depot effect seen in this study.

To date, one study has compared the intravenous, intraosseous, and endotracheal routes of lidocaine administration in a cardiac arrest model (Brickman et al, 1988). Serum lidocaine levels for the endotracheal route were significantly lower than for the other routes. As seen with epinephrine, the absorption and transport of endotracheal lidocaine during cardiopulmonary resuscitation are much slower than by the intravascular route in a normal subject with a functioning cardiovascular system.

Both animal and clinical studies have dem-

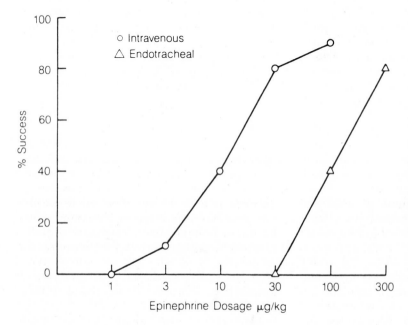

FIGURE 2–2. Cumulative dose-response relationships for recovery of animals from electromechanical dissociation following injection of epinephrine either intravenously or endotracheally. (Reproduced with permission from Ralston SH, Tacker WA, Shonen L, et al: Endotracheal versus intravenous epinephrine during electromechanical dissociation with CPR in dogs. Ann Emerg Med 14:1044–1048, 1985.)

onstrated that 2 to 3 mg/kg of lidocaine administered endotracheally produces therapeutic blood levels. There is, however, a discrepancy about when therapeutic levels are obtained (5 minutes in animal studies versus 5 to 20 minutes in human studies).

Further complicating our understanding of the pharmacokinetics is a lack of information about lidocaine absorption and transport from the tracheobronchial tree in such disease states as pulmonary edema, COPD, or heart failure resulting from arrhythmias. Until further data are available, an endotracheal dose of 2 to 3 mg/kg appears to be adequate to produce therapeutic serum levels of lidocaine.

Atropine

A case report by Greenberg and co-workers (1982) is the only clinical report on endotracheally administered atropine in recent literature. In this case, 1 mg of atropine was administered to an apneic, pulseless patient with a nodal rhythm of 30 complexes per minute; an electrocardiographic response was noted within 30 seconds, at which time the serum atropine level was less than 3 ng/ml. The patient improved and was discharged from the hospital.

Elam (1977) demonstrated that atropine was rapidly absorbed from the lungs of dogs that were bradycardic from hypoxia. He administered 2 mg of atropine in 10 ml of distilled water and observed an increase in the heart rate 11 to 21 seconds later. A depot effect was also noted.

Based on the report by Greenberg and associates, the dose of atropine for endotracheal use should probably be 1.0 mg, as is currently recommended for intravenous administration by the American Heart Association.

Diazepam

Diazepam is the most controversial of the drugs currently recommended for endotracheal administration. The results of two animal studies have clearly demonstrated that the drug is well absorbed, but recently questions have been raised about potential adverse effects on the lungs.

Barsan and co-workers (1982), using a dog model in a study in which diazepam 0.5 mg/kg was diluted in 95% ethanol, demonstrated that therapeutic serum levels could be attained within 30 seconds. More recently,

Rusli and associates (1987) demonstrated therapeutic blood levels within 60 seconds in a cat model wtih 0.1 mg/kg of undiluted diazepam. In the latter study, diazepam was used as commercially prepared in a suspension of propylene glycol. Most of the cats receiving diazepam in this study developed pneumonia within 2 days, raising questions about potential damage to the alveolar lining caused by the diazepam or its vehicle. As part of this study, the authors included a brief case report of endotracheal diazepam used to stop a seizure in a child. No adverse effects occurred, and the child was discharged from the hospital. Currently no clinical guidelines exist for the endotracheal administration of diazepam.

Naloxone

Despite only one clinical report of endotracheally administered naloxone, this route should be considered early in the management of a serious narcotic overdose. Because of the difficulty in obtaining intravenous access in the intravenous drug abuser, and because of the potential lethal effects of heroin and other narcotics, the endotracheal route may be lifesaving once an airway has been established. In the only reported case, 1.6 mg of endotracheal naloxone was administered for management of a heroin overdose and resulted in rapid reversal of the respiratory and mental depression. No known adverse effects occurred. The recommended endotracheal dose of naloxone is 2 mg, the same as that recommended for intravenous use.

Adverse Effects

No adverse effects of endotracheal drug administration have been reported to date. Several theoretical concerns, such as damage to the alveolar lining, destruction of surfactant, impaired oxygen diffusion, and adult respiratory distress syndrome (ARDS), have been raised but none has been demonstrated in humans. The drugs previously mentioned, with the possible exception of diazepam, are safe in the currently recommended doses. Drugs that should not be used for endotracheal absorption include glucose, sodium bicarbonate, bretylium, and calcium chloride. Glucose is hyperosmolar and may induce pneumonia. Calcium chloride and sodium bicarbonate are suspected of destroying surfactant and sclerosing the alveolar membranes. Bretylium is a polar molecule and not transported well across the alveolar membrane.

INTRAOSSEOUS

The intraosseous route provides a method of access to the cardiovascular system that is similar to the venous route. It was widely used in the 1940s for crystalloid, blood, and drug administration in children with poor vascular access. In recent years, it has been reintroduced as a method of emergency vascular access in the pediatric population. It is recommended for use when peripheral or central venous access is not readily available.

The most commonly used bone is the tibia, which has access sites at both the proximal and distal ends. The medullary cavity in the proximal and distal tibia is a spongy network of venous sinusoids that flow into a central venous channel. From there blood exits the bone through emissary and nutrient veins and drains into the large vessels of the leg.

The pharmacokinetics of intraosseous infusion are almost identical to those of the intravenous route. The transport time, peak serum levels, and rate of elimination are all similar. As early as 1940, Tocantins and O'Neil demonstrated that Congo Red dye injected into the tibia of a rabbit appeared in the right ventricle within 10 seconds. Other studies have shown that, with a normal car-

diovascular system, peak serum levels for diazepam and atropine occur within 60 seconds following intraosseous administration. In addition to producing similar serum levels, diazepam given by the intraosseous route has been demonstrated to be as effective in stopping seizures as that given by the intravenous route. The rate of elimination and decrease in serum levels of intraosseous drugs are similar to those given by the intravenous route. There does not appear to be a significant depot effect with this route.

The primary indication for intraosseous infusion is cardiac arrest in infants and children. The intraosseous route has been demonstrated to be an effective means to obtain access to the circulation and to provide rapid transport to the central circulation during cardiopulmonary resuscitation. In 1985, Spivey and co-workers compared the intraosseous, intravenous, and central venous routes for sodium bicarbonate administration during cardiac arrest in a swine model. The blood pH was significantly higher in the central venous and intraosseous groups than in the animals receiving sodium bicarbonate by the peripheral intravenous route (Fig. 2–3). The reason for this was postulated to be a rapid exit of sodium bicarbonate from the tibia and movement of the drug into the large vessels of the legs. More recently, Brickman and associates (1988) compared lidocaine administration by the endotracheal, central venous, and intraosseous routes. The

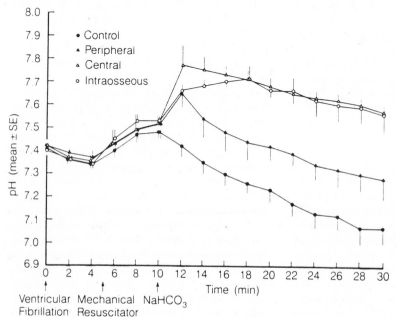

FIGURE 2–3. Comparison of the effect of sodium bicarbonate on pH of femoral artery blood when administered by different routes in a swine cardiac arrest model. Sodium bicarbonate 1 mEq/kg was administered after 10 minutes of arrest and 5 minutes of cardiopulmonary resuscitation by the peripheral (n = 6), central (n = 5), or intraosseous (n = 6) route. (Reproduced with permission from Spivey WH, Lathors CM, Malone DR, et al: Comparison of intraosseous, central and peripheral routes of sodium bicarbonate administration during CPR in pigs. Ann Emerg Med 14:1135–1140, 1985.)

results following intraosseous and central venous administration were similar and significantly better than those following administration by the endotracheal route.

Drugs that have been administered by the intraosseous route include vasopressors, sodium bicarbonate, atropine, diazepam, antibiotics, and anesthetic agents. Hypertonic drugs, such as glucose and sodium bicarbonate, should be injected slowly, as should drugs with a low pH, such as phenytoin. Marrow-toxic agents, such as chloramphenicol, are best avoided.

In addition to drugs, crystalloid and blood may be administered by the intraosseous route. The rate of fluid administration ranges from 10 to 40 ml/min, depending on the size of the marrow cavity and the pressure on the infusion bag. In animal studies, using a 13-gauge needle in a 15-kg animal, pressures of 300 mmHg have produced a flow of 40 ml/min. The flow rate of blood is about 60 to 75% as fast as that of crystalloid.

As with any technique, complications occur with intraosseous infusion. The most common problem is the inability to gain access to the bone, which occurs in approximately 20% of patients. Extravasation of drugs into the surrounding tissues may occur if the needle is not properly placed or if excess pressure is used during infusion. Drugs such as calcium and sodium bicarbonate may damage the tissues when given intraosseously.

Infection was reported in 0.6% of 4270 cases reviewed from 1942 to 1977 (Rossett et al, 1985). In many of these cases, the needle had been left in for several days. No data currently exist regarding the infection rate following emergency intraosseous infusions. Another potential complication is damage to the epiphyseal plate, but this has never been reported and is unlikely to occur if proper technique is used.

ENTERAL

Oral administration is the most common and most convenient method of giving non-emergency drugs. It utilizes the large absorptive surfaces of the stomach and small intestine and does not require special equipment. The onset of therapeutic effects for most drugs occurs within 30 minutes. Absorption may be affected by gastric pH, the presence of food in the stomach, lipid solubility of the drug, or presence of other drugs.

Drugs absorbed in the stomach are significantly affected by gastric pH. When drugs are not ionized, they diffuse freely across the mucosal surface of the stomach. However, when drugs are ionized, they are not absorbed. For instance, organic acids, such as salicylic acid, are well absorbed because they are almost completely nonionized. Bases, on the other hand, are ionized in the low pH of the stomach and therefore poorly absorbed. By buffering the stomach contents, absorption of bases may be improved.

Another factor that may affect absorption in the stomach is the presence of food. Food may complex with the drug and prevent absorption. An example is tetracycline, which is poorly absorbed in the presence of dairy products and other calcium-containing substances. Calcium complexes with tetracycline to form an insoluble calcium salt that is poorly absorbed.

Many drugs, electrolytes, and other molecules are actively transported across the mucosal surface of the gastrointestinal system. Others are not transported and do not diffuse across the membranes. Magnesium, which has recently been used to treat a variety of disorders such as arrhythmias secondary to myocardial infarction and acute asthma, must be administered parenterally because it is not absorbed by the gastrointestinal system. In fact, magnesium acts as a cathartic when given orally. Drugs that are actively transported by the gastrointestinal system may not be absorbed if the transport mechanism is inhibited. An example is folic acid, which is dependent on an enzyme for hydrolysis to the monoglutamate before it can be absorbed. Phenytoin inhibits the hydrolysis of folic acid and thus may cause megaloblastic anemia.

Many drugs commonly used in emergency situations are not absorbed or are destroyed by the gastrointestinal system. Epinephrine and insulin are both destroyed by gastrointestinal enzymes. Lidocaine is absorbed but is completely metabolized in a first pass through the liver and cannot be used to treat arrhythmias. Propranolol and hydralazine are also subject to first-pass metabolism by the liver, but not as completely as lidocaine.

Despite problems with absorption, many drugs used in emergency situations are well absorbed and produce a therapeutic response and blood levels similar to those obtained following intravenous administration. An example is theophylline, which may be administered orally to produce therapeutic

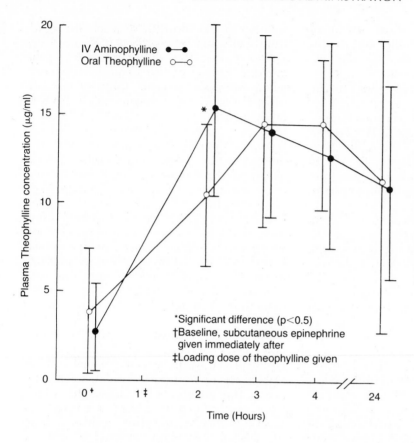

FIGURE 2–4. Plasma theophylline concentrations versus time in patients loaded with intravenous aminophylline compared with those of patients loaded with liquid theophylline by the oral route. (Reproduced with permission from Carrier JA, Shaw RA, Porter RS, et al: Comparison of intravenous and oral routes of theophylline loading in acute asthma. Ann Emerg Med 14: 1145–1151, 1985.)

blood levels. As seen in Figure 2–4, plasma levels and therapeutic responses are similar for patients given oral or intravenous theophylline.

SUBLINGUAL AND BUCCAL

Historically, the sublingual and buccal routes have been used as a means of administering drugs in situations or illnesses in which a rapid response is required. Morphine was commonly administered by these routes in the early 1900s. Today these routes are used for administering drugs such as nitroglycerin and nifedipine. The sublingual and buccal routes are tolerated well by most patients and offer a method of rapid absorption without the time and equipment required for intramuscular or intravenous administration.

The sublingual and buccal surfaces act like other lipoidal membranes. Absorption depends on the drug pKa, rate of partitioning of the un-ionized form of the drug, and passive diffusion. A change in any of these characteristics may alter absorption. For instance, increasing the pH of morphine sulfate from 4 to 10 will increase absorption over 200%, as shown in Figure 2–5. Another factor that increases absorption is an increase in surface area. The recent introduction of an isosorbide dinitrate and nitroglycerin spray has eliminated the time required for a tablet to dissolve and has increased the area for absorption of these drugs, resulting in a decrease in time of absorption and earlier onset of effects.

The sublingual and buccal routes have certain limitations. First, the patient must be able to hold the tablet in his mouth. This is not always possible in cases of obtundation, cerebrovascular accident, or vomiting. Second, the drug must be adequately absorbed by the sublingual or buccal mucosa. Sublingual nifedipine has recently become a common emergency treatment for hypertension. However, a recent report has demonstrated that very little of the drug is absorbed in the mouth. Instead, most absorption occurs in the stomach. Patients who swallow the drug have significantly higher blood levels of the drug than do those who keep it in the mouth (Fig. 2–6).

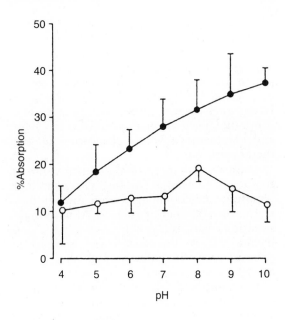

FIGURE 2–5. Percent buccal absorption of morphine sulfate *(solid circles)* and morphine-3-glucuronide *(open circles)* as a function of pH of the buccal membrane. (Reproduced with permission from Al-Sayed-Omar O, Johnston A, Turner P: Influence of pH on the buccal adsorption of morphine sulfate and its major metabolite, morphine-3-glucuronide. J Pharm Pharmacol 39:934–935, 1987.)

RECTAL

The rectal route has been well accepted as a method of drug administration in Europe for centuries. However, in the United States it has not gained popularity except in the administration of antipyretics such as acetaminophen. This is probably due to a combination of cultural influences and questions in the literature regarding absorption.

One advantage of the rectal route over the oral route is that it may produce higher serum concentrations of drugs that are destroyed by the liver. The rectum is drained by the superior, middle, and inferior rectal veins. The superior rectal vein drains into

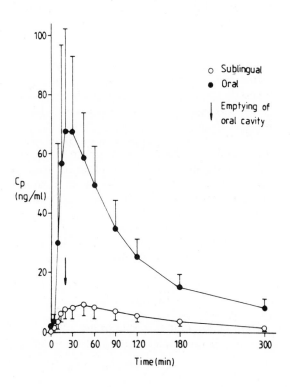

FIGURE 2–6. Plasma concentrations (Cp) of nifedipine after sublingual *(open circles)* and oral *(solid circles)* administration. The oral cavity was washed out after 20 minutes *(indicated by the arrow)* to prevent swallowing and gastric absorption. (Reproduced with permission from Van Harten J, Burggraaf K, Danhof M, et al: Negligible sublingual absorption of nifedipine. Lancet 2:1363–1364, 1987.)

the portal system, whereas the middle and inferior rectal veins drain directly into the inferior vena cava, thus bypassing the portal system and the liver. This allows a higher serum concentration of drugs that have a high rate of first-pass metabolism in the liver. Drugs such as morphine, hydralazine, and propranolol are all metabolized in the liver and may achieve better absorption by the rectal route.

Another advantage of the rectal route is that it can be used in patients with nausea or vomiting. It is commonly used for administration of antiemetics such as trimethobenzamide (Tigan) and prochlorperazine (Compazine). It is also useful for antipyretic administration in children and adults who are unable to take oral medications.

The most underutilized emergency indication for rectal administration is the use of anticonvulsants in status epilepticus. When intravenous access is not available, a solution of diazepam may be administered into the rectum. In one study, this was demonstrated to be 80% effective in the acute management of seizures. Of the 20% of patients who did not respond, half did not respond to diazepam by any route. The initial absorption is much more effective if the drug is administered as a solution than as a suppository. If a solution is used, therapeutic levels may be achieved within 5 minutes in both infants and newborns. The drug may be instilled into the rectum using a small 1-ml syringe or through a pediatric feeding tube. The dose used is the same as that recommended for intravenous administration. Paraldehyde is another anticonvulsant that may be administered by the rectal route and has been shown to be effective when other anticonvulsants fail.

Other drugs that may be administered by the rectal route include nifedipine and morphine. Nifedipine has been demonstrated to significantly decrease systolic and diastolic blood pressure within 30 minutes when administered intrarectally to patients with severe hypertension. Therapeutic effects are seen 7 hours after administration of the drug. Narcotics such as morphine are not commonly administered by the rectal route. They are, however, used by oncologists for cancer patients with pain who cannot tolerate oral medications.

One major concern that most physicians have about the rectal route is the reliability of absorption. Although most European literature supports its reliability, there have been studies that question it. If stool is present in the rectum or the patient is unable to retain the suppository or solution, adequate absorption may not occur. Underlying rectal disease may also prevent adequate absorption.

REFERENCES

Al-Sayed-Omar O, Johnston A, Turner P: Influence of pH on the buccal absorption of morphine sulfate and its major metabolite, morphine-3-glucuronide. J Pharm Pharmacol 39:934–935, 1987.

Arbeiter HI, Greengard J: Tibial bone marrow infusion in infancy. J Pediatr 25:1–12, 1944.

Barker W, Rodeheaver GT, Edgerton MT, et al: Damage to tissue defenses by a topical agent. Ann Emerg Med 11:307–310, 1982.

Barsan WG, Ward JT, Otten EJ: Blood levels of diazepam after endotracheal administration in dogs. Ann Emerg Med 11:242–247, 1982.

Bederka J, Takemori AE, Miller JW: Absorption rates of various substances administered intramuscularly. Eur J Pharmacol 15:132–136, 1971.

Boster SR, Danzl DF, Madden RJ, et al: Translaryngeal absorption of lidocaine. Ann Emerg Med 11:461–465, 1982.

Boyes RN, Scott DB, Jebson PJ, et al: Pharmacokinetics of lidocaine in man. Clin Pharmacol Ther 12:105–111, 1971.

Brickman K, Rega P, Guiness M: Comparison of intraosseous endotracheal and central venous administration of lidocaine in pigs. Ann Emerg Med 17(4):435, 1988.

Bromage PR, Robson JG: Concentrations of lidocaine in the blood after intravenous, intramuscular, epidural and endotracheal administration. Anesthesia 16:461–478, 1961.

Carrier JA, Shaw RA, Porter RS, et al: Comparison of intravenous and oral routes of theophylline loading in acute asthma. Ann Emerg Med 14:1145–1151, 1985.

Choonara IA: Giving drugs per rectum for systemic effect. Arch Dis Child 62:771–772, 1987.

Chu SS, Rah KH, Brannan MD, et al: Plasma concentration of lidocaine after endotracheal spray. Anesth Analg 54:438–441, 1975.

Courtice FC, Phipps PJ: The absorption of fluids from the lungs. J Physiol 105:186–190, 1946.

Curran J, Hamilton C, Taylor T: Topical analgesia before tracheal intubations. Anesthesia 30:765–768, 1975.

Delgado-Escueta AV, Treiman DM: The emergency treatment of status epilepticus. In Johnson RT (ed): Current Therapy in Neurological Disease 1985–1986. Toronto, BC Decker, 1986, pp. 51–60.

Dulac O, Aircardi J, Rey E, et al: Blood levels of diazepam after single rectal administration in infants and children. J Pediatr 93:1039–1041, 1978.

Elam JO: The intrapulmonary route for CPR drugs. In Safar P (ed): Advances in Cardiopulmonary Resuscitation. New York, Springer-Verlag, 1977, p 132.

Elias PM, Cooper ER, Korc A, et al: Importance of stratum corneum structural parameters vs. lipid composition for percutaneous absorption (abstr). Clin Res 28:134, 1980.

Elston JT, Jaynes RV, Kaump DH, et al: Intraosseous infusions in infants. Am J Clin Pathol 17:143–150, 1947.

Graeser JB, Rowe AH: Inhalation of epinephrine for the relief of asthmatic symptoms. J Allergy 6:415–420, 1935.

Greenberg MI, Mayeda DV, Chrzanowski R, Endotracheal administration of atropine sulfate. Ann Emerg Med 11:546–548, 1982.

Greenberg MI, Baskin SI, Kaplan AM, et al: Effects of endotracheally administered distilled water and normal saline on the arterial blood gases of dogs. Ann Emerg Med 11:600–604, 1982.

Greenberg MI, Roberts JR, Krusz JC, et al: Endotracheal epinephrine in a canine anaphylactic shock model. J Am Coll Emerg Physicians 8:500–503, 1979a.

Gueugniaud PY, Theurey O, Vaudelin T, et al: Peripheral versus central intravenous lines in emergency cardiac care (abstr). Lancet 2(8558):573, 1987.

Hallen B, Carlsson P, Uppfeldt: Clinical study of a lignocaine-prilocaine cream to relieve the pain of venipuncture. Br J Anaesth 57:326–328, 1985.

Harvey, SC: Pharmaceutical sciences. In Gennaro AR (ed): Drug Absorption, Action, and Disposition. Easton, PA, Mack Publishing Company, 1985, p 713–740.

Hedges JR, Barsan WB, Doan LA, et al: Central versus peripheral intravenous routes in cardiopulmonary resuscitation. Am J Emerg Med 2:285, 1984.

Hillestad L, Hansen T, Melsom H, et al: Diazepam metabolism in normal man. Clin Pharmacol Ther 16:479–484, 1974.

Hodge D, Delgado-Paredes C, Fleisher G: Intraosseous infusion flow rates in hypovolemic "pediatric" dogs. Ann Emerg Med 16:305–307, 1987.

Kaye W, Bircher NG: Access for drug administration during cardiopulmonary resuscitation. Crit Care Med 16(20):179–182, 1988.

Knepp, VM, Handgralt J, Gay RH: Transdermal drug delivery: Problems and possibilities. Crit Rev Ther Drug Carrier Syst 4(1):13–37, 1987.

Knudsen FU: Rectal administration of diazepam in solution in the acute treatment of convulsions in infants and children. Arch Dis Child 54:855–857, 1979.

Knudsen FU: Plasma-diazepam in infants after rectal administration in solution and by suppository. Acta Paediatr Scand 66:563–567, 1977.

Kurosawa S, Kurosawa N, Owada E: Rectal administration of nifedipine: Haemodynamic effects and pharmacokinetics in hypertensives. J Int Med Res 15:121–127, 1987.

Lubens HM, Ausdenmoore RW, Shafer AD, et al: Anesthetic patch for painful procedures. Am J Dis Child 128:192–194, 1974.

Lacy CR, Rodby RA, Insel J, et al: Comparison of central and peripheral venous routes of medication administration during closed-chest cardiopulmonary resuscitation in humans (abstr). Crit Care Med 15(4):369, 1987.

Langslet A, Meberg J, Bredesen JE, Lunde PKM: Plasma concentrations of diazepam and n-desmethyldiazepam in newborn infants after intravenous, intramuscular, rectal and oral administration. Acta Paediatr Scand 67:699–704, 1978.

Mace SE: The effect of dilution on plasma lidocaine levels with endotracheal administration. Ann Emerg Med 16:522–526, 1987.

McNamara RM, Spivey WH, Unger HD, et al: Emergency applications of intraosseous infusion. J Emerg Med 5:97–100, 1987.

Murphy MM, Caplen SM, Nowak RM, et al: Endotracheal bretylium tosylate in a canine model. Ann Emerg Med 13:87–91, 1984.

Prete MR, Hannan CJ, Burkle FM: Plasma atropine concentrations via the intravenous, endotracheal and intraosseous routes of administration (abstr). Ann Emerg Med 15:195, 1986.

Principles of Drug Action. Chapter 2, In Goldstein A, Aronow L, Kalman SM (eds): The Absorption, Distribution, and Elimination of Drugs. New York, John Wiley & Sons, 1974, pp 129–217.

Pryor G, Kilpatrick WR, Opp DR: Local anesthesia in minor lacerations: Topical TEC versus lidocaine infiltration. Ann Emerg Med 9:568–571, 1980.

Ralston SH, Tacker WA, Showen L, et al: Endotracheal versus intravenous epinephrine during electromechanical dissociation with CPR in dogs. Ann Emerg Med 14:1044, 1985.

Rebuck AS, Bracde AC: Assessment of drug deposition in the lung. Drugs 28:544, 1984.

Redding JS, Asuncion FS, Pearson JW: Effective routes of drug administration during cardiac arrest. Anesth Analg 46:253–258, 1967.

Reisin LH, Landau E, Darawshi A: More rapid relief of pain with isosorbide dinitrate oral spray than with sublingual tablets in elderly patients with angina pectoris. Am J Cardiol 61:2E–3E, 1988.

Roberts JR, Greenberg MI, Baskin SI: Endotracheal epinephrine in cardiorespiratory collapse. J Am Coll Emerg Physicians 8:515–519, 1979.

Roberts JR, Greenberg MI, Knaub MA, et al: Blood levels following intravenous and endotracheal epinephrine administration. J Am Coll Emerg Physicians 8:53–56, 1979b.

Roberts JR, Greenberg MI, Knaub MA, et al: Comparison of the pharmacological effects of epinephrine administered by the intravenous and endotracheal routes. J Am Coll Emerg Physicians 7:260–263, 1978.

Rossetti VA, Thompson BM, Miller J, et al: Intraosseous infusion: An alternative route of pediatric intravascular access. Ann Emerg Med 14:885–888, 1985.

Rusli M, Spivey WH, Bonner H, et al: Endotracheal diazepam: Absorption and pulmonary pathologic effects. Ann Emerg Med 16(3):314–318, 1987.

Russo J, Lipman AG, Comstock TJ, et al: Lidocaine anesthesia: Comparison of iontophoresis, injection and swabbing. Am J Hosp Pharm 37:843–847, 1980.

Schanker LS: Commentary: Drug absorption from the lungs. Biochem Pharmacol 27:381, 1978.

Schoffstall JM, Spivey WH, Lathers CM, et al: Comparison of intraosseous infusion in large and small swine (abstr). Ann Emerg Med 16:511, 1987.

Segal MS, Ryder CM: Penicillin aerosolization in the treatment of serious respiratory infections. N Engl J Med 233:747–756, 1945.

Shaw JE, Prevo ME, Amkraut AA: Testing of controlled release transdermal dosage. Arch Dermatol 123:1548–1556, 1987.

Sonander H, Arnold E, Nilsson K: Effects of the rectal administration of diazepam. Br J Anaesth 57:578–580, 1985.

Spivey WH: Intraosseous infusions. J Pediatr 111:639–643, 1987.

Spivey WH, Lathers CM, Malone DR, et al: Comparison of intraosseous, central and peripheral routes of sodium bicarbonate administration during CPR in pigs. Ann Emerg Med 14:1135–1140, 1985.

Spivey WH, Unger HD, Lathers CM, et al: Intraosseous diazepam suppression of pentylenetetrazol-induced epileptogenic activity in pigs. Ann Emerg Med 16:156–159, 1987.

Standards and Guidelines for Cardiopulmonary Resuscitation and Emergency Cardiac Care. JAMA 255(21):2841–3044, 1986.

Sweeney WM, Hardy SM, Dornbrush AC, Ruegsegger JM: Absorption of tetracycline in human beings as affected by certain excipients. Antibiot Med Clin Ther 4:642–656, 1957.

Tocantins LM, O'Neil JF: Infusion of blood and other fluids into circulation via the bone marrow. Proc Soc Exp Biol Med 45:782–783, 1940.

Trandberg D, Abercrombie D: Treatment of heroin overdose with endotracheal naloxone. Ann Emerg Med 11:443, 1982.

Vandenburg MJ, Griffiths GK, Brandman S: Sublingual nitroglycerin or spray in the treatment of angina. Br J Clin Pract 40(12):524–527, 1986.

vanHarten J, Burggraaf K, Danhof M, et al: Negligible sublingual absorption of nifedipine. Lancet 2:1363–1364, 1987.

Ward JT: Endotracheal drug therapy. Am J Emerg Med 1:71–82, 1983.

CHAPTER 3

Drug Therapy During Pregnancy and Lactation

LYNNETTE DOAN-WIGGINS, M.D.

Although the use of medications by gravid women has declined in recent years, it is estimated that, excluding vitamin and iron supplements, up to 75% of women take one or more medications at some time during their pregnancy. The agents most commonly used include the non-narcotic analgesics, cough and cold preparations, antacids, and antibiotics. Almost half of all drugs taken before labor are over-the-counter preparations, acetaminophen being the drug most commonly used by pregnant women.

Drug therapy during pregnancy must be considered in terms of its effect on the fetus and in terms of the effect that the multiple physiologic changes accompanying pregnancy will have on the pharmacokinetics of the drug.

EFFECT OF PREGNANCY ON DRUG PHARMACOKINETICS

Pregnancy is accompanied by many physiologic changes that may affect drug therapy. *Absorption* of drugs in the gastrointestinal tract during gestation has not been well studied but is believed to be similar to that in nonpregnant patients. Despite a progesterone-induced prolongation of gastric emptying and intestinal transit times, pregnancy has little effect on gastrointestinal secretion, digestion, and absorption.

The *distribution* of drugs during pregnancy is influenced by several factors. Total body water increases gradually throughout pregnancy as plasma volume expands by as much as 50%, edema fluid accumulates, and the fetoplacental unit develops. These changes significantly increase the volume of distribution of many drugs and decrease the serum concentration achieved after a given dose. Serum proteins relevant to drug binding also undergo considerable change. Despite an increase in albumin production, serum albumin concentration decreases due to a correspondingly greater rise in plasma volume. The actual albumin-binding capacity of drugs is thus reduced, allowing more unbound or "free" drug to accumulate and become available for placental transfer. For drugs that are highly protein bound, such as phenytoin, this reduction in binding capacity also leads to a decrease in total plasma concentration and an accelerated clearance of the drug.

Hepatic and renal *metabolism* of drugs is variably affected by pregnancy. Metabolism of drugs in the liver is influenced by increasing amounts of circulating steroid hormones, and direct metabolism by hepatic microsomal enzymes generally increases. Hepatic blood flow, on the other hand, remains relatively unchanged, and minimal centrilobular bile stasis occurs in the liver as pregnancy progresses. Therefore, drugs for which the rate of elimination is dependent on the activity of liver enzymes, such as phenytoin and theophylline, can show a large increase in clearance. In contrast, the clearance of drugs for which metabolism depends primarily on hepatic blood flow, such as propranolol, is relatively unaffected. The excretion of drugs eliminated primarily by the kidney is also altered during pregnancy and may be more rapid as a result of increased renal perfusion and glomerular filtration. Renal blood flow increases 25 to 50% during gestation because of increased cardiac output; glomerular filtration rate increases by 50%.

In general, the net effect of the physiologic changes of pregnancy is a decrease in maternal serum drug concentrations. For many drugs, the volume of distribution increases and total clearance rises during gestation as renal clearance and hepatic metabolism increase and drug half-life shortens.

EFFECTS OF DRUG THERAPY ON THE DEVELOPING FETUS

Drugs are believed to account for up to 5% of all fetal malformations, but currently their role in the etiology of fetal malformations is not entirely clear. The impact of maternal medication on the incidence of spontaneous abortion, fetal growth retardation, and other adverse sequelae is not accurately known.

Studies of fetal pharmacokinetics demonstrate that many drugs cross the placenta, primarily by simple diffusion but also by active transfer. With few exceptions, any drug in sufficient concentration will eventually cross the placenta if maternal therapeutic blood levels of the drug have been maintained for an extended period of time. Placental transfer of a drug is dependent on the relative concentration gradients of free drug and on the drug's molecular size, lipid solubility, electrical charge, and degree of protein binding. An unbound, un-ionized drug of molecular weight less than 1000 is usually lipid soluble and will rapidly penetrate the placental tissues that separate the maternal and fetal circulations. Drug transfer is greater during late gestation as a result of an increase in the maternal concentration of unbound drug available for transport, increased placental surface area, and greater physical disruption of placental membranes.

Fetal serum levels of drugs that cross the placental barrier frequently reach concentrations approaching 50 to 100% of that of maternal serum. A few drugs, such as diazepam and local anesthetics, may reach fetal concentrations at equilibrium that are greater than those in the mother.

The effects of a drug and its metabolites on the fetus are related to the dose and duration of administration of the drug and to the developmental stage of the fetus at the time of exposure. The total exposure of the fetus to a drug and its metabolites is more important than the rate of transplacental transfer; chronic drug exposure is much more likely to produce adverse fetal effects than is single-dose therapy.

The susceptibility of fetal organs to teratogenesis is greatest during the first 10 weeks postconception. Dysmorphogenic effects occurring during the first 2 to 3 weeks postconception typically result in death of the embryo and spontaneous abortion. The period of organogenesis when the embryo shows extreme sensitivity to teratogens and during which exposure results in major organ malformations and functional abnormalities occurs 3 to 8 weeks following conception. Physiologic defects and growth delay are the principal adverse effects resulting from exposure beyond the tenth week of gestation.

The lack of total reliability of results of animal testing to determine a drug's teratogenicity in humans was demonstrated in the 1960s when the association of thalidomide and phocomelia was first recognized in humans despite previous animal studies that had demonstrated the absence of congenital malformations associated with thalidomide use. The lack of interspecies reliability in determining a drug's teratogenic potential is believed to relate to distinct physiologic, pharmacologic, and functional anatomic differences among species and illustrates the difficulty in applying animal research to predict the safety of drug use in human pregnancy.

In 1977, the United States Food and Drug Administration (FDA) established five categories indicating a drug's potential for teratogenesis, and this information is now included in the precautions section of the drug's package insert. All prescription drugs absorbed systemically or known to have a potential for harm to the fetus are categorized according to the level of risk as follows:

Category A. Controlled studies in women have failed to demonstrate a risk to the fetus, and the possibility of fetal harm is remote.

Category B. Either (1) animal studies have not demonstrated a fetal risk but there are no adequate studies in women, or (2) animal studies indicate some risk to the fetus that has not been confirmed in well-controlled studies in women.

Category C. Either (1) studies in animals have revealed adverse effects on the fetus and there are no adequate controlled studies in women, or (2) studies in women and animals are not available.

Category D. Positive evidence of human fetal risk exists, but the benefits for pregnant women may be acceptable despite the risk. A Category D drug will generally be one indicated for use in a life-threatening situation or serious disease for which safer drugs cannot be used or are ineffective. If a Category D drug is given to a pregnant woman or if a woman becomes pregnant while taking it, the physician should inform her of the potential risks to the fetus.

Category X. Fetal abnormalities have been demonstrated in animal or human studies, and the potential risks clearly outweigh the potential benefits. Such drugs are contraindicated for use during pregnancy.

Because it is possible that all drugs represent a potential hazard to the fetus, both prescription and over-the-counter drugs should be used with caution throughout pregnancy and be given only for specific indications at the minimum effective dose for the shortest duration of time.

DRUG THERAPY DURING LACTATION

The number of women who breast-feed their infants has increased from 25% in 1975 to greater than 50% at present. Data on the long- and short-term effects and safety of maternal medications on the breast-feeding infant, however, remain incomplete.

The majority of drugs present in a woman's blood will be detectable in her breast milk. Drugs generally cross membranes by simple diffusion, and the degree to which a drug enters the maternal milk depends on the concentration of the drug in the maternal blood; the drug's molecular weight, lipid solubility, and degree of ionization; and whether it is actively secreted into the milk. Local blood flow in breast tissue is increased during lactation, and simple diffusion is facilitated.

With few exceptions, all drugs present in the maternal circulation are transferred into the breast milk. The maximum amount secreted into milk, however, seldom exceeds 1 to 2% of the maternal dose and does not reflect the total amount absorbed by the infant. Because most drugs given to the mother will affect the nursing infant, the same principles of drug administration that apply during pregnancy should be adhered to during lactation.

It is generally agreed that certain drugs, such as chloramphenicol, lithium, isotretinoin, phenindione, the antimetabolites, and radioactive pharmaceuticals, are contraindicated during breast-feeding. Drugs that are relatively contraindicated include the sulfonamides, nitrofurantoin, metronidazole, chlorthalidone, iodides, and antithyroid medications, with the possible exception of propylthiouracil.

REFERENCES

Abramowicz M (ed): Update: Drugs in breast milk. Med Lett Drugs Ther 21:21, 1979.

American Medical Association: Drug Evaluations, 6th ed. Prepared by the American Medical Association Department of Drugs, Division of Drugs and Technology. Philadelphia, WB Saunders, 1986, Chapters 2 and 3.

Bogaert MC, Thiery M: Pharmacokinetics and pregnancy. Eur J Obstet Gynecol Reprod Biol 16:229, 1983.

Doan LA: Drug therapy during pregnancy and lactation. In Farrell RG (ed): OB/Gyn Emergencies: The First 60 Minutes. Rockville, MD, Aspen, 1986, p 87.

Hill RM, Stern L: Drugs in pregnancy: Effects on the fetus and newborn. Drugs 17:182, 1979.

Iams JD, Rayburn WF, Zuspan FP: Drug effects on the fetus. In Rayburn WF, Zuspan FP (eds): Drug Therapy in Obstetrics and Gynecology. Norwalk, CT, Appleton-Century-Crofts, 1986, pp 13–23.

Niederhoff H, Zahradnik HP: Analgesics during pregnancy. Am J Med 14:117, 1983.

Pregnancy labeling. FDA Drug Bulletin, p 23, September, 1977.

Rayburn WF, Andresen BD: Principles of perinatal pharmacology. In Rayburn WF, Zuspan FP (eds): Drug Therapy in Obstetrics and Gynecology. Norwalk, CT, Appleton-Century-Crofts, 1986, pp 3–12.

Rayburn W, Wible-Kant J, Bledsoe P: Changing trends in drug use during pregnancy. J Reprod Med 27:569, 1982.

Rubin PC: Prescribing in pregnancy. Br Med J 293:1415, 1986.

Whipkey RR, Paris PM, Stewart RD: Drug use in pregnancy. Ann Emerg Med 13:346, 1984.

CHAPTER 4

Considerations in the Dosing of Pediatric Patients

BRYAN BLACKWELDER, Pharm.D.
JAY L. SCHAUBEN, Pharm.D., FABAT

INTRODUCTION

It is obvious, from both a diagnostic and therapeutic standpoint, that pediatric patients differ considerably from their adult counterparts. Size differences will understandably require a decrease in the amount of medication administered to pediatric patients, but the dose often cannot simply be scaled down on the basis of weight alone, especially when the drug being given has a narrow therapeutic window. When using medication in an emergent situation, those agents that impart their clinical effects immediately (e.g., dopamine, norepinephrine, nitroprusside) may be easily titrated to patient response. On the other hand, drugs that normally display reliable correlations between serum levels and clinical effect (i.e., theophylline, lidocaine, digoxin) have fostered attempts to calculate dosage based exclusively on what is necessary to attain adequate serum concentrations, without regard for a variety of factors that may justify a modification of this dose. The clinician should be forewarned that a simplistic approach to pediatric dosing may lead to a therapeutic failure or the precipitation of toxic or adverse side effects; both circumstances are undesirable and of no help to the patient.

For some time, children were labeled as "therapeutic orphans" to provoke interest in research involving the pharmacokinetics and pharmacodynamics of drugs in this age group. Although the necessity for safe and effective pediatric dosing regimens has enhanced both the quantity and quality of these studies in children, only 25% of all medications currently available carry Federal Drug Administration approval for pediatric use. This situation will not likely change owing to the increased liability incurred by the manufacturer of a pharmaceutical approved for pediatric use. It would therefore be advantageous to incorporate information on the maturational and disease-related changes influencing drug disposition into our thought processes.

PHARMACOKINETIC ALTERATIONS IN THE PEDIATRIC PATIENT

The presence of age-dependent variables will markedly influence the pharmacokinetic handling of drugs, which is further complicated by the variability and unpredictability with which the maturation process proceeds in the general pediatric population. Variations in gastric and intestinal pH, gastric emptying time, intestinal motility, absorptive surface area, biliary function, cell membrane permeability, and gut flora are factors known to influence the absorption of an orally administered compound. The distribution characteristics of a compound are known to be affected by changes in the proportion of body water and fat, protein and tissue binding, circulatory factors, and blood–brain barrier development. It is the interaction of these variables that will determine how much of the drug will actually reach the tissue receptor sites. In turn, these receptors may also exhibit age-related changes in their sensitivity and binding affinity. Drug effects may be further confounded by age-related changes in the amount of plasma protein binding. Various pathways for the biotransformation of compounds are known to be altered in different age groups as shifts in the metabolic degradation schemes parallel the maturation of enzyme subsystems.

The net effect of these age-dependent variables may translate into an increased or decreased ability to handle the prescribed dose. For this reason, physicians unfamiliar with pediatric dosing protocols should have resources readily available that allow for appropriate dosage selection and modification. Insensitivity to these inherent age-related, disease-related, and individual variables may lead to serious errors when dosing a child. It is beyond the scope of this chapter to discuss the pharmacokinetic changes in detail. Nevertheless, highlights of these age- and disease-related alterations in the pharmacokinetic handling of drugs are presented here to familiarize the non-pediatric-trained physician with specific parameters that may explain these differences.

As expected, age-related modifications in the absorption, distribution, metabolism, or excretion (ADME) of a compound may remarkably alter the elicited clinical effect. These modifications in the ADME appear to be most marked in the newborn, with a progressive trend over time toward the "normal adult situation." Pediatric patients demonstrate deviations in elimination-rate kinetics as a result of age-related differences in the amount of enzyme stores, enzyme activity, and hepatic and/or renal maturity.

Disease-related factors may also disturb normal pharmacokinetic handling of drugs.

Metabolic effects such as dehydration, fever, and acidosis, all common in the diseases of childhood, can markedly alter the effects of a drug. Metabolic acidosis can have a profound effect on the penetration and accumulation of compounds in the tissue compartment. The cellular uptake and concentration of weakly acidic drugs in this environment are increased; for weakly basic drugs, they are decreased. Plasma protein binding may also be affected. Hydration status will influence the volume of distribution of a drug, making predictions for reaching and maintaining therapeutic levels difficult. The presence of fever may modify the response to certain medications, possibly by accelerating the metabolic breakdown of the compound.

Alteration in the Absorption of Drugs

Gastrointestinal absorption of a drug is influenced by gastric acidity, gastric and intestinal motility, biliary function, enzymatic activity, permeability and maturation of the mucosal membrane, bacterial flora, and composition of the diet. These factors vary considerably from birth to adulthood. Considerable maturational changes in these variables occur within the first few days after birth and continue to change during the next few years of life.

Changes in gastric pH occur as early as the first 24 to 48 hours after delivery. Although the initial pH ranges from 6 to 8 at birth and decreases to 1 to 3 very rapidly, total acidity remains low for the first few months of life. Frequent formula feedings will also alter gastric pH during the first six months. Normal adult values for gastric acid secretion will not be reached for approximately two years. Consequently, a weakly acidic drug will be absorbed slowly, and a weakly basic drug absorbed preferentially.

Gastric emptying time may be as long as 6 to 8 hours in the newborn and will not approach adult values until 6 months of age. Diarrhea frequently decreases gastric transit time, conceivably impairing the absorption of certain drugs (e.g., ampicillin, digoxin).

There is an increased potential for dermal absorption in infants when compared to adults, apparently due to the presence of an immature stratum corneum and a thinner, more well hydrated epidermis. Percutaneous absorption of certain compounds, such as those related to hexachlorophene, aniline dyes, naphthalene, pentachlorophenol, boric acid, potent corticosteroids, and phenylmercury diaper rinses, are known to produce intoxication in infants.

Intramuscular absorption in neonates, infants, and children is often unpredictable due to variable blood flow, vasomotor activity, and tissue oxygenation. Onset of activity may be significantly delayed with this mode of administration.

Rectal administration of drugs in the pediatric patient has been considered an attractive alternative in the child who is vomiting or reluctant to take oral medication. Some clinicians use this route in an attempt to avoid the first-pass effect of the liver. Unfortunately, this route is not an ideal entry port for medication because of the considerable individual variation in rectal venous drainage and, therefore, overall drug absorption from the site.

Alteration in the Volume of Distribution

The distribution characteristics of a drug can be markedly affected by changes in the proportion of body water and fat, protein and tissue binding, circulatory factors, blood–brain barrier development, and other concurrent physiologic and pathologic conditions. Since drugs are distributed between extracellular water and fat according to the lipid/water partition coefficient, the relative variability of these parameters can alter drug distribution characteristics. Blood flow, tissue mass, and fat content will influence the amount of drug that actually reaches the tissue receptor sites. These receptors in turn may vary with age in their sensitivity and binding affinity characteristics. A relative change in the amount of tissue mass, especially lymphatic and renal tissue, which occurs throughout childhood, may further alter distribution characteristics.

Throughout infancy and childhood there is a continual change in the body's water compartment. Total body water may be responsible for as much as 85% of a premature infant's weight and 70 to 75% of a full-term infant's weight but accounts for only 55% of adult body weight. Intracellular water remains fairly constant throughout life. The most dramatic changes occur in the postnatal and infancy periods. Extracellular water accounts for 50% of body weight in premature newborns, 35% in the 4- to -6-month-old,

25% in the 1-year-old, and only 20% in adulthood, which is reached at approximately 13 to 15 years of age. Due to the comparatively larger extracellular fluid compartment found in the younger age group, lower plasma concentrations of water-soluble compounds (e.g., theophylline, the aminoglycosides) should be expected when children are given a proportionally similar dose. Conversely, the fraction of total body weight present as fat increases with age; therefore, the volume of distribution for lipid-soluble drugs is smaller in the neonate than in the adult.

Infants and young children will generally display reduced plasma protein binding when compared to their adult counterparts. Accordingly, a larger amount of free drug will be available for distribution to and interaction with tissue receptors, and this may have a profound effect on the interpretation of drug levels, since analytical techniques commonly measure the total drug concentration (both free and bound) with no regard to active (unbound) or inactive (bound) drug. In addition to the reduced plasma protein concentration, the serum albumin exhibits a qualitatively lower binding capacity for acidic drugs. This characteristic also results in an increased free fraction of drug (unbound) with an enhanced potential for toxicity.

Another aspect of drug binding is competition with endogenous substances in the body, such as bilirubin. A renowned example of this is sulfonamide's potential to displace bilirubin from its albumin binding sites in the jaundiced neonate, which results in an increased risk for kernicterus. The binding of basic drugs to alpha-1-glycoprotein also exhibits age-related effects. In neonates there is a reduced concentration of this protein, and adult values are usually not reached until 7 to 12 years of age.

The blood–brain barrier in newborns is developmentally incomplete, resulting in increased permeability for certain substances into the brain (e.g., lipid-soluble drugs). This increased permeability may make the infant or young child more "sensitive" to direct central nervous system effects than the older child or adult.

Alteration in the Metabolism of Drugs

Metabolic degradation enhances the water solubility of a compound to make it more easily excretable. The rate of oxidative metabolism (e.g., hydroxylation) and glucuronidation is often reduced in newborns, resulting in persistent drug-related effects of compounds metabolized via this pathway, whereas sulfate conjugation and demethylation seem to proceed at adult levels. Metabolic oxidation processes in newborns are approximately 50 to 70% of normal adult values. Compounds such as acetaminophen, phenobarbital, phenytoin, diazepam, lidocaine, nortriptyline, and theophylline may be metabolized to intermediate products that necessitate conjugation pathways for final elimination. Immaturity, specifically in the glucuronidation pathway, is known to influence the handling of chloramphenicol, salicylic acid, and nalidixic acid. Chloramphenicol may produce the "gray baby syndrome" when used in neonates exhibiting a decreased capacity for glucuronidation, especially when clinicians forego appropriate monitoring procedures. After approximately 1 month of age, the efficiency of glucuronidation increases dramatically, ultimately approaching adult levels at approximately 3 to 4 years of age. Acetaminophen, primarily metabolized by glucuronidation in adults, is biotransformed predominantly by sulfation in children under 9 to 12 years of age. This difference in metabolic profile may be responsible for their observed "hepato-tolerance" to acetaminophen overdose.

Compared to adults, drug metabolism is decreased in neonates, accelerated in children ages 1 to approximately 5 years, and then slowly reverts to adult values by puberty. The age-dependent metabolic pattern of theophylline biotransformation is a notable example of this effect. Premature infants, because of their limited ability to metabolize theophylline, can manifest theophylline half-lives of up to 30 hours. As the enzyme system matures, the elimination rate increases, reducing the observed theophylline half-life to approximately 4 hours by 1 year of age. This very rapid elimination is purportedly due to a greater liver-weight to body-weight ratio in comparison to adults. Upon reaching the ninth year of life, this ratio begins to normalize slowly toward adult standards. Consequently, the theophylline half-life returns to generally accepted adult values (approximately 8 hours).

The bioavailability of orally ingested compounds exhibiting high hepatic clearances may also display great individual variability consistent with alterations in hepatic first-pass metabolism (e.g., propranolol, propoxyphene). Phenobarbital, phenytoin, acetaminophen, and riboflavin are shown to have either decreased absorption or decreased bioavailability.

Although not considered an age-related phenomenon, pharmacogenetic variations in glucose-6-phosphate-dehydrogenase activity, oxidation, acetylation, and pseudocholinesterase activity also play a role in the predictability of clinical drug effects. If aberrations in metabolic pathways are suspected or present in a patient, modification in dosage will be required to avoid toxic effects.

Alteration in the Elimination of Drugs

Metabolic degradation renders a compound more water soluble and therefore more susceptible to renal elimination. Renal excretion may involve the elimination of both active and inactive metabolites, as well as unchanged parent compounds. Obviously, a decrease in the elimination rate for unchanged drug or active metabolite will prolong drug effect. Developmentally, renal function is incomplete at birth. Glomerular filtration rates for newborns are 35 to 50% of those exhibited by older children and adults (newborn 10 ml/min/m^2 versus 70 ml/min/m^2 for adults). Obviously, this will affect the elimination of a drug primarily dependent on the kidney for final excretion, such as vancomycin and the aminoglycoside antibiotics.

Renal tubular function at birth (both secretory and absorptive) is moderately decreased compared to adult standards, affecting elimination of such agents as the penicillin and cephalosporin congeners. Renal function comparable to that of an adult is not achieved until approximately 6 months to 1 year of age. Newborn renal plasma flow is reportedly only 2 to 40% of adult values and improves quickly by 4 weeks of age. Full adult capacity may not be realized until 12 months of age.

TECHNICAL FACTORS

The inability to access the systemic circulation via intravenous catheter placement in the pediatric patient is of considerable concern for the non-pediatric-trained physician. In addition to the use of the endotracheal tube for medication administration, the intraosseous route, popular in the 1940s before venous catheters became available, has been enjoying renewed interest. Its use has been advocated for administration of resuscitation drugs when peripheral venous access cannot be readily obtained in the pediatric patient. The procedure for intraosseous access is considered simple and has been adequately described in Chapter 2. With proper technique, access to the systemic circulation can be established in 60 to 90 seconds, whereupon crystalloids, blood, anticonvulsants, muscle relaxants, epinephrine, atropine, sodium bicarbonate, hypertonic glucose, antibiotics, or continuous infusions of dopamine and dobutamine can be used.

Another technological concern when initiating intravenous therapy in the pediatric patient involves the appropriate dilution of medication for intravenous administration. Obviously, adult protocols for infusion preparation will often result in a fluid-overloaded child. On the other hand, a too-concentrated solution may make it difficult to titrate dosage adequately. Many different formulas and protocols have been published to address this problem and may help the physician determine the proper dilution factor needed to customize patient management (Appendix I).

CONCLUSION

Much has been written concerning the need for more precise pediatric dosage regimens. Philosophies seem to revolve around the use of body weight (dosing on a mg/kg of body weight basis) or on the calculation of body surface area (dosing on a mg/m² of body surface area basis). Unfortunately, evidence to prove that these methods are indeed accurate is lacking. With the exception of calculating the dosage of the chemotherapeutic agents, the body weight method seems to be preferred. Recently, a method that correlates body length to body weight and drug dosage has been advocated for emergency use. The "Broselow tape" is currently being produced for the commercial market. Clearly, the drug dosage required for a desired therapeutic affect may be significantly altered by individual variation in

drug metabolism and by specific disease states. This dosage variation becomes particularly important when employing resuscitation and other emergency medications, most of which exhibit very narrow margins between their therapeutic and toxic ranges. Whichever method one uses to determine the appropriate dose for the specific patient, there is no substitute for good clinical judgment in identifying specific conditions requiring a deviation from the generally accepted protocols.

REFERENCES

Cavell B: Gastric emptying in preterm infants. Acta Pediatr Scand 68:725–730, 1979.

Friis-Hansen B: Body water compartments in children: Changes during growth and related changes in body composition. Pediatrics 28:169–175, 1961.

Krasner J, Giacoia P, Yaffe ST: Drug-protein binding in the newborn infant. Ann NY Acad Sci 226:101–114, 1973.

Lubitz DS, Seidel JL, Chameides L, et al: A rapid method for estimating weight and resuscitation drug dosages from length in the pediatric age group. Ann Emerg Med 17:576–581, 1988.

Milsap RL, Szefler SJ: Special pharmacokinetic considerations in children. In Evans WE, Schentag JJ, Jusko WJ (eds): Applied Pharmacokinetics: Principles of Therapeutic Drug Monitoring. Spokane, WA, Applied Therapeutics Press, 1986, pp 294–330.

Miner WF, Corneli HM, Bolte RG: Prehospital use of intraosseous infusion by paramedics. Pediatr Emerg Care 5:5–7, 1989.

Morselli PL: Clinical pharmacokinetics in neonates. Clin Pharmacokinet 1:81–98, 1976.

Morselli PL, Franco-Morselli R, Bossi L: Clinical pharmacokinetics in newborns and infants: age-related differences. Clin Pharmacokinet 5:485–527, 1980.

Plakogiannis FM, Cutie AJ: Basic Concepts in Biopharmaceutics: An Introduction. Brooklyn, NY, Brooklyn Medical Press, 1977.

Pratt J: Intraosseous infusion. International Pediatrics 4:19–23, 1989.

Rane E, Wilson JT: Clinical pharmacokinetics in infants and children. Clin Pharmacokinet 1:2–24, 1976.

Shirkey HC: Pediatric clinical pharmacology and therapeutics. In Shirky HC (ed): Pediatric Therapy, 5th ed. St Louis, CV Mosby, 1975.

Shirkey HC: Therapeutic orphans. J Pediatr 72:119–120, 1968.

Stewart CF, Hampton EM: Effect of maturation on drug disposition in pediatric patients. Clin Pharm 6:548–564, 1987.

Wallace S: Factors affecting drug-protein binding in the plasma of newborn infants. Br J Clin Pharmacol 3:510–512, 1976.

Wilson JT, Atwood GF, Shand DG: Disposition of propoxyphene and propranolol in children. Clin Pharmacol Ther 19:264–270, 1976.

CHAPTER 5

Fluid and Electrolyte Therapy

JONATHAN WARREN, M.D.

INTRODUCTION

Fluid and electrolyte homeostasis depends on adequate and continued intake and excretion of free water and solutes. Because these are often disrupted during illness, fluid and electrolyte disorders are common in acutely ill patients. Vomiting and diarrhea are especially troublesome in this regard.

Hypovolemia is perhaps the most common manifestation of disrupted water homeostasis, and its symptoms are caused mainly by intravascular volume depletion. Hypovolemia results in decreased tissue perfusion and, thus, a reduction in oxygen and nutrient transport. The decreased tissue perfusion causes anaerobic metabolism, which results in (1) the accumulation of toxic metabolites, such as lactic acid, with a precipitous fall in intracellular pH; and (2) a shift in the intracellular oxidation/reduction potential toward the reduced state. Irreversible tissue injury results if protein denaturation occurs. The brain and heart are particularly sensitive to this type of injury. The goal of fluid resuscitation is to normalize intravascular volume and restore tissue perfusion.

Disturbances in serum electrolyte concentrations, particularly in sodium and potassium concentrations, frequently accompany fluid losses during disease and can be life-threatening. The severity of the disturbance is related to both the rapidity with which it develops and the magnitude of deviation from normal values. Brain and/or cardiac dysfunction is the most common clinical manifestation of electrolyte abnormalities. Therefore, any patient presenting with seizures, altered mental status (including coma), or a cardiac dysrhythmia should be suspected of having an electrolyte disturbance until proved otherwise.

Therapy for electrolyte disorders depends mainly on correcting the abnormality by eliminating from or replacing into the circulation the appropriate chemical substance(s). The rate at which the abnormality is corrected is often of critical importance. Care must be taken to follow established guidelines of therapy to avoid unnecessary complications.

MAINTENANCE FLUID THERAPY

All patients must receive maintenance fluid, either orally or intravenously. The maintenance regimen must provide for insensible water losses and for water consumed through normal metabolism and tissue maintenance. In addition, maintenance fluid therapy must replace any abnormal ongoing fluid losses, such as those resulting from diarrhea, sweating, drainage from open wounds and burns, and abnormally high urine output.

Standard maintenance fluid therapy is simply approximated. For both adults and infants, 100 ml/kg/24 hours is provided for the first 10 kg of body weight, 50 ml/kg/24

35

hours for the next 10 kg of body weight, and 20 ml/kg/24 hours for each additional kilogram of body weight. For example, a patient weighing 16 kg would receive 1000 + 300 = 1300 ml/24 hours, or about 54 ml/hour as maintenance fluid. A patient weighing 70 kg would receive 1000 + 500 + 1000 = 2500 ml/24 hours, or about 104 ml/hour.

The choice of maintenance intravenous solution depends on the underlying disease state and preexisting pathology. The standard maintenance fluid recommended by most clinicians for hemodynamically stable patients is 5% dextrose/0.2% sodium chloride (NaCl) with 10 to 20 mEq potassium chloride (KCl) added per liter. The dextrose is provided to make the solution approximately isotonic with blood. The NaCl and KCl content can be adjusted as indicated by serum electrolyte measurements. The choice of intravenous solution is very important in young infants and in adults with renal insufficiency, in whom renal concentrating and diluting abilities are suboptimal. Healthy adults can usually compensate for inadequate or excessive solute and water loads by altering renal excretion.

A supplement must be added to maintenance fluids to compensate for abnormal ongoing fluid losses. Insensible fluid losses, normally 600 to 800 ml/day in the average adult, increase with hyperventilation, fever, high environmental temperature, and low humidity. These losses are extremely difficult to measure and are best estimated by changes in body weight. Diarrhea, nasogastric suction, and vomiting are common causes of abnormally increased fluid losses,

but these losses can be quantitated and replaced. By determining the electrolyte content of the fluid lost by these routes, the electrolyte losses can also be replaced. Abnormal losses of sodium, potassium, and water can occur through the urine in many disease states, and these can also be quantitated and replaced. Finally, clinical situations such as peritonitis, burns, and trauma can lead to third-spacing of large volumes of fluid. Third-space losses are difficult to estimate, and, under most circumstances, one must rely on the physical examination (e.g., blood pressure, pulse rate, moistness of the mucous membranes) to assess the extent of loss from the extracellular fluid (ECF) compartment. The pulmonary artery wedge pressure may be helpful in assessing the adequacy of intravascular volume in these patients.

CONDITIONS

Hypovolemia

Diagnosis

The fluid deficit in hypovolemia may be one primarily of free water (dehydration), an isotonic loss of water plus electrolytes (volume depletion), or a combination of the two, depending on the etiology of the depleted state (Table 5–1). Signs and symptoms of hypovolemia usually do not begin to manifest until a 5% water loss from the ECF compartment has occurred. Patients with this degree of fluid deficit generally present with tachycardia, dry mucous membranes, and a con-

TABLE 5–1. Etiology and Characteristics of Hypovolemia

Clinical Disorder	Primary (Secondary) Losses	Water and Electrolyte Disturbances
Vomiting	Water (HCl, K^+)	Dehydration, hypokalemia, metabolic alkalosis, hypernatremia
Diabetes insipidus	Water (K^+)	Dehydration, hypokalemia, hypernatremia
Diarrhea (acute)	Water (Na^+, K^+, HCO_3^-)	Dehydration and volume depletion, hypernatremia, hypokalemia, metabolic acidosis
Environmental heat injury (heat exhaustion, heat stroke)	Water° (NaCl)	Dehydration and volume depletion, hypernatremia
Diarrhea (chronic)	Na^+, K^+, water (HCO_3^-)	Volume depletion, hypokalemia, hyponatremia, metabolic acidosis
Hemorrhage	Whole blood	Volume depletion
Thermal injury	Serum	Volume depletion

°Through perspiration.

centrated urine. In the crying infant, production of tears may be poor. As the ECF deficit approaches 10%, oliguria develops, skin turgor becomes poor, and the eyeballs may appear sunken. In the young infant, the anterior fontanelle may appear depressed as well. ECF deficits become critical as they approach 15%. It is at this level of volume deficit that blood pressure begins to fall and lactic acid production rises, the latter resulting from the anaerobic metabolism caused by poor tissue perfusion. In these patients, capillary refill is usually poor, a physical finding helpful in determining this degree of volume deficit.

It should be noted that with hyponatremic (hypotonic) volume depletion, physical manifestations of hypovolemia appear with less total fluid loss. This is because the relatively greater intracellular osmotic forces tend to pull water from the relatively hypotonic ECF compartment, exacerbating the intravascular volume depletion. Conversely, with hypernatremic (hypertonic) volume depletion, signs and symptoms of hypovolemia occur later. This is because the relatively high ECF osmolarity tends to draw water from the relatively hypotonic intracellular space, reducing the net fluid lost from the ECF compartment. The circulating blood volume is thus preserved at the expense of cell water.

Indications for Treatment

The need for intravenous volume replacement in hypovolemia is determined by the degree of hypovolemia and the potential for ongoing fluid losses. Any individual with an estimated ECF deficit of 10% or greater should be rehydrated by the intravenous route. Patients with smaller estimated ECF deficits, particularly if due to a self-limited problem such as acute gastroenteritis, may be given a trial of oral rehydration with a simple electrolyte solution (Pedialyte for infants, Gatorade for older children and adults). If the oral fluid replacement is not tolerated, intravenous therapy will be necessary.

Individuals with an acute volume deficit due to a short, self-limited condition often feel much better after receiving 1 or 2 liters of replacement fluid and can then have intravenous fluid therapy discontinued. In situations in which ongoing fluid deficits are to be expected (e.g., diabetic ketoacidosis, Crohn's disease, burns, diabetes insipidus) or in which bowel function is not expected to return quickly (e.g., bowel obstruction, pancreatitis, ulcerative colitis), continued intravenous fluid therapy is necessary. In these situations, existing volume deficits should be replaced over the first several hours using Ringer's lactate. Ongoing intravenous therapy should then consist of normal maintenance needs plus an additional volume of fluid to replace additional abnormal losses resulting from fever, vomiting, diarrhea, osmotic diuresis, or drainage through wounds or other abnormal sources such as fistulas. The abnormal fluid losses should be measured directly, if at all possible, so replacement can be precisely quantified. It is also useful to measure the electrolyte content of the fluid losses as a guide to adjust the composition of the replacement fluids. (See box.)

Discussion

The goals of therapy in hypovolemia, in order of importance, are (1) to restore intravascular volume to normal, (2) to correct electrolyte disturbances, and (3) to replace extravascular water losses. Intravascular volume deficits should be corrected rapidly, using the intravenous route whenever possible, especially in the presence of shock or other symptoms of severe hypovolemia. This is accomplished by inserting a large-bore intravenous catheter and administering fluids at a maximal ("wide-open") rate until symptoms abate. In cases of life-threatening hypovolemia, two sites of intravenous access should be used simultaneously. In general, peripheral venous access is preferred because of its low risk, ease of access, and the high flow rates achievable with short, large-bore catheters. However, when peripheral access is impossible, as may be the case in hypovolemic shock, a large-bore central venous catheter may be used.

Patients not responding to reasonable fluid challenges should be considered for invasive monitoring by way of pulmonary artery catheterization. Measurement of the pulmonary artery wedge pressure (PAWP) is the best bedside technique currently available for estimating intravascular volume status. PAWP measurements of less than 5 mmHg indicate hypovolemia. Under these circumstances, fluids should be administered aggressively until oxygen consumption is maximized. Oxygen consumption is defined as the product of the cardiac output and the arterial-venous oxygen content difference. Central venous

---

DRUG TREATMENT: HYPOVOLEMIA

First-Line Therapy

Crystalloids (Ringer's Lactate, 0.9% NaCl)

Initial Dose	Adult: 250–500 ml IV over 15–30 minutes
	Pediatric: 20 ml/kg IV over 15–30 minutes
Repeat Dose	Every 15–30 minutes as indicated by clinical status
End-Point	Improved blood pressure, urine output, capillary refill, and saliva production; decreased heart rate

Second-Line Therapy

Colloids (5% Albumin, Plasma Protein Fraction, Hetastarch)

Initial Dose	Adult: 250 ml IV over 15–30 minutes
	Pediatric: 10 ml/kg IV over 15–30 minutes
Repeat Dose	Every 15–30 minutes as indicated by clinical status
End-Point	Improved blood pressure, urine output, capillary refill, and saliva production; decreased heart rate

---

pressure is often used as a crude estimate of intravascular volume. However, this value may be unreliable and should be interpreted with caution in the critically ill patient.

Much controversy exists regarding which type of fluid (colloid versus crystalloid) should be used for volume resuscitation, and many different fluid types for intravenous administration are currently marketed (Table 5–2). Studies in both animals and humans have claimed to show advantages or disadvantages of one type of fluid over the other. However, a critical assessment of many of these reports demonstrates problems in study design or in the interpretation of data. A recent well-designed study in humans by Kaufman and associates (1986) showed that although colloids are more efficient plasma volume expanders (on a per volume basis), crystalloids are equally efficacious when used in sufficient quantities. Efficacy was assessed by measuring PAWP, cardiac output, oxygen transport, and oxygen consumption. The only difference noted among therapies was the radiographic appearance of pulmonary edema in a significant number of the crystalloid-treated patients. However, hypoxemia was not reported. Some animal studies have demonstrated a mild decrease in arterial oxygenation with crystalloid resuscitation.

Some investigators have raised a concern over the possible leakage of administered colloidal proteins across leaky pulmonary capillaries in shock-induced adult respiratory distress syndrome (ARDS), possibly resulting in a worsening of the pulmonary dysfunction. Hauser and associates (1980) and Appel and Shoemaker (1981) addressed this

TABLE 5–2. Solutions Available for Intravenous Administration and Their Cost

Solution	Cost/500 ml° ($)
Crystalloids	
Ringer's lactate	7.96
0.9% NaCl ("normal" saline)	6.56
1%–5% NaCl (hypertonic saline)	8.16
5% Dextrose	6.65
Dextrose/saline combinations	
Colloids	
5%, 25% Albumin (25 g)	150.00
Plasma protein fraction (Plasmanate)	91.40
Fresh-frozen plasma	
Hetastarch (Hespan)	109.00
Dextran 40	91.22
Dextran 70	59.51

°Wholesale prices as listed in the "Blue Book," American Druggist. Data from First Databank. Annual Directory of Pharmaceuticals. New York, Hearst Corporation, 1989.

TABLE 5–3. Causes of Edema and Third-Space Fluid Accumulation

Organic Causes
Right heart failure
Liver failure
Renal failure
Hypoproteinemia
Positive end-expiratory pressure (PEEP)

Capillary Leak Syndromes
Sepsis
Peritonitis/postoperative abdomen
Burns
Soft tissue trauma
Allergic reactions (angioedema)

issue by randomly treating patients having ARDS with either colloids or crystalloids. Colloids were shown to improve hemodynamic and respiratory function, as measured by cardiac output, oxygen transport, and oxygen consumption.

In summary, either colloids or crystalloids may be used in acute volume resuscitation. Colloids are more efficient plasma volume expanders than are crystalloids, but because of the high cost of the former, most physicians prefer to use crystalloids. Ringer's lactate and normal saline are the preferred crystalloid solutions. Human albumin, plasma protein fraction, and hetastarch are the preferred colloid solutions. Fresh-frozen plasma should be reserved for patients with deficiencies in plasma coagulation factors and given in conjunction with red blood cell transfusions in patients with hemorrhagic shock.

Once intravascular volume has been repleted, the intracellular fluid compartment should be assessed, and fluid disturbances within this compartment should be corrected. This goal should be met gradually, over a period of 48 hours, and may be carried out either orally or intravenously, depending on clinical circumstances. One must be certain to provide adequate fluid and electrolytes, not only for the repletion of existing deficits but also for ongoing losses and normal body maintenance.

Body weight is the best estimate of the adequacy of total body water. Exceptions occur in disease states in which tissue edema or other third-space fluid is prominent (Table 5–3). Under these circumstances, substantially increased volumes of extravascular water can be present in the face of intravascular volume depletion. One must rely on physical findings, such as skin turgor, tear production, and the moistness of mucous membranes, or on invasive hemodynamic monitoring to assess intravascular water under these conditions.

Some physicians use the initial serum sodium measurement as a rough guide to estimating the total body water deficit. This method is most useful following acute water losses, such as those resulting from vomiting or acute diarrheal states. With dehydration that has developed more slowly, sodium ion shifts and sodium losses render the serum sodium measurement less valid as an estimate of total body water.

Hypernatremia

Diagnosis

Hypernatremia is a condition found mainly in the very young and the very old and can be classified into three groups based on etiology (Table 5–4): (1) pure water loss, (2) pure solute gain, and (3) water loss in excess of solute loss. The diagnosis is made when the serum sodium concentration rises to greater than 150 mEq/liter. Symptoms generally do not appear, however, until the concentration approaches 160 mEq/liter. Most symptoms of hypernatremia are referable to the central nervous system and correlate with both the degree and the rate of rise of the serum sodium. Patients are initially irritable and/or restless and may have increased muscle tone. With worsening hypernatremia, patients may progress to develop lethargy, stupor, and coma. Permanent neurologic deficits occur in at least 11 to 15% of patients presenting with a serum sodium concentration of greater than 160 mEq/liter. The injury usually results from shrinkage of the brain, stretching of subdural vessels and resulting subdural hemorrhage, or, more commonly, from red blood cell sludging that

TABLE 5–4. Classification of Hypernatremia

Pure Water Loss
Diabetes insipidus (central, nephrogenic)
Essential hypernatremia

Pure Solute Gain
Concentrated infant formula feedings
Excessive $NaHCO_3$ administration (cardiac resuscitation)

Water Loss in Excess of Solute Loss
Diarrhea (acute)
Vomiting
Osmotic diuresis (glucosuria, mannitol, etc.)
Excessive sweating

causes small vessel occlusion or sinus thrombosis. Seizures may result from these occlusive phenomena. Children with sickle cell anemia are particularly susceptible to these complications, and exchange transfusions may be a necessary part of therapy.

Indications for Treatment

Hypernatremia, defined as a serum sodium concentration above 150 mEq/liter, must be treated as soon as it is diagnosed because of its potential for causing permanent neurologic damage. A serum sodium concentration greater than 160 mEq/liter should be considered an acute life- and brain-threatening emergency requiring immediate action. Alert, cooperative patients with intact thirst mechanisms and a mild degree of hypernatremia (150 to 155 mEq/liter) can be allowed a trial of oral free water repletion while the underlying etiology of the hypernatremia is being identified and treated. When oral therapy is used, the serum sodium must be monitored every 4 to 6 hours and intravenous therapy instituted if it continues to rise. Those patients with serum sodium concentrations greater than 155 mEq/liter should have intravenous free water therapy instituted at the time of diagnosis and continued until the serum sodium is below 150 mEq/liter and the underlying cause has been corrected or the patient has demonstrated the ability to maintain adequate oral free water intake. (See box.)

Discussion

The serum sodium concentration should be corrected over a period of 48 hours. This requires estimating the water deficit and choosing an appropriate electrolyte solution. The best method of estimating the total body water deficit is by determining the loss in body weight. If the baseline weight is known, one can crudely estimate the total body water deficit from the above equation. Note that this latter method has no value in patients with pure solute gain, and it underestimates the fluid deficit in patients with water loss in excess of solute loss.

Patients with hypernatremia of the pure water loss type have a deficient or nonexistent antidiuretic hormone (ADH) production or a renal insensitivity to the hormone. Since the latter is rare, most patients will respond to exogenous hormone therapy with 1-dea-

---

DRUG TREATMENT: HYPERNATREMIA

First-Line Therapy

Free Water (Low-Sodium Solutions)
(0.45% NaCl, 5% Dextrose, 5% Dextrose/0.3% NaCl, 2.5% Dextrose/0.45% NaCl, etc.)

Dose   Volume of any of the above solutions equal to the free water deficit

Free water deficit determined by:

1. Body weight (1 kg weight loss = 1 liter deficit)
2. Serum sodium measurement

$$\text{Water deficit (liters)} = \frac{[Na^+] - 140}{140} \times BW \times 0.6$$

$[Na^+]$ = serum sodium concentration (mEq/liter)
BW   = body weight
0.6   = the body's fractional content of water

Administer over 48 hours; initial rate to decrease the $[Na^+]$ by 2 mEq/hour until symptoms resolve or $[Na^+] < 160$ mEq/liter; then at a rate to provide the rest of the deficit over 48 hours

End-Point   Normal serum sodium

mino-(8-D-arginine)-vasopressin (DDAVP) and free water administration. Patients with pure solute gain must have the offending substance(s) discontinued. The subsequent administration of free water will allow the renal excretion of excess solute. Patients with water loss in excess of solute loss have deficits of both free water and solute that must be replaced from exogenous sources. In all cases, the hypernatremia must be corrected *slowly*. Of course, the presence of severe hypovolemia and shock necessitates rapid fluid resuscitation. However, this scenario is rare with hypernatremia because, as discussed previously, the extracellular fluid compartment in these patients is relatively spared at the expense of cell water.

In choosing a replacement fluid, one must be sure to provide free water. Specifically, the sodium content of the replacement fluid should be less than 140 mEq/liter. Dextrose is added to the fluid to prevent hypotonicity. Thus, any of the solutions listed above are acceptable choices. (*Note:* The amount of free water provided by each of these solutions is different. For example, 1 liter of 5% dextrose provides 1 liter of free water, whereas 1 liter of 0.45% NaCl provides only 500 ml of free water. These variations must be taken into account when determining type and rate of fluid replacement.)

The single most important complication of rehydration therapy is cerebral edema. This complication is manifested clinically by stupor, increased intracranial pressure (e.g., hypertension, decreased mental status), and seizures. In almost all cases it follows the excessively rapid administration of fluid that is hypotonic relative to the patient's serum. The pathogenesis of the cerebral edema remains unknown. It has been shown that during the development of hypernatremia, osmotically active particles appear within the intracellular compartment of brain cells. These "idiogenic osmols" have not been characterized but may act as a compensating mechanism to minimize the brain shrinkage that occurs when fluid is shifted from the body's intracellular fluid compartment to the extracellular fluid compartment in hypernatremic states. During rehydration therapy, the brain's intracellular osmotic forces remain high, resulting in an inappropriately high influx of water and, hence, cerebral edema.

During rehydration therapy, one can anticipate cerebral edema and seizures by closely monitoring patients for signs of increased intracranial pressure. Fluid therapy can be slowed as indicated. In the event that seizures do occur, an infusion of mannitol or hypertonic saline should be considered. This produces a prompt decompression of the brain and control of the seizures. Rehydration therapy can subsequently be restarted at a reduced rate.

Hyponatremia

Diagnosis

In most patients, hyponatremia is mild and asymptomatic. Vague and nonspecific symptoms such as nausea or vomiting may develop as the serum sodium level falls below 125 mEq/liter. More severe hyponatremia results in abdominal cramps, muscle weakness, and myoclonus. Symptoms may progress to the cerebral manifestations of restlessness, confusion, seizures, and coma as the serum sodium falls below 115 mEq/liter. Permanent neurologic damage or death is not uncommon with severe hyponatremia.

Three clinical categories of hyponatremia are defined according to the status of the extracellular fluid volume (Table 5–5): hypervolemic, hypovolemic, and euvolemic. Patients with hypervolemic hyponatremia are characterized by having pitting edema and/or ascites. This is generally caused by a reduced renal perfusion that results in a decrease in glomerular filtration rate and an increase in proximal tubule sodium and water reabsorption. Although total body sodium is increased, total body water is increased even more because these patients usually have increased thirst and water intake.

TABLE 5–5. Classification of Hyponatremia

Hypervolemic
Congestive heart failure
Cirrhosis
Myxedema
Iatrogenic (intravenous therapy)

Hypovolemic
Chronic diuretic therapy
Chronic diarrhea
Salt-wasting nephropathy
Adrenal insufficiency

Euvolemic
Inappropriate antidiuretic hormone syndromes
Primary polydypsia
Iatrogenic (intravenous therapy)

Hypovolemic hyponatremia is characterized by extracellular volume depletion. Most patients have losses of both free water and sodium but have replaced part of the free water because of increased thirst. However, total body water is not brought back to normal, usually because of continued pathologic fluid losses or because a balance is reached between low plasma volume and hypotonicity. The urine is almost always hypertonic with respect to plasma, and urine sodium excretion is low (except in patients with salt-losing states).

Euvolemic hyponatremia is an uncommon disorder characterized by euvolemia, normal renal function, and the absence of edema. Since the administration of ADH plus water to normal subjects can produce the syndrome of euvolemic hyponatremia, it is postulated that these patients have an obligatory secretion of ADH independent of their intravascular volume status. The syndrome has been reported as a paraneoplastic phenomenon, as a drug side effect, and in certain neurologic disorders. The most common cause of euvolemic hyponatremia is iatrogenic, namely intravenous fluid therapy with excess free water and/or insufficient sodium content.

Indications for Treatment

Any patient with a serum sodium concentration less than 130 mEq/liter should have this electrolyte disturbance treated. Asymptomatic patients with a serum sodium between 120 and 130 mEq/liter should be treated with restriction of free water, identification and management of the underlying cause of the hyponatremia, and, in most cases, sodium replacement with intravenous normal saline given at a rate that will replace the deficit over several days. An approximation of the sodium deficit can be calculated using the following formula:

$$Na^+ \text{ deficit (in mEq)}$$
$$= TBW \times (140 - [Na^+])$$

$[Na^+]$ = serum sodium concentration
TBW = total body water
      $0.6 \times$ lean weight (kg) in males
      $0.5 \times$ lean weight (kg) in females

Patients who have symptoms of hyponatremia, such as altered mental status or seizures, and a serum sodium concentration lower than 120 mEq/liter, should be given intravenous hypertonic saline as the initial therapy at a rate that will increase the serum sodium concentration to 121 to 134 mEq/liter over 5 to 6 hours. Then the hypertonic saline should be stopped and management continued with normal saline and definitive therapy of the underlying cause of the hyponatremia. (See box.)

Discussion

Much controversy exists concerning the optimal therapy for hyponatremia. Excessively slow therapy appears to result in increased mortality, but rapid treatment has been reported to cause a fatal osmotic demyelinating syndrome that frequently in-

---

DRUG TREATMENT: HYPONATREMIA

First-Line Therapy
Hypertonic Saline (3% NaCl)

    Dose   50–100 ml/hour via central line. Determine serum sodium concentration every 2 hours during infusion.

    End-Point   Serum sodium 121–134 mEq/liter

Second-Line Therapy
Normal Saline (0.9% NaCl)

    Dose   Infuse at a rate that will return serum sodium concentration to normal over 48 hours.

    End-Point   Normal serum sodium

volves the pons ("central pontine myelinolysis"). This syndrome is manifested by persistent coma with brain stem signs after correction of the hyponatremia. Scanning by computed tomography or magnetic resonance imaging shows characteristic cystic lesions in the brain stem. A recent study by Ayus and colleagues (1987) suggested that it is best to correct severe symptomatic hyponatremia rapidly with hypertonic saline, but only *partially*, to within the range of 121 to 134 mEq/liter. The remainder of the correction should take place over several days. All patients so treated did well and had no neurologic complications. Demyelinating lesions were observed only with rapid *total* correction (or overcorrection) of the serum sodium concentration or when correction was associated with insults such as hypoxia/anoxia or hepatic coma.

Hyperkalemia

Diagnosis

The diagnosis of hyperkalemia is made when the serum potassium concentration exceeds 5.5 mEq/liter, although serious complications rarely occur at concentrations

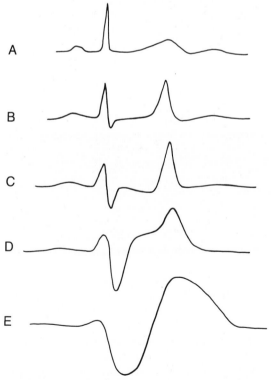

FIGURE 5–1. Sequential ECG changes with increasing serum potassium levels.

lower than 6.5 mEq/liter. Manifestations include muscle weakness, paresthesias, and cardiac arrhythmias (including bradycardia, ventricular fibrillation, and asystole). As the serum potassium rises, characteristic changes are seen on the electrocardiogram (ECG) (Fig. 5–1). These include loss of the P wave, peaking of the T wave, and widening of the QRS complex to a classic "sine wave" pattern. An ECG should be obtained immediately on suspicion of hyperkalemia, and therapy must be instituted as rapidly as possible if the tracing suggests an elevated serum potassium level.

Hyperkalemia can be attributed to an increased potassium load (e.g., increased oral intake of potassium, muscle injury, hemolysis), decreased potassium excretion (e.g., acute renal failure, potassium-sparing diuretics, adrenal insufficiency), or acute metabolic or respiratory acidosis. Under the latter circumstances, intracellular potassium ions undergo exchange with extracellular hydrogen ions to simultaneously buffer the acidosis and maintain charge neutrality. There is no net potassium gain.

Indications for Treatment

Hyperkalemia, defined as a serum potassium concentration greater than 5.5 mEq/liter, should be treated as soon as it is diagnosed. The aggressiveness of the therapy depends on the degree of hyperkalemia and its ECG manifestations. Asymptomatic patients with a serum potassium level in the 5.5 to 6.0 mEq/liter range and an ECG pattern similar to *A* and *B* in Figure 5–1 can be treated with potassium restriction, discontinuation of potassium-containing (e.g., some penicillins) or potassium-sparing (e.g., spironolactone) medications, and careful observation with continuous ECG monitoring and frequent serum potassium measurements. Patients with symptoms, ECG changes similar to *C*, *D*, or *E* in Figure 5–1, or a serum potassium level above 6.0 mEq/liter require the above measures as well as active intervention to both counteract the cardiac effects of hyperkalemia and hasten the elimination of potassium from the body. (See box.)

Discussion

The treatment for severe hyperkalemia is multifaceted, the goals being, in order of importance, (1) to antagonize the cardiac and neuromuscular effects of potassium with cal-

DRUG TREATMENT: HYPERKALEMIA

First-Line Therapy (Five Phases)

Phase I—CaCl₂ or Calcium Gluconate

Initial Dose	5–10 ml 10% solution IV over 2–5 minutes
Repeat Dose	5–10 ml 10% solution IV over 2–5 minutes if ECG abnormalities persist
End-Point	Normalization of ECG

Phase II—Sodium Bicarbonate

Initial Dose	50–100 mEq IV over 10 minutes
Repeat Dose	50–100 mEq IV over 10 minutes if ECG abnormalities persist
End-Point	Normalization of ECG

Phase III—Insulin

Initial Dose	10 u regular insulin by IV bolus; should be followed by 25 g glucose IV unless hyperglycemia present
Repeat Dose	10 u regular insulin by IV bolus at 30 minutes if ECG abnormalities persist
End-Point	Normalization of ECG

Phase IV—Albuterol (Alternate Therapy)

Initial Dose	20 mg by nebulizer inhaler over 10 minutes
Repeat Dose	Same as initial dose in 2 hours
End-Point	Normalization of ECG

Phase V—Kayexalate (Sodium Polystyrene Sulfonate)

Initial Dose	15–50 g orally, depending on degree of hyperkalemia
	or
	30–50 g as retention enema
Repeat Dose	15–50 g orally every 3–4 hours
	or
	20–50 g as retention enema every 6 hours
	Monitor serum potassium levels.
End-Point	Serum potassium less than 5.5 mEq/liter

Second-Line Therapy

Hemodialysis

cium ions, (2) to force potassium intracellularly, and (3) to remove potassium from the body (except if the hyperkalemia is secondary to acidosis, in which case there is no actual total body potassium increase).

Calcium should be administered urgently in severe hyperkalemia because it competitively antagonizes the cardiac and neuromuscular effects of potassium. One can safely administer 5 to 10 ml of 10% calcium chloride or calcium gluconate intravenously over 2 to 5 minutes. This dose can be repeated after 5 minutes if ECG abnormalities persist. Caution must be used when administering calcium to patients receiving digitalis preparations, because the sudden fall in serum potassium can cause digitalis-toxic cardiac rhythm disturbances. Hyperkalemic patients on digitalis therapy should be monitored continuously by ECG while receiving calcium.

Three agents may be used to temporarily force potassium ions intracellularly. The first is sodium bicarbonate, which functions by the exact opposite mechanism that results in the hyperkalemia of metabolic acidosis. Specifically, hydrogen ions leave the intracellular compartment to buffer the administered bicarbonate. Potassium ions enter cells to conserve charge. Generally, 50 to 100 mEq of bicarbonate can be administered over 10 minutes while continuously monitoring the ECG. Since this represents a large sodium load, caution should be used when administering this agent to patients susceptible to pulmonary edema.

The second agent used to temporarily force potassium ions intracellularly is insulin. A dose of 10 units of regular insulin administered as an intravenous bolus will usually result in a rapid reduction in the serum potassium level. Unless significant hyperglycemia is present, dextrose (25 g as 50 ml of a 50% solution) should be administered concomitantly with the insulin bolus to prevent hypoglycemia.

Beta$_2$-adrenergic stimulation has been discovered to cause a lowering of the serum potassium level, probably due to intracellular potassium shifts. In a recently reported study, inhaled albuterol, given by nebulization, produced a 0.6 mmol/liter drop in the serum potassium level after a 10-mg dose and a 0.98 mmol/liter drop after a 20-mg dose. When intravenous access is a problem, this therapy provides an alternative regimen that can be immediately instituted and that produces a significant fall in the serum potassium level within 30 minutes.

The definitive method of decreasing total body potassium, especially in the setting of renal failure, is peritoneal dialysis or hemodialysis. When hyperkalemia is not life-threatening, enteral cation-exchange resins will usually suffice. Kayexalate (sodium polystyrene sulfonate), the most commonly used commercially available product, is a sodium-based resin that exchanges approximately 1.3 to 1.7 mEq Na$^+$ for each 1 mEq K$^+$ removed. The usual dosage is 15 to 60 g orally per day in divided doses. A single dose of 20 to 50 g may be given for severe hyperkalemia, and this may be repeated every 3 to 4

hours as indicated by the serum potassium level. When given orally, each gram of Kayexalate can be expected to remove 1 mEq K$^+$ from the body. If the oral route is not feasible, one can give 30 to 50 g Kayexalate every 6 hours as a retention enema. Because of the large sodium load that results from the use of this agent, it should be administered with caution to patients with hypervolemia and those susceptible to cardiogenic pulmonary edema.

Therapy for hyperkalemia due to metabolic or respiratory acidosis should be directed toward the cause of the acidosis. Simple bicarbonate therapy may be all that is indicated for metabolic acidosis. In either case, dialysis and/or Kayexalate therapy is not indicated.

Hypokalemia

Diagnosis

Symptoms of hypokalemia rarely occur with serum potassium concentrations greater than 3.0 mEq/liter. When present, they include weakness, hyporeflexia, and, with severe hypokalemia, even paralysis or tetany. ECG abnormalities include inverted T waves, prominent U waves, depressed ST segments, and ventricular ectopy. Hypokalemia increases cardiac sensitivity to digitalis and may be associated with digitalis-toxic arrhythmias at therapeutic digitalis blood levels. Hypokalemia is a cause of nephrogenic diabetes insipidus, resulting from a decreased renal sensitivity to ADH and, thus, a decrease in urine-concentrating ability. When hypokalemia leads to the unavailability of potassium ions in the distal nephron, hydrogen ions substitute for potassium in the Na$^+$/K$^+$ ATPase exchange, and metabolic alkalosis may result. This situation is aggravated when volume depletion is present, due to the stimulation of ATPase by aldosterone. Last, serum potassium concentrations of less than 2.5 mEq/liter can lead to rhabdomyolysis.

Hypokalemia can be attributed to a decreased potassium intake, an increase in renal or gastrointestinal potassium losses, or acute metabolic or respiratory alkalosis. Under the latter circumstances, extracellular potassium ions undergo exchange for intracellular hydrogen ions to simultaneously buffer the alkalosis and maintain charge neutrality. There is no net potassium loss.

Decreased potassium intake is a rare cause

of hypokalemia. It can occur because, unlike sodium, there are obligatory gastrointestinal (10 to 15 mEq/day) and renal (5 mEq/day) potassium losses. Thus, dietary potassium deficiency can cause hypokalemia. However, most vegetables and meats contain substantial amounts of potassium, rendering this cause of hypokalemia uncommon.

Losses of potassium from the upper gastrointestinal tract are usually small. For example, gastric secretions contain less than 10 mEq/liter of potassium. However, vomiting results in volume contraction and metabolic alkalosis. Since hypovolemia is a strong stimulant for renin secretion, a secondary hyperaldosteronism occurs that enhances renal losses of potassium. Further, the metabolic alkalosis shifts potassium ions intracellularly. Thus, vomiting can lead to severe hypokalemia. Diarrheal fluid contains substantial amounts of potassium and can lead directly to hypokalemia.

Renal losses of potassium are enhanced under many circumstances, the most common being diuretic use, primary hyperaldosteronism, and salt-wasting nephropathies. Both postobstructive diuresis and the diuretic phase of acute tubular necrosis can be associated with large potassium losses in the urine. In all of these pathologic situations, renal losses of potassium are often substantial.

Indications for Treatment

Hypokalemia should be treated when the serum potassium level is less than 3.0 mEq/liter or if the patient has symptoms attributable to hypokalemia at a higher potassium level. The initial therapy should include oral or intravenous potassium supplementation while sources of potassium loss are being identified and corrected. Patients receiving digitalis preparations represent an important exception to these guidelines. Such patients should ideally have serum potassium levels maintained in the 4.5 to 5.0 mEq/liter range and should receive replacement therapy whenever the level falls below 4.0 mEq/liter. (See box.)

Discussion

Under severe circumstances, potassium can be given intravenously at rates of up to 40 mEq/hour. However, rates of 10 mEq/hour are sufficient in most instances. Intravenous solutions containing more potassium than 60 mEq/liter must be given by central vein, since potassium at high concentrations can cause pain and phlebitis when given by peripheral vein. When oral potassium re-

---

DRUG TREATMENT: HYPERKALEMIA

First-Line Therapy
Potassium Replacement

Initial Dose	40 mEq KCl orally
	or
	10 mEq KCl IV over 1 hour (can give up to 40 mEq IV over 1 hour for life-threatening hypokalemia)
Repeat Dose	40 mEq KCl orally every 3–4 hours
	or
	10 mEq KCl IV/hour
	Monitor serum potassium levels.
End-Point	Serum potassium level greater than 3.5 mEq/liter

placement is feasible, 40 mEq KCl as a 10% aqueous solution can be given every 3 to 4 hours as tolerated. Since the serum potassium concentration does not accurately reflect total body potassium stores, frequent serum potassium measurements and ECG evaluation should take place during replacement therapy to determine the adequacy of repletion and to avoid overshoot hyperkalemia.

Therapy for hypokalemia due to metabolic or respiratory alkalosis should be directed toward the cause of the alkalosis. Potassium replacement therapy is not indicated under these circumstances.

SPECIFIC AGENTS

Crystalloids

Dextrose in Water

Pharmacology

Composition

5%—5 g dextrose in each 100 ml
10%—10 g dextrose in each 100 ml

pH

Variable, 3.5 to 6.5

Osmolarity

5%—252 mOsm/liter
10%—505 mOsm/liter

Indications

5%—hypernatremia as hypotonic replacement fluid; vehicle for many intravenous drug infusions; keep-vein-open solution for sodium-sensitive patients (cardiac, renal, etc.)
10%—hypoglycemia; weaning from total parenteral nutrition

Cautions

Not appropriate for volume resuscitation
Not appropriate as maintenance IV solution
Not compatible with blood transfusions (causes hemolysis)

Toxicity

Hyponatremia
Hyperglycemia (especially 10%)
Increased brain edema

Ringer's Lactate

Pharmacology

Composition

	mEq/liter
Calcium	3
Chloride	109
Lactate	28
Potassium	4
Sodium	130

	mg/liter
Sodium chloride	6000
Sodium lactate	3100
Potassium chloride	300
Calcium chloride	200

Ringer's lactate is also available containing 5% dextrose (50 g/liter).

pH

6.5

Osmolarity

273 mOsm/liter

Indications

Preferred crystalloid resuscitation fluid for rapid intravascular volume expansion
May be used as maintenance IV fluid

Cautions

Not compatible with blood transfusion (causes clotting)
Contains potassium, so use with caution in renal failure or hyperkalemia
Lactate may accumulate in hepatic failure

Note: Shock-induced lactic acidosis is *not* a contraindication to use of Ringer's lactate. At physiologic pH, the dissociation equilibrium between lactate, a base, and lactic acid is strongly in favor of lactate. Hepatic metabolism via the Krebs tricarboxylic acid cycle converts lactate to bicarbonate. Thus, Ringer's lactate actually provides buffering capacity in the face of a metabolic acidosis.

Toxicity

Hyperkalemia

Peripheral edema is to be expected with large-volume crystalloid resuscitation but should be considered an expected result of therapy rather than toxicity.

Saline Solutions

Pharmacology

Composition

	0.2%	0.45%	0.9%	3.0%
mEq Na$^+$/ liter	34	77	154	513
mEq Cl$^-$/ liter	34	77	154	513
mg NaCl/ liter	2000	4500	9000	30,000
pH	4.0	4.0	5.0	5.0
Osmolarity mOsm/ liter	67	150	300	1027

The 0.2, 0.45, and 0.9% solutions are also available with 5% dextrose (50 g/liter).

Indications

0.2% (usually with dextrose)—treatment of hypernatremia or maintenance IV solution

0.45% (with or without dextrose)—maintenance IV therapy; hypernatremia

0.9% (without dextrose)—rapid volume resuscitation; companion solution for blood transfusions; hyponatremia; eye irrigation

3.0%—correction of severe hyponatremia ([Na$^+$] < 120 mEq/liter); hypertonic burn resuscitation

Cautions

0.2 and 0.45%—not appropriate for rapid volume resuscitation

0.9%—not appropriate as maintenance IV solution

3.0%—beware of too rapid an overcorrection of hyponatremia

Toxicity

0.2 and 0.45%—hyponatremia

0.9%—hyperchloremic acidosis

3.0%—hypernatremia; central pontine myelinolysis; phlebitis

Sodium Polystyrene Sulfonate (Kayexalate)

Pharmacology

Cation exchange resin

Mechanism of Action

Releases sodium and binds potassium with an in vitro capacity of binding 3.1 mEq potassium in exchange for 4.1 mEq sodium

In vivo action variable and unpredictable and should not be expected to be more than 33% of in vitro activity

Also binds calcium and magnesium

Kinetics

Variable, depending on bowel function

Enemas should be allowed to dwell for at least 60 minutes.

Indications

Hyperkalemia

Cautions

Contraindications

Patients unable to tolerate a sodium load

Bowel perforation

Oral—bowel obstruction, mechanical or functional

Rectal—acute diverticulitis

Dosage adjustment in organ failure—none

Use in pregnancy—yes, as it is not absorbed

Use in lactation—yes

Use in childhood—yes; but reduce dose in proportion to patient's size

Dosage

Oral—15 g every 6 hours with 30 g of sorbitol to prevent impaction

Enema—30 to 50 g in 100 ml water or sorbitol by retention enema every 6 hours

Cleansing enema (non–sodium-containing) should precede and follow each dose of Kayexalate.

Toxicity

Drug Interactions

Metabolic alkalosis with antacids and laxatives such as magnesium hydroxide

Side Effects

No systemic absorption occurs.

Local effects: gastric irritation, anorexia, nausea, vomiting, constipation, impaction with bowel obstruction

Systemic effects: congestive heart failure, hypertension, edema, hypocalcemia, hypomagnesemia

Treatment of Toxicity

Local upper GI effects—give as enema.

Constipation—add sorbitol.

Impaction—stop drug; disimpact by manual and chemical means.

Systemic—stop drug; provide oxygen, vasodilators, diuresis; replace calcium; replace magnesium.

REFERENCES

Allon M, Dunlay R, Copkney C: Nebulized albuterol for acute hyperkalemia in patients on hemodialysis. Ann Intern Med 110:426–429, 1989.

Appel PL, Shoemaker WC: Fluid therapy in adult respiratory failure. Crit Care Med 9:862–869, 1981.

Ayus JC, Krothapalli RK, Arieff AI: Treatment of symptomatic hyponatremia and its relation to brain damage. N Engl J Med 317:1190–1195, 1987.

Baylis PH: Hyponatremia and hypernatremia. Clin Endocrinol Metab 9(3):625–637, 1980.

Fluid and electrolyte therapy. In Rowe PC (ed): The Harriet Lane Handbook. A Manual for Pediatric House Officers, 11th ed. Chicago, Year Book Medical Publishers, 1987, pp 230–238.

Haddow JE, Cohen DL: Understanding and managing hypernatremic dehydration. Pediatr Clin North Am 21(2):435–441, 1974.

Haupt MT, Teerapong P, Green D, et al: Increased pulmonary edema with crystalloid compared to colloid resuscitation of shock associated with increased vascular permeability. Circ Shock 12:213–224, 1984.

Hauser CJ, Shoemaker WC, Turpin I, Goldberg SJ: Hemodynamic and oxygen transport responses to body water shifts produced by colloids and crystalloids in critically ill patients. Surg Gynecol Obstet 150:811–816, 1980.

Hogan GR: Hypernatremia—Problems in management. Pediatr Clin North Am 23(3):569–574, 1976.

Kaufman BS, Rackow EC, Falk JL: Fluid resuscitation in circulatory shock. Colloids versus crystalloids. Curr Stud Hematol Blood Transfus 53:186–198, 1986.

Lutz H, Georgieff M: Effects and side effects of colloid plasma substitutes as compared to albumin. Curr Stud Hematol Blood Transfus 53:145–154, 1986.

Monafo WW, Halverson JD, Schechtman KS: The role of concentrated sodium solutions in the resuscitation of patients with severe burns. Surgery 95:129–135, 1984.

Ross AD, Angaran DM: Colloids vs crystalloids—A continuing controversy. Drug Intell Clin Pharm 18:202–212, 1984.

Sterns RH: Severe symptomatic hyponatremia: Treatment and outcome. Ann Intern Med 107:656–664, 1987.

Sterns RH, Riggs JE, Schochet SS: Osmotic demyelination syndrome following correction of hyponatremia. N Engl J Med 314:1535–1542, 1986.

CHAPTER 6

Plasma and Volume Expanders

Steven C. Dronen, M.D.

INTRODUCTION

History

Throughout recorded history there exists evidence of mankind's appreciation of the life-sustaining properties of blood. Older civilizations considered blood to be a source of life and vigor and often associated disease with poisoning or contamination of the victim's blood. Thus, ancient Egyptians bathed the sick in blood, and the Romans drank the blood of dying gladiators in the hope of thus acquiring their strength and courage. Actual transfusions of blood did not occur until the Middle Ages, often with disastrous results for both donors and recipients. There was not even a basic understanding of the function of blood in the cardiovascular system, and transfusion was primarily regarded as the giving of a potion capable of restoring health. There was, of course, no understanding of the immune system. Donors were chosen based on their overall health, and in some cases animal donors were used. For some recipients, clinical deterioration occurred in conjunction with "black urine," suggesting that immunologic incompatibility resulted in massive hemolysis. The overall results were sufficiently dismal that in the late 16th century the governments of both England and France outlawed further human

blood transfusions. James Blundell is credited with elevating the understanding of blood from a mysterious tonic to an essential physiologic material. He was the first to express an understanding of the detrimental effects of blood loss, and in 1818 he revived the practice of human blood transfusion. Progress was slow until the early 20th century when Landsteiner first described the ABO blood groups. This was followed in 1914 by the discovery that blood coagulation could be prevented by the addition of citrate and in 1916 by the discovery that the addition of dextrose to stored blood prolonged its viability. Transfusion therapy truly entered the modern age with the development of the plastic storage container. This device has permitted blood collection to occur in a completely closed system, thereby decreasing the risk of bacterial contamination. More importantly, however, it has facilitated the separation of whole blood into several fractions and has led to the now standard practice of transfusing only the needed blood component. Components currently available for use include packed red cells, platelets, fresh-frozen plasma, albumin, plasma protein fraction, cryoprecipitate, and Factor VIII and IX concentrates. In addition, a number of asanguineous products have been developed for use as volume expanders to supplement and, in some cases, replace blood-derived products. Those currently in clinical use include dextran and hetastarch.

Risks of Therapy

Modern blood banking practices have greatly reduced the risks associated with transfusion therapy. A number of immune-mediated reactions may occur in response to the infusion of foreign proteins, but these are not generally severe or life-threatening. Most of the life-threatening reactions can be eliminated by strict adherence to well-established protocols for the collection and typing of blood specimens and the administration of blood products. At the present time the most significant concern associated with the transfusion of blood-derived products is the transmission of communicable diseases. Those that have been linked to transfusion include hepatitis, both B and non-A/non-B (C); acquired immunodeficiency syndrome (AIDS); syphilis; cytomegaloviral infections; mononucleosis; bacteremia; malaria; toxoplasmosis; trypanosomiasis; leishmaniasis; and filariasis. In the United States hepatitis and AIDS pose the greatest threat.

Hepatitis

Although it has been known since 1883 that hepatitis can be transmitted parenterally, it was first documented in 1943 that clinical cases of hepatitis occurred after transfusion of blood and plasma. Outbreaks of hepatitis during the Second World War led to intensification of the search for a causative agent, and ultimately both hepatitis A and B viruses were identified. After the parenteral pattern of hepatitis B transmission was recognized, tests were developed to detect the presence of the carrier state. Improvements in the sensitivity of these tests, coupled with conversion from a paid to a volunteer donor system, led many to assume that the risk of post-transfusion hepatitis could be eliminated. Unfortunately this assumption proved to be incorrect. Although the incidence of post-transfusion hepatitis B has decreased, there has been only a small reduction in the *overall* incidence of post-transfusion hepatitis. It has since been recognized that in about 90% of the cases of post-transfusion hepatitis the etiologic agent is not the B virus. These cases are referred to as non-A/non-B or C, and an adequate test to identify the presence of C has recently been developed. Incubation period clustering at 8

and 12 weeks suggests that more than one agent is responsible. Since 1987 donors have been screened for alanine aminotransferase, an enzyme commonly elevated in the acute phase of the disease. This practice is likely to result in the rejection of donors who do not have hepatitis as well as some of those who do. At this time, the overall effect cannot be predicted with certainty. The primary screening test for hepatitis B is the hepatitis B surface antigen. This test is specific but unfortunately not completely sensitive. Recently the hepatitis B core antigen has been added to the donor screening panel.

Because of changes in donor screening practices as well as the geographic variation in the incidence of hepatitis it is impossible accurately to predict the risk of contracting hepatitis following transfusion. It is currently estimated that the risk of contracting non-A/non-B (C) hepatitis is 1% per unit of single-donor product transfused. Pooled-donor products carry a much greater risk. The only blood products for which an effective method has been developed for removal or inactivation of the hepatitis virus are albumin and purified protein fraction. Factor VIII concentrate is currently heat-treated, but the effectiveness of this process is unproved.

AIDS

The ongoing AIDS epidemic has heightened awareness of the risk of transfusions in both the lay and medical communities. This is of some benefit in that it has decreased the incidence of unnecessary transfusion. Unfortunately it has also caused considerable anxiety that has probably led some patients to refuse necessary transfusions. The actual risk of contracting AIDS is quite low. As of 1987, there were 802 post-transfusion cases of AIDS reported to the Centers for Disease Control. The true number is undoubtedly higher because of the long incubation period of the disease, but it is still likely to represent only a tiny fraction of the total number of blood products transfused. Hemophiliacs are the group at greatest risk because of their frequent use of pooled-donor products. Since 1985 all donors have been screened for the HIV antibody, and members of high-risk groups have been asked to refrain voluntarily from donating blood. The antibody test is highly sensitive. Its primary limitation is that it detects antibody rather than antigen and thus will be negative in the interval between infection and antibody formation. It is very likely, however, that the measures that have been adopted will be effective in protecting recipients of blood products from spread of the AIDS virus.

CONDITIONS

Hemorrhagic Shock

Diagnosis and Indications for Treatment

Hemorrhagic shock is defined as a state of impaired tissue perfusion occurring secondary to acute blood loss. Signs and symptoms vary with the degree of blood loss and the underlying physical condition of the patient (Table 6–1). Although it is commonly thought that a blood volume loss of up to 25% may occur without symptoms, it is more likely that subtle symptoms of early shock frequently go undetected. Early symptoms are in large part caused by catecholamine release and reflect physiologic compensatory mechanisms. Blood is shunted away from the skin and distal extremities, causing cool clammy skin and delayed capillary refill. Cardiovascular compensation includes an increased heart rate and constriction of the capacitance vessels, resulting in a narrowing of the pulse pressure.

As shock progresses beyond the initial compensatory phase, the clinical manifestations become much more apparent. Hypotension, marked tachycardia, diminished peripheral pulses, pallor, tachypnea, agitation, and decreased urine output are characteristic findings of this stage. Finally, when death is imminent, the patient becomes lethargic or comatose, respirations become irregular or absent, and the blood pressure is unmeasurable by standard techniques.

Conditions causing hemorrhagic shock include blunt and penetrating trauma, ruptured or dissecting aortic aneurysm, gastrointestinal hemorrhage, ruptured ectopic pregnancy or ovarian cyst, massive vaginal bleeding, and retroperitoneal hemorrhage. In victims of trauma it is important to distinguish hypotension secondary to blood loss from hypotension secondary to impaired cardiac filling or contractility. Typically the latter group will have elevated central venous pressure, demonstrated clinically by distended external jugular veins. (See box.)

TABLE 6–1. Signs and Symptoms of Hemorrhagic Shock

Compensatory Shock
Blood pressure: usually in "normal" range; orthostatic changes present; pulse pressure narrowed
Pulse: normal or elevated; orthostatic changes present
End-organ function: usually normal; urine output decreased
Physical signs: ± cool clammy skin

Decompensated Shock
Blood pressure: decreased
Pulse: increased
End-organ function: decreased urine output; myocardial ischemia; ± central nervous system dysfunction
Physical signs: cool clammy skin; agitation; diminished peripheral pulses; tachypnea

End-Stage Shock
Blood pressure: often unobtainable
Pulse: marked tachycardia or bradycardia
End-organ function: no urine output; marked central nervous system dysfunction; myocardial ischemia
Physical signs: lethargy or coma; irregular or absent respirations; cold skin; absent signs of life

Discussion

Management of the hemorrhagic shock victim begins with a rapid assessment of the adequacy of ventilation and circulation. Specific items to be assessed include patency of the airway, rate and depth of respirations, level of consciousness, skin color and temperature, pulse rate and amplitude, and blood pressure. During this brief examination, two or more large-bore intravenous lines should be started. As the lines are started, blood samples should be drawn for typing and cross-matching, a complete blood count, prothrombin time and partial thromboplastin time determinations, and a platelet count. Continuous monitoring of the hemorrhagic shock victim is essential. Although cardiac monitoring is commonly used, it provides relatively little useful information. It is far more valuable to monitor parameters that reflect the adequacy of perfusion, oxygen delivery, and volume status such as the central venous pressure, urine output, and noninvasive oximetry measurements.

Major goals in the early management of hemorrhagic shock are (1) control of hemorrhage, (2) restoration of circulating blood volume, and (3) maintenance of oxygen delivery. The first of these goals may be easily accomplished if the hemorrhage is superficial and accessible to manual compression. Generally this is not the case, and surgical in-

DRUG TREATMENT: HEMORRHAGIC SHOCK

Compensated Phase

First-Line Therapy
Crystalloid (0.9% Saline, Lactated Ringer's)

Initial Dose	Up to 30 ml/kg
Repeat Dose	10–15 ml/kg boluses as indicated by clinical status
End-Points	Signs of improved peripheral perfusion, decreased heart rate

Second-Line Therapy
Cross-matched Packed Cells

Initial Dose	7–10 ml/kg
Repeat Dose	As indicated by clinical status. Consider surgical intervention if repeat doses are needed.
End-Points	Signs of improved peripheral perfusion; return to normal heart rate, blood pressure, and urine output

Decompensated Phase

First-Line Therapy
Crystalloid (0.9% Saline, Lactated Ringer's)

Initial Dose	At least 30 ml/kg infused rapidly
Repeat Dose	Continue rapid fluid infusion

AND

Type-Specific Blood (Cross-matched Blood When Available)

Initial Dose	7–10 ml/kg
Repeat Dose	3–5 ml/kg as indicated by clinical status. Consider urgent surgical intervention if repeat doses needed!
End-Points	Improved mental status, urine output, skin perfusion; increased blood pressure; decreased heart rate

End-Stage Shock

First-Line Therapy
Crystalloid (0.9 Normal Saline, Lactated Ringer's); Type O Packed Cells (Type-Specific Blood When Available)

Initial Dose	Crystalloid: at least 30 ml/kg Blood: at least 10 ml/kg
Repeat Dose	Crystalloid: run wide open; titrate to clinical response. Blood: 3–5 ml/kg as indicated by clinical status; switch to cross-matched blood when available. Consider urgent surgical intervention!
End-Points	Improved vital signs and mentation

tervention will be required. Thus the emergency management usually is focused on restoration of circulation. Equally important, but sometimes neglected, is maintenance of oxygen delivery.

The amount and type of volume expander used depend primarily on the clinical status of the patient and to a lesser extent on individual or institutional preference. In most hospitals isotonic saline solutions (0.9% NaCl or lactated Ringer's) are the asanguineous agents of choice for the initial management of acute hemorrhage. In the compensated shock patient, isotonic saline should be rapidly infused. If the patient continues to show signs of impaired perfusion after a total of 30 ml/kg has been administered, it is likely that blood loss exceeds 15% of the total blood volume. At this point, it is appropriate to begin red cell transfusions, particularly if blood loss has not been controlled. In this situation it is usually possible to wait for fully cross-matched blood, but that decision must be individualized based on the assessment of ongoing blood loss and the efficiency of the local blood bank in performing cross-matches. When in doubt, it is advisable to use type-specific blood. Several studies have shown this to be a very safe practice, and delays in providing needed oxygen-carrying capacity are potentially more harmful to the patient.

More aggressive therapy is mandated in the uncompensated shock patient. These patients almost always require blood transfusions, and it is appropriate to begin type-specific blood early unless there is a prompt and steady improvement in perfusion with saline alone. Administration of large volumes of saline to patients who have sustained major blood loss may result in profound dilution of the remaining red cell mass. Volume restored at the expense of oxygen-carrying capacity is of questionable therapeutic value, and therefore type-specific blood should be given in conjunction with asanguineous fluids.

The moribund patient requires even more prompt restoration of circulating red cell mass. In this case, type O blood should be used if it is available. Type O negative blood should be given to females of child-bearing age. In most other situations, type O positive blood is preferred because of its greater availability. A type and cross-match should always be drawn before administration of type O blood. Autologous whole blood may also be given to these patients if the hemorrhage is intrathoracic or intra-abdominal (without fecal contamination) and the capabilities for autotransfusion exist. In the majority of cases, blood transfused for the treatment of hemorrhagic shock is provided as packed red cells rather than as whole blood. There remains in practice today proponents of the old adage that whole blood should be replaced with whole blood. There is, however, no convincing evidence of the superiority of whole blood over packed red cell transfusions. Much of the debate on this issue has been rendered mute by the widespread conversion to component therapy in most modern blood banks.

Although isotonic saline is most commonly used in the initial management of hemorrhagic shock, the debate over the asanguineous fluid of choice (i.e., crystalloid versus colloid) is no closer to resolution than ever. Albumin has recently fallen into disfavor, but purified protein fraction and fresh-frozen plasma continue to be recommended and used. Central to the issue are the effects of fluid resuscitation on the pulmonary interstitium. Proponents of protein replacement argue that saline resuscitation following hemorrhage results in a fall in intravascular oncotic pressure and a reversal of the normal gradient favoring intravascular fluid retention. Theoretically this may lead to pulmonary edema and impaired tissue oxygenation. Colloid administration is advocated because it raises oncotic pressure in the pulmonary capillary bed. This argument ignores the fact that the pulmonary capillary endothelium permits considerable flow of fluids, including plasma proteins, between the capillaries and the interstitium. A fall in intravascular oncotic pressure is compensated by a fall in pulmonary interstitial oncotic pressure, thereby minimizing changes in the pressure gradient. It appears likely that pulmonary capillary hydrostatic pressure (measured as pulmonary artery wedge pressure) is far more important than pulmonary capillary oncotic pressure in determining the amount of fluid flowing to the interstitium. Maintenance of the wedge pressure below 15 mmHg is probably the most important factor in preventing pulmonary edema. Despite the above information, it seems likely that proponents of protein replacement will continue to recommend its use. To date there are little data to show that albumin is harmful, but the inability to convincingly demonstrate beneficial effects in scores of animal and clinical studies certainly suggests that benefits are minimal. Clinicians inclined to use albumin, purified protein fraction, or fresh-frozen plasma in the resuscitation of hemorrhagic shock should question whether the undocumented benefits of this therapy are worth the 1800% cost differential compared to normal saline or, in the case of fresh-frozen plasma, the risk of disease transmission.

Alternatives to the use of naturally occurring colloid preparations include synthetic colloid solutions such as hydroxyethyl starch and dextran. The volume-expanding properties of hydroxyethyl starch are equivalent to those of 5% albumin. Hydroxyethyl starch differs significantly from albumin, however, in that it remains predominately in the intravascular space because of its high molecular weight. Interstitial edema is not a concern as it is with albumin. Furthermore, the plasma-expanding effects of hydroxyethyl starch are more prolonged than those of albumin.

The volume-expanding properties of dextran 70 are slightly better than those of 5% albumin. Like hydroxyethyl starch, dextran remains predominately in the intravascular space because of its large highly branched molecular structure. Interstitial edema is not a concern with dextran as it is with albumin. Dextran 40 is also an excellent volume expander, but its use is not indicated in the initial resuscitation of the hypovolemic patient. Unlike dextran 70, dextran 40 has a short duration of action, causes significant dilution of plasma proteins, and markedly increases urine viscosity. In the hypovolemic patient with decreased urine output, this may lead to renal failure. Dextran 70 is therefore preferred as a volume expander.

Anemia

Diagnosis

Anemia is defined as a deficit in either the serum concentration of hemoglobin or the volume of red cells that places the patient outside the statistical norms for a given population. Normal levels vary among patients of different age, sex, and habitat. Normal hemoglobin levels for males living at sea level are 15.5 g/dl and for females are 14.0 g/dl.

Although the laboratory diagnosis of anemia is relatively straightforward, its clinical diagnosis is not. There are no specific symptoms, and the disease typically has an almost imperceptible onset. There is considerable variation in the hemoglobin level at which patients begin to complain of symptoms. Most often the initial complaint is fatigue. Because of the nonspecific nature of this complaint, it is likely to be attributed to other causes. As the disease progresses, decreased exercise tolerance, dyspnea, and high-output cardiac failure may develop. Patients with even mild anemia and underlying atherosclerotic vascular disease may experience symptoms (e.g., angina, claudication) that are incorrectly attributed to progression of the primary disease.

Causes of Anemia

I. Decreased red cell production
   A. Aplastic anemia (unicellular or pancellular)
   B. Marrow infiltration (malignancy, granulomatous disease, storage disease, myelofibrosis)
   C. Erythropoietin deficiency (liver or renal disease, chronic disease, malnutrition, endocrine disorders)

II. Abnormal red cell or hemoglobin production
   A. Microcytic anemias
      1. Iron deficiency
      2. Lead poisoning
      3. Chronic disease
      4. Thalassemia
      5. Sideroblastic anemia
   B. Macrocytic anemias
      1. Folate deficiency
      2. B_{12} deficiency

III. Increased red cell destruction
   A. Congenital hemolytic disorders
      1. Membrane disorders (spherocytosis)
      2. Abnormal hemoglobin (sickle cell disease, thalassemia)
      3. Enzyme defects (glucose-6-phosphate dehydrogenase)
   B. Acquired hemolytic disorders
      1. Immune complex mediated
      2. Drug or toxin induced
      3. Metabolic disorders
      4. Traumatic (burns, cardiac valves)
      5. Infection
      6. Splenic sequestration

Indications for Treatment

1. Signs of end-organ oxygen deprivation (chest pain, dyspnea, syncope)
2. Hemoglobin 8 g/dl or lower in the perioperative period
3. Asymptomatic patient with hemoglobin 7 g/dl or lower (See box.)

DRUG TREATMENT: ANEMIA

First-Line Therapy

Correction of underlying disorder and replacement of vitamin or mineral deficiencies

Second-Line Therapy

Packed Red Blood Cells

Initial Dose	7–10 ml/kg
Repeat Dose	3–5 ml/kg
End-Points	Hemoglobin >8 g/dl and resolution of symptoms of end-organ oxygen deprivation (chest pain, dyspnea, claudication, syncope)

Discussion

A gradual loss of red cell mass is compensated for by an increase in heart rate and cardiac output, thereby maintaining oxygen delivery. Also, an increase in 2,3-diphosphoglycerate favors oxyhemoglobin dissociation at the tissue level. The presence of these mechanisms, as well as a considerable reserve capacity for oxygen delivery, permits most patients to tolerate anemia without the need for red cell replacement. Correction of the underlying disorder (e.g., vitamin or mineral deficiency, blood loss, hemolysis) is the principal and often the only therapy required for chronic anemias. The transfusion of packed red cells is indicated in the presence of symptoms of end-organ oxygen deprivation, such as chest pain, dyspnea, or syncope. Transfusion is also indicated if the patient is undergoing a physiologically stressful event such as general surgery. It has been widely accepted that a hemoglobin level of no less than 10 g/dl is required prior to general surgery, although there are no studies supporting this recommendation. A recent National Institutes of Health consensus conference on perioperative red cell transfusion recommends that a value of 8 g/dl be used.

There is no generally accepted hemoglobin level below which it is recommended that the asymptomatic nonstressed patient be transfused. Frequently transfusions are given when the hemoglobin is 7 g/dl or lower, but if the patient is truly asymptomatic or has only fatigue, this is probably not necessary. The threshold for transfusion should be lowered in patients with significant atherosclerotic vascular disease. The potential benefit to the patient should always be weighed against the potential for complications associated with transfusion. It is also important to remember that the patient with chronic anemia is generally normovolemic. Administration of blood to these patients must be done slowly to avoid volume overload.

The anemia associated with some disease states may be quite severe and not amenable to correction of the underlying disorder. Two examples commonly encountered are chronic renal failure and sickle cell disease. A hemoglobin level in the range of 5 to 7 mg/dl is not uncommon in chronic renal failure, and patients tolerate these levels quite well without the need for transfusions.

Sickle cell patients generally maintain serum hemoglobin levels above 6 to 7 mg/dl without the need for transfusions. Because of the life-long nature of this disease, transfusion should be given very selectively. The body's ability to excrete iron is limited, and repeat transfusions therefore carry the additional risk of hemosiderosis. Transfusion may be indicated for the treatment of aplastic or splenic sequestration crisis, high-output congestive heart failure, and symptoms of end-organ oxygen deprivation. Partial exchange transfusions are used for treatment of prolonged vaso-occlusive episodes, for priapism, for acute symptoms of vascular insufficiency (e.g., cerebrovascular accident), and prior to major surgical procedures.

Hemophilia

Diagnosis

Hemophilia A (Factor VIII deficiency) and hemophilia B (Factor IX deficiency) are diseases associated with impaired hemostasis and a sex-linked pattern of inheritance. Both occur almost exclusively in males, although mild manifestations of the disease may occur in female carriers of hemophilia A. Homozygous females with hemophilia are distinct rarities.

Factor VIII deficiency may be qualitative or quantitative, and the disease is therefore graded according to the percent of normal Factor VIII activity present. The disease is characterized as severe, moderate, or mild, correlating with <1%, 1 to 5%, and 5 to 25% of normal activity, respectively. Factor VIII is a large molecule confined predominately to the intravascular space. One unit of activity is defined as the amount present in 1 ml of normal plasma. Given the average plasma volume of about 40 ml/kg, a 70-kg man has roughly 2800 units of activity. Levels of 50 to 80% of normal may be required to control hemorrhage, depending on the source.

Factor IX deficiency is generally quantitative. Much lower levels are sufficient to achieve hemostasis, and therefore the clinical manifestations tend not to be as severe. Levels of <1% generally correlate with moderate disease and levels of 1 to 5% with mild disease. Factor IX is a small molecule that is distributed in a space about 1.5 to 2.0 times the plasma volume. Larger doses per unit of body weight are therefore required to reach a desired level, but levels of 25% are usually adequate to control hemorrhage.

The diagnosis of hemophilia is suggested by clinical evidence of impaired hemostasis and a family history of bleeding disorders. It should be distinguished from von Willebrand's disease, which has an autosomal dominant inheritance pattern. Coagulation studies will reveal a prolonged partial thromboplastin time. Failure of the partial thromboplastin time to return to normal when the sample is mixed with plasma known to be deficient in Factor VIII or IX confirms the diagnosis as hemophilia A or B.

Soft tissue hematomas and hemarthroses are by far the most common clinical manifestations of the disease. Hematuria and bleeding after dental extractions are also common. Life-threatening hemorrhage may occur from the gastrointestinal tract. More problematic are hemorrhages occurring adjacent to vital structures such as the brain or upper airway. Occult hemorrhages occurring in the cranial vault and retroperitoneum are not uncommon and should always be suspected.

Indications for Treatment

1. Prophylactic replacement therapy
2. Anticipated surgical procedure
3. Any active bleeding other than that associated with superficial soft tissue injuries
4. Suspected or potential hemorrhage adjacent to a vital structure

(See boxes, Drug Treatment: Hemophilia A and Drug Treatment: Hemophilia B.)

Discussion

Management of the hemophiliac patient requires a team approach, including the patient's regular physician or a clinical nurse coordinator, the treating physician, and, most important, the patient himself. It is helpful if emergency departments maintain a file of known local hemophiliacs, including information such as the severity of their factor deficiency and the presence of inhibitors. In recent years, emphasis has been placed on home self-care in order to reduce the potentially great costs associated with this disease. The patients therefore tend to be well educated about their disease and familiar with therapy and its potential complications.

Blood products available for the treatment of hemophilia include fresh-frozen plasma, cryoprecipitate, antihemophilia factor, and Factor IX concentrate. The decision to use a particular product is based on the age of the patient, the history of prior product use, the degree of factor deficiency, and the desired increase in factor levels.

Treatment of Hemophilia A

The desired Factor VIII level varies depending on the site of bleeding. Levels of 80 to 100% are recommended prior to major surgical procedures; for the treatment of major wounds or injuries; for potentially life-threatening hemorrhage (e.g., gastrointestinal bleed, hemoptysis); for hemorrhage potentially involving vital structures such as the brain, spinal cord, or retropharyngeal space; and for deep hemorrhage into the retroperitoneal space or iliopsoas sheath. Levels of 30 to 50% are recommended for minor surgical procedures (e.g., dental extractions) and for hemorrhage of moderate severity (deep muscle hemorrhages near vital structures). Levels of 20% are recommended for treatment of hemarthroses and for minor muscle hemorrhages involving the extremities. Because of the large amount of Factor VIII re-

DRUG TREATMENT: HEMOPHILIA A

First-Line Therapy

Antihemophilia factor

(If large doses [>2000–3000 units] are required or the patient has previously received this product)

Second-Line Therapy

Cryoprecipitate*

(If small doses are required [<2000—3000 units] and the patient has not previously received antihemophilia factor)

Dose   Calculate Factor VIII dose as follows:

$$\text{(Body weight in kg)} \times \text{(desired Factor VIII level} - \text{current Factor VIII level)} \times (0.5)\dagger$$

Determine the desired Factor VIII level as follows:
80–100%
  Anticipated major surgery
  Major wound or injury
  Potential life-threatening hemorrhage
  Hemorrhage potentially involving brain, spinal cord, airway
  Retroperitoneal hemorrhage
30–50%
  Anticipated minor surgery
  Deep muscle hemorrhages
20%
  Hemarthroses
  Minor muscle hemorrhages

End-Points   Cessation of clinical signs of impaired hemostasis
            Normal coagulation profile
            Measured Factor VIII level at desired level

*Contains 80 to 100 units per single donor bag.
†Doses may be significantly higher if Factor VIII inhibitor levels are 5% or greater.

quired in most cases, Factor VIII concentrate (antihemophilia factor [AHF]) is the most practical product available. It does not require cross-matching, can be stored without refrigeration, is easily prepared, and contains a known quantity of Factor VIII. For these reasons it is commonly used in home care programs. Drawbacks of therapy with AHF are cost and, more important, disease transmission. Although donors are now screened for both hepatitis B surface antigen and HIV antibody, and the product is heat treated to attenuate viruses, the effectiveness of these measures is unproved. The incidence of exposure to hepatitis or HIV viruses in hemophiliacs who received AHF before these measures were instituted is very high. Ironically, AHF can now be used in these same patients with minimal risk of further infectivity.

Cryoprecipitate is not as convenient to use as AHF and is not practical when very large amounts of Factor VIII activity are needed or when very rapid replacement is indicated. It must be frozen until use and administered in lots of 20 or more single-donor units in the adult. The major advantage of cryoprecipitate is that it is collected from far fewer donors, thereby significantly decreasing the risk of viral disease transmission. Young hemophiliacs may be treated with cryoprecipitate collected from a single known donor, further decreasing their risk. Patients who have received multiple prior treatments with AHF have been exposed to so many thousands of donors that cryoprecipitate offers them little advantage other than lower cost.

Fresh-frozen plasma contains at most 1 unit of Factor VIII activity per milliliter,

DRUG TREATMENT: HEMOPHILIA B

First-Line Therapy

*Fresh-Frozen Plasma**

(If desired level can be reached without risk of volume overload)

Second-Line Therapy

Factor IX Concentrate

(Indicated only for treatment of major hemorrhages and prior to major surgery when doses exceed that which can be safely administered with fresh-frozen plasma)

Dose Calculate the Factor IX dose as follows:

(Body weight in kg) × (desired Factor IX level − measured Factor IX level)

Determine the desired Factor IX level as follows:
50–60%
  Anticipated major surgery
  Major wound or injury
  Potential life-threatening hemorrhage
  Hemorrhage potentially involving brain, spinal cord, airway
  Retroperitoneal hemorrhage
25%
  Anticipated minor surgery
  Deep muscle hemorrhages
  Hemarthroses

End-Points Cessation of clinical signs of impaired hemostasis
  Normal coagulation profile
  Measured Factor IX level at desired level

*0.4 ml/kg of fresh-frozen plasma will raise the Factor IX level about 1%.

making it impractical for use as a replacement product unless the patient is also significantly hypovolemic. It should only be used if no other therapy is available, and the patient's volume status should be monitored carefully.

Another strategy in the management of hemophilia is stimulation of endogenous coagulation factor production. The intravenous infusion of 1-deamino-8-D-arginine vasopressin (DDAVP), a synthetic analogue of vasopressin, is associated with a dose-dependent increase in the activity of Factors VIII:c and VIII:vWF. The increase in Factor VIII activity typically ranges from three- to sixfold. DDAVP can therefore be used to achieve moderate Factor VIII levels in patients with pretreatment levels of greater than 5%.

DDAVP may be used for prophylaxis prior to minor surgical procedures and for the treatment of minor hemorrhages such as hemarthroses, muscle hematomas, and mucosal

bleeding. It should not be used in patients with severe or life-threatening hemorrhages, in patients with pretreatment levels of 5% or lower, or in patients who have developed Factor VIII inhibitors. If the pretreatment factor level is unknown, one should assume a level of < 1%.

Hemophilia A with Factor VIII Inhibitors

About 10% of patients repeatedly exposed to Factor VIII infusion develop inhibitors in the form of neutralizing antibodies. Inhibitor levels are measured in Bethesda units, with 1 unit representing the ability to neutralize 1 unit of Factor VIII/ml of plasma. As the inhibitor level increases, the cost and risk of therapy escalate dramatically. Inhibitor levels above 5 units/ml require either huge doses of AHF or alternate therapies, including plasmapheresis, exchange transfusion, and, recently, administration of anti-inhibitor coagulant complex. Factor IX complex may be given in large doses in an attempt to bypass the function of Factor VIII in the coagulation pathway. This strategy is frequently successful but may be complicated by undesired thrombotic events.

Treatment of Hemophilia B

Factor IX levels required to achieve hemostasis are generally no more than 25% of normal. In contrast to hemophilia A, adequate factor levels can usually be achieved with fresh-frozen plasma. Factor IX concentrate is indicated only for the treatment of major hemorrhages and in the perioperative period. In these situations it is recommended that levels be attained that are two-thirds as high as those recommended for hemophilia A.

Thrombocytopenia

Diagnosis

Thrombocytopenia is defined as a platelet count of less than $100,000/\mu l$. This number defines a level below the statistical norm for the population but has relatively little clinical significance. Assuming that the remaining platelets are functional, spontaneous bleeding does not generally occur unless levels fall below $20,000/\mu l$. Bleeding with surgical procedures is likely to occur at levels below $40,000$ to $50,000/\mu l$.

Severe thrombocytopenia commonly presents with signs of mucosal or cutaneous hemorrhage. Clinical symptoms include gingival and dental extraction bleeding, epistaxis, gastrointestinal hemorrhage, menorrhagia, ecchymoses, and petechiae. A bleeding time determination should be ordered to document that a low platelet count is the cause of abnormal bleeding.

Causes of Thrombocytopenia

1. Increased platelet consumption: disseminated intravascular coagulation, infections
2. Decreased platelet production: marrow hypoplasia (drugs, toxins, infection, radiation), marrow infiltration (myelofibrosis, malignancy)
3. Sequestration of platelets: splenomegaly
4. Increased platelet destruction: idiopathic thrombocytopenic purpura (ITP), drug related, infections, posttransfusion

Indications for Treatment

1. Platelet count <20,000 with abnormal bleeding and increased bleeding time
2. Platelet count <50,000 in perioperative period

Discussion

Treatment of the thrombocytopenic patient with platelet transfusions seems relatively straightforward, but there are controversies over the appropriate indications for use of this product. There is not a simple test to document either need for or efficacy of treatment, and it is generally assumed that platelet transfusions are overused.

Determination of appropriate indications is difficult in the emergency setting because the patient is not well known to the physi-

---

DRUG TREATMENT: THROMBOCYTOPENIA

First-Line Therapy
Platelet Concentrate*

Dose	6 units
Repeat Dose	Same
End-Points	Cessation of bleeding, normal bleeding time, platelet count >20,000 (>50,000 in perioperative period or after massive transfusion)

*Platelets may not be effective in patients with thrombocytopenia caused by increased platelet destruction.

cian and the cause of thrombocytopenia may be unrecognized. Perhaps the most controversial issue surrounding platelet use concerns the treatment of dilutional thrombocytopenia.

Dilutional thrombocytopenia is a major cause of diffuse microvascular bleeding that occurs during massive transfusion of banked blood. The term is somewhat misleading in that platelet counts cannot be accurately predicted from the amount of blood replaced, implying that factors other than simple dilution are involved. Increased platelet consumption is believed to occur with trauma and hemorrhage and may be a major factor. In general, dilutional thrombocytopenia of clinical significance does not occur until at least two blood volumes have been replaced. Platelet transfusions are indicated for the treatment of active bleeding not responsive to standard surgical therapy when the platelet count is 50,000 or lower. Prophylactic treatment protocols calling for a fixed ratio of platelet to red cell transfusions are not recommended. These generally lead to unnecessary platelet transfusions.

Other conditions for which platelets may be indicated include decreased platelet production, increased platelet consumption, and platelet destruction and sequestration. Trauma, burns, sepsis, shock, malignancies, and the postoperative period may be associated with increased utilization of clotting factors and platelets, leading to diffuse bleeding. Correction of the thrombocytopenia may help control the bleeding, but correction of the underlying disorder is the primary goal of therapy.

Patients with myeloproliferative disorders are likely to present with thrombocytopenia either as a primary manifestation of the disease or secondary to chemotherapy. Platelet transfusions are indicated when there are clinical signs of impaired hemostasis and the platelet count is 20,000 or lower. These patients are likely to have developed platelet antibodies from prior platelet transfusions, and single-donor HLA-compatible platelets may be indicated.

Patients with hepatosplenomegaly may sequester platelets in the spleen, leading to chronic thrombocytopenia. Their ability to develop platelet levels adequate to control acute hemorrhage is limited. Platelets are indicated when there is active bleeding and the platelet count is 20,000 or lower.

Platelet destruction may be associated with idiopathic thrombocytopenic purpura (ITP), drug therapy (e.g., quinidine), acute infection, or the post-transfusion development of platelet antibodies. As a general rule, platelet transfusions are either unnecessary or ineffective in treating these disorders. It is recommended that a hematologist be consulted prior to initiating platelet transfusions in these patients.

Clotting Factor Deficiencies

Diagnosis

Although a large number of coagulation factor deficiencies exist, few are likely to need emergency treatment. Those that are most common include anticoagulation secondary to coumadin use, the coagulopathy of liver disease, and dilutional coagulopathy.

Indications for Coumadin Reversal or Treatment of Coagulopathy of Liver Disease

1. Anticipated surgical procedures
2. Major hemorrhage
3. Suspected occult hemorrhage (intracranial, intraperitoneal, retroperitoneal)
4. Hemorrhage threatening vital structures (brain, spinal cord, airway, pericardium)

Indications for Treatment of Dilutional Coagulopathy

1. Abnormal prothrombin time or partial thromboplastin time, *and*
2. Clinical evidence of impaired hemostasis

(See box.)

Discussion

With the exception of hemophilia A, coagulation factor deficiencies are most commonly treated with fresh-frozen plasma, which contains normal amounts of the stable and labile coagulation factors. Because of limitations on the volume of fresh-frozen plasma that can be infused in normovolemic patients, it is useful only if hemostasis can be achieved by a low level of the desired factor. Fresh-frozen plasma is efficacious for the replacement of Factors II, VII, X, and XI; it may be used for replacement of Factor IX if the deficiency is not severe. Fresh-frozen plasma cannot effectively replace Factor VIII because the high levels of this factor re-

---

DRUG TREATMENT: CLOTTING FACTOR DEFICIENCY
(FACTORS II, VII, X, XI)

First-Line Therapy
Fresh-Frozen Plasma*

Initial Dose	15–20 ml/kg
Repeat Dose	6–10 ml/kg
End-Points	Cessation of active bleeding and improvement in coagulation studies

Second-Line Therapy
Vitamin K

Initial Dose	5–10 mg IV at rate < 1 mg/min
Repeat Dose	May be repeated in 6–8 hours
End-Point	Clinical response or correction of prothrombin time

*Vitamin K is indicated for reversal of coumadin anticoagulation if the need for reversal is not urgent.

---

quired to achieve hemostasis mandate the use of excessively large volumes.

Treatment with coumadin is associated with a deficiency of the coagulation Factors II, VII, IX, and X, as well as proteins C and S. Levels of 30% or lower for each of these factors or proteins will achieve hemostasis, and these levels can generally be provided with fresh-frozen plasma without risk of volume overload. Fresh-frozen plasma is the treatment of choice for reversal of coumadin effects in patients who are actively bleeding or in need of emergency surgery. Vitamin K is preferred when the need for reversal is not urgent.

Liver disease may be associated with impaired synthesis of coagulation Factors I, II, V, VII, IX, and X. Most often this does not result in clinically significant bleeding. However, in the presence of hemorrhage or prior to a major surgical procedure, correction of abnormal coagulation with fresh-frozen plasma is indicated. Again, it should be noted that platelet abnormalities are common in these patients and are frequently the cause of impaired hemostasis.

Rapid replacement of more than one blood volume may be associated with a clinically significant dilutional coagulopathy. Altered hemostasis is not, however, a universal consequence of massive transfusion, and there is neither a sound theoretical basis nor existing clinical data to support the routine use of

fresh-frozen plasma in this setting. Several studies have shown that there is not a predictable relationship between the number of units of blood transfused and the levels of the labile clotting factors V, VIII, and IX or the values for the prothrombin time and partial thromboplastin time. Depending on the age of the blood transfused, the levels of the labile clotting factors may be adequate to achieve hemostasis. Furthermore, there is evidence from animal studies that plasma proteins, including coagulation factors, are infused from the interstitial space into the intravascular space during times of need. Current data support the use of fresh-frozen plasma only when there is clinical evidence of impaired hemostasis and when the prothrombin time and partial thromboplastin time suggest that the bleeding is due to a coagulation factor deficiency. It is important to recognize that platelet abnormalities (thrombocytopenia or impaired platelet function due to storage) are far more common causes of bleeding in the setting of massive transfusion.

Massive transfusion is also frequently associated with a consumptive coagulopathy. The appearance of this disorder seems to correlate more directly with the duration of the shock state and the severity of the tissue injury rather than the amount of blood transfused. Correction of the underlying triggering mechanism is the first priority in treatment, but replacement of depleted coagulation factors with fresh-frozen plasma may also be indicated.

SPECIFIC AGENTS

Albumin

Pharmacology

Preparations: 5% albumin; 25% albumin; plasma protein fraction (5% albumin); derived from pooled plasma

Indications

Burn injury (selected cases)
Chronic hypoalbuminemia (selected cases)
Hemorrhagic shock (selected cases)

Cautions

Renal failure—increased plasma volume may exacerbate volume overload.
Cardiac failure—increased plasma volume may exacerbate volume overload.
Hepatic failure—no contraindications
Pregnancy—may be used.
Childhood—may be used.

Dosage and Administration

Dosage in shock is 250 to 500 ml rapidly IV.
Maintain serum albumin >2.5 g/dl in burns.

Toxicity

Allergic Reactions

Fever, chills, flushing, headache, urticaria, nausea, vomiting
Hypotension may occur after rapid infusion.

Treatment

Discontinue infusion; give antihistamines.

Disease Transmission

Heat pasteurization kills hepatitis virus; probably effective against AIDS virus

Cryoprecipitate

Pharmacology

Volume—20 ml/single-donor bag
Good source of Factors VIII, VIIIc, XIII, von Willebrand's factor, fibrinogen
80 to 100 units Factor VIII/single-donor bag

80 to 100 units Factor VIIIc/single-donor bag

Indications

Hemophilia
von Willebrand's disease
Hemorrhage or major surgery with uremia
Coagulopathy of uremia

Cautions

Same as for fresh-frozen plasma (see p 65)

Dosage and Administration

See Drug Treatment: Hemophilia A
Limits: large doses increase risk of disease transmission and transfusion reaction.

Toxicity

Febrile transfusion reaction: same as for whole blood (see p 67)
Allergic transfusion reaction: same as for whole blood (see p 67)
Disease transmission: because multiple units are usually required, the risk of disease transmission will increase.

Desmopressin Acetate (DDAVP, Stimate)

Pharmacology

A synthetic analogue of the antidiuretic hormone 8-arginine vasopressin
Has a potent and prolonged antidiuretic effect
Causes a dose-related increase (up to three- to sixfold) in Factor VIII levels that begins within 30 minutes of intravenous infusions and peaks at 120 minutes

Indications

Hemorrhage prophylaxis prior to minor surgical procedures or for the treatment of minor hemorrhages such as hemarthroses, muscle hematomas, or mucosal bleeds
Indicated only in patients with hemophilia A or Type I von Willebrand's disease with Factor VIII levels greater than 5%
Coagulopathy of uremia

Cautions

Cardiovascular—desmopressin has both antidiuretic and vasopressor activities. Its use may result in hyponatremia and volume overload as well as hypertension.

Use in pregnancy—Category B; safety of desmopressin in pregnancy has not been established.

Use in children—should not be used in infants <3 months of age for hemophilia A or von Willebrand's disease

Dosage and Administration

The dose is 0.3 μg/kg in 50 ml 0.9% saline, infused over 15 to 30 minutes. In children weighing 10 kg or less, the volume of diluent should be decreased to 10 ml. Monitor vital signs during the infusion.

When used for hemorrhage prophylaxis, administer desmopressin 30 minutes prior to the anticipated time of surgery. The patient's clinical condition and coagulation profile should be used to determine the need for repeat doses or supplemental blood product administration.

Toxicity

Hypertension: high doses may cause mild to moderate elevation in blood pressure.

Allergic reactions: erythema, swelling, facial flushing, nausea, and abdominal cramping have been reported.

Dextran

Pharmacology

Composition—glucose polymerized into branched-chain polysaccharides

Dextran 40—molecular weight 40,000 daltons

Dextran 70—molecular weight 70,000 daltons

Half-life—dextran 40, 3 hours; dextran 70, 24 hours

Indications

Volume expansion

Cautions

Same as for hydroxyethyl starch (see p 66)

Dosage and Administration

Dose adjusted to desired hemodynamic effects

Initial dose: 500 ml at 20 to 40 ml/min

Upper limit: 20 ml/kg

Toxicity

Volume overload—see Cautions

Allergic reactions—urticaria, flushing, chest tightness, bronchospasm, hypotension

Fatal reactions have been reported.

Gastrointestinal disturbances—nausea, vomiting, involuntary defecation

Coagulation abnormalities—same as for hydroxyethyl starch (see p 66)

Laboratory abnormalities—may interfere with Rh and ABO blood typing

May falsely elevate serum glucose

Treatment

Stop infusion; provide supportive care.

Factor VIII: Antihemolytic Factor (Koate, Monoclate, Humak-P, Factorate)

Pharmacology

Derivation—fractionation of pooled human plasma

Kinetics—half-life = 12 hours (4 to 24 hours)

Clearance—biphasic

Preservation

Stable after reconstitution for 24 hours at room temperature

Indications

Bleeding episodes with Factor VIII deficiency

Cautions

Should always be administered through a needle filter

Renal failure—no contraindications

Cardiac failure—no contraindications

Hepatic failure—no contraindications

Pregnancy—may be used

Childhood—may be used

Dosage and Administration

Total dose = (body weight in kg) × (desired Factor VIII level − current Factor VIII level) (0.5)

Assume current level = 0 if unknown

Larger doses are required if Factor VIII inhibitor is present.

Toxicity

Development of Factor VIII inhibitor occurs 10% of the time in frequently treated patients.

Hemolysis may occur with large or repeated doses.

Allergic Transfusion Reaction

Fever, chills, urticaria, headache, vomiting, flushing, bronchospasm, reaction to murine antigens

Treatment

Slow the infusion rate.

Disease Transmission

Viral contamination risk high
Screening and heat treatment do not eliminate risk.

Factor IX Complex (Konyne, Proplex, Profilnine)

Pharmacology

Derivation—pooled plasma proteins; contains Factors II, VII, IX, X
Kinetics—half-life = 24 hours
Clearance—biphasic

Preservation

Stable for 12 hours after reconstitution

Indications

Bleeding due to Christmas disease (hemophilia B)
Bleeding in hemophilia A with Factor VIII inhibitors
Reversal of coumarin anticoagulation (selected cases)

Cautions

Should always be given with needle filter
Renal failure—no contraindications
Hepatic failure—no contraindications
Cardiac failure—no contradications
Use in pregnancy—may be used
Use in childhood—may be used

Dosage and Administration

Dosage (units) = (body weight in kg)
× (desired Factor IX level
− measured Factor IX level)

Factor VIII inhibitors—75 units/kg
Coumarin anticoagulation—15 units/kg

Toxicity

Thrombosis: simultaneous heparin administration may be indicated in patients at risk for thrombosis.
Allergic transfusion reaction: same as for Factor VIII, above
Hemolysis: same as for Factor VIII, p 64

Disease transmission: same as for Factor VIII, above

Fresh-Frozen Plasma

Pharmacology

Volume—200 to 250 ml (1 unit)
Single donor

Preservation

12 months frozen
2 hours thawed

Indications

Replacement of isolated coagulation factor deficiencies (Factors II, VIII, IX, X, XI)
Reversal of anticoagulation due to coumarin use
Correction of coagulopathy due to massive transfusion
Correction of coagulopathy due to liver disease
Antithrombin III deficiency
Treatment of thrombotic thrombocytopenic purpura

Cautions

Use only type-specific fresh-frozen plasma.
Renal failure—may contribute to volume overload
Cardiac failure—may contribute to volume overload
Hepatic failure—no contraindications
Use in pregnancy—may be used
Childhood—may be used

Dosage and Administration

Initial Dose

6 to 8 ml/kg for isolated coagulation factor deficiencies
10 ml/kg will increase Factor IX level by 25%.
15 to 20 ml/kg administered rapidly for severe coagulopathies
1 to 2 units for coumarin reversal

Repeat Dose

6 to 10 ml/kg every 8 to 12 hours if severe coagulation defect persists
3 to 4 ml/kg for isolated factor deficiencies
Need for continued treatment should be determined by presence of active bleeding.

Toxicity

Febrile transfusion reaction: same as for whole blood (see p 67)

Allergic transfusion reaction: same as for whole blood (see p 67)

Disease transmission: same as for whole blood (see p 67)

Hydroxyethyl Starch (Hetastarch)

Pharmacology

Heterogeneous mixture of branched amylopectin molecules

Average molecular weight = 450,000 daltons

Half-life = 17 days

Actions—increased colloidal oncotic pressure, expansion of plasma volume

Indications

Volume expansion

Cautions

Cardiac failure—may precipitate circulatory overload

Renal failure—may precipitate circulatory overload

Hepatic failure—may raise indirect serum bilirubin; close monitoring advised

Use in pregnancy—has not been adequately studied; use contraindicated unless benefits clearly outweigh the risks.

Childhood—may be used

Dosage and Administration

Dosage adjusted to desired hemodynamic effects

Usual dose = <20 ml/kg over 1 hour

Toxicity

Volume overload: see Cautions, above

Allergic reactions: uncommon; treatment is supportive.

Coagulation abnormalities: may dilute platelets

May dilute plasma proteins, including coagulation factors

Packed Red Cells

Pharmacology

Volume—250 ml

Preservation

Shelf life, 35 to 42 days at 4°C

Indications

Acute hemorrhage—acute blood loss >15% of total blood volume (may be less in compromised patients)

Anemia—symptomatic patients with hemoglobin <8 g/dl

Cautions

Renal failure—same as whole blood (see p 67)

Cardiac failure—same as whole blood (see p 67)

Hepatic failure—same as whole blood (see p 67)

Use in pregnancy—same as whole blood (see p 67)

Dosage and Administration

See Drug Treatment.

Toxicity

Same as whole blood (see p 67)

Platelet Concentrate

Pharmacology

Volume—50 to 60 ml/unit

Pooled plasma unless specifically stated otherwise

Preservation

70% platelet viability for 5 days at 22°C

Indications

Thrombocytopenia due to increased platelet consumption, decreased platelet production, platelet sequestration, platelet destruction, nonfunctional platelets

Cautions

Renal failure—transfusion volume may exacerbate volume overload.

Cardiac failure—transfusion volume may exacerbate volume overload.

Hepatic failure—may require two to three times normal dose due to sequestration

Pregnancy—Rh-negative females of childbearing age should receive Rh-compatible transfusion.

Childhood—may be used

Dosage and Administration

Standard dose: 1 unit/10 kg, up to 6 to 8 units total

Repeat dose: based on response to initial dose

Toxicity

Alloimmunization: very likely if recipient exposed to >20 donors. Immunization period lasts 6 weeks.

Febrile transfusion reaction: same as for whole blood (see below)

Bacterial contamination: same as for whole blood (see below)

Disease transmission: same as for cryoprecipitate (see p 63)

Whole Blood

Pharmacology

Volume—450 to 500 ml
Single donor

Preservation

Shelf life, 35 to 42 days at 4°C
Factor VIII—function decreased 50% at 7 to 14 days
Factor V—function decreased after 1 to 2 weeks; function decreased to 10% at 21 days
Platelets—function decreased 50% after 24 hours; function decreased <90% after 72 hours

Indications

Neonatal exchange transfusion
"Fresh" whole blood—massive hemorrhage

Cautions

Renal failure—high potassium level in stored blood may worsen hyperkalemia.
Cardiac failure—may precipitate or aggravate congestive heart failure with rapid infusion of whole blood
Hepatic failure—none
Use in pregnancy—avoid incompatible blood in Rh-negative females of childbearing age.
Childhood—may be used

Dosage and Administration

See Drug Treatment: Hemorrhagic Shock.

Toxicity

Hemolytic Transfusion Reaction

Fever, anxiety, tachycardia, infusion site pain, back pain, hypotension, bronchospasm

May produce acute renal failure or disseminated intravascular coagulation

TREATMENT

Discontinue transfusion.
Maintain urine output 1 to 2 ml/kg/hour with IV fluids, furosemide, mannitol.

Febrile Transfusion Reaction

Fever, urticarial rash
More common after multiple transfusions

TREATMENT

Discontinue transfusion if severe or if hemolytic reaction is possible.
Treat with antipyretics and antihistamines.

Allergic Transfusion Reaction

Urticaria most common
Bronchospasm, nausea, vomiting, hypotension possible

TREATMENT

Discontinue transfusion if allergic reaction is severe or if hemolytic reaction is possible.
Treat with antihistamines.

Bacterial Contamination

Rare

Rh Incompatibility

Rare

Citrate Toxicity

May produce hypocalcemia
Uncommon

TREATMENT

IV calcium if indicated

Disease Transmission

Same risk as with other single-donor products

Other Reactions

Hypothermia
Hemosiderosis

REFERENCES

Bove JR: Transfusion–associated hepatitis and AIDS. N Engl J Med 4:242–245, 1987.

Braunstein AH, Oberman HA: Transfusion of plasma components. Transfusion 4:281–286, 1984.

Brzica SM: Complications of transfusion. Int Anesthesiol Clin 20:171–193, 1982.

Consensus Conference: Fresh frozen plasma: Indications and risks. Transfusion Medicine Reviews 3:201–204, 1987.

Consensus Conference: Perioperative red blood cell transfusion. JAMA 18:2700–2703, 1988.

Consensus Conference: Platelet transfusion therapy. JAMA 13:1777–1780, 1987.

Fisher M: Transfusion-associated acquired immunodeficiency syndrome—What is the risk? Pediatrics 1:157–159, 1987.

Harrigan C, Lucas C, Ledgerwood A, Mammen E: Primary hemostasis after massive transfusion for injury. American Surgeon 48:393–396, 1982.

Heaton A, Miripol R, Aster P, et al: Use of Adsol® preservation solution for prolonged storage of low viscosity AS-1 red blood cells. Br J Haematol 57:467–478, 1984.

Honig CL, Bove JR: Transfusion-associated fatalities: Review of bureau of biologics reports 1976–1978. Transfusion 6:653–661, 1980.

Hougie C: Disorders of hemostasis—congenital disorders of blood coagulation factors. In Williams JW, Beutler E, Erslev AJ, et al (eds): Hematology, ed 3. New York, McGraw-Hill, 1983, pp 1563–1583.

Johnson AJ, Aronson DL, Williams WJ: Preparation and clinical use of plasma and plasma fractions. In Williams JW, Beutler E, Erslev AJ, et al (eds): Hematology, ed 3. New York, McGraw-Hill, 1983, pp 1529–1548.

Kruskall MS, Mintz PD, Bergin JJ, et al: Transfusion therapy in emergency medicine. Ann Emerg Med 17:327–335, 1988.

Masouredis SP: Preservation and clinical use of erythrocytes and whole blood. In Williams JW, Beutler E, Erslev AJ, et al (eds): Hematology, ed 3. New York, McGraw-Hill, 1983, pp 1529–1548.

Nilsson L, Hedner V, Nilsson IM, Robertson B: Shelf-life of bank blood and stored plasma with special reference to coagulation factors. Transfusion 23:377–381, 1983.

Peters RM, Hargens AR: Protein vs. electrolytes and all of the Starling forces. Arch Surg 116:1293–1298, 1981.

Reed RL, Ciavarella D, Heimbach DM, et al: Prophylactic platelet administration during massive transfusion. Ann Surg 203:40–48, 1986.

Richter AW, Hedin HI: Dextran hypersensitivity. Immunology Today 5:132–138, 1982.

Schwab CW, Shayne JP, Turner J: Immediate trauma resuscitation with type O uncrossmatched blood: A 2-year prospective experience. J Trauma 26(10):897, 1986.

Strautz RL, Nelson JM, Meyer EA, et al: Compatibility of Adsol–stored red cells with intravenous solutions. Am J Emerg Med 2:162–164, 1989.

Timberlake GA, McSwain NE: Autotransfusion of blood contaminated by enteric contents: A potentially lifesaving measure in the massively hemorrhaging trauma patient? J Trauma 6:855–857, 1988.

Tranbaugh RF, Lewis F: Crystalloid versus colloid for fluid resuscitation of hypovolemic patients. Adv Shock Res 9:203–216, 1983.

Tullis JL: Albumin: Background and use. 4:355–360, 1977.

Tullis JL: Albumin: Guidelines for clinical use. JAMA 5:460–463, 1977.

Weaver DW, Ledgerwood AM, Lucas CE, et al: Pulmonary effects of albumin resuscitation for severe hypovolemic shock. Arch Surg 113:387–392, 1978.

Yacobi A, Stoll R, Sum C, et al: Pharmacokinetics of hydroxyethyl starch in normal subjects. J Clin Pharmacol 33:206–212, 1982.

CHAPTER 7

Injected Anesthetics

JOHN I. GERSON, M.D.

INTRODUCTION

It is well to remember the medical dictum *primum non nocere* ("first do no harm") when considering the use of anesthetics. Anesthetics are not in themselves therapeutic; rather, they are toxic agents given to facilitate other therapies. Thus, before they are used, the physician should ask himself or herself whether the proposed therapy can be accomplished without them.

The pathophysiology induced by the anesthetic drugs themselves must be understood before looking at the pathophysiology of medical conditions in which they are used. Indeed, inexperienced anesthetists are often struck by the similarity between the induction of anesthesia and the onset of a cardiopulmonary crisis. The American Heart Association's ABCs of cardiopulmonary resuscitation is a useful guide to the pathophysiology produced by general anesthetics.

The physician must be prepared, both by skill and with the appropriate equipment, to manage the following anesthetic-induced effects before using anesthetic agents.

Anesthetic Effects Related to the Airway

Obstruction of the non–gas-exchanging passages through which air must travel on its way from the environment to the alveoli is usually induced by anesthetics and often by sedatives. Brief periods of airway obstruc-

tion may be managed with standard airway positioning maneuvers (head tilt, chin lift, or jaw thrust) or with an oral or nasopharyngeal airway. Endotracheal intubation is the preferred method of airway management when a long-acting agent is used.

Anesthetics, narcotics, and sedatives often either produce vomiting or allow passive regurgitation of gastric contents. Thus, suction and airway-protecting equipment and maneuvers should be known and immediately available when these drugs are used. Regurgitation or vomiting will likely occur on loss of consciousness in patients with full stomachs unless specific precautions are taken; such precautions include rapid endotracheal intubation with a cuffed tube while an assistant provides firm pressure on the cricoid (not the thyroid) cartilage to occlude the esophagus.

Anesthetic Effects Related to Breathing

Functional residual capacity is reduced by about 500 cc after induction of anesthesia with the patient in the supine position. This reduction begins within 30 seconds after intravenous thiopental induction and does not increase with time. Thus, any interruption of ventilation in the anesthetized state will more quickly result in arterial hypoxemia than in the awake state, since the functional residual capacity is the lung's main reserve store of oxygen.

Hypoventilation is to be expected during general anesthesia. The anesthetized patient produces approximately 10% less carbon dioxide than does an awake patient with a normal metabolic rate, and most injected anesthetics depress minute ventilation more than this, leading to hypercarbia. The ventilatory response to carbon dioxide is depressed in a dose-related fashion by most anesthetics.

Worse, the ventilatory response to hypoxia is depressed to about 25% of control by low, sedating-only concentrations of inhaled anesthetics, and narcotics and injected sedatives are believed to have similar effects. An increase in the paO_2-paO_2 gradient is seen during anesthesia, especially in older patients. This is likely caused by increased transpulmonary shunt and/or increased ventilation/perfusion mismatching.

The clinical implications of the adverse changes in respiration are clear: supplemental oxygen must be provided and ventilation may need to be assisted when sedative doses of anesthetics are administered. Furthermore, ventilation should be controlled and supplemental oxygen given when sleep-producing doses of injected anesthetics are administered. A greater margin of safety against hypoxia is provided if patients are given a high concentration of oxygen to provide an oxygen store in the functional residual capacity prior to drug administration.

Anesthetic Effects Related to Circulation

In general, the effects of injected anesthetics on the circulation are adverse but far more variable than the respiratory effects. This variability is partly due to the drugs themselves and partly due to the amount the circulation is being supported by the sympathetic nervous system in stressful pathologic states, such as multiple trauma.

Thiopental lowers blood pressure and cardiac output and work, largely as a result of its depressant effect on myocardial contractility, whereas benzodiazepines depress blood pressure through vasodilation, with minimal effects on cardiac contractility. Both thiopental and the benzodiazepines probably decrease the tone of capacitance vessels, whereas ketamine stimulates the sympathetic nervous system to increase venous and arterial tone. Tachycardia is commonly seen with all these drugs. On the other hand, narcotics (except meperidine) generally slow the pulse. Vasodilation is seen with mor-

phine but not with the synthetic opiates of the fentanyl class. It is best to assume that none of the intravenous anesthetics may be relied on to produce a stable circulation in the emergency setting. Removal or lessening of anxiety and pain by producing anesthesia or sedation will most likely depress the blood pressure, regardless of the agent used. Correction of hypovolemia, combined with cautious incremental titration of anesthetics, will reduce but not eliminate this circulatory depression.

CONDITIONS

Endotracheal Intubation

Diagnosis

Many medical conditions of unrelated pathophysiology require endotracheal intubation for management. It is convenient to divide these conditions into operational rather than pathophysiologic headings, since these will more readily help the physician recall the indication for intubation. Intravenous anesthetics may or may not be required to perform intubation (as may muscle relaxants, which are discussed in Chapter 25).

The problem of maintaining a patent airway may be solved by intubating the patient with facial or cervical trauma; bleeding from the upper respiratory or gastrointestinal tract; unconsciousness from metabolic, neoplastic, toxic, or traumatic cause; or obstruction by tumor, hematoma, or foreign body.

Ventilatory failure, whose hallmark is an elevated pCO_2, may be treated by intubation and mechanical ventilation. Such diverse conditions as central nervous system (CNS) disease (structural, traumatic, or toxic), neuromuscular disorders (including respiratory muscle fatigue in chronic lung disease), thoracic or upper abdominal trauma, ascites, or pleural effusions may result in ventilatory failure requiring intubation.

Intubation and mechanical ventilation may be needed in any condition causing hypoxemia that is not corrected by inhalation of oxygen by face mask. Such conditions may be generally subdivided into primarily pulmonary or primarily cardiac disorders. Intubation may also be necessary for pulmonary toilet, since mechanical removal of secretions or blood is facilitated by intubation and endotracheal suctioning.

Combative or uncooperative patients may

need short-term sedation to facilitate diagnostic studies or to protect them from harming themselves. A good example is the agitated, intoxicated head-injured patient with a neck fracture who needs a computed tomographic (CT) scan. These patients are best managed by endotracheal intubation for ventilatory support so they can be controlled with anesthesia or neuromuscular paralysis during the scan.

Indications for Treatment

Although all of the foregoing conditions may require intubation, most patients do not require intravenous anesthesia while being intubated. In general, anesthesia should be reserved for those patients in whom intubation is impossible or dangerous without it. Combative or uncooperative patients or patients having seizures with deteriorating ventilation and/or oxygenation are the most common example. Head-injured patients in whom coughing, straining, and hypertension are undesirable are another. Recognizing the anesthetics' deleterious effect on respiration, the practitioner must realize that these drugs will make respiration worse in the short term (indeed may well cause apnea) and *never* undertake their use for intubation without assuring himself or herself that he or she has the necessary equipment and skill for bag-valve-mask ventilation at hand. (See box.)

DRUG TREATMENT: ENDOTRACHEAL INTUBATION

First-Line Drug
Midazolam

Initial Dose	0.5 mg IV over 1 minute
Repeat Dose	0.25 mg every 2–5 minutes until desired level of sedation is reached
End-Points	Sedated, relaxed patient without loss of spontaneous respirations
	Endotracheal intubation

Second-Line Drug
Morphine

Initial Dose	2 mg IV
Repeat Dose	1–2 mg every 5 minutes until desired level of sedation is achieved
End-Points	Sedated, relaxed patient without loss of spontaneous respirations
	Endotracheal intubation

Third-Line Drug
Ketamine

Initial Dose	1 mg/kg IV
Repeat Dose	Usually not necessary
End-Points	Sedated, relaxed patient without loss of spontaneous respirations
	Endotracheal intubation

Fourth-Line Drug
Thiopental

Initial Dose	2–3 mg/kg IV
Repeat Dose	Usually not necessary
End-Points	Sedated, relaxed patient without loss of spontaneous respirations
	Endotracheal intubation

Discussion

Before endotracheal intubation is attempted, the patient should be preoxygenated with 100% oxygen. It is a good idea to determine the feasibility of bag-and-mask ventilation, which may be necessary if the intubation fails, before eliminating the patient's own respirations with anesthetics. The majority of emergency intubations can be performed without any anesthesia or by using topical anesthesia alone. Intravenous lidocaine, 1 mg/kg given several minutes before the intubation, will blunt the hypertensive response to intubation in patients in whom hypertension might be detrimental, particularly those with cerebral pathology such as head injury or subarachnoid hemorrhage.

When an intravenous anesthetic is needed to facilitate endotracheal intubation, midazolam is an excellent agent. It has a rapid onset of action, producing sedation and amnesia within several minutes after intravenous injection. Midazolam's effects usually last for only 30 to 60 minutes. This short duration of action represents a distinct advantage over diazepam in acute situations, particularly if untoward effects occur. The manufacturer has issued numerous warnings to physicians about overdosages with midazolam. These have occurred with use of preset, rather than titrated, doses; with rapid injection, rather than with slow infusion over several minutes; and as a result of the increased sensitivity of elderly and debilitated patients to this drug. Midazolam should be administered by incremented titration of small doses, which is facilitated by using the 1 mg/ml concentration diluted to 10 ml with normal saline or 5% dextrose and water (D_5W). Give 0.5 mg IV over 1 minute, wait 2 to 3 minutes to assess the clinical effect, and give additional doses of 0.25 mg over 1 minute at 2- to 5-minute intervals until the desired level of sedation is achieved, which usually occurs when the patient's speech becomes slurred. Expect the desired response at a lower dose in patients who are debilitated or older than 60 years, or who have received other sedatives, such as ethanol or narcotics.

Morphine may also be used to achieve sedation for endotracheal intubation but is more likely than midazolam to cause hypotension, especially in hypovolemic trauma patients. On the other hand, morphine's venodilating properties are advantageous in the cardiac patient needing intubation for pulmonary edema. The benzodiazepines do not produce analgesia, so morphine might be preferred in those patients who require analgesia in addition to sedation. Morphine, and indeed all injectable anesthetics, should be given by slow incremental titration rather than by rapid injections of "standard doses." Give 2 mg IV over 30 to 60 seconds, wait 5 minutes to assess both desired and toxic effects, and give repeated doses of 1 to 2 mg every 5 minutes until the desired level of sedation occurs. Hypotension results from venous dilation and will usually respond to a fluid bolus. Severe toxicity can be rapidly reversed with naloxone, 0.4 to 0.8 mg IV.

Ketamine, a phencyclidine derivative, when first released in the late 1960s, appeared to represent a significant advance over the barbiturates. It may be given by the intramuscular (5 to 10 mg/kg) or intravenous (1 to 2 mg/kg) route; it stimulates the sympathetic nervous system (unless this is already maximally stimulated by disease) so that blood pressure, pulse, and cardiac index generally increase by about 30%; it does not depress ventilation ($paCO_2$ rises < 3 mmHg); and airway-protective reflexes are often maintained. The drug is an excellent analgesic and may be given in so-called subdissociative doses (0.2 to 0.5 mg/kg). Consciousness is lost in about 1 minute after intravenous administration and in 3 to 5 minutes after intramuscular administration. The awakening period is longer than that of barbiturates, with about 10 to 15 minutes required after a single intravenous dose. Allergy and organ toxicity occur rarely, if ever.

Patients receiving ketamine can experience upper airway obstruction or vomiting and aspiration, and patients near shock may become hypotensive. Cerebral blood flow increases, causing elevated intracranial pressure in patients with space-occupying lesions. However, the main reason for ketamine's relative lack of popularity is the vivid, hallucinatory, and often morbid dreams that persist for about 24 hours after its administration. In fact, the anesthetic state itself is called "dissociative," reflecting that the grimacing, contorted facies exhibited by patients means they are "dissociated" from their surroundings. The parent compound, phencyclidine, is abused as the street drug PCP, or "angel dust."

A special acute situation in which ketamine may prove useful is in providing anesthesia for endotracheal intubation of asthmatic patients. Intubation itself may worsen bronchospasm, and ketamine relieves bronchospasm both in animal models and in humans. However, seizures manifested by extensor posturing have been reported with the combination of aminophylline and ketamine.

Thiopental is the anesthetic agent used for routine induction of anesthesia and endotracheal intubation in the controlled environment of the operating suite. However, this setting is very different from an emergency intubation of a critically ill patient. In the operating room, the patients have been premedicated with an anticholinergic agent to counteract the airway secretions that are often troublesome with barbiturates, and they can be adequately preoxygenated and also given neuromuscular paralysis, which facilitates both intubation and bag-and-mask ventilation, if needed. Usually, none of these indications exists in the acute setting. Thiopental is more likely than the other recommended drugs to totally abolish the patient's spontaneous respirations, thus removing the only, albeit often poor, safety net these patients have if intubation fails.

Agitation Control

Diagnosis

Diverse pathologic conditions can produce an agitated mental state. Possible etiologies include primary CNS pathology (e.g., head injury, encephalitis, meningitis, brain tumor, seizures), metabolic disturbances (e.g., hypoxia, hypercarbia, renal or hepatic encephalopathy, various electrolyte imbalances), endocrinopathies, ingestion of a drug or toxin, drug withdrawal, infections, shock, and psychotic illnesses. The immediate assessment of an acutely agitated patient should be focused on finding historical (e.g., a diabetic patient taking insulin) and physical (e.g., a bruise on the forehead) clues that will provide an immediate diagnosis and thus lead to definitive treatment. Particular attention should be paid to airway, breathing, and circulation, both as causes of an altered mental state and because of the effect of the drugs used to control agitation on these crucial physiologic functions.

Indications for Treatment

An agitated mental state may prevent the diagnostic evaluation necessary to identify the underlying etiology, thus delaying specific treatment, and may cause further harm to the patient. For example, agitation can produce dangerous increases in intracranial pressure in a head-injured patient. Thus, agitated patients may need sedation on a short-term basis to facilitate diagnostic studies such as CT scanning or on a longer-term basis as a therapeutic modality. Intravenous anesthetic agents are used therapeutically for agitated patients with increased intracranial pressure, to control patients who are not tolerating mechanical ventilation, to manage some patients with drug withdrawal or delirium tremens, and to manage status epilepticus. When intravenous anesthetic agents are used in these settings, the patient *must* have an endotracheal tube in place and mechanical support of ventilation and be in a setting that provides intensive monitoring of cardiovascular and respiratory functions. (See box.)

Discussion

Control of agitation for short diagnostic procedures and ongoing control of an acutely ill patient not requiring endotracheal intubation are best accomplished by major or minor tranquilizers, as described in Chapter 9. Patients who need endotracheal intubation for other reasons or who do not respond to tranquilizers are best managed with intravenous anesthetic techniques. An excellent way of managing the patient needing long-term sedation for agitation control is with a regimen of rapid sedation by incremental intravenous titration of an injectable anesthetic followed by continuous infusion of the same agent to maintain the desired mental status. With the appropriate choice of drug and careful monitoring and titration, it is possible to achieve any mental status, ranging from deep general anesthesia to an awake, comfortable, cooperative patient. It is important to emphasize that this approach requires endotracheal intubation, mechanical support of ventilation, and ongoing physiologic monitoring and support in an intensive care unit.

Morphine is the best agent to use when the mental status desired is that of a relatively awake but calm, cooperative, and comfortable patient. Morphine has both sedative and analgesic effects. Since a variety of painful procedures are an inherent part of the intensive care unit experience, morphine's analgesic actions are appreciated by the patient. Morphine depresses the cough reflex, which is another beneficial effect in patients needing sedation because they are not tolerating

DRUG TREATMENT: INTUBATED, AGITATED PATIENT

First-Line Drug
Morphine

Initial Dose	1–2 mg IV bolus every 5 minutes until desired mental status is achieved
Maintenance Dose	Continuous infusion of 1–5 mg/hour
End-Points	Calm, manageable patient
	No circulatory compromise
	Desired suppression of respiratory drive

Second-Line Drug
Thiopental

Initial Dose	2–3 mg/kg IV over 1–2 minutes; may repeat one-half of this dose in 5 minutes
Maintenance Dose	Continuous IV infusion of 1–5 mg/kg/hour
End-Points	Calm, manageable patient
	No circulatory compromise
	Desired suppression of respiratory drive

Third-Line Drug
Diazepam

Initial Dose	3–5 mg IV; may repeat one-half of initial dose
Maintenance Dose	2.5 mg IV every 2–4 hours
End-Points	Calm, manageable patient
	No circulatory compromise
	Desired suppression of respiratory drive

endotracheal intubation and mechanical ventilation.

Immediate control is achieved by using the incremental titrated loading regimen, described earlier. Ongoing control is maintained by administering a continuous infusion of morphine, with the dose titrated to the desired effects and to the individual variability in response. As a rough guide, a continuous morphine infusion in the range of 1 to 5 mg/hour can be expected to produce drowsiness with normal arousal, calmness during awakening, analgesia, and some suppression of spontaneous respiration. Higher doses will produce apnea and coma but also more side effects. When a patient being managed by a continuous morphine infusion needs additional sedation, this can be provided either by adding a single dose of a benzodiazepine or by giving an additional 1- to 2-mg bolus of morphine and increasing the infusion rate.

Hypotension and respiratory depression are the acute side effects of concern when using morphine anesthesia. The respiratory depression is not a problem, since these patients should be intubated and ventilated anyway. The hypotension usually responds to volume infusion and often does not necessitate a reduction in dose after the expanded venous capacitance bed is repleted. Severe hypotension can be reversed with naloxone, 0.4 to 0.8 mg by IV push, but this will also reverse the sedative and analgesic effects of morphine. Parasympathetic inhibition occurs with long-term narcotic use and may manifest as urinary retention, nausea and vomiting, constipation with the potential for acute toxic dilation of the colon (Ogilvie's syndrome), and biliary colic. Addiction is a concern but does not seem to occur for at least several weeks. With continuous infusion the "wooden chest" syndrome is an unusual but life-threatening complication occurring when near-anesthetic levels of narcotics cause marked skeletal muscle rigidity, which prevents ventilation. This syndrome is treated by neuromuscular paralysis with pancuronium, 0.1 mg/kg IV.

Thiopental, rather than morphine, is the preferred intravenous anesthetic agent in selected circumstances, including conditions associated with increased intracranial pressure (i.e., head injury, Reye's syndrome, subarachnoid hemorrhage), status epilepticus, and drug withdrawal (including delirium tremens), and when complete suppression of respiratory drive is desired. Thiopental is beneficial in some brain insults because it decreases cerebral metabolic demands and may lower intracranial pressure. However, a recent large prospective study has shown that it does not improve outcome following global brain ischemia. A small subset of patients with narcotic withdrawal or delirium tremens will need endotracheal intubation for other reasons (e.g., concomitant pneumonia or unstable spine fractures that require immobility). This regimen gives deep anesthesia with no danger of inadvertent movement by the patient. After 5 to 7 days, the patient will awaken with the withdrawal syndrome resolved and no recall of the experience. I prefer to use thiopental rather than the combination of a sedative and neuromuscular paralyzing agent when total control of ventilation is desired. With neuromuscular paralysis, it is possible to be awake and paralyzed, which is a very psychologically traumatizing condition. This is not a concern with the thiopental technique, since thiopental both sedates and stops ventilation.

Acute control is achieved by giving a 2 to 3 mg/kg IV bolus of thiopental over 1 to 2 minutes. Patients who are elderly or hypovolemic or who have recently received other sedating drugs should be given a smaller loading dose. A second loading bolus of one-half the initial dose may be given in 5 minutes if the desired level of sedation has not been achieved. Anesthesia is maintained by a continuous infusion of thiopental, which is titrated to the findings of the neurologic examination and the patient's cardiovascular status. A good starting rate is 2.5 mg/kg/hour and will provide the desired sedation in most patients. If the patient is too awake, give an additional IV bolus of 1 to 1.5 mg/kg and increase the infusion rate by 1 mg/kg/hour. Thiopental is an ultra–short-acting barbiturate when given as a single IV bolus because of its rapid redistribution into other tissues. However, when given by prolonged continuous infusion, its elimination half-life is quite prolonged at approximately 24 to 36 hours. Thus, the dose required to maintain the desired level of sedation will be less after the first day of the infusion, and awakening may be delayed for several days after discontinuing the infusion.

Thiopental is both a vasodilator and a negative inotropic agent with the potential for causing severe circulatory collapse. However, neither of two recent articles describing this regimen reported any serious hemodynamic compromise when the drug, and especially the loading dose, was carefully titrated.

Diazepam has a long-standing tradition of use for controlling patients requiring mechanical ventilation. When used for this purpose, it is given as intermittent boluses of 1 to 5 mg IV at 1- to 4-hour intervals. As these broad dosing ranges indicate, there is considerable individual variation in responsiveness, which makes the drug's effectiveness somewhat unpredictable. Diazepam's long half-life tends to cause a cumulative effect with repetitive dosing, resulting in deepening of the level of sedation and prolongation of awakening time. Morphine is much easier to titrate when the goal is a level of unconsciousness at the awake end of the spectrum, and thiopental is more reliable in producing deep coma. Midazolam has pharmacokinetic properties that might make it a suitable agent for use by continuous infusion to maintain a constant level of sedation. However, the current experience base with this regimen is too limited to allow any specific recommendations.

SPECIFIC AGENTS

Diazepam (Valium)

Pharmacology

Clinical Formula

7-chloro-1,3-dihydro-1-methyl-5-phenyl-2H-1,4-benzodiazepin-2-one

Mechanism of Action

Binds to specific benzodiazepine receptors in cortical and limbic areas of CNS

Enhances inhibitory properties of the neurotransmitter gamma-aminobutyric acid (GABA)

Kinetics

	PO	IV
Onset	20–30 minutes	1–2 minutes
Peak	45–60 minutes	2–5 minutes
Duration	4–6 hours	4–6 hours
Half-life	43 hours	43 hours

Metabolism

Initial—redistribution into adipose tissue

Elimination by hepatic biotransformation—microsomal oxidation, glucuronide conjugation

---

Note: **Bioavailability is poor after intramuscular injection. This route of administration should not be used due to unpredictable absorption and high incidence of sterile abscess formation.**

Clinical Effects

Reduction in anxiety

Anticonvulsant

Reduction in arousal and alertness

Skeletal muscle relaxation

Amnesia

Preservation of autonomic and endocrine responses to emotions and nervous stimuli

Indications

Sedation

Muscle relaxation

Anxiety reduction

Anticonvulsant

Management of drug withdrawal

Dosage

IV: adults, 3- to 5-mg bolus by slow push; children, 0.1 mg/kg bolus by slow push (maximum dose of 2.5 mg)

PO: 5 to 10 mg

Cautions

Dosage adjustment in organ failure: none

Use in pregnancy—Category D

Use in lactation—no

Use in childhood—yes; dose 0.1 mg/kg to maximum single dose of 2.5 mg

Toxicity

Drug Interactions

Increased CNS depression with alcohol, narcotics, barbiturates

Increased effect with acetaminophen, beta-blockers, cimetidine, oral contraceptives, disulfiram, isoniazid, valproic acid

Decreased effect with caffeine, rifampin, ranitidine (oral diazepam only), theophylline

Enhances toxicity of amiodarone, digoxin, lithium (combination causes hypothermia), succinylcholine (prolonged paralysis)

Side Effects

Common: sedation and impairment of psychomotor and intellectual function; reduced memory and recall; increased intraocular pressure (do not use in acute glaucoma)

Uncommon: paradoxical excitement

Dangerous: prolonged coma with repetitive doses; impaired ventilatory drive; hypotension

Treatment of Toxicity

Ventilatory support

Volume infusion

Flumazenil (available in Europe as Anexate) is a specific benzodiazepine antagonist currently undergoing clinical trials in the United States. It should be available for the specific treatment of diazepam toxicity soon.

Ketamine (Ketalar)

Pharmacology

dl 2-(o-chlorophenyl)-2-(methylamino) cyclohexanone hydrochloride

Mechanism of Action

Interrupts association pathways of CNS, producing a state termed "dissociative anesthesia"

Kinetics

	IV	IM
Onset	30–60 seconds	3–4 minutes
Peak	1 minute	4 minutes
Duration	5–10 minutes	12–25 minutes
Half-life		
Redistribution	15 minutes	15 minutes
Metabolism	2.5 hours	2.5 hours

Metabolism

Initially a redistribution into adipose tissue terminates the anesthetic effect.
Hepatic metabolism

Clinical Effects

Analgesia
At low doses, cataleptic state without unconsciousness
Preservation of pharyngeal and laryngeal reflexes
Bronchodilation
Sympathetic stimulation
No muscle relaxation

Indications

Endotracheal intubation of asthmatic patients
Short painful procedures not requiring muscle relaxation

Dosage

IV: 1 to 2 mg/kg over 60 seconds
IM: 10 mg/kg

Cautions

Dosage adjustments in organ failure: none; do not use if intracranial pressure is elevated.
Use in pregnancy—Category C
Use in lactation—no
Use in childhood—yes

Toxicity

Drug Interactions

Prolonged sedation with other CNS depressants (e.g., ethanol, narcotics, barbiturates)

Side Effects

Common: emergence reactions consisting of diverse and often unpleasant psychologic manifestations occurring in 12% of patients, tachycardia, increased secretions

Uncommon: hypotension, bradycardia, respiratory depression, nausea and vomiting, rash, tonic-clonic motor activity

Treatment of Acute Toxicity

Emergence reactions: minimal stimulation; if reaction is severe, 1.5 mg/kg thiopental
Respiratory depression: assisted ventilation

Midazolam (Versed)

Pharmacology

Imidazobenzodiazepine derivative

Mechanism of Action

Benzodiazepine receptor binding

Kinetics

	PO	IM or IV
Onset	20–30 minutes	1–2 minutes
Peak	45–60 minutes	3–5 minutes
Duration	0.5–2 hours	0.5–2 hours
Half-life	1.5–3 hours	1.5–3 hours

Metabolism

Hepatic oxidation to its 1-hydroxymethyl metabolite (potency half of parent compound)
Excreted in urine as glucuronide conjugates

Indications

Preoperative sedation
Sedation
Anticonvulsant
Anesthesia induction
Significant advantages over diazepam and lorazepam: (1) it reduces pain/phlebitis associated with oil-based injectable benzodiazepines; (2) it produces profound amnesia; (3) it may be combined in the same syringe with other water-soluble agents (e.g., morphine or meperidine); (4) it has a shorter duration of action; and (5) it may be equally efficacious when administered IM or IV.

Dosage

PO: 0.08 mg/kg, to maximum of 3 to 5 mg
IV or IM: 0.1 mg/kg, to maximum of 2.5
  mg (1.5 mg in patients $\geq$ 60 years of
  age)

Cautions

Dosage adjustments in pulmonary, cardiac, or renal failure: careful titration
  using the lowest effective dose
Use in pregnancy—no; category D
Use in lactation—no
Use in childhood—yes. Midazolam has
  been used for the sedation of infants and
  children for various procedures (although not approved by the Food and
  Drug Administration for use in children
  in the United States), in combination
  with nalbuphine for outpatient sedation,
  for sedation of children receiving artificial ventilation following cardiac surgery, and widely as a preoperative and
  induction agent for anesthesia.
Maximum single dose 1.5 mg; titrate
  slowly and carefully

Toxicity

Drug Interactions

Same as other benzodiazepines

Side Effects

Common and uncommon: same as diazepam
Dangerous: respiratory depression and
  cardiac arrest reported before dosage
  guidelines revised

Treatment of Toxicity

Ventilatory support
Volume infusion
Flumazenil (available in Europe as Anexate) is a specific benzodiazepine antagonist currently undergoing clinical trials
  in the United States. It should be available for the specific treatment of midazolam toxicity soon.

Morphine

Pharmacology

Opium alkaloid

Mechanism of Action

Agonist that binds to stereospecific receptors widely distributed in the CNS and
  on smooth muscle

Kinetics (IV Bolus)

Onset	1–2 minutes
Peak	30 minutes
Duration	2–3 hours
Half-life	1.5–2 hours

Metabolism

Hepatic conjugation to glucuronide
Renal (90%) and gastrointestinal (10%) excretion of the glucuronide metabolite

Clinical Effects

Analgesia
Sedation
Decreased respiratory drive
Venous dilation
Bradycardia

Indications

Sedation of the agitated, intubated patient
Pain control

Dosage

Only the intravenous route should be used
  for acute situations.

Loading Dose

1 to 2 mg IV every 5 minutes until desired
  effect achieved

Maintenance Dose

Preferred: continuous infusion of 1 to 10
  mg/hour based on patient response
Alternative: repeat IV bolus of one-half
  total amount required for initial loading
  every 2 hours

Cautions

Dosage adjustments in organ failure—
  loading, none; maintenance, reduce in
  renal or hepatic failure
Use in pregnancy—yes; Category B
Use in lactation—no
Use in childhood—yes. Reduce dose in
  proportion to size.

Toxicity

Drug Interactions

Additive CNS depression with ethanol,
  barbiturates, other narcotics, antihistamines, beta-blockers, cimetidine, phenothiazines, tricyclic antidepressants,
  butyrophenones

Side Effects

Common: nausea and vomiting, urinary retention, constipation, pruritus, respiratory depression

Uncommon: dysphoria, hypotension, biliary colic
Dangerous: hypotension, respiratory failure

Treatment of Acute Toxicity

Fluid infusion
Ventilatory support
Naloxone, 0.4 to 0.8 mg IV. Remember morphine has a longer duration of action than naloxone, so symptoms should be expected to recur, requiring repeated doses of naloxone.

Thiopental (Pentothal)

Pharmacology

Sodium 5-ethyl-5-(1-methylbutyl)-2-thiobarbiturate

Mechanism of Action

Blocks reticular activating system

Kinetics (IV Bolus)

Onset	10–15 seconds
Peak	30–40 seconds
Duration	5–10 minutes
Half-life	3 minutes (redistribution)
	5–12 hours (elimination)

Metabolism

Anesthetic effect initially disappears due to redistribution.
Final elimination by hepatic degradation to inactive metabolites that are excreted by the kidney

Note: When administered as a single IV bolus, thiopental is an ultra–short-acting barbiturate because redistribution from brain to other tissues (primarily muscle) rapidly causes brain concentrations to become subtherapeutic.

When thiopental is administered as a continuous infusion, all body tissues become saturated and act as a reservoir that maintains plasma and brain concentrations at anesthetic levels. Thiopental then becomes a long-acting barbiturate with a half-life of 24 to 36 hours because its removal from the brain is dependent on metabolism and not redistribution.

Clinical Effects

Coma
Respiratory depression/apnea
Venous dilation
Analgesia relatively poor

Indications

Induction of anesthesia
Deep anesthesia for short procedures
Prolonged sedation for drug withdrawal, status epilepticus, ventilator control, increased intracranial pressure

Dosage

IV bolus: 3 to 5 mg/kg over 1 to 2 minutes
Maintenance infusion: 1 to 5 mg/kg/hour

Cautions

Dosage adjustments in organ failure: reduce dose if cardiac, hepatic, or renal failure, or patient's age > 60 years
Higher loading dose per kilogram of body weight required with obesity
Porphyria—causes death
Status asthmaticus: contraindicated
Hypersensitivity to barbiturates
Use in pregnancy—no; Category C
Use in lactation—no
Use in childhood—yes; dose based on weight

Toxicity

Drug Interactions

Thiopental effect increased by other CNS depressants, reserpine (hypotension), sulfonamides, chloramphenicol, probenecid
Effect decreased by thiopental (increased metabolism): oral anticoagulants, tricyclic antidepressants, beta-blockers, cimetidine, oral contraceptives, corticosteroids, cyclosporine, digitoxin, haloperidol, phenothiazines, quinidine, tetracyclines, theophylline, methadone (may cause withdrawal syndrome)
Thiopental increases hepatic toxicity of acetaminophen.

Side Effects

Common: respiratory depression, hypotension, coughing, shivering during emergence
Uncommon: laryngospasm, bronchospasm, arrhythmias, tissue necrosis with extravasation
Dangerous: apnea, laryngospasm, bronchospasm, hypotension, arrhythmias

Treatment of Toxicity

Stop drug
Ventilatory support
Volume infusion
Vasopressor
Antiarrhythmic drugs per American Heart
  Association protocols
Laryngospasm—neuromuscular paralysis
Extravasation—infiltrate site with 1% pro-
  caine; apply heat to site.

REFERENCES

Albrion-Sotelo R, Flint LS, Kelly KJ, et al: Healthcare
  Provider's Manual for Basic Life Support. Dallas, TX,
  American Heart Association, 1988.
Bovill JG, Sebel PS, Stanley TH: Opioid analgesics in anesthesia. Anesthesiology 61:731–755, 1984.
Carlon GC, Kahn RC, Goldiner WH, et al: Long term
  infusion of sodium thiopental. Crit Care Med 6:311–
  316, 1978.
Cilip M, Chelluri L, Jastremski MS, Baily R: Continuous
  intravenous infusion of sodium thiopental for managing drug withdrawal syndromes. Resuscitation
  13:243–248, 1986.
Corssen G, Reves JG, Stanley TH: Intravenous Anesthesia and Analgesia. Philadelphia, Lea & Febiger, 1988,
  pp 99, 175–176.
Dripps RD, Eckenhoff JE, Vandam LD: Introduction to
  Anesthesia, 6th ed. Philadelphia, WB Saunders, 1982,
  pp 146–152.
Gal TJ, DiFazio CA, Moscicki J: Analgesic and respiratory depressant activity of nalbuphine: A comparison
  with morphine. Anesthesiology 57:367–374, 1982.
Goodman LS, Gilman A (eds): The Pharmacologic Basis
  of Therapeutics. New York, Macmillan, 1985.
Halford FJ: A critique of intravenous anesthesia in war
  surgery. Anesthesiology 4:67, 1943.
Hirshman CA, Krieger W, Littlejohn G, et al: Ketamine-
  aminophylline-induced decrease in seizure threshold.
  Anesthesiology 56:464–467, 1982.
Homer TD, Stanski DR: The effect of increasing age on
  thiopental disposition and anesthetic requirement.
  Anesthesiology 62:714–724, 1985.
Hornbein TF: Anesthetics and ventilatory control. In
  Covino BG, Fozzard HA, Rehder K, et al (eds): Effects
  of Anesthesia. Bethesda, MD, The American Physiological Society, 1985, p 79.
Lee CM, Yeakell AE: Patients' refusal of surgery following Innovar premedication. Anesth Analg 54:224–
  226, 1975.
Montgomery WH, Donegan J, McIntyre KM, et al: Standards and guidelines for cardiopulmonary resuscitation and emergency cardiac care. JAMA 255:2841–
  3044, 1986.
Nunn JF: Anesthesia and pulmonary gas exchange. In
  Covino BG, Fozzard HA, Rehder K, et al (eds): Effects
  of Anesthesia. Bethesda, MD, The American Physiological Society, 1985, pp 137–147.
Nunn JF: Applied Respiratory Physiology, 3rd ed. Boston, Butterworths, 1987, p 350.
Price HL Kornat PJ, Safar, JN, Gonnor EH, The uptake
  of thiopental by body tissues and its relation to the duration of narcosis. Clin Pharmacol Ther 1:16–22,
  1960.
Rehder K: Anesthesia and the mechanics of respiration.
  In Covino BG, Fozzard HA, Rehder K, et al (eds): Effects of Anesthesia. Bethesda, MD, The American
  Physiological Society, 1985, p 92.
Reves JG, Fragen RJ, Vinik HR, et al: Midazolam: Pharmacology and uses. Anesthesiology 62:310–324,
  1985.
Reves JG, Gelman S: Cardiovascular effects of intravenous anesthetic drugs. In Covino BG, Fozzard HA,
  Rehder K, et al (eds): Effects of Anesthesia. Bethesda,
  MD, The American Physiological Society, 1985, pp
  185–189.
Rizack MA, Hillman CD: Handbook of Adverse Drug Interactions. New Rochelle, NY, The Medical Letter,
  1987.
Roscow CE: Cardiovascular effects of narcotics. In Covino BG, Fozzard HA, Rehder K, et al (eds): Effects of
  Anesthesia. Bethesda, MD, The American Physiological Society, 1985, pp 195–205.
Stanski DR, Mihm FG, Rosenthal MH, Kalman SM:
  Pharmacokinetics of high-dose thiopental used in cerebral resuscitation. Anesthesiology 53:169–171,
  1980.
Stanski DR, Watkins WD: Drug Disposition in Anesthesia. New York, Grune & Stratton, 1982, pp 72–83.
Stoelting RK: Pharmacology and Physiology in Anesthetic Practice. Philadelphia, JB Lippincott, 1987, pp
  69–114, 117–137, 141–143, 347–353.

CHAPTER 8

Analgesics

SUSAN M. DUNMIRE, M.D.
PAUL M. PARIS, M.D.

INTRODUCTION

Analgesia has long been one of the most challenging, frustrating, and poorly understood entities in medicine. Of over 80 million visits to emergency departments in the United States per year, the most common symptom is pain. Although pain relief is of primary importance to the patient, proper analgesia is often delayed until evaluation and diagnosis of the underlying medical problem are completed. During our years of medical training we become tolerant to the pain of others, rationalizing our insensitivity by excuses such as "I can't treat the pain until I know the cause of the pain"; "If I treat the pain before I have completed the evaluation, I may mask physical findings"; or "They shouldn't really have that much pain." While these may be true concerns of the physician, they have no scientific basis. The appropriate administration of analgesia by a skilled physician will provide adequate pain relief to the patient without confounding the diagnosis.

Physiology of Pain

Throughout history there have been many theories on the pathophysiology of pain. The most recently accepted mechanism is the "gate theory" proposed by Melzach and Wall in 1965. This theory postulates a "neural gate" in the dorsal horn of the spinal cord, which modulates nociceptive input before it reaches the central nervous system (CNS). In theory, when input arrives at the dorsal horn via large myelinated A fibers, there is negative feedback to the transmission cell and the gate is closed. Sensory input via small unmyelinated C fibers opens the gate, and painful sensory information is transmitted to the CNS. Substance P is the neurotransmitter released by the C fibers in the dorsal horn. Pain impulses exit the dorsal horn and ascend in either the spinothalamic or spinoreticulothalamic tracts to the cerebral cortex. The final degree of pain perception is believed to be a balance between the number of C fibers versus the number of A fibers stimulated. Despite shortcomings, this theory explains a number of clinical phenomena such as the pain relief obtained with transcutaneous electrical nerve stimulation (TENS) and acupuncture, in which the large A fibers are stimulated and thus inhibit transmission through the "gate."

The most exciting development for pain management in recent years has been the discovery of opiate receptors and endogenous opiate peptides. Currently five classes of opiate receptors have been demonstrated to exist (Table 8–1). The unique activity of an opiate is due to the specific opiate receptors with which it binds. The newer class of narcotic agonist/antagonist analgesics combines opiate agonist and antagonist properties by selective actions on various opiate re-

TABLE 8–1. Classes of Opiate Receptors

Receptor Class	Function
Kappa	Spinal analgesia
	Miosis
	Sedation
Mu	Respiratory depression
	Euphoria
	Physical dependence
Sigma	Hallucinations
	Dysphoria
Delta	Unknown
Epsilon	Unknown

TABLE 8–2. Disadvantages of Intramuscular Narcotic Administration

1. Painful injection
2. Variation in plasma level depending on site of injection.
3. Delayed onset of action (10–30 minutes)
4. Difficult to titrate

ceptors. These drugs offer some significant advantages over the traditional pure agonist class, including less respiratory depression and abuse potential. While great advances have already been made in delineating the pathophysiology of pain, it is hoped that within the next decade advances will be made in new therapies such as analgesics that selectively bind to certain classes of opiate receptors.

Principles of Analgesia

Narcotic analgesics are often improperly administered. Common mistakes clinicians make include prescribing an inadequate dose, using the wrong route of administration, prescribing improper frequency of dosing and choosing the wrong analgesic for a particular clinical situation.

Dosage

The most important factor in achieving adequate analgesia with narcotics is the proper dose. There is wide intersubject variability in effective analgesic serum concentrations. Dahlstrom found that effective serum concentrations of meperidine in postoperative patients varied from 94 μg/ml to 754 μg/ml, and effective concentrations of morphine ranged from 6 μg/ml to 33 μg/ml. The best method to achieve proper dosage is careful intravenous titration. Some patients may require more than 200 mg of intravenous meperidine or 25 mg of morphine whereas others may need only one-fourth of these doses. There is little correlation of dose with weight or sex; there is, however, a trend for lower dose requirements in the elderly.

Route of Administration

Although the intramuscular route is popular for administration of narcotic analgesics in the emergency setting, this route has many disadvantages (Table 8–2). The major disadvantage is that it is not possible to easily and reliably titrate the chosen analgesic to maximal patient comfort. Once the drug is administered intramuscularly, the physician and patient must wait 20 to 30 minutes to determine if effective analgesia has been achieved. If the dose was inadequate, the patient must undergo another painful injection. Studies have also shown that serum levels obtained with a given intramuscular dose vary with the time of day, site of injection, and disease process. Considering these disadvantages, intramuscular narcotic administration should not be used when rapid and reliable analgesia is desired. Intravenous injection is clearly the superior route of administration. It provides rapid onset of action, reliable serum drug levels, ease of titration, and a less painful injection for the patient.

Frequency of Administration

A prolonged dosing interval is a common cause of inadequate analgesia. Meperidine, one of the most popular analgesics, has a relatively short half-life and requires repeated dosing every 2 to 3 hours. The individual dosing interval should be based on the subjective comfort of the patient. It is important to remember that it takes less analgesia to prevent pain than to treat well-established pain.

CONDITIONS

Analgesia for Short Procedures

When selecting the appropriate analgesic(s) for short procedures, the clinician must take several factors into consideration. Most short procedures are performed in an outpatient setting. For most short procedures such as joint relocation or incision and drainage of abscesses, severe pain occurs during the procedure and is significantly alleviated after its completion. In such cases, a short-acting agent that offers a rapid onset of action is preferable to longer-acting narcotics that prolong the patient observation period. (See Figure 8–1.) If significant sedation remains after completion of the procedure, a small dose of naloxone may be indicated. Longer-acting narcotics are indicated for procedures that will produce pain for a significant period after their completion. For example, insertion of a thoracostomy tube requires long-term analgesia, and since most patients will be admitted for further management, use of a longer-acting narcotic analgesic makes sense. All patients receiving parenteral titration of narcotic agents should be closely monitored, and airway equipment must be near the bedside. The clinician should also consider using nitrous oxide or benzodiazepines as adjuncts to narcotic analgesia for short procedures. Nitrous oxide is available in a 50% nitrous oxide, 50% oxygen mixture that is self-administered by the patient. This agent can potentiate opiate analgesia and is a valuable anxiolytic. Relative contraindications include impaired mental status, pneumothorax, severe lung disease, or abdominal pain with suspected obstruction (see Chapter 26). Benzodiazepines offer relief from some of the anxiety that accompanies pain. There may be an increased risk of respiratory depression when an opiate is combined with a benzodiazepine. Midazolam (Versed) has become a popular adjunct to narcotic analgesia because of its potent amnestic properties (see Chapter 9).

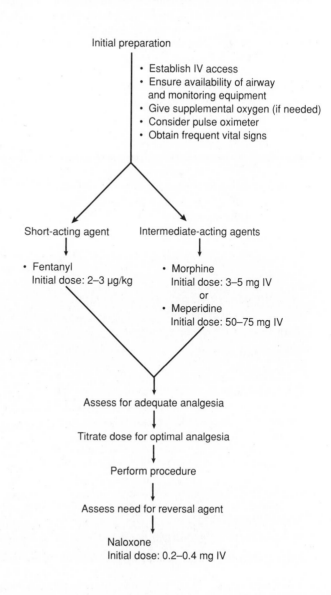

FIGURE 8–1. Treatment algorithm: analgesia for short procedures.

Diagnosis and Indications for Treatment

See box, Drug Treatment: Analgesia for Short Procedures.

Joint Relocation

Joint relocation is a relatively painful procedure, with minimal residual pain following successful relocation. Intravenous titration with a short-acting agent such as fentanyl or its derivatives is ideal for this situation. Morphine and meperidine are good alternatives.

Fracture Reduction

Fracture reduction is usually an outpatient procedure, with moderate residual pain after reduction. Intravenous titration with morphine or meperidine offers slightly more prolonged analgesia than fentanyl in this setting. Local anesthesia including hematoma blocks and intravenous regional anesthesia (Bier block) are other useful methods of pain control in this situation.

Incision and Drainage of Abscesses

Local anesthesia is frequently inadequate for this procedure, making intravenous titration with a short-acting agent such as fentanyl or its derivatives a valuable adjunct.

Suturing

Although local anesthesia is often adequate for suturing, if the laceration is quite extensive or complex and requires prolonged cleansing and suturing, intravenous administration of a short-acting narcotic may be useful. Fentanyl has become increasingly popular in the pediatric population when suturing of a facial laceration requires short-acting sedation and analgesia.

Thoracostomy Tube Insertion

Local anesthesia is often not adequate for this exquisitely painful procedure. A longer-acting narcotic is advisable because of the significant residual pain. Intravenous meperidine, morphine, hydromorphone (Dilaudid), nalbuphine, or butorphanol are all viable analgesics.

Dressing Changes/Repacking Abscesses

For outpatient dressing and packing changes, intravenous narcotics are rarely

---

DRUG TREATMENT: ANALGESIA FOR SHORT PROCEDURES

Short-Acting Agent

Fentanyl

Initial Dose	2–3 μg/kg IV
Repeat Dose	1 μg/kg IV every 5 minutes
End-Point	Patient sedated but arousable to painful stimuli

Intermediate-Acting Agents

Morphine Sulfate

Initial Dose	3–5 mg IV
Repeat Dose	3–5 mg IV every 10 minutes
End-Points	Patient should be sedated but arousable to painful stimuli. Dose may be limited by respiratory depression or hypotension.

OR

Meperidine

Initial Dose	50–70 mg IV
Repeat Dose	25–50 mg IV every 15 minutes
End-Points	Patient should be sedated but arousable to painful stimuli. Dose may be limited by respiratory depression or hypotension.

needed. Having the patient take an oral narcotic such as oxycodone approximately 1 hour prior to the procedure is frequently helpful. For dressing changes of extensive burns, intravenous titration with fentanyl, morphine, or meperidine is necessary.

Discussion

Desired duration of pain relief should be the determining factor in choosing a first-line narcotic analgesic. For short, painful procedures after which the patient is relatively pain free (e.g., joint relocation, incision and drainage, pediatric suturing), fentanyl should be the first-line agent considered. For procedures that may be accompanied by significant pain of longer duration (e.g., fracture reduction, chest tube insertion), morphine is a good first-line agent. Meperidine is an alternative agent when intermediate duration of analgesia is required.

In addition to narcotic agents, nitrous oxide and/or sedative hypnotic agents can be used for painful procedures. Sedative hypnotic agents can be useful in procedures where muscle relaxation or amnesia is desired. (See Chapters 9 and 26.)

Analgesia for Severe Pain of Longer Duration

Analgesia for the patient in severe pain poses a challenge to the physician. Proper selection of a narcotic with an intermediate to long half-life coupled with careful intravenous titration should result in optimal pain relief. Frequently, specific actions of these drugs on the cardiovascular and other organ systems can be used to the patient's advantage in a particular situation (e.g., morphine reducing preload in an acute myocardial infarction). The clinician should be familiar with the actions and potential side effects of any drug that is chosen.

Analgesia for patients experiencing severe pain is often delayed while the physician completes the evaluation and formulates a diagnosis. A common worry, particularly in the setting of abdominal pain in which surgery is contemplated, is that the accuracy of physical examination will be clouded if narcotic analgesia is administered. Careful titration of analgesia to achieve patient comfort has not been shown to alter the findings of guarding or rebound or to delay the diagnosis of a surgical abdomen. Once the initial evaluation of the patient has been rapidly completed, there is no excuse for prolonging this painful state by withholding analgesia.

Analgesia in Acute Myocardial Infarction

Diagnosis and Indications for Treatment

The mechanism of pain production from myocardial ischemia remains unclear. One theory suggests that a chemical mediator is released by ischemic myocardium and subsequently stimulates nerve endings. Another theory postulates that the pain is a result of abnormal stretch of ischemic muscle. Regardless of the etiology of the pain, myocar-

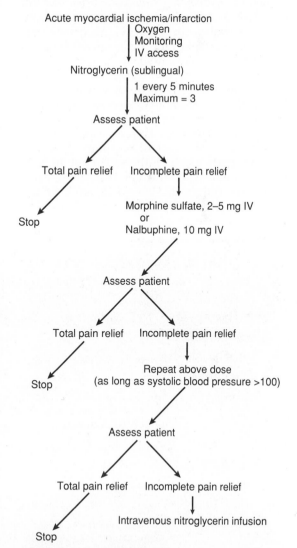

FIGURE 8–2. Treatment algorithm: management of pain from acute myocardial ischemia.

dial ischemia reflects an imbalance of oxygen supply and demand to the heart muscle.

In treating the severe pain of myocardial ischemia, the clinician must address not only the pain itself, but also the accompanying anxiety, which results in catecholamine release, increased systemic vascular resistance, and possibly further myocardial damage. The standard initial therapy consists of oxygen and sublingual nitroglycerin. If 2 to 3 nitroglycerin tablets are unsuccessful in alleviating the pain, narcotic analgesia provides a valuable adjunct (Fig. 8–2; see also box, Drug Treatment: Narcotic Analgesia for Pain from Acute Myocardial Ischemia.)

Discussion

Narcotic analgesia is indicated for the pain of acute myocardial infarction that has not resolved after institution of oxygen or sublingual nitroglycerin therapy. Morphine has long been the narcotic analgesic of choice in the setting of acute myocardial infarction. It offers the potential advantage of a decrease in systemic vascular resistance, thereby decreasing myocardial oxygen consumption. In addition, its sedative effects make it an ideal agent in this setting. Hypotension can be a significant side effect of morphine administration, particularly in the setting of an inferior wall infarction in which high filling pressures are required. Careful titration of the intravenous morphine dose will limit the incidence of hypotension. However, if the blood pressure falls, it should respond rapidly to fluids and placing the patient in the Trendelenburg position.

Nalbuphine, a narcotic agonist/antagonist, is a potentially valuable alternative to morphine in the setting of acute myocardial infarction. It is an effective analgesic that offers the advantage of less hypotension than morphine and a "plateau effect" of respiratory depression.

Abdominal Pain

Diagnosis and Indications for Treatment

Analgesia for the patient with abdominal pain and a possible surgical problem has always been controversial. As discussed previously, the clinician would like to maintain patient comfort without losing the reliability of the physical examination. This can be achieved with careful intravenous titration of a chosen agent. Once a diagnosis has been established and a decision to proceed with surgical intervention has been made, the reliability of the physical examination becomes much less important. Analgesia in doses sufficient to relieve the patient's pain should be administered in an expeditious manner.

DRUG TREATMENT: NARCOTIC ANALGESIA FOR PAIN FROM ACUTE MYOCARDIAL ISCHEMIA

First-Line Agent

Morphine Sulfate

Initial Dose	3–5 mg IV
Repeat Dose	3–5 mg IV every 10 minutes
End-Point	Complete pain relief. If after 2 to 3 doses of morphine sulfate the patient has obtained little pain relief, a continuous intravenous infusion of nitroglycerin should be considered.

OR

Nalbuphine

Initial Dose	10 mg IV
Repeat Dose	10 mg IV in 30 minutes if no pain relief has been obtained
End-Point	Complete pain relief. If pain relief is minimal after 2 doses of nalbuphine, a continuous intravenous infusion of nitroglycerin should be considered.

The characteristics of the pain may influence the choice of drug therapy. Pancreatitis and biliary tract disease are frequently accompanied by colicky pain, which can be exacerbated by an agent that has spasmogenic effects. (See box, Drug Treatment: Abdominal Pain.)

Discussion

Meperidine and morphine have traditionally been the narcotic analgesics of choice for abdominal pain. Although effective, they both have the potential disadvantage of increased intrabiliary pressure secondary to spasmogenic effects. In biliary colic and pancreatitis, this increased biliary pressure can actually worsen the pain. The newer agonist/antagonist analgesics (butorphanol, nalbuphine) do not produce the same rise in biliary pressure and may be more desirable analgesics for acute abdominal pain. These agents also offer the advantage of less respiratory depression and less abuse potential for the patient with recurrent pain (e.g., chronic pancreatitis). The end-point for narcotic analgesia administration when the diagnosis remains in doubt is not complete pain relief. Rather, patient comfort should be maintained while allowing continued assessment.

Migraine Headache

Diagnosis and Indications for Treatment

Migraine headache is a common painful condition seen by physicians. Some estimates report that as many as 29% of all women and 19% of men are affected by migraines. Controversy still exists as to the pathophysiology of the pain during these headaches. It is now believed that in the initial phase serotonin released from platelets enters the brain, resulting in increased vascular permeability and a lower pain threshold. A variety of neurotransmitters have been implicated in the painful phase of the migraine.

Classic migraine headaches are characterized by visual changes (blind spots or scintillating scotomas) or neurologic symptoms (paresthesias, speech changes, etc.) preced-

---

DRUG TREATMENT: ABDOMINAL PAIN

Colicky Pain

First-Line Agent

Butorphanol

Initial Dose	1–2 mg IV
Repeat Dose	1–2 mg IV every 30–60 minutes as needed
End-Point	Pain relief

Second-Line Agent

Nalbuphine

Initial Dose	10 mg IV
Repeat Dose	10 mg every 30–60 minutes as needed
End-Point	Pain relief

Noncolicky Pain

Meperidine

Initial Dose	50–100 mg IV
Repeat Dose	50–75 mg every 60 minutes as needed
End-Point	Pain relief

ing the onset of a severe, throbbing, unilateral headache. Common migraines frequently do not have these heralding symptoms. Both types are often accompanied by nausea, vomiting, and photophobia. The presence of a severe unilateral headache should suggest the diagnosis of migraine. Other conditions with similar presentations (i.e., acute sinusitis, acute glaucoma, temporal arteritis, ear or jaw pathology) should be ruled out. Since migraine headaches are recurrent, many patients can reliably characterize their symptoms as similar to previous attacks. Special care should be taken to rule out other conditions when a patient presents with these symptoms for the first time or when a patient reports that the symptoms are "different" from his or her typical migraine.

Treatment is indicated for migraine headaches when the symptoms have failed to respond to conservative measures. These headaches often resolve with rest in a quiet, dark environment, with or without acetaminophen or aspirin. By the time most patients seek medical care, they have usually attempted these measures without obtaining relief. (See box, Drug Treatment: Analgesia for Migraine Headaches.)

DRUG TREATMENT: ANALGESIA FOR MIGRAINE HEADACHES

First-Line Agents

Butorphanol

Initial Dose	1–2 mg IV
Repeat Dose	1–2 mg IV after 60 minutes
End-Point	Headache relief

OR

Nalbuphine

Initial Dose	10 mg IV
Repeat Dose	10 mg IV after 60 minutes
End-Point	Headache relief

OR

Prochlorperazine

Initial Dose	10 mg IV over 2–3 minutes
Repeat Dose	5 mg IV in 30 minutes if no relief
End-Points	Pain relief *or* total dose 15 mg

OR

Dihydroergotamine

Initial Dose	1 mg IM or IV
Repeat Dose	1 mg after 60 minutes
End-Point	Relief of headache *or* total dose of 2 mg

Second-Line Agent

Meperidine

Initial Dose	50–75 mg IV
Repeat Dose	50 mg IV after 60 minutes
End-Point	Headache relief

Discussion

Parenteral pure narcotic agonists are effective in the treatment of pain associated with migraine headaches, but they should not be considered first-line therapy. For those patients experiencing frequent headaches, dependence on narcotic analgesia becomes a concern. The agonist/antagonist narcotics (butorphanol, nalbuphine), with their lower abuse potential, are valuable first-line agents in this situation. For patients with nausea and vomiting as prominent symptoms, an antiemetic/phenothiazine may be an appropriate first-line agent. Ergotamines have long been recognized as effective abortive drugs if given early in the course of the headache. Dihydroergotamine, a parenteral ergotamine with strong vasoconstrictive properties, has shown promise in aborting well-established headaches. Dihydroergotamine is contraindicated in the presence of significant peripheral vascular disease, coronary artery disease, hypertension, and pregnancy. Its use is usually limited to otherwise young, healthy patients with early severe migraine symptoms.

Renal Colic

Diagnosis and Indications for Treatment

The diagnosis of renal colic is frequently obvious on initial presentation. Acute onset of severe flank pain radiating to the groin and accompanied by hematuria is a hallmark of this disease. The diagnosis can be confirmed by radiographic contrast studies or ultrasonography. The severe pain associated with renal colic requires rapid and effective treatment. Analgesia can be administered while the examination and work-up are in progress and while awaiting the laboratory results and personnel, which may delay intravenous pyelography. Although narcotic analgesia frequently does not completely alleviate the pain, one dose usually makes the patient significantly more comfortable. Since these patients commonly have associated nausea and vomiting, the addition of an antiemetic is often necessary. (See box, Drug Treatment: Renal Colic.)

Discussion

An antiemetic should be administered in addition to the narcotic whenever nausea or vomiting is present (see Chapter 14). Recent studies using nonsteroidal anti-inflammatory drugs such as indomethacin in the treatment of acute renal colic are promising. The mechanism of action is thought to be secondary to prostaglandin inhibition, which results in relaxation of the ureteral spasm. The initial Scandinavian studies using intravenous indomethacin reported complete relief of symptoms in 76% of patients within 20 minutes of the first dose. Although indomethacin is not approved by the Food and Drug Administration for intravenous use in renal colic, some studies have shown that indomethacin rectal suppositories may provide

---

DRUG TREATMENT: RENAL COLIC

First-Line Agents

Meperidine

Initial Dose	50–100 mg IV
Repeat Dose	25–50 mg IV every 15 minutes
End-Point	Patient should have pain relief but remain arousable to verbal stimuli. Dose is limited by hypotension or respiratory depression.

OR

Morphine Sulfate

Initial Dose	3–5 mg IV
Repeat Dose	3–5 mg IV every 10 minutes
End-Point	As for meperidine, above

an effective alternative. Future studies are needed to delineate the value of this therapy.

Vaso-occlusive Crisis of Sickle Cell Anemia

Diagnosis

Vaso-occlusive crisis is a diagnosis of exclusion. Other manifestations of sickle cell disease, including anemic crisis, pulmonary events, septicemia, splenic infarction, and cholecystitis, can present with acute pain and may be confused with vaso-occlusive crisis. Vaso-occlusion is caused by plugs of sickled erythrocytes in the distal capillary beds. Episodes of vaso-occlusion may be precipitated by hypoxia, cold, infections, or altitude exposure. The musculoskeletal system is the most common site involved. Pain is usually constant and may last hours to weeks.

The first step in evaluating a patient with acute pain and sickle cell anemia is to eliminate causes other than vaso-occlusive crisis. The patient will often recognize the pain as characteristic of previous crises. A temperature greater than 102°F suggests an infectious etiology rather than vaso-occlusion. The presence of abdominal or chest pain as the predominant symptom should prompt a search for a pulmonary event or cholecystitis. No single laboratory test can confirm the diagnosis of vaso-occlusive crisis. Once other possibilities have been excluded, a sickle cell patient with a history of musculoskeletal pain typical of previous crises should receive appropriate therapy.

Indications for Treatment

In most cases, the patient will already have taken oral narcotics prior to seeking care. Appropriate therapy for sickle cell crisis includes analgesia, hydration, and oxygenation. Most patients tolerate oral fluids well and do not require intravenous hydration. Patients with acute vaso-occlusive crisis or crisis not responsive to oral analgesia will require parenteral narcotic analgesia. Occasionally, this can become a particularly frustrating problem for the physician. As their disease progresses, these patients experience more frequent crises and often become dependent on prescribed narcotics to control their pain. This situation often culminates in the physician feeling frustrated and angry and labeling the patient a "drug seeker."

The agonist/antagonist group of narcotics may be a valuable alternative in this patient population. Initially, the patient may not be as happy with this new drug because he or she does not experience the same euphoria as with other narcotics, but adequate analgesia can be obtained with careful intravenous titration. In patients who are dependent on narcotics, the agonist/antagonist group can precipitate withdrawal. It is important in conditions associated with chronic pain, such as sickle cell disease, that the patient be followed closely by one physician and one hospital and that a unified plan for pain therapy be developed. (See box, Drug Treatment: Vaso-occlusive Crisis of Sickle Cell Anemia.)

Discussion

The agonist/antagonist narcotics are first-line drugs that may precipitate withdrawal symptoms in patients who are dependent on narcotics. A second-line drug (pure narcotic agonist) should be used in narcotic-addicted patients. Patients who receive parenteral morphine may also be treated with simultaneous administration of oral sustained-release morphine (MS-Contin or Roxanol) to maintain stable blood levels for a prolonged period. Oxygenation and hydration should be initiated in addition to the administration of analgesics. Most patients with vaso-occlusive crisis can be adequately rehydrated by oral intake of fluids. Vaso-occlusion does not resolve in a matter of hours. For this reason, the end-point of therapy is not complete pain relief. Rather, the goal is to maintain patient comfort at a level where outpatient therapy is possible. Continued severe pain in spite of parenteral analgesia may require longer in-hospital therapy.

Reversal of Narcotics

Diagnosis

Narcotic analgesics can produce life-threatening respiratory depression and profound sedation when used therapeutically or illicitly. The syndrome is usually easy to recognize because other signs of opiate use are present, including miosis. In patients presenting with decreased level of consciousness of unknown etiology, intentional or accidental intoxication with opiates should be suspected even in the absence of other physical signs of opiate ingestion.

DRUG TREATMENT: VASO-OCCLUSIVE CRISIS OF SICKLE CELL ANEMIA

First-Line Drugs

Butorphanol

Initial Dose	1–2 mg IV
Repeat Dose	1–2 mg IV 60 minutes after initial dose
End-Point	Substantial pain reduction

OR

Nalbuphine

Initial Dose	10 mg IV
Repeat Dose	10 mg IV after 60 minutes
End-Point	Substantial pain reduction

Second-Line Drug

Morphine Sulfate

Initial Dose	3–5 mg IV or 10–15 mg IM
Repeat Dose	3–5 mg IV (after 15 minutes)
	10 mg IM (after 1–2 hours)
End-Point	Substantial pain reduction

Indications for Treatment

In a patient presenting with a decreased level of consciousness of unknown etiology, administration of naloxone is indicated as a diagnostic and therapeutic agent to detect the presence of narcotics and their contribution to the altered level of consciousness. Although naloxone is a specific antagonist for opiate receptors, it has been reported anecdotally to reverse sedation from ethanol, benzodiazepines, and other sedating drugs. Because opiates and naloxone have varying affinities for different opiate receptors, the dose of naloxone required to reverse sedation and respiratory depression may vary depending on the specific opiate ingested.

If significant respiratory depression results from therapeutically administered opiates, or if sedation is profound, naloxone may be administered. The dose should be smaller than that used for ingestions of unknown substances. (See boxes, Drug Treatment: Depressed Level of Consciousness from Suspected Opiate Ingestion and Drug Treatment: Reversal of Therapeutically Administered Opiates.)

Discussion

If the drug ingested is unknown, the ABCs (airway, breathing, circulation) of emergency care should always be the first priority. After the initial evaluation and stabilization, naloxone administration should proceed. When intravenous access is difficult, naloxone may be given in the same dosage by the intramuscular, sublingual, or endotracheal route. If methadone, methadone derivatives, or propoxyphene has been ingested, the naloxone dose required for reversal may approach 10 mg, and frequent repeated doses or intravenous infusion may be necessary to maintain reversal. If 10 mg of naloxone is given with no effect on sedation or respiratory depression, narcotic overdosage can be excluded as a cause for coma. The actions of naloxone may last only 20 to 40 minutes, and vigilance is necessary to prevent recurrent respiratory depression and

---

DRUG TREATMENT: DEPRESSED LEVEL OF CONSCIOUSNESS FROM SUSPECTED OPIATE INGESTION

First-Line Drug

Naloxone

Initial Dose	2 mg IV
Repeat Dose	2 mg every 2 minutes
End-Points	Reversal of sedation or 10 mg total dose given without effect
	Intravenous infusion of 0.4–4 mg/hour may be given to maintain reversal.

DRUG TREATMENT: REVERSAL OF THERAPEUTICALLY ADMINISTERED OPIATES

First-Line Drug

Naloxone

Initial Dose	0.1 mg IV
Repeat Dose	0.1–0.2 mg every 2 minutes
End-Point	Desired reversal of sedation

---

coma. Patients should not be discharged until they have been observed for at least 90 minutes after naloxone administration with no recurrence of respiratory depression. Naloxone will produce a withdrawal state in patients addicted to opiates.

When using naloxone for the reversal of therapeutically administered opiates, small doses should be used and titrated to the desired effect. Rapid reversal of opiate analgesia after surgery has been documented to produce hypertension, cardiac arrhythmias, and even death in rare cases.

SPECIFIC AGENTS

Alfentanil (Alfenta)

Pharmacology

Distribution

Alfentanil is similar to fentanyl in that it is highly lipophilic, but it offers the advantages of a more rapid onset and shorter duration. It is also metabolized in the liver. Serum half-life is approximately 30 minutes.

Excretion

Alfentanil is excreted by the kidney.

Actions

RESPIRATORY. Unlike morphine and many other narcotics, alfentanil does not stimulate histamine release, which makes it a more attractive analgesic for patients with a history of chronic obstructive pulmonary disease or asthma. Respiratory depression can occur but is easily reversed with naloxone.

CARDIOVASCULAR. Alfentanil produces less hypotension than morphine and no myocardial depression (even in high doses), which is probably related to the lack of histamine release. It is a popular analgesic in cardiac surgery for this reason. There is actually a slight increase in the cardiac index with alfentanil.

Indications

Short procedures—alfentanil is an ideal drug for short, painful procedures. It has been used frequently for joint relocation, orthopedic reductions, and extensive lacerations requiring prolonged suturing.

Cautions

Hepatic failure—alfentanil should be administered with caution to patients with a history of cirrhosis or hepatic dysfunction. A reduced dose should be given initially.

Renal failure—since alfentanil is excreted primarily renally, both a reduced dose and an increase in dosing interval may be necessary in patients with renal dysfunction.

Use in pregnancy—Category C. Alfentanil has been shown to impair fertility and to have embryocidal effects in rats. No controlled human studies have been performed. It should only be used in pregnancy when its potential benefit outweighs the risk to the fetus.

Use in children—not recommended. Experience is limited.

Onset and Duration of Action

Dosage

Initial dose: 10 to 15 μg/kg IV over 3 to 5 minutes

Repeat dosing: every 30 minutes as needed

Toxicity

Nitrous oxide can produce cardiovascular depression when used in combination with higher doses of alfentanil.

Some patients may exhibit respiratory depression at therapeutic doses of alfentanil. When alfentanil is being administered, the patient should be monitored closely. Respiratory depression responds rapidly to naloxone.

Higher doses of alfentanil can produce muscle rigidity, which may become so severe that ventilation is difficult. This muscle rigidity can be treated with naloxone and muscle relaxants.

Buprenorphine (Buprenex)

Pharmacology

Distribution

Buprenorphine is well absorbed by the oral, sublingual, intramuscular, and intravenous routes. Kinetics following oral administration are not currently known, but there does seem to be a significant first-pass effect in the liver. This is a highly lipid-soluble, protein-bound compound that undergoes significant enterohepatic circulation.

Elimination

Buprenorphine is metabolized in the liver via dealkylation. The metabolites are excreted primarily by the kidney.

Actions

CNS—buprenorphine causes sedation in up to 45% of patients.

Respiratory—peak respiratory depression may be delayed for as long as 3 hours after intramuscular administration. It is not clear whether buprenorphine exhibits the same "plateau" effect on respiratory depression as do the other agonist/antagonist analgesics.

Cardiovascular—buprenorphine has similar hemodynamic effects to morphine with a decrease in heart rate and blood pressure.

Indications

Moderate to severe pain in which a long-acting agent is required—buprenorphine is 25 to 30 times more potent than morphine on a weight basis.

Biliary colic—one study has shown buprenorphine to be significantly less spasmogenic than morphine and pentazocine in the treatment of biliary colic.

Cautions

Renal or hepatic insufficiency—use is not recommended as there is currently limited information on the pharmacokinetics of buprenorphine.

Use in pregnancy—Category C. No information is available on the safety of buprenorphine during pregnancy, and its use if not recommended at this time.

Use in children—not recommended. Experience is limited.

Onset and Duration of Action

Dosage

Intravenous/intramuscular: 0.3 to 0.6 mg

Repeat Dosing

Although the serum half-life of buprenorphine is 2 to 3 hours, the analgesic effects last 6 to 8 hours secondary to the drug binding tightly to the mu opiate receptor.

Toxicity

Respiratory depression—reversal of respiratory depression may require large doses of naloxone (10 to 15 mg).
Sedation—occurs in 45% of patients
Nausea/vomiting—occurs in 10 to 15% of patients
Narcotic withdrawal symptoms—the narcotic antagonist properties of buprenorphine can precipitate withdrawal symptoms in patients who have chronically received narcotic agonists.

Butorphanol (Stadol)

Pharmacology

Distribution

Butorphanol is well absorbed when given orally. However, 80% of the drug undergoes a first-pass metabolism in the liver.

Elimination

Butorphanol is metabolized in the liver via hydroxylation, dealkylation, and conjugation. The metabolites are excreted primarily by the kidney, but some biliary excretion does occur.

Actions

Cardiovascular—the hemodynamic effects of butorphanol are similar to those of pentazocine in that it increases blood pressure, resulting in an increased cardiac workload.

Indications

Butorphanol is 3 to 7 times as potent as morphine on a weight basis. It is used for alleviation of moderate to severe pain. As with nalbuphine, it may offer advantages in the treatment of biliary colic and vascular headaches. It increases myocardial workload and thus is not recommended for angina or myocardial infarction.

Cautions

Hepatic or renal insufficiency—butorphanol should be administered with caution. Although clinical studies have not been performed, laboratory studies indicate that decreased doses may be necessary in both conditions.
Use in pregnancy—Category C. The safety of butorphanol during pregnancy has not been established.

Use in children—experience is limited. Use is not recommended.

Onset and Duration of Action

Dosage

Intravenous: 0.5 to 4.0 mg
Oral: 4 to 16 mg

Repeat Dosing

Every 3 to 4 hours

Toxicity

Acetaminophen has been found to enhance the analgesic activity of butorphanol.

Sedation—occurs in 35% of patients
Dizziness/vertigo—occurs in 5% of patients
Nausea/vomiting—occurs in 6% of patients
Dysphoric reaction—dysphoric reactions have been reported with butorphanol, but are rare. They can be treated with large doses of naloxone (10 to 15 mg).
Narcotic withdrawal—in patients who have had a prolonged course of narcotic agonists for chronic pain, butorphanol can precipitate withdrawal symptoms
Hypersensitivity—butorphanol contains sodium metabisulfite (a common preservative in many drugs), which can cause an allergic reaction in sensitive individuals. There is an increased incidence of allergic reactions in patients with a history of asthma.

Fentanyl (Sublimaze)

Pharmacology

Distribution

Fentanyl is rapidly absorbed and highly lipid soluble, allowing it to pass the blood–brain barrier. It undergoes extensive first-pass metabolism in the liver. Fentanyl is metabolized in the liver to a polar metabolite. Serum half-life is 90 minutes.

Elimination

Fentanyl is excreted by the kidneys.

Actions
RESPIRATORY. Unlike morphine and many other narcotics, fentanyl does not stimulate histamine release, which makes it a more attractive analgesic for patients with a history

of chronic obstructive pulmonary disease or asthma. Respiratory depression can occur but is easily reversed with naloxone.

CARDIOVASCULAR. Fentanyl produces less hypotension than morphine and no myocardial depression (even in high doses), which is probably related to the lack of histamine release. It is a popular analgesic in cardiac surgery for this reason. There is actually a slight increase in the cardiac index with fentanyl.

Indications

Short procedures—fentanyl is an ideal drug for short, painful procedures. It has been used frequently for joint relocation, orthopedic reductions, and extensive lacerations requiring prolonged suturing.

Pediatric procedures—fentanyl is gaining popularity over the traditional "cocktails" frequently used for analgesia in pediatric short procedures. It offers the advantages of rapid onset and short duration.

Cautions

Hepatic failure—fentanyl should be administered with caution to patients with a history of cirrhosis or hepatic dysfunction. A reduced dose should be given initially.

Renal failure—since fentanyl is excreted primarily renally, both a reduced dose and an increase in dosing interval may be necessary in patients with renal dysfunction.

Use in pregnancy—Category C. Fentanyl has been shown to impair fertility and to have embryocidal effects in rats. No controlled human studies have been performed. It should only be used in pregnancy when its potential benefit outweighs the risk to the fetus.

Use in children—may be used

Onset and Duration of Action

Dosage

Fentanyl is 75 to 200 times more potent than morphine due to its lipid solubility.

Initial dose: 2 to 3 μg/kg over 3 to 5 minutes IV

Repeat dosing: the dosing interval for fentanyl is 1 to 2 hours, but a repeat dose should rarely be necessary since it is primarily used for short procedures.

Toxicity

Nitrous oxide can produce cardiovascular depression when used in combination with higher doses of fentanyl.

Some patients may exhibit respiratory depression at therapeutic doses of fentanyl. When fentanyl is being administered, the patient should be monitored closely. Respiratory depression responds rapidly to naloxone.

Higher doses of fentanyl can produce muscle rigidity, which may become so severe that ventilation is difficult. This muscle rigidity can be treated with naloxone and muscle relaxants.

Hydromorphone (Dilaudid)

Pharmacology

Distribution

Hydromorphone is highly soluble and well absorbed following oral, subcutaneous, intravenous, intramuscular, and rectal suppository administration. The onset of action occurs within 15 minutes of parenteral administration and 30 minutes following oral dosing. The half-life is approximately 2.5 hours. Hydromorphone is metabolized in the liver in a fashion similar to morphine.

Elimination

Hydromorphone is excreted via the kidney.

Actions

Hydromorphone has actions very similar to those of morphine. It has the advantage of oral administration.

Indications

Hydromorphone is used in the treatment of moderate to severe pain. It has become a popular analgesic in chronic pain associated with cancer.

Cautions

Renal failure—dosage adjustment will be necessary in patients with renal failure due to the primary renal excretion of hydromorphone.

Hepatic failure—adjustment of both dose and dosing interval may be necessary in patients with hepatic failure.

Use in pregnancy—Category C. No human studies are available to support the safety of the use of hydromorphone during pregnancy. It should only be used in pregnancy when the potential benefit to the patient outweighs the risk to the fetus.

Use in children—experience is limited. Use is not recommended.

Onset and Duration of Action

Dosage

Oral: 1 to 5 mg every 1 to 2 hours
Subcutaneous, intramuscular, intravenous: 1 to 5 mg every 1 to 2 hours

Repeat Dosing

Hydromorphone has a half-life of 2.5 hours. Dosage is usually repeated every 2 hours.

Toxicity

Gastrointestinal—hydromorphone can produce nausea and vomiting, which is readily treated with phenothiazines.
Respiratory—hydromorphone will produce a dose-related respiratory depression, which can be reversed by naloxone.
Cardiovascular—orthostatic hypotension can occur after intravenous administration of hydromorphone.

Meperidine (Demerol)

Pharmacology

Metabolism

Meperidine is metabolized in the liver via demethylation. The only active metabolite is normeperidine. Meperidine's plasma half-life is 2.5 hours.

Elimination

Meperidine is renally excreted.

Actions

Many of the actions of meperidine are similar to those of morphine (see Morphine, later in this chapter, for details). Only those actions that differ from morphine are discussed below.

CARDIOVASCULAR. There are significant differences between meperidine and morphine with respect to their effects on the cardiovascular system. While morphine has no effect or may decrease heart rate due to its vagotonic actions, meperidine may increase heart rate due to its atropine-like effects. Meperidine may also decrease cardiac contractility to a small degree.

GASTROINTESTINAL. Meperidine and morphine increase biliary pressure to a similar degree. Meperidine is less constipating than morphine, but still slows gastrointestinal motility.

URINARY TRACT. Some authors believe that there is a lower incidence of urinary retention with meperidine and that it may offer an advantage over morphine in the patient with prostatic hypertrophy.

Indications

Meperidine is the most widely used narcotic analgesic in the United States. Some of the more common uses include the following:

Abdominal pain: intestinal obstruction, appendicitis, pancreatitis, sickle cell crisis, ischemic bowel (Note: If biliary colic is suspected, one of the agonist/antagonist group of analgesics, which are less spasmogenic, may be preferable.)
Short procedures with moderate to severe pain, e.g., incision and drainage, orthopedic relocations, chest tube placement, debridement
Renal colic
Vascular headaches

Cautions

Renal failure—elevated serum levels of the active metabolite normeperidine occur under conditions of renal failure and can lead to an increased incidence of CNS toxicity (i.e., seizures).
Hepatic failure—the half-life of meperidine can be significantly prolonged in the patient with hepatic failure. Morphine is a preferred analgesic under these conditions.
Use in pregnancy—meperidine has no known teratogenic effects. The major concern with its use during pregnancy is the possibility of fetal respiratory depression. The half-life of meperidine in the fetus may be as long as 18 hours due to underdeveloped metabolic pathways.
Use in Children—may be used. Dosage is 1 mg/kg.

Dosage

The *intravenous* route is preferred because it gives reliable blood levels, and accurate titration of analgesia is more easily accomplished.

Initial dose: 25 to 50 mg IV. The dose for children is 1 mg/kg.
Repeat dose: 2 to 3 hours

The *intramuscular* route is popular for administration of meperidine. This route, however, results in unpredictable blood levels.

Initial dose: 50 to 200 mg IM
Repeat dose: 2 to 3 hours

Toxicity

Monoamine oxidase (MAO) inhibitors interfere with the metabolism of meperidine and thus increase the chance of toxicity. In addition, the combination of meperidine and an MAO inhibitor can result in MAO inhibitor crisis.

CNS toxicity, including nervousness, tremors, disorientation, hallucinations, psychosis, and seizures, can occur and is thought to be due to accumulation of normeperidine. Treatment is supportive.

In case of respiratory depression, the treatment is naloxone.

For nausea and vomiting, the treatment is phenothiazines.

Morphine

Pharmacology

Distribution

Morphine, a basic amine, is approximately 35% protein bound in plasma and is rapidly absorbed into body tissues. It has a large volume of distribution of 3 to 4 times body weight. The distribution half-life when administered parenterally is 1.65 minutes.

Metabolism

The major metabolic pathway of morphine is conjugation with glucuronic acid in the liver. The glucuronide form is believed to be pharmacologically inactive. The hepatic enzyme system responsible for conjugation is not saturated by large doses of morphine.

Elimination

Eighty-five percent of morphine is excreted via glomerular filtration of the glucuronide form, and only 10 to 50% is excreted either unchanged in the urine or as the conjugated form in the feces. The elimination half-life is 2 to 3 hours in young healthy adults and 4 to 5 hours in the elderly. The terminal elimination half-life is 18 to 60 hours.

Actions

Morphine is classified as a pure agonist of opiate receptors. It is the standard to which all other narcotic analgesics are compared. Morphine has a variety of effects on many organ systems. The pathophysiology of these effects is similar for many of the narcotics discussed in this chapter.

CENTRAL NERVOUS SYSTEM. The most prominent CNS action is analgesia. At routine doses there is little impairment of intellectual function. Morphine can induce a sense of euphoria, which accounts for its abuse potential.

Respiratory effects. Morphine has a direct effect on the pontine and medullary respiratory centers, resulting in respiratory depression. It decreases the sensitivity of the brain stem chemoreceptors to carbon dioxide, resulting in a decreased respiratory rate and tidal volume. Respiratory depression is a dose-dependent phenomenon. Maximum respiratory depression occurs within minutes of intravenous administration of morphine but may be delayed for 30 minutes after intramuscular injection and as long as 90 minutes after subcutaneous injection. Respiratory depression is easily reversible with naloxone.

Pupils. Morphine causes pupillary constriction (miosis). Tolerance to pupillary constriction does not occur.

Nausea/vomiting. Morphine causes nausea by direct stimulation of the chemoreceptor trigger zone (CTZ) in the medulla.

PULMONARY. Bronchoconstriction may occur with the use of morphine as a result of histamine release.

GASTROINTESTINAL. Morphine decreases the motility of the stomach and increases antral tone, resulting in decreased gastric emptying. It can cause spasm of the sphincter of Oddi, resulting in drastic increases in biliary pressure. This increase in pressure occurs within minutes of the drug's administration but can persist for 2 hours or longer. Morphine decreases peristalsis and increases resting tone in both the large intestine and anal sphincter. This leads to significant constipation.

CARDIOVASCULAR. Morphine may cause small decreases in mean arterial pressure due to a decrease in peripheral vascular resistance. It causes venodilation by an unknown mechanism that is not blocked by narcotic antagonists. In patients with marginal left ventricular filling pressures, morphine can cause a decrease in cardiac output. In therapeutic doses morphine causes little change in heart rate, but in higher doses it can decrease the heart rate.

URINARY TRACT. Morphine has been found to cause urinary urgency and retention due to an increase in smooth muscle tone in the ureters, bladder, and vesical sphincter.

Indications

Morphine is an ideal analgesic for treatment of moderate to severe pain. It is frequently used for short procedures, including joint reductions, incision and drainage, and so forth. Other specific indications include (1) acute myocardial infarction, (2) pulmonary edema, and (3) abdominal pain.

Cautions

Renal failure—morphine is primarily metabolized by the liver to inactive metabolites that are excreted by the kidney. With renal failure, significant accumulation of the active form of the drug is unlikely. In repetitive dosing, however, the physician must be aware that smaller doses at less frequent intervals may be necessary.

Hepatic failure—in the past morphine was reported to precipitate hepatic encephalopathy in patients with cirrhosis. Morphine is conjugated by the liver and thus is less affected by hepatic failure than are drugs that are oxidized, such as meperidine.

Congestive heart failure—patients in congestive heart failure may require less frequent dosing of morphine.

Use in pregnancy—there are no well-controlled studies investigating the safety of morphine during pregnancy, but clinical experience has not indicated any adverse effects in short-term usage. Infants born to mothers who are chronic users of morphine may manifest withdrawal symptoms.

Use in children—may be used. Dosage is 0.1 mg/kg.

Dosage

Intravenous use of morphine initially will allow the physician to titrate analgesia to the patient's needs.

Initial dose: 3 to 5 mg. Titrate upward as necessary. Dose will be limited only by hypotension or respiratory depression, and some patients may require doses as high as 25 mg. The dose for children is 0.1 mg/kg.
Repeat dosing: every 2 to 3 hours

Intramuscular administration of morphine leads to unpredictable blood levels secondary to variable absorption.

Initial dose: 5 mg
Repeat dosing: every 2 to 3 hours

Subcutaneous administration is less painful than intramuscular administration but has the same disadvantage of variable absorption. Onset is rapid.

Initial dose: 5 to 10 mg
Repeat dose: 2 to 3 hours

Buccal tablets that dissolve over 6 hours are new on the market and give excellent plasma levels.

Oral morphine has been used in the Brompton's cocktail for chronic pain of cancer. It is an effective analgesic when given orally, but the dose must be increased secondary to the first-pass effect in the liver.

Toxicity

Respiratory depression may occur and is treated with naloxone, 0.4 to 2.0 mg IM or IV.

Nausea/vomiting can be treated with phenothiazines.

Increased intracranial pressure has been reported with morphine secondary to respiratory depression and an elevation in pCO_2. This effect combined with a possible decrease in the level of consciousness makes morphine an unattractive drug in the treatment of patients with head injuries.

Nalbuphine (Nubain)

Pharmacology

Distribution

There is extensive first-pass liver metabolism with nalbuphine, which makes oral administration one-fifth as potent as parenteral usage.

Elimination

Details of the pharmacokinetics of nalbuphine are not completely known. It is metabolized in the liver by an unknown mechanism and excreted renally. The half-life is approximately 3.5 hours.

Actions

CNS—sedation occurs in approximately 35% of patients.

Respiratory—nalbuphine and morphine have equal potential for respiratory depression. The major advantage of nalbuphine is that at therapeutic doses, there is a "plateau" effect above which an increase in dose will not increase respiratory depression.

Cardiovascular—a major advantage of nalbuphine is its lack of cardiovascular side effects.

Gastrointestinal—the effects of nalbuphine on the gastrointestinal tract have not been studied. However, it appears to cause less constipation than morphine.

Indications

Nalbuphine is indicated in the treatment of moderate to severe pain. It has approximately 80 to 90% the analgesic potency of morphine and is three times as potent as pentazocine on a weight basis.

Angina—nalbuphine, with further study, may prove to be a valuable drug in the treatment of angina. It offers the advantage of less hypotension than seen with morphine and the "plateau" effect of respiratory depression.

Biliary colic—although no study has been done specifically with nalbuphine, the narcotic agonist/antagonist group has been found to cause less of an increase in biliary pressure than the pure agonists.

Vascular headaches—nalbuphine may offer some advantages over the traditional narcotics in the therapy of vascular headaches because it produces less habituation.

Chronic pain—a study of the chronic pain of cancer patients showed nalbuphine to be effective for up to 186 days with fewer side effects and development of less tolerance to its effects than with morphine.

Cautions

The pharmacokinetics of nalbuphine are not yet well known; and thus its use should be avoided in the patient with renal or hepatic insufficiency.

Use in pregnancy—Category C. Use is not recommended.

Use in children—experience is limited. Use is not recommended.

Onset and Duration of Action

Dosage

The initial recommended dose is 10 mg. It can be administered intravenously, intramuscularly, or subcutaneously.

Repeat Dosing

Doses can be repeated every 3 to 4 hours or sooner if indicated.

Toxicity

Sedation—occurs in 35% of patients

Dizziness/vertigo—occurs in 5% of patients

Nausea/vomiting—occurs in 6% of patients

Dysphoric reaction—dysphoric reactions have been reported with nalbuphine, but are rare. They can be treated with large doses of naloxone (10 to 15 mg).

Narcotic withdrawal—in patients who have had a prolonged course of narcotic agonists for chronic pain, nalbuphine can precipitate withdrawal symptoms.

Hypersensitivity—nalbuphine contains sodium metabisulfite (a common preservative in many drugs), which can cause an allergic reaction in sensitive individuals. There is an increased incidence of allergic reactions in patients with a history of asthma.

Naloxone (Narcan)

Pharmacology

Distribution

Naloxone is widely distributed and highly lipid soluble. It enters the brain rapidly and thus has a rapid onset of action.

Elimination

Naloxone undergoes hepatic metabolism. Extensive first-pass metabolism excludes oral use. The mean half-life is 64 minutes, although clinical effects of narcotic reversal may last only 15 to 30 minutes.

Receptor Actions

Naloxone has high affinity for the mu opiate receptor and less for the kappa and sigma receptors.

Indications

Reversal of narcotic-induced sedation and respiratory depression

Cautions

Renal failure—no dosage adjustment necessary

Cardiac failure—no dosage adjustment necessary

Hepatic failure—elimination of naloxone may be prolonged. A reduction in dosage is probably not necessary although the effects may last longer.

Use in pregnancy—Category B. There is no evidence of impaired fertility or fetal harm in animal studies.

Use in children—may be used. Dosage is 0.01 mg/kg.

Onset and Duration of Action

Dosage

May be given by the intravenous, intramuscular, subcutaneous, or intrapulmonary route

0.1 to 2 mg initially by any route

Children: 0.01 mg/kg initially

Limits

If sedation or respiratory depression is not reversed with 10 mg, further naloxone is not indicated.

Repeat Dosing

The initial dose may be repeated as often as necessary to maintain narcotic reversal. An intravenous infusion can be maintained at 0.4 to 4 mg/min in reversal of long-acting narcotics.

The repeat dose in children is 0.1 mg/kg.

Toxicity

Opiate Withdrawal

Naloxone should be given with caution to patients suspected of being opiate addicted. Acute abstinence syndrome can result although the effects should dissipate within 1 hour.

Recurrent Sedation

The effects of naloxone on sedation and respiratory depression may be short-lived.

Patients should be observed for at least 90 to 120 minutes for recurrent sedation.

Postoperative Patients

Small doses should be used initially in the reversal of sedation of postoperative patients. Cases of severe hypertension, cardiac arrhythmias, and pulmonary edema have been reported after abrupt reversal with large doses.

Treatment of Toxicity

Supportive care until the effects have dissipated

Oxymorphone (Numorphan)

Pharmacology

The pharmacology of oxymorphone is similar to that of morphine. Administered parenterally, 1 mg of oxymorphone is equivalent in analgesia to 10 mg of morphine. Its onset of action occurs within 5 to 10 minutes of administration, and duration of action is approximately 3 to 6 hours. It undergoes hepatic metabolism and is excreted renally.

Indications

Oxymorphone is indicated in the setting of moderate to severe pain.

Cautions

Renal failure—oxymorphone is primarily metabolized by the liver to inactive metabolities that are excreted by the kidney. With renal failure, significant accumulation of the active form of the drug is unlikely. In repetitive dosing, however, the physician must be aware that smaller doses at less frequent intervals may be necessary.

Hepatic failure—in the past oxymorphone was reported to precipitate hepatic encephalopathy in patients with cirrhosis. Oxymorphone is conjugated by the liver and thus is less affected by hepatic failure than are drugs that are oxidized, such as meperidine.

Congestive heart failure—patients in congestive heart failure may require less frequent dosing of oxymorphone.

Use in pregnancy—there are no well-controlled studies investigating the safety of oxymorphone during pregnancy, but clinical experience has not indicated any adverse effects in short-term usage. Infants born to mothers who are chronic users of oxymorphone may manifest withdrawal symptoms.

Use in children—experience is limited. Use is not recommended.

Onset and Duration of Action

Dosage

Intravenous: 0.5 mg initially (titrate as necessary)

Intramuscular/subcutaneous: 1.0 to 1.5 mg initially

Repeat Dosing

Every 4 to 6 hours

Toxicity

As with morphine, the primary adverse side effects are respiratory depression and sedation. These effects are easily reversed with naloxone, 0.4 to 2.0 mg.

REFERENCES

Andriaensen H, Van De Walle J: Clinical use of buprenorphine in chronic administration. Acta Anaesthesiol Belg 27:187, 1976.

Barash PG, Kopriva CJ: Narcotics and the circulation. In Kitahata LM, Collins JG (eds): Narcotic Analgesics in Anaesthesiology. Baltimore, Williams & Wilkins, 1982, pp 91–132.

Barsan WG, Seger D, Danzl D, et al: Duration of antagonistic effects of nalmefene and naloxone in opiate-induced sedation for emergency department procedures. Am J Emerg Med 7(2):155–161, 1989.

Beaver WT, McMillan D: Comparison of the analgesic effect of acetaminophen and codeine and their combination in patients with postoperative pain. Clin Pharmacol Ther 21:108, 1978.

Beaver WT, Feise GA, Robb D: Analgesic effect of intramuscular nalbuphine and morphine in patients with postoperative pain. J Pharmacol Exp Ther 204:487–496, 1978.

Benthuysen JL, Smith NT, Sanford TJ, et al: Physiology of alfentanil-induced rigidity. Anesthesiology 66:440–446, 1986.

Bentley J: Pharmacokinetic approach. In Smith G, Covino BG (eds): Acute Pain. Boston, Butterworths, 1985, pp 42–67.

Billmire DA, Neale HW, Gregory RO: Use of IV fentanyl in the outpatient treatment of pediatric facial trauma. J Trauma 25:1079–1080, 1985.

Bowman WC, Rand MJ (eds): Drugs used to relieve pain. In Textbook of Pharmacology. Oxford, Blackwell, 1980.

Bowsher D: Pain mechanisms. Res Staff Physicians 29:26–34, 1983.

Bullingham RES, McQuay HJ, Moore RA: Clinical pharmacokinetics of narcotic agonist-antagonist drugs. Clin Pharmacokinet 8:332–343, 1983.

Buprenorphine. Medical Letter 28:56, 1986.

Colsanti BK: Narcotic analgesics and antagonists. In Stitzel RE, Craig CR (eds): Modern Pharmacology. Boston, Little, Brown & Co, 1986.

Dahlstrom B, Tamson A, Paalzow L, et al: Patient-controlled analgesic therapy. Part IV: Pharmacokinetics and analgesic plasma concentrations of morphine. Clin Pharmacokinet 7:266–279, 1982.

Errick JK, Heel RC: Nalbuphine: A preliminary review of its pharmacologic properties and therapeutic efficacy. Drugs 26:191–211, 1983.

Fleiss D: Pentazocine-induced fibrous myopathy. JAMA 232:1126, 1975.

Foldes EF, Nagashima H, Daramanian AV, et al: Double blind comparison of the respiratory and circulatory effects of intravenous butorphanol and morphine. Proceedings of the 37th Annual Scientific Meeting, Committee on Problems of Drug Dependence. Washington, DC, May 19–21, 1975, p 373.

Gould RJ, Van Kley H, Knight WN: Elevation of serum amylase levels after narcotic administration. South Med J 75:711–712, 1982.

Grabinski PY, Kaiko RF, Rogers AG, Houde RW: Plasma levels of analgesia following deltoid and gluteal injections of methadone and morphine. J Clin Pharmacol 23:48–55, 1983.

Graves DA, Foster TS, Batenhorst RL, et al: Patient-controlled analgesia. Ann Intern Med 99:360–366, 1983.

Greene NM, Hug CC: Pharmacokinetics. In Kitahata LM, Collins JG (eds): Narcotic Analgesics in Anaesthesiology. Baltimore, Williams & Wilkins, 1982, pp 1–36.

Heel RC, Brogden RN, Speight TM, et al: Buprenorphine: A review of its pharmacological properties and therapeutic efficacy. Drugs 17:81–110, 1979.

Heel RC, Brogden RN, Speight TM, et al: Butorphanol: A review of its pharmacological properties and therapeutic efficacy. Drugs 16:473–505, 1978.

Jaffe JH, Martin WR: Opioid analgesics and antagonists. In Goodman and Gillman's The Pharmacological Basis of Therapeutics, 6th ed., New York, Macmillan, 1985, pp 491–531.

Jasinski DR, Mansky DA: Evaluation of nalbuphine for abuse potential. Clin Pharmacol Ther 13:78–90, 1972.

Kitahata LM, Collins JG, Robinson CJ: Narcotic effects on the nervous system. In Kitahata LM, Collins JG (eds): Narcotic Analgesics in Anaesthesiology. Baltimore, Williams & Wilkins, 1982, pp 57–89.

Kliman A, Lipson MJ, Warren R, et al: Clinical experience with intramuscular butorphanol for the treatment of a variety of chronic pain syndromes. Curr Ther Res 22:105, 1977.

Lang DW, Pilon RN: Naloxone reversal of morphine-induced biliary colic. Anesth Analg 59:619–620, 1980.

Leaman DM, Nellis SH, Zelis F, Field JM: Effects of morphine sulfate on human coronary blood flow. Am J Cardiol 41:324–326, 1978.

Marks RM, Sachar EJ: Undertreatment of medical inpatients with narcotic analgesics. Ann Intern Med 78:173–181, 1973.

Meyer D, Halfin V: Toxicity secondary to meperidine in patients on monamine oxidase inhibitors: A case report and review. Brief Rep 1:319–321, 1981.

Momose Y: Potentiation of postoperative analgesic agents by hydroxyzine. Anesth Analg 59:22–27, 1980.

Nagle RE, Pilcher J: Respiratory and circulatory effects of pentazocine. Br Heart J 34:244–251, 1972.

Ouellette RD, Mod MS, Gilbert MS, et al: Comparison of buprenorphine and morphine: A multidose, multicenter study in patients with severe postoperative pain. Contemp Surg 28:1–7, 1986.

Paris PM, Stewart RD: Pain Management in Emergency Medicine. Norwalk, CT, Appleton & Lange, 1988.

Pasternak GW: Opiate, enkephalin and endorphin analgesia: Relations to a single subpopulation of opiate receptors. Neurology 31:1311–1315, 1981.

Patwardhan RV, Johnson RF, Hoyumpa A, et al: Normal metabolism of morphine in cirrhosis. Gastroenterology 81:1006–1008, 1981.

Pert CB, Pasternak GW, Snyder SH: Opiate agonists and antagonists discriminated by receptor binding in the brain. Science 1359–1361, 1973.

Radney PA, Brodman E, Mankikar D, Duncalf D: The effect of equi-analgesic doses of fentanyl, morphine, meperidine and pentazocine on common bile duct pressure. Anaesthetist 29:26–29, 1980.

Rafferty TD: Respiratory effects of narcotic analgesics. In Kitahata LM, Collins JG (eds): Narcotic Analgesics in Anaesthesiology. Baltimore, Williams & Wilkins, 1982, pp 133–141.

Roebel LE, Cavanaugh RL, Buyniski JP: Comparative gastrointestinal and biliary tract effects of morphine and butorphanol. J Med 10:225–238, 1979.

Romagnoli A, Keats AS: Ceiling effect for respiratory depression by nalbuphine. Clin Pharmacol Ther 27:478–485, 1980.

Romagnoli A, Keats AS: Comparative hemodynamic effects of nalbuphine and morphine in patients with coronary disease. Bull Tex Heart Inst 5:19–24, 1978.

Roscow CE: Newer synthetic opioid analgesics. In Smith G, Covino BG (eds): Acute Pain. London, Butterworths, 1985, pp 68–103.

Roscow CE, Moss J, Philbin DM, Savarese JJ: Histamine release during morphine and fentanyl anesthesia. Anesthesiology 56:93–96, 1982.

Rosenfeldt FL, Houston B, Dussek J, et al: Haemodynamic effects of a new analgesic agent, buprenorphine. Br J Clin Pharmacol 5:362, 1978.

Ruskis AF: Effects of narcotics on the gastrointestinal tract, liver and kidneys. In Kitahata LM, Collins JG (eds): Narcotic Analgesics in Anaesthesiology. Baltimore, Williams & Wilkins, 1982, pp 143–156.

Rutter PC, Murphy F, Dudley HA: Morphine: Controlled trial of different methods of administration for postoperative pain relief. Br Med J 280:12–13, 1980.

Semenkovich CF, Jaffe AS: Adverse effects due to morphine sulfate. Am J Med 79:325–330, 1985.

Stanski DR, Greenblatt DJ, Lowinstein E: Kinetics of intravenous and intramuscular morphine. Clin Pharmacol Ther 24:52–59, 1978.

Stimmel B: Narcotic analgesics I: Narcotic agonists. In Pain, Analgesia and Addiction. New York, Raven, 1983, pp 97–133.

Sugioka K, Boniface KJ, Davis DA: The influence of meperidine on myocardial contractility in the intact dog. Anaesthesiology 18:622–623, 1957.

Tammisto T, Tigerstedt I: Comparison of the analgesic effects of intravenous nalbuphine and pentazocine in patients with postoperative pain. Acta Anaesth Scand 21:390–394, 1977.

Thomas M, Malcrona R, Fillmore S: Haemodynamic effects of morphine in patients with acute myocardial infarction. Br Heart J 27:863–875, 1965.

Vatner SF, Marsh JD, Swain JA: Effects of morphine on coronary and left ventricular dynamics in conscious dogs. J Clin Invest 55:207–217.

Zola EM, McLeod DC: Comparative effect and analgesic efficacy of the agonist-antagonist opioids. Drug Intell Clin Pharm 17:411–417, 1983.

CHAPTER 9

Sedative-Hypnotics

THOMAS E. TERNDRUP, M.D.

INTRODUCTION

Simply defined, a sedative drug is one that decreases activity, moderates excitability, and calms the recipient. A hypnotic drug is one that produces drowsiness and facilitates the onset and maintenance of a state of sleep. Drug-induced hypnosis resembles natural sleep in its electroencephalographic characteristics and allows the recipient to be easily aroused.

The development of safe and effective sedative-hypnotic agents for clinical use has been plagued by several problems. Many of these agents have had an unacceptably low therapeutic-to-toxic ratio; others have led to tolerance and accumulation in body tissues, prolonging their undesirable effects; some agents have a significant abuse potential; and many have led to the induction of drug withdrawal phenomena following chronic administration. Despite these flaws, the use of sedative-hypnotic medications remains widespread in the general population. Use of these agents for therapeutic purposes and to enhance diagnostic efforts is frequent in acute care situations. Complication rates and efficacy can be improved by applying a thorough understanding of the indications, side effects, drug interactions, and contraindications to sedative-hypnotic administration. However, inappropriate selection or administration of these drugs to patients may increase morbidity and mortality.

The traditional categories of sedative-hyp-notic agents are the benzodiazepines, the barbiturates, and the nonbarbiturates. The nonbarbiturate group includes paraldehyde, chloral hydrate, hydroxyzine, promethazine, and diphenhydramine. Selected antipsychotic agents are also used to produce rapid tranquilization or chemical sedation of violent or agitated patients. Haloperidol, traditionally an antipsychotic agent, is a model drug used for rapid calming of these patients. Although other agents, such as the opioids and certain anesthetics, have sedative and hypnotic properties, they will only be mentioned in this chapter in the context of their sedative properties. These agents are discussed further in Chapters 7 and 8.

Although there are many benzodiazepine agents available for sedative-hypnotic indications (Table 9–1), only diazepam, midazolam, and lorazepam are reviewed in detail in this chapter. The reasons for reviewing only these three agents largely relate to their applicability in acute treatment. These agents have a relatively rapid onset of action and generally predictable levels of sedation; can be administered intravenously, allowing titration of dosage to produce desired clinical effects; and have a variable duration of activity, allowing for selection of the appropriate agent.

Several considerations or cautions must be addressed prior to sedative-hypnotic administration in unselected patients. This is particularly true for patients with head trauma, acutely agitated elderly patients without

TABLE 9-1. Characteristics of Benzodiazepines

Benzodiazepine (Trade Name; Year Available)	Onset (PO) Route(s)	Half-life (Hours)	Active Substances	Elimination Rate	Equivalent Dosage (mg)	Approved Indications
Alprazolam (Xanax; 1981)	Intermediate PO	11	Alprazolam	Intermediate	0.75–1.5 (usual daily dose)	Anxiety, anxiety-depression
Chlordiazepoxide (Librium; 1960)	Slow PO, IM, IV	5–30	Desmethylchlordiazepoxide, chlordiazepoxide	Slow	25	Anxiety, alcohol withdrawal, preoperative sedation
Clonazepam (Clonopin; 1974)	Intermediate PO	25	Clonazepam	Intermediate	Not applicable	Seizure disorders
Clorazepate (Tranxene; 1972)	Rapid PO	30–200	Desmethyldiazepam	Slow	7.5	Anxiety, alcohol withdrawal, seizure disorders
Diazepam (Valium; 1962)	Rapid PO, IV	20–100	Desmethyldiazepam, diazepam	Slow	5	Anxiety, alcohol withdrawal, preoperative sedation, muscle spasm, status epilepticus
Flurazepam (Dalmane; 1970)	Rapid to intermediate PO	74	Flurazepam aldehyde, desalkylflurazepam	Slow	30	Insomnia
Halazepam (Paxipam; 1981)	Intermediate to slow PO	14	Desmethyldiazepam, diazepam	Slow	60–160 (usual daily dose)	Anxiety
Lorazepam (Ativan; 1977)	Intermediate PO, IM, IV	10–20	Lorazepam	Intermediate	1	Anxiety, anxiety-depression, preoperative sedation
Midazolam (Versed; 1987)	Rapid PO, IM, IV	1–12	1-OH, methylmidazolam, midazolam	Rapid	1–1.5	Preoperative sedation, anesthesia induction
Oxazepam (Serax; 1963)	Intermediate PO	5–15	Oxazepam	Intermediate to rapid	15	Anxiety, anxiety-depression, alcohol withdrawal
Prazepam (Centrax; 1977)	Slow PO	30–200	Desmethyldiazepam	Slow	10	Anxiety
Temazepam (Restoril; 1981)	Intermediate to slow PO	13	Temazepam	Intermediate	15–30	Insomnia
Triazolam (Halcion; 1983)	Intermediate PO	2.3	Triazolam	Rapid	0.25–0.5	Insomnia

documented psychiatric histories, patients with any alteration in vital signs (including body temperature), children, patients with suspected poisoning or drug overdose, and patients with any metabolic disorder. Prior to the administration of sedative-hypnotic drugs, it is essential for the physician to ensure the adequacy of the airway, ventilation, and hemodynamic stability of these patients.

Historical Development of Sedative-Hypnotic Agents

The development of the benzodiazepines revolutionized the outpatient treatment of anxiety and insomnia. Prior to the development of chlordiazepoxide (Librium) and diazepam (Valium) in the early 1960s, only relatively inadequate agents were available. Early in this century, the bromides, paraldehyde, and chloral hydrate were the most widely used sedative-hypnotic drugs. Although generally effective, these agents had unacceptable side effects, a high rate of drug misuse, and administration inconveniences. The major disadvantage of the bromides was that they had an extraordinarily long half-life and tended to accumulate in the body with repeated doses. Paraldehyde was often the preferred drug for treating alcohol withdrawal states; however, it has an offensive odor, and frequent use leads to tolerance and dependency. Chloral hydrate remains in common clinical use and is one of the few hypnotics that does not cause major disturbances in the normal pattern of sleep. Also, although tolerance to this agent may develop, abuse and withdrawal reactions are virtually unknown. Unfortunately, chloral hydrate has a slow onset of action, significant gastrointestinal toxicity, and broad dosage recommendations, limiting its applicability in emergency situations.

The barbiturates increased in popularity during the 1930s and 1940s, when they occupied a position quite comparable to that of the benzodiazepines today. The barbituric acid structure permitted many different chemical substitutions, which allowed the development of agents with tailored onsets and durations of action. The barbiturates remain in active clinical use, largely for the induction of anesthesia (thiopental) and for anticonvulsant therapy (phenobarbital) and, less commonly, as sedative-hypnotic agents (phenobarbital or pentobarbital). The major problem encountered with the use of the barbiturates is their high rate of abuse, tolerance, and dependency, which limits their outpatient clinical applicability.

The era of the benzodiazepines began with the development of chlordiazepoxide in 1960 and diazepam in 1962. Although these drugs were initially developed as antianxiety agents, it was soon apparent that they had excellent prospects for other indications. Their advantages were that they had a spectrum of indications comparable to that of the barbiturates and limited toxicity in the setting of overdosage, without the high rate of abuse associated with barbiturates. Various benzodiazepines were developed that had considerably different pharmacokinetic profiles, allowing for tailored drug administration. Finally, several investigators identified a specific benzodiazepine receptor, thus facilitating the development of a benzodiazepine antagonist. The major disadvantage of the benzodiazepines is the potential for significant respiratory depression when they are administered rapidly intravenously or mixed with other sedative-hypnotic drugs.

General Indications for Use of Sedative-Hypnotic Agents

The indications for sedative-hypnotic drug administration in the emergency situation are somewhat different from their general clinical indications in other settings. In the nonemergency department clinical environment, the most frequent indications for sedative-hypnotics are anxiety and insomnia. Less commonly, they are administered for preoperative sedation, skeletal muscle relaxation, and anxiety-depressive disorders. In emergent situations, the most frequent indications are for the initial management of psychosis, for violent or disruptive patients, for various withdrawal states, as intravenous anesthetic agents, and to facilitate various diagnostic and therapeutic procedures. In general, the acute indications and goals for sedative-hypnotic administration are the following:

1. To provide chemical control of violent or disruptive patients who are dangerous to themselves or others
2. To provide pain relief and amnesia during procedures that are difficult and traumatic

3. To enhance quality diagnostic testing in uncooperative patients
4. To promote the rapid stabilization of patients undergoing drug withdrawal
5. To facilitate the rapid assessment and stabilization of patients who are uncooperative and unstable (e.g., a multiple trauma patient who is intoxicated, uncooperative, and severely injured)
6. To calm the psychotic patient who is disruptive, threatening, or self-destructive

Very young and very old patients should be approached with particular caution because they may require lower dosages. Likewise, patients with underlying renal or hepatic disease may need reduced dosage of some sedative-hypnotic agents. The general contraindications to emergency administration of sedative-hypnotic drugs include the inability to establish and ensure a patent airway and ventilation, marked hemodynamic instability, hypersensitivity to the specific agent being considered, and serious drug interactions (e.g., a monoamine oxidase [MAO] inhibitor and meperidine). The administration of phenothiazines in patients with hypotension or seizure disorders should be strongly discouraged because of the increased incidence of exacerbation of these conditions. Relative contraindications to sedative-hypnotic use include an altered mental status of unknown origin; a suspected concurrent acute medical problem (e.g., a patient with chronic obstructive pulmonary disease exacerbation) or an acute surgical problem; patients with drug dependency or drug-seeking behavior; pregnancy (particularly during the first trimester); and patients at the extremes of age. Relative contraindications allow the administration of sedative-hypnotics to patients with these disorders as long as resuscitative equipment and personnel are available should the patient deteriorate clinically.

CONDITIONS

Agitation Control

Diagnosis
The diagnostic considerations in patients with an undifferentiated, agitated, or uncooperative state include respiratory disorders (hypoxemia and hypercarbia); head injury; seizure disorder; cerebrovascular accidents; metabolic disorders, including encephalopathy (hepatic or renal), endocrinopathy (hypothyroidism, hyperthyroidism, adrenal insufficiency), electrolyte abnormalities (hypoglycemia, hypocalcemia, hypercalcemia, hyponatremia, and hypernatremia); concurrent drug ingestion, both therapeutic and illicit; drug withdrawal manifestations; infections, both central nervous system (CNS) and generalized; and psychosis or other psychiatric presentations.

The rapid assessment of these patients should include analysis of the patient's airway, ventilation, and vital signs and a rapid neurologic examination. Blood for arterial blood gas determinations and appropriate testing should be obtained simultaneously with initial resuscitative measures. Rapid intervention should be undertaken to correct any abnormalities of vital signs. Empiric intravenous administration of 50 g of dextrose and 2 mg of naloxone should be considered, although rapid bedside testing of blood glucose and the lack of signs of opioid overdosage may occasionally modify this routine treatment. The history and a rapid neurologic assessment may allow differentiation of organic and functional disorders. Every effort should be made to identify reversible causes of agitation prior to administration of sedatives or other psychoactive drugs. However, the decision to initiate sedative-hypnotic therapy emergently should be based not only on a specific diagnosis but also on the urgency and effectiveness with which treatment can or should be initiated.

Indications for Treatment
Occasionally, it may be necessary to administer a rapidly acting sedative-hypnotic agent to control the patient during the initial assessment. This should be done only when careful monitoring of vital signs, electrocardiogram, and mental status is possible. A patient who is endangering himself or herself by failing to adhere to the cautions and interventions advised by the staff should be considered for rapid chemical control and sedation. For example, the multiple trauma patient whose cervical spine has not been adequately evaluated and who refuses to cooperate with attempts to immobilize the cervical spine is in need of physical and chemical restraint.

Adjuncts for control of certain disruptive, violent, and uncooperative patients should be used early in initiating diagnostic and therapeutic procedures. These include, when possible, a quiet, dimly lit room with limited outside stimuli from other patients or staff members; the application of secure leather restraints on the patient's extremities; and, finally, a calm, caring demeanor portrayed by the staff. However, despite these adjuncts to patient control, it may be necessary to administer rapidly acting sedative-hypnotic agents to facilitate immediate evaluation and stabilization. A protocol for coordinated management of violent and disruptive patients should be developed.

Patients with signs of *drug withdrawal*, such as piloerection, disorientation, visual or tactile hallucinations, anxiety, irritability, abdominal pain, nausea and vomiting or diarrhea, yawning, rhinorrhea, tremulousness, tachycardia, and diaphoresis, with a history (or strong suspicion) of drug misuse, should receive an agent designed to reverse the withdrawal state. (See boxes, Drug Treatment: Control of the Violent Disruptive, or Psychotic Adult, and Drug Treatment: Control of the Traumatized or Medically Unstable Adult.)

Discussion

For patients with undifferentiated agitation, uncooperativeness, hostility, or violence, these drug regimens provide a graduated approach to management. Initially, patients should be physically restrained to

DRUG TREATMENT: CONTROL OF THE VIOLENT, DISRUPTIVE, OR PSYCHOTIC ADULT

First-Line Drug

Haloperidol

Initial Dose	5–10 mg IM
Repeat Dose	Double the prior dose every 30 minutes until agitation is controlled; then 2–10 mg maintenance dose every 2–8 hours based on the patient's clinical status
End-Points	Calm, cooperative patient
	Further diagnostic evaluation possible
	Stable respiratory and hemodynamic status

Second-Line Drug

Diazepam

Initial Dose	3–5 mg IV
Repeat Dose	1–2.5 mg IV in 10 minutes
End-Points	Calm, cooperative patient
	Further diagnostic evaluation possible
	Stable respiratory and hemodynamic status

Third-Line Drug

Lorazepam

Initial Dose	1–2 mg IV
Repeat Dose	0.5–1 mg IV in 10 minutes
End-Points	Calm, cooperative patient
	Further diagnostic evaluation possible
	Stable respiratory and hemodynamic status

DRUG TREATMENT: CONTROL OF THE TRAUMATIZED OR MEDICALLY UNSTABLE ADULT

First-Line Drug
Diazepam

Initial Dose	3–5 mg IV
Repeat Dose	1–2.5 mg IV in 10 minutes
End-Points	Calm, cooperative patient
	Further diagnostic evaluation possible
	Stable respiratory and hemodynamic status

Second-Line Drug
Midazolam

Initial Dose	1–2.5 mg IV over 2 minutes
Repeat Dose	1–2 mg IV in 5 minutes
End-Points	Calm, cooperative patient
	Further diagnostic evaluation possible
	Stable respiratory and hemodynamic status

Third-Line Drug
Haloperidol

Initial Dose	2–5 mg IV
Repeat Dose	Double the prior dose every 20 minutes until patient is calm; then IM maintenance dose of 2–10 mg every 2–8 hours based on clinical status of patient
End-Points	Calm, cooperative patient
	Further diagnostic evaluation possible
	Stable respiratory and hemodynamic status

Fourth-Line Drug
Atracurium

	Endotracheal intubation must be achieved before using this drug, and ventilation must be supported.
Initial dose	0.4–0.5 mg/kg IV
Repeat Dose	0.4–0.5 mg/kg IV in 20–30 minutes as effect of previous dose wanes
End-Point	Motor paralysis

prevent harm to themselves or to staff while verbal attempts are undertaken to calm them. If an intravenous line cannot be safely established, they should be rapidly controlled physically by multiple staff members, followed by the intramuscular administration of haloperidol. Haloperidol is a butyrophenone antipsychotic agent and is effective in achieving rapid tranquilization of acutely psychotic patients. It has also been demonstrated to be safe and effective for unselected agitated patients. Haloperidol does not appear to decrease the seizure threshold or increase the risk of hypotension, as do the phenothiazines. The onset of action after intramuscular administration is 15 to 20 minutes, whereas intravenous administration (not approved by the Food and Drug Administration but widely practiced) promotes much more rapid sedation. The duration of clinical effects varies from 1.5 to 4 hours. Advantages to haloperidol administration include relatively few side effects (predominantly extrapyramidal or dystonic reactions), rapid sedation, and few cardiorespiratory depressant side effects. Disadvantages associated with its use include the induction of dystonic reactions, the neuroleptic malignant syndrome, and the dyskinetic syndrome. If an intravenous line can be established, diazepam, 3 to 5 mg IV, is an acceptable alternative. Both haloperidol and diazepam promote rapid sedation, allowing for further assessment of the patient's condition, but diazepam has a greater tendency to induce respiratory depression. Although midazolam and lorazepam may be used intramuscularly, their use in the management of unselected agitated or hostile patients has not been studied.

In the traumatized or medically unstable patient who is also agitated and uncooperative, sedative-hypnotics may be useful to calm the patient for protection of the cervical spine and facilitation of diagnostic or therapeutic procedures. However, these patients are also more likely to develop the adverse hemodynamic or respiratory effects possible from these drugs. Neuromuscular paralysis with atracurium may be necessary to facilitate diagnostic studies in those patients who remain agitated and uncooperative despite repeated doses of sedative-hypnotics and who have been endotracheally intubated for airway control and ventilation.

Patients undergoing presumed opioid withdrawal should receive methadone, 10 mg IM. It is difficult to estimate initial doses for heroin addicts. Patients on methadone maintenance programs should receive two-thirds of their usual dosage intramuscularly divided twice a day, when unable to tolerate oral medication. Methadone achieves appreciable plasma concentrations within 15 to 20 minutes after intramuscular administration. It is extensively metabolized by hepatic enzymes. The elimination half-life is 1 to 1.5 days.

Patients undergoing barbiturate or alcohol withdrawal should receive intravenous diazepam in 5- to 10-mg increments until withdrawal symptoms and signs stabilize. Large doses of diazepam are frequently required,

particularly for ethanol withdrawal. Frequent reassessment allows individual titration to minimize withdrawal complications and the side effects of medication. Alternatively, intramuscular or intravenous phenobarbital should be used in patients hypersensitive to the benzodiazepines or undergoing benzodiazepine withdrawal. Doses of 10 to 15 mg/kg, with a maximum initial dose of 120 mg, are generally recommended. Seizures resulting from withdrawal should be managed in the usual fashion, with intravenous lorazepam or diazepam as the initial therapeutic agent. Compared to diazepam, lorazepam has similar efficacy and perhaps produces less respiratory depression when administered to patients in status epilepticus.

The intravenous route of administration is preferable in hemodynamically unstable patients, since absorption is more reliable by this route. However, in occasional disruptive, violent patients, the intramuscular administration of haloperidol may be the only option possible. Intramuscular absorption depends primarily on adequate muscular perfusion and on the vehicle in which the medication is suspended. Intramuscular drug administration is distinctly contraindicated in patients in shock with peripheral vasoconstriction, and in patients with peripheral vascular disease or other pathology impairing muscular perfusion. Although not popular in the United States, rectal administration of diazepam, lorazepam, midazolam, paraldehyde, methohexital, and other sedative-hypnotic agents has been shown to deliver comparable serum levels in most patients, when compared with intravenous administration, and is an option for pediatric patients. Careful attention to technique, elimination of patients with acute or chronic rectal pathology, and the use of drugs in solution should increase uniform drug levels and the clinical efficacy of rectally administered drugs.

Sedation for Diagnostic or Therapeutic Purposes

Diagnosis and Indications for Treatment

When painful or uncomfortable procedures need to be performed in alert patients, short-term sedation may be used to ensure that the procedure may be performed effectively and without causing undue discomfort. This would include patients requiring conscious endotracheal intubation, tube thoracostomy insertion, reduction of large joint dislocations, reduction of fractures, incision and drainage of abscesses, laceration repair, cardioversion, anoscopy, endoscopy, and other such procedures. Adjuncts to these short, painful procedures include the use of topically applied anesthetics; local anesthesia by nerve blocks, infiltration, or regional techniques; psychologic measures, such as playing calming music or story-telling for younger patients; and physical restraint. Proper technique and allowing sufficient time for local measures to take effect will en-

hance the efficacy of these adjunctive measures. (See boxes, Drug Treatment: Short, Painful Procedures—Cooperative Adult Patient, and Drug Treatment: Short, Painful Procedures—Pediatric Patient.)

Discussion
Adult Patients

The drug treatment flow sheet outlines a graduated approach to the drug therapy of *cooperative* adult patients undergoing painful procedures or diagnostic tests. For most adults, administration of a sedative-hypnotic is unnecessary. However, in the occasional adult or, more commonly, in the pediatric patient, the administration of sedatives, mus-

---

DRUG TREATMENT: SHORT, PAINFUL PROCEDURES— COOPERATIVE ADULT PATIENT

First-Line Drug
Nitrous Oxide

Initial Dose	50:50 with oxygen by continuous inhalation
Repeat Dose	Maximum usage time—30 minutes
End-Points	Successful procedure
	No respiratory or cardiac side effects

Second-Line Drugs
Midazolam and Morphine

Initial Dose	Midazolam, 1–2 mg IV
	and
	Morphine, 3–5 mg IV (in same syringe over 5 minutes)
Repeat Dose	Midazolam, 1–2 mg IV in 30–40 minutes
	Morphine, one-half of initial dose in 10 minutes
End-Points	Successful procedure
	No respiratory or cardiac side effects

Third-Line Drugs
Meperidine and Hydroxyzine

Initial Dose	Meperidine, 1–1.5 mg/kg IM
	Hydroxyzine, 25–50 mg IM
Repeat Dose	50% of initial dose of both drugs in 45 minutes
End-Points	Successful procedure
	No respiratory or cardiac side effects

DRUG TREATMENT: SHORT, PAINFUL PROCEDURES— PEDIATRIC PATIENT

First-Line Drugs

Meperidine, Promethazine, and Chlorpromazine

Initial Dose	Meperidine, 2 mg/kg IM ($\leq$ 50 mg)
	Promethazine, 1 mg/kg IM ($\leq$ 25 mg)
	Chlorpromazine, 1 mg/kg IM ($\leq$ 25 mg)
Repeat Dose	Not recommended
End-Points	Successful procedure
	No respiratory or cardiac side effects

Second-Line Drug

Fentanyl

Initial Dose	0.001 mg/kg by slow IV push
Repeat Dose	One-half the initial dose in 10 minutes
End-Points	Successful procedure
	No respiratory or cardiac side effects

Third-Line Drugs

Meperidine and Diazepam

Initial Dose	Meperidine, 1–1.5 mg/kg IM (maximum dose, 50 mg)
	Diazepam, 0.1 mg/kg by slow IV push (maximum dose, 2.5 mg)
Repeat Dose	One-half the initial dose of only diazepam in 15 minutes IV
End-Points	Successful procedure
	No respiratory or cardiac side effects

cle relaxants, and analgesics may be necessary. In general, for diagnostic testing, the administration of sedatives is all that is required. For short, painful procedures or diagnostic testing in patients not responding to sedative administration alone, the combination of a sedative and an analgesic is required. When skeletal muscle relaxation is essential, such as in the reduction of a large joint dislocation, diazepam or midazolam should be administered intravenously.

For the cooperative adult, nitrous oxide is an attractive, efficacious, and rapidly reversible inhalation agent that can be self-administered. Its rapid onset and short duration of action allow patient-controlled titration of effects. It has been demonstrated to be safe and effective for use during incision and drainage of abscesses, musculoskeletal trauma, and abdominal pain without distention, among other indications. It has been used effectively by prehospital personnel as well. Nitrous oxide should be delivered at <70% concentration with oxygen to prevent asphyxia. Delivery in ambulances and the emergency department is straightforward with a commercially available system that delivers a 50:50 mix of nitrous oxide and oxygen and incorporates a scavenger system to reduce ambient contamination. Side effects are generally mild and include nausea and vomiting, dizziness, and lightheadedness. Contraindications to use of nitrous oxide include head injury, pneumothorax, chronic lung disease, bowel obstruction, decompression sickness, and an altered mental status.

For short, painful procedures requiring an analgesic *and* muscle relaxation, a combination of midazolam and morphine sulfate is effective. Both of these agents have a rapid onset of action, are short acting, and have relatively predictable clinical effects. Midazolam is a water-soluble benzodiazepine that facilitates deep sedation and produces profound amnesia. Initial doses of 1 to 2 mg IV can be repeated in 30 to 40 minutes as needed. Onset of action after intravenous administration is 1 to 2 minutes, with peak activity in 7 to 10 minutes. Duration of activity is approximately 20 to 30 minutes (25% of diazepam's duration). Midazolam is not currently approved for use in pediatric patients. Morphine sulfate is a potent narcotic that has significant analgesic, anxiolytic, and sedative properties. Dosages of 3 to 5 mg IV (0.1 mg/kg in pediatric patients) can be repeated in 7 to 10 minutes when delivered by slow intravenous infusion through a rapidly running peripheral line. The duration of action of morphine sulfate is 0.5 to 1.5 hours.

Dosage requirements of benzodiazepines are reduced and analgesia is added when they are administered with opioids. However, the risk of respiratory depression can be substantial with this combination. By administering these agents (midazolam and morphine may be given in the same syringe) via slow infusion over 5 to 7 minutes, the risk of respiratory depression is reduced. The risk of complications is increased in the elderly, in intoxicated patients, and in patients with head injury, chronic lung disease, or an altered mental state. Resuscitation equipment, including suction, oxygen, bag-valve-mask, and resuscitative drugs and defibrillator, should be immediately available. Naloxone, a specific narcotic antagonist, will reverse the respiratory, hemodynamic, and CNS depression associated with opioids. Generally, in the nonoverdose setting, 0.4 to 0.8 mg IV will rapidly reverse these side effects. The onset of action of naloxone after intravenous administration is rapid (1 to 3 minutes) but short-lived (10 to 15 minutes). Therefore, following intravenous administration of naloxone for narcotism, continued monitoring and management of the depressive side effects of opioids are indicated.

As a *third-line* agent for the cooperative adult patient when intravenous access is not available, meperidine, combined with hydroxyzine or promethazine, may be administered intramuscularly. Meperidine is a phenylpiperidine; 85 to 100 mg of meperidine is equivalent in potency to 10 mg of morphine. The onset of action of this combination is 20 to 30 minutes, with peak activity occurring at 45 to 60 minutes. The duration of activity is variable but is generally 2 to 3 hours. Doses of meperidine needed to achieve the same clinical effects vary among individuals. I recommend 75 to 150 mg (1.5 to 2 mg/kg for pediatric patients) IM of meperidine when given with 25 to 50 mg (0.5 to 1 mg/kg for pediatric patients) of hydroxyzine or promethazine. A repeat dose may be given after 45 minutes if sufficient sedation is not achieved, but the total dose of meperidine should not exceed 3 mg/kg. The advantages of this combination are a decreased incidence of nausea and vomiting, compared with isolated meperidine administration. It can be given safely to patients who are hypersensitive to morphine, its longer activity may facilitate procedures requiring prolonged effects, and it does not require intravenous access. However, no skeletal muscle relaxation is achieved; amnestic effects are minimal; dosages cannot be titrated to clinical effect; the duration of activity is longer than is generally required for the majority of emergency procedures; there may be no reduction in significant side effects when compared to slowly delivered intravenous medication; side effects may include seizures, tremor, and local wheal and flare reactions (related to histamine release); intramuscular drug administration is often unreliable; and the injection is painful.

End-points for successful therapy include successful completion of the procedure, stable vital signs, and an alert mental status. Occasionally emergency attempts to reduce a large joint dislocation may fail, and the patient may require general anesthesia, with muscular paralysis induced with succinylcholine or pancuronium. Skeletal muscle paralysis for other short, painful procedures is inappropriate.

Pediatric Patients

For short painful procedures in *pediatric patients* (generally ≤ 12 years old), one may use a combination of meperidine (Demerol), promethazine (Phenergan), and chlorpromazine (Thorazine) (DPT) in a ratio of 2/1/1 mg/kg, respectively, given by intramuscular injection. Maximum doses of 50/25/25 mg should not be exceeded. Doses must be based on body weight measured during the emergency department visit. The onset of action of DPT is generally 30 minutes and the duration of action can be quite long (4 to 24 hours). However, many of these patients can be observed in the emergency department for 3 to 4 hours and sent home with appropriate discharge precautions, assuming there will be reliable caretakers at the home. These patients should take nothing by mouth (NPO) and should sleep in the left lateral decubitus position under direct parental observation until they are alert. Advantages of DPT are relatively deep sedation, analgesia, efficacy, and few serious complications. Side effects include extrapyramidal signs (dystonic reactions), transient changes in vital signs, paradoxical hyperactivity, respiratory depression, apnea, and cardiac arrest. DPT should not be administered to patients with neurologic abnormalities (including seizure disorders) or an abnormal initial mental status examination, because of the increased risk of complications.

In the pediatric patient with an intravenous line established or with a head injury who must undergo a short painful procedure or diagnostic test, fentanyl may be the preferred agent. Fentanyl is an extremely potent, ultra–short-acting synthetic narcotic that appears efficacious in pediatric patients undergoing short procedures. Doses of 1 to 2 μg/kg are indicated, with repeat dosage titrated to clinical effect. Note that 200 μg of fentanyl is equivalent to 10 mg of morphine. It is reversible with naloxone and has predictable side effects, a rapid onset of action (1 to 2 minutes), and short duration of action (30 minutes). Cautions and contraindications to the use of fentanyl are identical to those of other narcotic agents. In addition, fentanyl may induce muscular rigidity, occasionally interfering with procedures or ventilation. Disadvantages to this agent are similar to those of other narcotic agents, plus an intravenous line must be established, which, in this age group, may be more traumatic than the intended procedure itself. Fentanyl undergoes hepatic metabolism and is eliminated with a half-life of 3.5 hours. Repeat doses may lead to drug accumulation, resulting in prolonged sedation and respiratory depression.

For pediatric patients undergoing large joint reduction or when marked skeletal muscle relaxation is required, a combination of diazepam, 0.1 mg/kg IV (maximum initial dose 2.5 mg), and meperidine, 1 to 1.5 mg/kg IM (maximum initial dose 50 mg), may be quite effective. I prefer intramuscular administration of meperidine about 20 minutes prior to the intended procedure, followed by intravenous administration of diazepam 1 to 2 minutes prior to the procedure itself. This combination may lead to profound respiratory and CNS depression. Therefore, I recommend frequent monitoring of blood pressure, respiratory rate, and mental status. Advantages to this combination are profound amnesia, skeletal muscle relaxation, and analgesia. Disadvantages are the potential for substantial respiratory depression and the prolonged duration of action of intramuscular meperidine.

SPECIFIC AGENTS

Benzodiazepines

Diazepam (Valium)
See Table 9–1 for a summary of other benzodiazepines.

Pharmacology

Clinical Formula
7-chloro-1,3-dihydro-1-methyl-5-phenyl-2H-1,4-benzodiazepin-2-one

Mechanism of Action
Binds to specific benzodiazepine receptors in cortical and limbic areas of the CNS
Enhances inhibitory properties of the neurotransmitter gamma-aminobutyric acid (GABA)

Kinetics

	PO	IV
Onset	20–30 minutes	1–2 minutes
Peak	45–60 minutes	2–5 minutes
Duration	4–6 hours	4–6 hours
Half-life	43 hours	43 hours

Metabolism
Initial: redistribution into adipose tissue
Elimination: by hepatic biotransformation, microsomal oxidation, glucuronide conjugation

Note: Bioavailability is poor after intramuscular injection. This route of administration should not be used because of unpredictable absorption and high incidence of sterile abscess formation.

Clinical Effects

Reduction of anxiety
Anticonvulsant
Reduction in arousal and alertness
Skeletal muscle relaxation
Amnesia
Preservation of autonomic and endocrine responses to emotions and nervous stimuli

Indications

Sedation
Muscle relaxation
Anxiety reduction
Anticonvulsant
Management of drug withdrawal

Dosage

IV: adults, 3 to 5 mg bolus by slow push; children, 0.1 mg/kg bolus by slow push (maximum dose of 2.5 mg)
PO: 5 to 10 mg

Cautions

Dosage adjustment in organ failure—none
Use in pregnancy—no; Category D
Use in lactation—no
Use in childhood—yes; dose 0.1 mg/kg to maximum single dose of 2.5 mg

Toxicity

Drug Interactions

Increased CNS depression with alcohol; narcotics, barbiturates
Increased diazepam effect with acetaminophen, beta-blockers, cimetidine, oral contraceptives, disulfiram, isoniazid, valproic acid
Decreased diazepam effect with caffeine, rifampin, ranitidine (oral diazepam only), theophylline
Diazepam enhances toxicity of amiodarone, digoxin, lithium (combination causes hypothermia), succinylcholine (prolonged paralysis)

Side Effects

Common: sedation and impairment of psychomotor and intellectual function, reduced memory and recall, increased intraocular pressure (do not use in acute glaucoma)
Uncommon: paradoxical excitement
Dangerous: prolonged coma with repetitive doses, impaired ventilatory drive, hypotension

Treatment of Toxicity

Ventilatory support
Volume infusion
Flumazenil (available in Europe as Anexate) is a specific benzodiazepine antagonist currently undergoing clinical trials in the United States.

Lorazepam (Ativan)

Pharmacology

Clinical Formula

7-chloro-5-(o-chlorophenyl)-1,3-dihydro-3-hydroxy-2H-1,4-benzodiazepin-2-one
The injectable form contains 0.18 ml polyethylene glycol in propylene glycol with 2% benzyl alcohol as a preservative.

Mechanism of Action

Benzodiazepine receptor binding

Kinetics (PO, IV, IM)

Intramuscular administration appears to result in more consistent drug delivery, when compared to diazepam.

Onset	PO, 45–60 minutes
	IV, 1–2 minutes
Peak	60–90 minutes
Duration	6–8 hours
Half-life	14 hours

Metabolism

75% of the dose excreted in the urine as the lorazepam glucuronide

Clinical Effects

Clinical effects are nearly identical to those of diazepam; however, skeletal muscle relaxation is poor. When compared to diazepam, there appears to be less chance of respiratory depression in patients treated with equivalent doses of lorazepam.

Indications

Preoperative sedation
Anxiolytic
Hypnotic
Anticonvulsant

Dosage

PO: 1 to 2 mg
IM or IV: 0.04 mg/kg, maximum 2 mg IV and 4 mg IM. Doses of one-half the ini-

tial IV dose may be repeated, if needed, after 15 to 20 minutes.

Cautions

Renal failure—reduce dose by 50% if glomerular filtration rate <10
Hepatic, cardiac failure—no dosage adjustments
Use in pregnancy—no; Category D
Use in lactation—no
Use in childhood—yes

Toxicity

Drug Interactions

Uncommon; same as for other benzodiazepines

Side Effects

Common and uncommon: same as for diazepam
Dangerous: respiratory depression

Treatment of Toxicity

Ventilatory support
Volume infusion
Flumazenil (available in Europe as Anexate) is a specific benzodiazepine antagonist currently undergoing clinical trials in the United States.

Midazolam (Versed) (Imidazobenzodiazepine Derivative)

Pharmacology

Mechanism of Action

Benzodiazepine receptor binding

Kinetics (PO, IM, IV)

Onset	PO, 20–30 minutes
	IM or IV, 1–2 minutes
Peak	PO, 45–60 minutes
	IM or IV, 3–5 minutes
Duration	0.5–2 hours
Half-life	1.5–3 hours

Metabolism

Hepatic oxidation to its 1-hydroxymethyl metabolite (potency half of parent compound)
Excreted in urine as glucuronide conjugates

Indications

Preoperative sedation
Sedation
Anticonvulsant
Anesthesia induction

Advantages

Significant advantages over diazepam and lorazepam include the following:

Reduction of pain/phlebitis associated with oil-based injectable benzodiazepines
Produces profound amnesia
May be combined in the same syringe with other water-soluble agents (e.g., morphine or meperidine)
Shorter duration of action
May be equally efficacious when administered IM or IV

Dosage

PO: 0.08 mg/kg, maximum of 3 to 5 mg
IV or IM: 0.1 mg/kg, maximum of 2.5 mg (1.5 mg in patients ≥ 60 years of age)

Cautions

Renal failure, cardiac failure, respiratory failure—reduce maximum single dose to 1.5 mg
Use in pregnancy—no; Category D
Use in lactation—no
Use in childhood—yes. Midazolam has been used for the sedation of infants and children for various procedures (although not approved by the Food and Drug Administration for use in children in the United States), it has been used in combination with nalbuphine for outpatient sedation, for sedation of children receiving artificial ventilation following cardiac surgery, and widely as a preoperative and induction agent for anesthesia.

Toxicity

Drug Interactions

Same as for other benzodiazepines

Side Effects

Common and uncommon: same as those for diazepam
Dangerous: respiratory depression and cardiac arrest reported before dosage guidelines revised

Treatment of Toxicity

Ventilatory support
Volume infusion

Flumazenil (available in Europe as Anexate) is a specific benzodiazepine antagonist currently undergoing clinical trials in the United States.

Haloperidol (Haldol)

Pharmacology

Clinical Formula

Butyrophenone 4-[4-(P-chloro-phenyl)-4-hydroxy-piperidino]-4'-fluorobutyrophenone

Mechanism of Action

Unknown

Kinetics

	IV or IM	PO
Onset	5–20 minutes	30–60 minutes
Peak	15–45 minutes	2–6 hours
Duration	Variable	8–12 hours

Metabolism

Biliary excretion
Renal excretion

Clinical Effects

Calming
Sedation—mild
Trivial hemodynamic and respiratory effects

Indications

Acute agitation
Various psychotic disorders
Tourette's syndrome
Hyperactivity in children

Dosage

IM: 5 to 10 mg
IV: 2 to 5 mg

For acute control of the agitated patient, double the initial dose every 20 minutes (IV) or 30 minutes (IM) until calming begins.

Maintenance dose requirements are variable, depending on patient response. It is important to give the drug at regular intervals rather than waiting for agitation to recur.

Cautions

Cardiac failure—use lower end of dosing range
Renal, hepatic failure—no dosage adjustment necessary

Use in pregnancy—no; Category C
Use in lactation—no; excreted in breast milk
Use in childhood—yes, if older than 3 years

Toxicity

Drug Interactions

Decreased haloperidol effect with barbiturates, carbamazepine, phenytoin
Toxicity with beta-blockers (hypotension), lithium (encephalopathy), methyldopa (dementia), indomethacin (coma)

Side Effects

Common: extrapyramidal reactions
Uncommon: rash, anticholinergic syndrome (dry mouth, blurred vision, urinary retention), GI upset, lactation, sexual dysfunction, gynecomastia, leukopenia, jaundice, headache, paradoxical agitation with chronic use, sedation
Dangerous: seizures, hypotension, laryngospasm, bronchospasm, agranulocytosis, neuroleptic malignant syndrome, extrapyramidal reactions, tardive dyskinesia with chronic use

Treatment of Acute Toxicity

Neuroleptic malignant syndrome: stop haloperidol; rapid cooling; intensive respiratory and cardiovascular support and monitoring
Extrapyramidal reactions (including laryngospasm): stop haloperidol; give diphenhydramine, 50 mg IV or IM
Hypotension: fluid bolus
Seizures: stop haloperidol; give diazepam, 5 mg IV

Hydroxyzine (Vistaril)

Pharmacology

Clinical Formula

1-(P-chlorobenzhydryl)4-[z-hydroxyethoxy)ethyl]piperazine

Mechanism of Action

H_1-receptor blocker

Kinetics (IM)

Onset	20–30 minutes
Peak	60 minutes
Duration	4–6 hours

Metabolism

Hepatic

Clinical Effects

Sedation
Antiemetic
Antispasmodic
Antihistaminic

Indications (with Meperidine)

Short, painful procedures in adults to enhance sedative effects and to block
emetic effects of coadministered meperidine

Dosage

IM: 25 to 30 mg
May repeat one-half of initial dose in 45
minutes

Cautions

Dosage adjustments in organ failure—
none
Use in pregnancy—yes, after first trimes-
ter
Use in lactation—no
Use in childhood—yes; dose is 1 mg/kg

Toxicity

Drug Interactions

Additive sedation with other CNS depressants—ethanol, narcotics, barbiturates

Side Effects

Common: dry mouth
Uncommon: prolonged sedation, seizures
(with prolonged high doses), tissue necrosis with subcutaneous injection
Dangerous: none

Treatment of Toxicity

Supportive care

Meperidine, Promethazine, and Chlorpromazine (Demerol, Phenergan, and Thorazine)

Pharmacology

Meperidine: synthetic narcotic; phenylpiperidine class. For further discussion of
this agent see Chapter 8.
Promethazine: H_1-receptor blocking antihistamine and phenothiazine

Chlorpromazine: prototype phenothiazine
(i.e., two benzene rings linked by a sulfur atom and a nitrogen atom).

Kinetics (IM only)

Onset	25–45 minutes
Peak	60–90 minutes
Duration	3–18 hours

Metabolism

Meperidine: hepatic hydrolysis and N-de-
methylation; one-third undergoes urinary excretion; normeperidine metabolite may accumulate in overdose setting
and induce seizures.
Promethazine: hepatic transformation
Chlorpromazine: hepatic hydroxylation;
excreted in urine and feces; 7-hydroxy
metabolite is active metabolite.

Clinical Effects

Sedation
Analgesia
Amnesia
Somnolence
Anxiolytic
Antimotion sensation properties
Histamine antagonism

Dosage (All IM)

Meperidine, 2 mg/kg; promethazine, 1
mg/kg; chlorpromazine, 1 mg/kg
Do not exceed 50, 25, 25 mg of meperidine, promethazine, and chlorpromazine, respectively.

Cautions

Repeat dosing not recommended
Do not use in hepatic failure
Reduce dose of meperidine by 50% in se-
vere renal failure.
Use in pregnancy—no
Use in lactation—no
Use in childhood—yes

Toxicity

Interactions

Effects enhanced by any sedative/hypnotic
agent, ethanol, head injury, or underlying neurologic disorder

Side Effects

Common: hypotension
Uncommon: respiratory depression,
extrapyramidal side effects (dystonic re-

actions), nausea and vomiting, paradoxical hyperactivity

Dangerous: respiratory arrest

Treatment of Toxicity

Ventilatory support
Volume infusion for hypotension
Diphenhydramine for dystonic reactions

REFERENCES

Ampel L, Hott KA, Sielaff GW, et al: An approach to airway management in the acutely head-injured patient. J Emerg Med 6:1–7, 1988.

Anderson WH, Kuehnle JC: Diagnosis and early management of acute psychosis. N Engl J Med 305:1128–1130, 1981.

Atkinson JH Jr: Psychopharmacologic treatment of anxiety. Postgrad Med 44:12–18, 1983.

Atkinson JH: Managing the violent patient in the general hospital. Postgrad Med 71:193–201, 1982.

Ayd FJ Jr: Benzodiazepine dependence and withdrawal. J Psychoactive Drugs 15:67–70, 1983.

Bell GD, Reeve PA, Moshiri M, et al: Intravenous midazolam: A study of the degree of oxygen desaturation occurring during upper gastrointestinal endoscopy. Br J Clin Pharmacol 23(6):703–708, 1987.

Bell GD, Spickett GP, Reeve, PA, et al: Intravenous midazolam for upper gastrointestinal endoscopy: A study of 800 consecutive cases relating to dose to age and sex of patient. Br J Clin Pharmacol 23(2):241–243, 1987.

Benforado JM, Houden D: The use of haloperidol to control agitation/violence during admission to an alcohol detoxification center. Curr Alcohol 7:331–338, 1979.

Boralessa H, Senior DF, Whitwam JG: Cardiovascular response to intubation: A comparative study of thiopentone and midazolam. Anaesthesia 38:623–627, 1983.

Briggs GS, Bodendorfer TW, Freeman RK, et al: Drugs in Pregnancy and Lactation: A Reference Guide to Fetal and Neonatal Risk. Baltimore, Williams & Wilkins, 1983.

Choonara IA: Giving drugs per rectum for systemic effect. Arch Dis Child 62:771–772, 1987.

Clinton JE, Sterner S, Stelmachers Z, et al: Haloperidol for sedation of disruptive emergency patients. Ann Emerg Med 16:319–322, 1987.

Colon GA, Gubert N: Lorazepam and fentanyl for outpatient office plastic surgical anesthesia. Plast Reconstr Surg 78:486–488, 1986.

Crawford TO, Mitchell WG, Snodgrass SR: Lorazepam in childhood status epilepticus and serial seizures: Effectiveness and tachyphylaxis. Neurology 37(2):190–195, 1987.

Darragh A, Lambe R, Scully M, et al: Investigation in man of the efficacy of a benzodiazepine antagonist, Ro 15-1788. Lancet 2:8–10, 1981.

Disclafani A, Hall RCW, Gardner ER: Drug-induced psychosis: Emergency diagnosis and management. Psychosomatics 22:845–855, 1981.

Dubin WR, Weiss KJ, Zeccardi JA: Organic brain syndrome: The psychiatric imposter. JAMA 249:60–62, 1983.

Dudley DL, Rowlett DB, Loebel PJ: Emergency use of intravenous haloperidol. Gen Hosp Psychiatry 1:240–246, 1979.

Ellison JM, Jacobs D: Emergency psychopharmacology: A review and update. Ann Emerg Med 15:962–968, 1986.

Franzoni E, Carboni C, Lambertini A: Rectal diazepam: A clinical and EEG study after a single dose in children. Epilepsia 24:35–41, 1983.

Gay GR: Clinical management of acute and chronic cocaine poisoning. Ann Emerg Med 11:562–572, 1982.

Gerle B: Clinical observations of the side effects of haloperidol. Acta Psychiatr Scand 40:65–76, 1964.

Goldfrank LR, Flomenbaum NE, Lewin NA, et al: Toxicologic Emergencies, 3rd ed. Norwalk, CT, Appleton-Century-Crofts, 1986.

Greenblatt DJ, Shader RI, Abernethy DR: Current status of benzodiazepines (Part 1). N Engl J Med 309:354–358, 1983.

Greenblatt DJ, Shader RI, Abernethy DR: Current status of benzodiazepines (Part 2). N Engl J Med 309:410–416, 1983.

Hillbom ME, Hjelm-Jager M: Should alcohol withdrawal seizures be treated with anti-epileptic drugs? Acta Neurol Scand 69:39–42, 1984.

Jacobs D: Evaluation and management of the violent patient in emergency settings. Psychiatr Clin North Am 6:259–269, 1983.

Khantzian EJ, McKenna GJ: Acute toxic and withdrawal reactions associated with drug use and abuse. Ann Intern Med 90:361–372, 1979.

Koch-Weser J, Thompson TL, Moran MG, et al: Psychotropic drug use in the elderly (Part 1). N Engl J Med 308:134–138, 1983.

Koch-Weser J, Thompson TL, Moran MG, et al: Psychotropic drug use in the elderly (Part 2). N Engl J Med 308:194–199, 1983.

Lacey DJ, Singer WD, Horwitz SJ, et al: Lorazepam therapy of status epilepticus in children and adolescents. J Pediatr 108:771–774, 1986.

Lenehan GP, Gastfriend DR, Stetler C: Use of haloperidol in the management of agitated or violent, alcohol-intoxicated patient in the emergency department: A pilot study. J Emerg Nurs 11:72–79, 1985.

Leonard F: Pain control: Anesthesia and analgesia. In Rosen P, Baker FJ, Barkin RM, et al (eds): Emergency Medicine: Concepts and Clinical Practice. St Louis, CV Mosby, 1988, pp 295–308.

Leppik IE, Derivan AT, Homan RW, et al: Double-blind study of lorazepam and diazepam in status epilepticus. JAMA 249:1452–1454, 1983.

McMicken D: Seizures in the alcohol-dependent patient: A diagnostic and therapeutic dilemma. J Emerg Med 1:311–316, 1984.

Resnick M, Burton BT: Droperidol vs. haloperidol in the initial management of acutely agitated patients. J Clin Psychiatry 45:298–299, 1984.

Reves JG, Fragen RJ, Vinik HR, et al: Midazolam: Pharmacology and uses. Anesthesiology 62:310–324, 1985.

Roberts DJ, Clinton JE, Ruiz E: Neuromuscular blockade for critical patients in the emergency department. Ann Emerg Med 15:152–156, 1986.

Rodrigo MR, Rosenquist JB: The effect of Ro15-1788 (Anexate) on conscious sedation produced with midazolam. Anaesth Intensive Care 15(2):185–192, 1987.

Rosenbaum JF: The drug treatment of anxiety. N Engl J Med 306:401–404, 1982.

Rouiller M, Forster A, Gemperle M: Assessment of the efficacy and tolerance of a benzodiazepine antagonist (Ro 15-1788). Ann Fr Anesth Reanim 6(1):1–6, 1987.

Sage DJ, Close A, Boas RA: Reversal of midazolam sedation with anexate. Br J Anaesth 59(4):459–464, 1987.

Schauben JL: Benzodiazepines. Topics in Emergency Medicine 7(3):39–45, 1985.

Smith DE, Wesson DR: The Benzodiazepines: Current Standards for Medical Practice. Boston, MTP Press, 1985.

Sury MRJ, Cole PV: Nalbuphine combined with midazolam for outpatient sedation. Anaesthesia 43:285–288, 1988.

Telintelo S, Kuhlman TL, Winget C: A study of the use of restraint in a psychiatric emergency room. Hosp Community Psychiatry 34:164–165, 1983.

Terndrup TE, Cantor RM, Madden CM: Intramuscular meperidine, promethazine, and chlorpromazine: Analysis of use and complications in 487 pediatric emergency department patients. Ann Emerg Med 18:528–533, 1989.

Tesar EG, Stern TA: Rapid tranquilization of the agitated intensive care unit patient. J Int Care Med 3:195–201, 1988.

CHAPTER 10

Anticonvulsants

MICHELLE H. BIROS, M.S., M.D.

INTRODUCTION

A seizure is the clinical manifestation of a sudden disordered excessive discharge of cerebral neurons. Its presentation depends on the location of the neuronal activity. Although most seizures are idiopathic, acute central nervous system insults, such as trauma or infection, or systemic metabolic disorders can also cause seizures. Occasionally, seizures may be the initial symptom of the acute pathology.

Since patients' medical admission records frequently list the underlying cause of the seizure as the primary diagnosis and often do not record the seizure itself, the exact incidence of seizures is difficult to determine. It has been estimated, however, that the incidence of new single seizures may be as high as 115/100,000 population/year (including febrile seizures). About 5% of patients with new single seizures will go on to develop recurrent, intermittent seizures (epilepsy). Any age group is susceptible to the development of seizures, but infants (<1 year) and older adults (>50 years) have a higher incidence of new seizures each year. There is a slightly higher incidence of new seizures in males than in females. The total incidence of epilepsy is estimated at 1% of the total population.

Seizures arise from a population of epileptogenic neurons that are subjected to certain pathologic states. These neurons can be located in either normal or abnormal brain tissue; they become hyperexcitable due to an alteration of their resting membrane potential, perhaps because of changing concentrations of neurotransmitters that alter sodium–potassium ion flux. Many local, systemic, and environmental factors can precipitate electrical activity of the epileptogenic focus. Once the focus has been stimulated to discharge, the electrical activity spreads until a critical mass of activated neurons has been reached. The propagation of the impulse through corticothalamic regions then occurs, resulting in the clinical manifestation of the seizure. Termination of seizure activity may occur because of the development of inhibitory impulses in the corticothalmic pathways. Depletion of neuronal metabolic substrates, energy stores, or neurotransmitters may also play a role in the termination of the seizure.

The causes of seizures are multiple and vary with age. Some common causes are listed in Table 10–1. As this list suggests, seizure patients represent a potentially large population of patients requiring emergent or critical care. In patients with preexisting epilepsy due to any cause, predisposing factors have been identified that make seizures more likely to occur. These include withdrawal or rapid tapering of anticonvulsants, use of alcohol, sleep deprivation (especially if coupled with another factor), infections, and fever. The scope of the problem is immense, and maximal therapy requires an understanding of the pathology, diagnosis, and

TABLE 10–1. Selected Causes of Seizures

Infections
Central nervous system
  Meningitis, encephalitis, abscess
Febrile illnesses
Metabolic Disorders/Toxins
Electrolyte imbalances
  Hypocalcemia, hypomagnesemia, hyponatremia,
    hypernatremia, hypoglycemia, nonketotic
    hyperglycemia
Inherited metabolic disorders
  Maple syrup disease, organic acidemias, etc.
Accidental/intentional toxic exposure/ingestion
  Heavy metals, drugs
Drug withdrawal
Hypoxia from any cause
Reye's syndrome
Trauma
Depressed skull fractures
Closed or open head trauma
Subdural/epidural hematoma
Structural Lesions
Tumor
Central nervous system malformations
Cerebrovascular disease
Intracerebral hematoma
Miscellaneous Causes
Idiopathic
Degenerative diseases

classification of seizures. Timely management is essential and most easily achieved with established treatment protocols.

Table 10–2 lists the International Classification of Epileptic Seizures. In general, if the event has been witnessed, it is relatively easy to obtain the historical information needed to determine that a seizure has occurred. Physical evidence of previous seizure activity includes tongue or lip biting, in-

TABLE 10–2. International Classification of Epileptic Seizures

I. Generalized seizures
  Tonic–clonic (grand mal)
  Absence (petit mal)
  Bilateral myoclonus
  Infantile spasms
  Akinetic
II. Partial seizures
  Simple
    Motor (including jacksonian)
    Sensory
    Affective
  Complex (temporal lobe or psychomotor)
III. Partial seizures with secondary generalization

continence of bowel or bladder, flaccidity immediately after the event, and a postictal state. Patients in the immediate postictal state often demonstrate a transient positive Babinski's sign. Physical examination should be directed toward the cause of the seizure. Laboratory studies may be useful in determining the precipitating or underlying cause of the seizure and should be ordered selectively. The most frequently occurring laboratory abnormality is probably subtherapeutic serum levels of anticonvulsant in patients on anticonvulsant medications, and these levels should be evaluated whenever appropriate.

A partial differential diagnosis of seizures is listed in Table 10–3. Pseudoseizures occurring in patients with known seizures are particularly difficult to differentiate from true seizures and can fool even the most experienced neurologists. Often, pseudoseizures are predicted by the patient, occur in situations in which the patient is likely to benefit from the attention the seizure would receive, and are associated with emotional extremes. Patients often cry, scream, or lash out during the pseudoseizure, and directed assaultive behavior is frequent. Postictal confusion is often not observed. Pseudoseizures are associated with a normal electroencephalogram (EEG), and, when possible, an EEG should be obtained to aid in the diagnosis. However, if this is impossible, it is best to treat the pseudoseizure as a real seizure and allow the diagnosis to be made at a later time under more controlled conditions.

TABLE 10–3. Differential Diagnosis of Seizures

Children
Infantile spasms
Breath holding
Spasmus nutans
Pavor nocturnus
Adults
Pseudoseizures
Syncope
Transient ischemic attack
Narcolepsy
Tics
Hyperventilation syndrome
Dissociative reactions
Fugue states
Drug/alcohol withdrawal
Cerebrovascular accident
Heat stroke
Coma (due to any cause)

CONDITIONS

Convulsive Status Epilepticus

Diagnosis

Convulsive status epilepticus is a condition in which a patient has had two or more generalized tonic–clonic seizures with no intervening recovery to neurologic baseline or interictal wakening. Approximately 60,000 to 120,000 patients develop convulsive status epilepticus each year, and in approximately 75% of these cases, a cause can be determined. Convulsive status epilepticus is rarely the initial presentation of an idiopathic seizure disorder, and it is not an expected event in the natural history of epilepsy. Less than 10% of patients with idiopathic seizure disorders will experience an episode of convulsive status epilepticus. The rapid or sudden withdrawal of anticonvulsants can precipitate status epilepticus seizures in patients with long-standing seizure disorders. Status epilepticus can occur in a number of primary disease states, including drug abstinence or withdrawal syndromes, hypoxic encephalopathy from any cause, meningitis, herpes encephalitis, hypertensive emergencies, intoxications or poisonings, or diseases resulting in hyponatremia or hypernatremia, hypoglycemia or hyperglycemia, and uremia. From 5 to 15% of chronic alcoholic patients experience seizures after the onset of drinking.

Despite advances in therapy, mortality from convulsive status epilepticus or its underlying cause remains at 10%. Immediate systemic complications of untreated convulsive status epilepticus include cardiac arrhythmias, respiratory dysfunction, systemic and cerebral acidosis, autonomic dysfunction resulting in hyperpyrexia, and excess fluid secretion resulting in dehydration. Delayed complications include aspiration syndromes, kidney failure due to rhabdomyolysis, disseminated intravascular coagulation, and hypoglycemia. When death is caused by the status epilepticus condition itself, it usually occurs from cardiovascular collapse, respiratory arrest, and ultimately cardiac arrest.

Prolonged seizure activity also has devastating cerebral effects. The cerebral metabolic rate is increased, and the depletion of energy stores and substrates for metabolism can result in cell death within 60 minutes after the start of the seizure; regional oxygen insufficiency may arise within as little as 20 minutes, leading to significant and sometimes permanent neuronal damage.

The dramatic presentation of patients in status epilepticus usually makes the diagnosis obvious, and events leading to morbidity and mortality from status epilepticus are well defined. Nonconvulsive status epilepticus can occur as petit mal (absence), complex partial (temporal lobe, psychomotor) status, and electromechanical disconnection (EMD), in which the motor activity of a generalized tonic–clonic seizure has ceased but the neuronal discharge continues. Continuous prolonged neuronal activity will result in cell damage even in the absence of motor activity. Clinically measurable memory deficits have been demonstrated in patients following prolonged partial complex status epilepticus. It is therefore essential to terminate this condition as quickly as possible in order to prevent subsequent neurologic deficit. Since clinical observation of these nonconvulsive states is often difficult, EEG monitoring can assist in the diagnosis and can also determine the effect of therapy in terminating the seizure activity. The EEG can also establish the presence of EMD and should be considered in all patients who have an extremely prolonged postictal state following the cessation of motor activity.

Initial laboratory assessment of the patient in status epilepticus should be directed toward detection of reversible causes of seizures. The most frequent laboratory abnormality is subtherapeutic anticonvulsant serum levels in patients with known seizure disorders. A urine toxicology screen and determination of blood electrolytes and magnesium, calcium, and phosphorus levels may be indicated in evaluation of the patient with status epilepticus. After termination of the seizure, the search for the precipitating cause may require a lumbar puncture, computed tomography (CT) of the head, and an EEG. If trauma has occurred secondary to the seizures, cervical spine x-ray evaluation may be indicated.

Indications for Treatment

Most seizures of any type occur singly and are short-lived; these situations usually do not require parenteral drug therapy. Emergent management of single seizures consists of maintenance of a patent airway and adequate oxygenation, hemodynamic stabilization, and evaluation for the cause of the seizure. Reversible causes, such as hypoglycemia, should be promptly treated.

Status epilepticus is a neurologic emergency, and rapid termination of seizures is best achieved by an established protocol using parenteral drug therapy. Most authorities believe that a seizure lasting longer than 5 to 10 minutes requires emergent drug intervention. Additional supportive measures, such as airway protection and hemodynamic support, should occur simultaneously with medical therapy.

The patient with frequently occurring intermittent seizures who never recovers to baseline between seizures should also be treated with parenteral drugs to prevent the recurrence of seizures. Emergent drug therapy is also indicated if a nonconvulsive status state is suspected or diagnosed.

Known seizure patients will occasionally experience an increase in the frequency of seizures because of inadequate prior medical therapy, medical noncompliance, progressive neurologic disease, or new neurologic insult. If these seizures are occurring so frequently (i.e., several times each day) that oral loading of drugs cannot be achieved safely, parenteral drug therapy is necessary to ensure that adequate anticonvulsant serum levels are quickly reached as the evaluation for precipitating causes proceeds. (See box.)

DRUG TREATMENT: CONVULSIVE STATUS EPILEPTICUS

First-Line Drugs
Diazepam (Valium)

Initial Dose	Adults, 2–5 mg IV over 1 minute
	Children, 0.1–0.3 mg/kg (up to 5 mg) IV over 1 minute
Repeat Dose	Every 5 minutes
End-Points	Termination of seizure activity
	Clinical signs of toxicity (e.g., respiratory depression, hypotension)
	Adults total dose = 20 mg
	Children <5 years, total dose = 5 mg; 5–10 years, total dose = 10 mg

OR

Lorazepam (Ativan)

Initial Dose	Adults, 2–4 mg IV over 1 minute
	Children, 1.5 mg IV over 1 minute
Repeat Dose	Every 5 minutes
End-Points	Termination of seizure activity
	Adults, total dose = 8 mg
	Children, total dose = 3.0 mg

Second-Line Drugs
Phenytoin (Dilantin)

Initial Dose	Adults, 15 mg/kg at no more than 50 mg/min
	Children, 15 mg/kg at no more than 3 mg/kg/min
Repeat Dose	5 mg/kg (total dose = 20 mg/kg) in 20 minutes

DRUG TREATMENT: CONVULSIVE STATUS EPILEPTICUS (continued)

End-Points   Termination of seizure

Adults, total dose = 1.5 g

Children, total dose = 20 mg/kg

Phenobarbital (Luminal)

Initial Dose   Adults, 10 mg/kg at no more than 60 mg/min

Children, 10 mg/kg at no more than 20 mg/min

Repeat Dose   10 mg/kg (to total of 20 mg/kg) after 30 minutes

End-Points   Termination of seizure

Adults, total dose = 600 mg acutely or 1.5 g over 24 hours

Children, total dose = 400 mg acutely

Third-Line Drugs

Lidocaine (Xylocaine)

Initial Dose   1.5–2.0 mg/kg at no more than 50 mg/min

Repeat Dose   0.5–1.0 mg/kg in 2–5 minutes (to total of 3.0 mg)

End-Points   Termination of seizure

Adults, total dose = no more than 300 mg

Children, total dose = 3 mg/kg

Paraldehyde (Paral)

Initial Dose   Adults: IM, 0.1–0.2 ml/kg (usually 5–10 ml); IV, 5 ml diluted 1:20 with normal saline, at a rate of 1 ml/min; per rectum, 4–8 ml delivered with normal saline flush; by nasogastric tube, 12 ml diluted with normal saline

Children: IM, 0.15 ml/kg; IV, 0.1–0.15 ml/kg diluted 1:20 with normal saline; per rectum, 0.3 ml/kg delivered with normal saline flush; by nasogastric tube, 0.3 ml/kg diluted with normal saline

Repeat Dose   Once in 20–30 minutes

End-Points   Termination of seizure

Total IM dose = 5–10 ml

Total IV dose = 0.3 ml/kg

Discussion

The goals of emergent management of status epilepticus are (1) to stop both the clinical and electrical seizure activity as soon as possible, (2) to prevent seizure recurrence by appropriate continued drug therapy, (3) to ensure adequate cardiovascular and respiratory status and adequate cerebral perfusion and oxygenation, (4) to identify and correct reversible precipitating factors, and (5) to readjust the metabolic and systemic detrimental effects of prolonged seizures. These goals are met simultaneously with airway and hemodynamic stabilization and parenteral drug therapy according to a preestablished logical protocol.

Simultaneously with drug therapy, the underlying cause of the seizure is sought and corrected if possible. The supply of oxygen and substrates for energy metabolism of the activated neurons is soon less than the demand because seizures increase the cerebral metabolic rate. Adequate oxygenation and cerebral perfusion are therefore essential to prevent prolonged hypoxia or substrate depletion at the epileptogenic site. Therefore, all seizure patients should receive supplemental oxygen and, if necessary, assisted ventilation or endotracheal intubation. An intravenous infusion of normal saline should be established as soon as possible in order to initiate drug therapy. An additional intravenous infusion containing 5% dextrose may be useful in the delivery of a steady supply of energy substrate to the brain tissue. Fluid administration should be kept to a minimum to avoid compounding the cerebral edema that is known to occur after prolonged seizure activity. Some reversible causes of seizures can be treated with 50% dextrose, thiamine, naloxone, and, in neonates, pyridoxine. These agents should be considered and, if appropriate, administered intravenously.

Drugs used in the emergency treatment of seizures must rapidly reach brain tissue in order to be effective. Drug delivery to brain tissue is influenced by cerebral blood flow. The ability of a drug to penetrate the blood–brain barrier depends on its lipid solubility, which is in turn influenced by the degree of ionization of the drug. Brain tissue levels of a drug depend on the binding and washout of the drug from the brain tissue, drug binding by biochemical compounds produced by cerebral metabolism, and the distribution half-life of the drug in the blood. Intravenous administration of most anticonvulsants used in emergency therapy of seizures will result in measurable drug levels within brain tissue within 10 seconds, and the drug is distributed through the entire blood volume within 1 minute after a single intravenous dose. Although many of these drugs can be given by other routes if necessary, intravenous administration is preferred because of predictable rapid distribution through the blood volume. In order to be maximally effective, adequate cerebral blood flow and oxygenation must be ensured with supportive measures during the seizure and in the postictal period. Since penetration of the drug through the blood–brain barrier depends on its pKa, serum pH can influence the ability of the drug to distribute to its site of action. Attempting to maintain serum pH at near-normal levels is therefore important in achieving maximal benefit of anticonvulsants.

Detrimental metabolic effects probably occur to discharging neurons within 20 minutes of the start of a seizure; therapy is therefore aimed at stopping the seizure within this time. If a selected drug has not been effective within this allotted time, another agent should be employed. The treatment of status epilepticus begins with administration of a rapidly acting benzodiazepine to stop the seizure completely, while simultaneously a parenteral loading dose of a longer-acting anticonvulsant is initiated. The first-line agent most widely used is diazepam: 33% of all seizures stop within 3 minutes after administration of the appropriate dose, and 80% stop within 5 minutes of the initial dose. Since the volume of distribution is great and the serum half-life of the drug is short, seizures are likely to recur within 20 minutes unless a longer-acting anticonvulsant is employed. Lorazepam is another benzodiazepine that is employed as a first-line anticonvulsant. It has been shown in animal studies to be up to five times more effective than diazepam in terminating prolonged seizure activity. It is less lipid-soluble than diazepam and therefore has a longer serum half-life. The effectiveness of lorazepam in terminating status epilepticus in humans has not been well studied, but preliminary reports suggest that it may be at least as effective as diazepam.

Phenytoin (Dilantin) has been used as an anticonvulsant since 1938 and is the drug of choice in prophylaxis of recurrent seizures. If first-line drugs are not effective in controlling status epilepticus or frequently recurring seizures within 20 minutes of their administration, phenytoin is employed for acute seizure control. It is effective for almost all seizures, is not sedating, and does not alter the neurologic examination. Hypotension is noted to occur occasionally during intravenous administration of phenytoin; this effect is due at least in part to the vehicle in which the drug is supplied. If hypotension occurs during the infusion, the rate of infusion should be slowed or the infusion discontinued. Fluids and/or vasopressors should be employed if additional hemodynamic support is needed. In addition to its use as an anticonvulsant, phenytoin is used for the treatment of cardiac dysrhythmias resulting from digitalis toxicity. Phenytoin has a direct effect on cardiac ventricular automaticity, and patients receiving phenytoin should be hemodynamically monitored. The decision to give loading doses of phenytoin to a patient who may have previously taken the drug should be directed by serum drug levels. If serum levels are not available, some clinicians recommend giving a full loading dose, since the immediate side effects of the drug (e.g., nystagmus, ataxia) are transient, mild, and not clinically significant. Others advise against this and express concern about the possibility of inducing potentially harmful cardiac or central nervous system (CNS) problems. These clinicians advocate a small intravenous dose (200 to 300 mg) pending serum drug level determinations.

Phenobarbital is a long-acting second-line anticonvulsant employed for prophylaxis against recurrence of seizures or for acute seizure control when first-line drugs have failed to terminate seizure activity. It is usually used after a trial of phenytoin but is occasionally used instead of phenytoin. Because of limited lipid solubility and relatively low concentrations of un-ionized drug at physiologic pH, phenobarbital penetrates the blood–brain barrier slowly, and after a single intravenous dose brain tissue levels may not be measurable for up to 20 minutes. Delayed sedative effects may be explained by this observation. Despite undetectable brain tissue levels, phenobarbital's anticonvulsant effect is felt within 5 minutes, leading to the speculation that CNS benefits may be present at very low CNS drug concentrations. It has also been postulated that phenobarbital concentrates in areas of the brain that have become acidic (i.e., the rapidly discharging epileptogenic focus) where more drug may be in the un-ionized state. At these sites, the concentration of the active drug would be higher than at other sites in the brain, and this could account for anticonvulsant action even when drug levels are undetectable in brain tissue in general. High *local* tissue drug levels but low overall tissue drug levels would also explain why patients receiving phenobarbital for acute seizure control benefit from its anticonvulsant effect without being affected by its sedative properties; these patients usually regain consciousness soon after the postictal state. Phenobarbital should be used cautiously in patients who have received benzodiazepines because the sedative effect may be additive. Respiratory support should be available to patients who receive phenobarbital.

In those rare instances in which the first- and second-line drugs have failed to terminate seizure activity, tertiary agents should be employed. Lidocaine has been successfully used in this fashion. The anticonvulsant activity of lidocaine was first noted about 25 years ago. Specific adverse effects of lidocaine administration are rare unless patients have underlying hepatic or renal disease. Paraldehyde is also employed occasionally as a third-line anticonvulsant. This drug may become of historical interest only, since its manufacturer may remove it from the market for economic reasons. Paraldehyde has a narrow therapeutic window between levels of drug that stop seizures and levels that cause sedation. Additionally, it can cause a metabolic acidosis, which is additive to the acidosis already present. For these reasons, its use is declining in favor of other drugs.

When standard drug therapy fails to stop seizure activity, therapy should be reassessed with consideration of the following. (1) Was adequate oxygenation and cerebral perfusion maintained during drug administration? (2) Was the dosing adequate? (3) Was the drug administered by the appropriate route? (4) Was appropriate therapy continued after the initial success? By the time first- through third-line drugs have been tried, the patient probably has been seizing for 60 minutes. If seizures persist, general anesthesia with neuromuscular blockade may be necessary to terminate the seizure.

The end-point of emergency parenteral drug therapy is not necessarily therapeutic serum drug levels but rather termination of acute seizure activity. Monitoring the clinical status of the patient and not the serum drug level is essential for appropriate management. If one anticonvulsant has been ineffective, a second should be employed, and serum drug levels of the first are meaningless in directing continued therapy of a seizing patient.

Prolonged Focal Status Epilepticus

Diagnosis

Focal status epilepticus is usually the result of a specific cerebral lesion. Although not as dramatic as convulsive status epilepticus and not as prone to significant medical complications, focal seizures often generalize to convulsive status. Additionally, as in convulsive status epilepticus, cerebral damage occurs even in the absence of motor activity unless neuronal electrical discharge is stopped as soon as possible.

Focal motor seizures (jacksonian seizures) frequently begin with tonic contractions of the fingers, face, or foot on one side of the body. The activity soon becomes clonic and spreads from the starting place to adjacent muscles. If the seizure stays confined to a particular group of muscles on the same side of the body, no alteration in consciousness occurs.

Focal motor status epilepticus is termed *epilepsia partialis continua.* The distal muscles of the arm or leg, particularly the flexor groups, are more affected than are the proximal groups. In most cases, an underlying abnormality such as a focal scar is identifiable as the seizure focus, although frequently the precipitating factor for focal status cannot be determined. Focal seizures may be the presenting sign of an intracranial mass, abscess, or hemorrhage. Metabolic abnormalities will not usually cause focal seizures.

An EEG will show focal abnormalities, and a CT scan may define the lesion. Additional laboratory work-up should be directed by historical and physical findings.

Although focal seizures by themselves are not life threatening, prolonged motor activity will produce lactic acidosis, electrolyte abnormalities, and potential renal damage from muscle anaerobic metabolism and tissue breakdown. Shifting electrolytes and acid–base status are potentially dangerous to cardiac muscle action and can precipitate fatal dysrhythmias.

Indications for Treatment

Focal status epilepticus is a neurologic emergency requiring rapid therapy to terminate the seizure activity. As with any seizure, the continuous neuronal discharge can rapidly deplete energy and oxygen stores of cerebral tissue, and detrimental biochemical effects occur within 20 minutes. Therefore, drug therapy should be given to terminate focal seizures that have persisted longer than 15 to 20 minutes. (See box.)

DRUG TREATMENT: FOCAL STATUS EPILEPTICUS

First-Line Drugs

Diazepam (Valium)

Initial Dose	Adults, 2–5 mg IV over 1 minute
	Children, 0.1–0.3 mg/kg IV (up to 5 mg) over 1 minute
Repeat Dose	Every 5 minutes
End-Points	Termination of seizure activity
	Clinical signs of toxicity (respiratory depression, hypotension)
	Adults, total dose = 20 mg
	Children <5 years, total dose = 5 mg; 5–10 years, total dose = 10 mg

OR

Lorazepam (Ativan)

Initial Dose	Adults, 2–4 mg IV over 1 minute
	Children, 1.5 mg IV over 1 minute
Repeat Dose	Once in 5 minutes
End-Points	Termination of seizure activity
	Adults, total dose = 8 mg
	Children, total dose = 3.0 mg

Second-Line Drugs

Phenytoin (Dilantin)

Initial Dose	Adults, 15 mg/kg at no more than 50 mg/min
	Children, 15 mg/kg at no more than 3 mg/kg/min

DRUG TREATMENT: FOCAL STATUS EPILEPTICUS (continued)

Repeat Dose   5 mg/kg (total dose = 20 mg/kg) in 20 minutes

End-Points   Termination of seizure

Adults, total dose = 1.5 g

Children, total dose = 20 mg/kg

OR

Phenobarbital (Luminal)

Initial Dose   Adults, 10 mg/kg at no more than 60 mg/min

Children, 10 mg/kg at no more than 20 mg/min

Repeat Dose   10 mg/kg (to total of 20 mg/kg) after 30 minutes

End-Points   Termination of seizure

Adults, total dose = 600 mg acutely or 1.5 g over 24 hours

Children, total dose = 400 mg acutely

Third-Line Drugs

Lidocaine (Xylocaine)

Initial Dose   1.5–2.0 mg/kg at no more than 50 mg/min

Repeat Dose   0.5–1.0 mg/kg in 2–5 minutes (to total of 3.0 mg)

End-Points   Termination of seizure

Adults, total dose = no more than 300 mg

Children, total dose = 3 mg/kg

Paraldehyde (Paral)

Initial Dose   Adults: IM, 0.1–0.2 mg/kg (usually 5–10 ml); IV, 5 ml diluted 1:20 with normal saline, at a rate of 1 ml/min; per rectum, 4–8 ml delivered with normal saline flush; by nasogastric tube, 12 ml diluted with normal saline

Children: IM, 0.15 mg/kg; IV, 0.1–0.15 ml/kg diluted 1:20 with normal saline; per rectum, 0.3 ml/kg delivered with normal saline flush; by nasogastric tube, 0.3 ml/kg diluted with normal saline

Repeat Dose   Once in 20–30 minutes

End-Points   Termination of seizure

Total IM dose = 5–10 ml

Total IV dose = 0.3 ml/kg

Discussion

As with all convulsing patients, attention to airway and hemodynamic parameters is essential for initial emergent therapy. Oxygen should be given and intravenous access obtained. A search for a precipitating cause should be initiated as therapy is begun. Particular attention should be paid to the metabolic status of the patient, which can be markedly abnormal as a result of the pro-longed muscle contraction and subsequent acidosis.

The general principles of drug therapy described under the section on convulsive status epilepticus hold true for the treatment of focal convulsive status epilepticus. As with convulsive status epilepticus, the first-line anticonvulsant employed for stopping seizures is diazepam. The dosing, route, and timing of administration are the same as for the treatment of convulsive status epilepticus. The success of lorazepam in the treatment of focal status epilepticus is not well described, but on a theoretical basis it should be effective. Phenytoin is the long-acting drug of choice for prophylaxis against recurrence of focal seizures or for termination of focal seizures not responsive to first-line therapy.

About 65% of focal seizures respond to the combination of diazepam and phenytoin. The use of additional parenteral therapy is not well described but should be considered if seizures persist despite adequate drug treatment. Surgical therapy directed at the causative lesion (in the case of an intracranial mass, hematoma, or abscess) usually will reduce the frequency of seizures. Surgical ablation of the epileptogenic focus has been performed in cases of intractable seizures.

Complex Febrile Seizures

Diagnosis

Febrile seizures occur primarily in children less than 6 years of age who have experienced a rapid change in body temperature as a result of an infectious process. Approximately 4% of all children will have one or more febrile seizures by 5 years of age. Most febrile seizures are generalized and occur singly; only 2 to 3% of children with febrile seizures will have more than one seizure within the same febrile illness. About 30% of children who have had a febrile seizure in the past will have another febrile seizure during a subsequent febrile illness.

Simple febrile seizures occur most frequently between the ages of 9 and 18 months, last less than 15 minutes, and are nonfocal. Following the seizure, complete neurologic recovery is the rule. A simple febrile seizure probably does not predispose to the later development of a seizure disorder. A febrile seizure is considered complex if it lasts longer than 20 minutes, is focal in nature, recurs within the same febrile episode, or is followed by a residual neurologic deficit. Subsequent development of a seizure disorder is more likely to occur following a complex febrile seizure than following a simple febrile seizure. Patients who have a recurrent seizure within 24 hours of the febrile seizure, have a family history of seizures or febrile seizures, or have a prior neurologic deficit are also at increased risk of developing epilepsy.

The diagnosis of febrile seizure can be made only if the patient is younger than 6 years of age, was previously seizure free, and has no primary neurologic illness or acute systemic metabolic disorder that could have caused the seizure. Seizures during febrile illness in children with preexisting neurologic or developmental abnormalities cannot be considered benign febrile seizures. Febrile seizures usually occur within 2 to 6 hours of the onset of the fever and are most often associated wtih body temperatures greater than 39°C.

Evaluation of the child with a febrile seizure is directed toward identifying the infectious source. The cause of the fever is usually extracranial; only 1% of patients younger than 7 years of age with febrile seizures have CNS infections. The most common infections are otitis media and pharyngitis/tonsillitis. However, up to 13% of cases of meningitis may present as a febrile seizure, especially in children younger than 2 years of age.

Laboratory evaluation should be directed by the history and physical examination. A complete blood count is useful in predicting bacteremia in children younger than 2 years of age with temperatures greater than 39°C. Electrolyte studies may occasionally show hypoglycemia, hyponatremia, or hypernatremia; these abnormal electrolyte levels could be the primary cause of a seizure regardless of the presence of a fever and should be ruled out. Electrolyte determinations are also useful in the assessment of the degree of hydration of the child. Calcium, magnesium, and phosphorus levels are rarely helpful in evaluation of seizures in previously healthy children. An EEG done at the time of the febrile seizure will be abnormal, but it should normalize within one week.

A chest x-ray and urinalysis may be indicated as part of the septic work-up if the fever source has not been identified by physical examination. The decision to perform a lumbar puncture (LP) must take into consideration the age and presentation of the child and the duration of the illness. Most authorities include an LP in a septic work-up if the child is younger than 2 years of age and/or is unable to demonstrate meningeal signs on examination. An LP should also be considered if there is no history of febrile seizures, recovery from the current seizure episode is prolonged, the current seizure was focal, or the child has been ill for longer than 48 hours. The index of suspicion for meningitis should be high in those patients who have had more than one seizure in the same febrile episode.

Indications for Treatment

Simple febrile seizures often occur at home or during emergency evaluation of the febrile child. The seizure is of short duration and stops spontaneously. Drug therapy in both the short and long run is usually not necessary.

With complex febrile seizures, prolonged focal or generalized seizure activity should be stopped immediately with parenteral drug therapy. Evaluation for other possibly reversible causes of seizures should be initiated concurrently with the acute management of the seizure. An active search for the infectious source should be initiated as soon as possible after the seizure has terminated. After acute management, continued long-term prophylactic anticonvulsant therapy is done at the discretion of the primary physician after discussion with the family. (See box.)

DRUG TREATMENT: PROLONGED COMPLEX FEBRILE SEIZURES

First-Line Drugs
Diazepam (Valium)

Initial Dose	0.1–0.3 mg/kg IV (up to 5 mg) over 1 minute
Repeat Dose	Every 5 minutes
End-Points	Termination of seizure activity
	Clinical signs of toxicity (respiratory depression, hypotension)
	Children <5 years old, total dose = 5 mg
	Children 5–10 years, total dose = 10 mg

OR

Lorazepam (Ativan)

Initial Dose	1.5 mg IV over 1 minute
Repeat Dose	Once in 5 minutes
End-Points	Termination of seizure activity
	Children, total dose = 3 mg

Second-Line Drugs
Phenobarbital (Luminal)

Initial Dose	IV, 10 mg/kg, mixed in 30–50 ml normal saline, over 5–10 minutes; IM, 10 mg/kg
Repeat Dose	Once in 30 minutes
End-Points	Termination of seizure activity
	Children, total dose = 400 mg acutely

Phenytoin (Dilantin)

Initial Dose	10–15 mg/kg IV, mixed in 30–50 ml normal saline, at no more than 3 mg/kg/min
Repeat Dose	5 mg/kg IV in 20 minutes
End-Points	Termination of seizure activity
	Children, total dose = 20 mg/kg

Discussion

The general principles of drug action and therapy described in the section on convulsive status epilpeticus also apply to the parenteral drugs used for the treatment of complex febrile seizures. Because a febrile seizure is usually an isolated event, subsequent treatment decisions are not as clear-cut as in the management of adult seizures. As with all seizures, prolonged neuronal discharge must be terminated to preserve normal cell function, and therefore prolonged

febrile seizures are treated with the goal of stopping seizure activity within 20 minutes.

A suggested management plan is presented in Figure 10–1. Although this plan is designed with the evaluation and management of febrile seizures in mind, it can be applied to all seizures in children, regardless of their cause. As with all critical patients, initial management steps are directed toward cardiopulmonary support. The airway of the child can usually be maintained by jaw-thrust or chin-lift manuevers or the place-

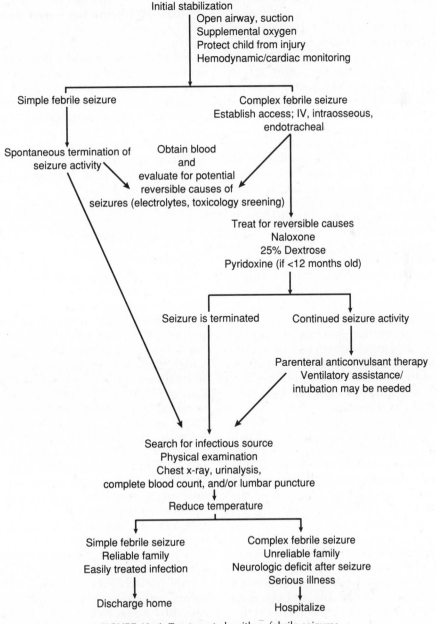

FIGURE 10–1. Treatment algorithm: febrile seizures.

ment of a nasopharyngeal airway. Intubation of children is difficult for clinicians who have little experience with children, and this intervention may be nearly impossible in the presence of seizures. It is therefore advisable to attempt to terminate the seizure activity, assist ventilation, and reassess the need for emergent intubation after the seizure has been terminated. On the other hand, actively discharging neurons rapidly deplete energy substrate stores, and conversion to anaerobic metabolism results in detrimental tissue lactic acidosis. If the seizure is prolonged, intubation may be the only method of providing adequate oxygenation to the brain.

Difficulty in establishing intravenous access in seizing children can delay essential anticonvulsant administration. The best route for drug administration is through an intravenous line; scalp veins and external jugular veins should not be overlooked in the search for peripheral intravenous access sites. All drugs used for acute control of seizures can be safely and effectively delivered by the intraosseous route. This technique allows rapid drug infusion into the marrow space. Measurable serum drug levels occur within a matter of minutes following intraosseous administration. Rectal administration of diazepam and paraldehyde has been used effectively if no other access site for drug delivery is available. A small feeding tube is placed in the rectum and the drug is flushed through with normal saline. If the patient has an endotracheal tube in place, diazepam can be delivered through it. The required amount of diazepam is diluted in about 3 ml of normal saline and delivered through the endotracheal tube. The patient is then rapidly ventilated for a few seconds to disperse the drug through the bronchial tree for rapid absorption.

Reversible causes of seizures in children should be considered, and dextrose and naloxone (Narcan) should be administered if indicated. Pyridoxine deficiency can present as late as 12 months after birth and frequently manifests only as seizures. Therefore, the administration of pyridoxine, 100 mg IV, should be considered.

Prolonged seizures unresponsive to initial stabilization should be treated with diazepam by any of the routes discussed earlier. Intramuscular injections are not indicated because absorption is variable and too slow to be of clinical benefit. Most complex fe-

brile seizures are very responsive to diazepam. Many clinicians use lorazepam as the benzodiazepine of choice for febrile seizures because it has less sedating and respiratory depressant effects than does diazepam. If benzodiazepines do not control the seizure, phenobarbital is usually the next drug administered. Phenobarbital should be used with caution if the patient has received a benzodiazepine because depressant and sedating effects are additive. It is relatively rapidly absorbed after intramuscular injection. Phenytoin is also an effective second-line drug for febrile seizures that can be used if first-line therapy has failed.

Once the seizure has been terminated, the search for the infectious source should begin. Persistent elevated temperatures should be lowered and treatment of the infection begun as soon as possible. The decision to continue anticonvulsant therapy is complex and depends on the patient's past medical history, family history, and the CNS status prior to and after the complex febrile seizure. However, most clinicians agree that children with a complex febrile seizure require hospitalization for subsequent observation and work-up.

Neonatal Seizures

Diagnosis

Seizures in neonates (infants 1 to 21 days of age) constitute a neurologic emergency, since the immature CNS of the newborn is highly susceptible to injury during stressful periods. The etiology of neonatal seizures can be determined in 70% of all cases, with a high incidence of underlying metabolic abnormalities as the precipitating cause. Other causes of neonatal seizures include anoxic cerebral injury, intracranial hemorrhage, cerebral anomalies, central nervous system infections, pyridoxine deficiency, and disorders of amino acid metabolism. A neonatal seizure can be a nonspecific sign of any severe illness that compromises cerebral blood flow or metabolism or a manifestation of acute drug withdrawal in infants born to mothers who used narcotics or other physiologically addicting drugs during pregnancy.

Seizures in the newborn are difficult to diagnose. Frequently, the first manifestation is a brief period of apnea. Tonic–clonic movements are rarely seen; tonic spasms, preceded by a few clonic jerks, may be the extent of the clinical presentation. The infant's pupils may dilate, the neck may become rigid, and the infant may drool excessively. Nystagmus, pallor, persistent staring, or hypotonia with no other signs or symptoms may be the only manifestation of a seizure in a newborn. Focal seizures may present as a few irregular jerky movements or as any other asymmetric sign. The poor differentiation of the seizure may be due to the lack of organization or myelinization of the immature CNS of the newborn.

Laboratory investigation must include evaluation of electrolyte and blood glucose levels. Magnesium, calcium, and phosphorus levels, although rarely useful in older children and adults, are essential studies in evaluation of a neonatal seizure. Additional laboratory studies may be warranted. These include a drug toxicology screen if drug ingestion by the mother is suspected; a CT scan or ultrasound study of the head, especially if the delivery was difficult and there is a potential for intracranial damage; and a septic work-up, including a lumbar puncture. An EEG will also provide useful information but is sometimes technically difficult to perform in newborns.

Hypoglycemia (blood glucose <30 mg/dl) is common among infants of diabetic mothers and can cause seizures that usually occur within the first 72 hours of life, especially if the infant is a poor feeder. Low blood glucose is also associated with sepsis and intracranial hemorrhage. Hypocalcemia occasionally causes neonatal seizures, usually between the fourth to the eighth days of life. Decreased magnesium, elevated glucose, and hyponatremia or hypernatremia are rare causes of neonatal seizures but must be evaluated in the initial work-up. Pyridoxine deficiency is a rare inherited disease that often is manifested clinically only by the occurrence of seizures within the first year of life. Seizures due to birth injury frequently develop between the second to the fifth days of life. Meningitis and sepsis must be considered in the differential diagnosis of all neonates with seizures.

Indications for Treatment

The occurrence of seizures in the newborn period signals the presence of a serious cerebral insult. The immature neonatal CNS cannot tolerate the seizure state for long before ischemic injury and neuronal death occur. Neonatal seizures therefore require emergent therapy to terminate seizure activity and prevent a recurrence. Reversible causes should be presumed; if seizures persist after administration of glucose, naloxone, and pyridoxine, parenteral anticonvulsant therapy should be given. (See box.)

Discussion

General principles of drug action and use are described in the section on convulsive status epilepticus. A protocol for the evaluation and management of neonatal seizures is presented in Figure 10–2. Immediate attention to oxygenation and airway control is essential. If possible, peripheral intravenous access should be obtained. Scalp and external jugular veins should not be overlooked as possible sites for intravenous access. An umbilical venous catheter, intraosseous line, saphenous venous cutdown, or endotracheal tube may be alternative routes for drug delivery if attempts at peripheral intravenous lines fail. Since reversible metabolic causes of seizures are common in neonates, initial management presumes their presence and dictates treatment. Intravenous access is therefore essential. Pyridoxine, 100 mg IV bolus, is given to treat seizures resulting from pyridoxine deficiency. The effect is immediate, and the drug is not associated with any reported adverse reactions. If the seizure stops, the diagnosis is presumed to be pyridoxine deficiency, and continuous daily therapy is started. Dextrose is administered at a concentration of 25% to avoid chemical irritation to the vasculature. The dose is 2 ml/kg, given as an IV bolus. Naloxone, 0.01 mg/kg IV, IM, by intraosseous infusion, or by endotracheal tube, will reverse drug-related seizures in neonates born to drug-abusing mothers.

Continued seizures require anticonvulsant therapy. Although diazepam is frequently listed as the first-line drug to terminate seizures, it must be used cautiously. In addition to its potential respiratory and CNS depressant effect, its chemical vehicle may interfere with bilirubin binding and alter the protein binding of the diazepam compound or other drugs given to the infant. Because of this, phenobarbital is sometimes the preferred first-line drug. In neonates, phenobarbital has a prolonged half-life of 40 to 100 hours, and therefore the dosing is somewhat lower than when it is used in older patients. Clinical signs of toxicity should be constantly sought when neonates receive phenobarbi-

DRUG TREATMENT: NEONATAL SEIZURES

First-Line Drugs

Phenobarbital (Luminal)

Initial Dose	10–15 mg/kg by slow IV push
Repeat Dose	One-half initial dose once in 20–30 minutes
End-Points	Termination of seizure
	Signs of clinical toxicity
	Total dose = 15–20 mg/kg

Diazepam (Valium)

Initial Dose	0.1–0.3 mg/kg by slow IV push
Repeat Dose	Every 5 minutes
End-Points	Termination of seizure
	Signs of clinical toxicity
	Total dose = 3–5 mg

Second-Line Drug

Phenytoin (Dilantin)

Initial Dose	10–15 mg/kg by slow IV push
Repeat Dose	5–10 mg/kg once in 20–30 minutes
End-Points	Termination of seizure
	Signs of clinical toxicity
	Total dose = 20 mg/kg

Third-Line Drugs

Lidocaine (Xylocaine)

Initial Dose	1.0–2.0 mg/kg by slow IV push
Repeat Dose	0.5–1.0 mg/kg once in 2–5 minutes
End-Points	Termination of seizure
	Signs of clinical toxicity
	Total dose = 3 mg/kg

Paraldehyde (Paral)

Initial Dose	0.2 ml/kg IM, per rectum, or IV
Repeat Dose	Once in 60 minutes
End-Points	Termination of seizure
	Signs of clinical toxicity
	Total dose = 0.4 mg/kg

tal. Phenytoin is employed if seizures have not responded to diazepam or phenobarbital. Phenytoin should be used with caution in jaundiced patients because it competes with bilirubin binding to albumin. High levels of bilirubin displace phenytoin from albumin and result in increased free active drug concentration in the serum.

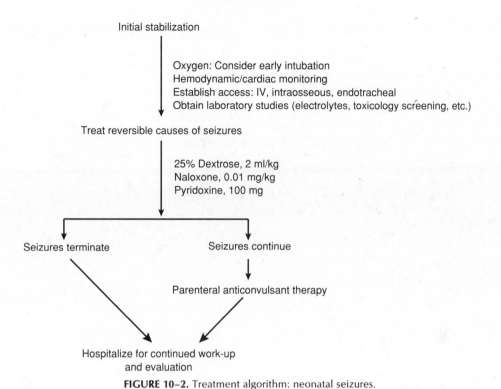

Initial stabilization

Oxygen: Consider early intubation
Hemodynamic/cardiac monitoring
Establish access: IV, intraosseous, endotracheal
Obtain laboratory studies (electrolytes, toxicology screening, etc.)

Treat reversible causes of seizures

25% Dextrose, 2 ml/kg
Naloxone, 0.01 mg/kg
Pyridoxine, 100 mg

Seizures terminate   Seizures continue

Parenteral anticonvulsant therapy

Hospitalize for continued work-up
and evaluation

FIGURE 10–2. Treatment algorithm: neonatal seizures.

Neurosurgical Problems and Prophylaxis

Diagnosis

Seizure control and prophylaxis are therapeutic concerns in certain neurosurgical emergencies and following certain neurosurgical procedures. The onset of first-time seizures in adults may be the initial manifestation of significant neurosurgical disease.

Seizures following head trauma account for 5 to 15% of acquired seizures, with peak incidence at age 20 to 40 years. The initial injury to the cerebral tissue may consist of shearing, crushing, and tearing forces. Shortly after trauma, cerebral edema and focal ischemia compound the tissue injury. The occurrence of seizures after head trauma depends on the severity of injury and degree of edema formation and is increased if the dura is disrupted. Most patients who develop seizures after penetrating head trauma will develop seizures within 1 hour after trauma is sustained. In this group, there is an equal incidence of focal and generalized seizures. Patients with open head trauma to the frontal region are three times more likely to develop generalized seizures than are other head trauma patients. Delayed seizures after head trauma (occurring more than 3 months after injury) are usually generalized.

Of new-onset seizures in adults, 10% are due to brain tumors, and up to 40% of tumors may present as a first-time seizure. The likelihood of seizures in brain tumor patients depends on the tumor type and growth rate and on the location of the mass. Tumor-related seizures are usually generalized. Metastatic disease to the brain can cause seizures and may be the first sign of the primary cancer.

Neurosurgical procedures that require incision of the dura result in increased risk of the development of postoperative seizures; prophylaxis is frequently initiated in the immediate postoperative period.

Indications for Treatment

Patients with known neurosurgical pathology who present actively convulsing require immediate first-line parenteral drug therapy to terminate the seizure activity as quickly as possible. Postictal patients should also receive anticonvulsants to reduce the risk of recurrent seizures.

Parenteral drug therapy for seizure prophylaxis is indicated in certain high-risk neurosurgical patients in whom oral drug loading is not possible, such as postoperative patients who remain obtunded after surgery. Patients who have sustained open head trauma are usually given parenteral drug prophylaxis for seizures. This is especially important if the trauma patient is to be transferred to another institution or if diagnostic studies, such as a CT scan, are to be performed outside of the emergency department or the intensive care unit in an area where close observation is not possible. (See box.)

DRUG TREATMENT: NEUROSURGICAL PROBLEMS AND PROPHYLAXIS

First-Line Drugs
Diazepam (Valium)

Initial Dose	Adults, 2–5 mg IV over 1 minute
	Children, 0.1–0.3 mg/kg (up to 5 mg) IV over 1 minute
Repeat Dose	Every 5 minutes
End-Points	Termination of seizure activity
	Clinical signs of toxicity (respiratory depression, hypotension)
	Adults, total dose = 20 mg
	Children <5 years, total dose = 5 mg; 5–10 years, total dose = 10 mg

OR

Lorazepam (Ativan)

Initial Dose	Adults, 4 mg IV over 1 minute
	Children, 1.5 mg IV over 1 minute
Repeat Dose	Once in 5 minutes
End-Points	Termination of seizure activity
	Adults, total dose = 8 mg
	Children, total dose = 3.0 mg

Second-Line Drug
Phenytoin (Dilantin)

Initial Dose	Adults, 15 mg/kg at no more than 50 mg/min
	Children, 15 mg/kg at no more than 3 mg/kg/min
Repeat Dose	5 mg/kg (total dose = 20 mg/kg) in 20 minutes
End-Points	Termination of seizure
	Adults, total dose = 1.5 g
	Children, total dose = 20 mg/kg

Third-Line Drugs
Lidocaine (Xylocaine)

Initial Dose	1.5–2.0 mg/kg; no more than 50 mg/min
Repeat Dose	0.5–1.0 mg/kg in 2–5 minutes (to total of 3.0 mg)

DRUG TREATMENT: NEUROSURGICAL PROBLEMS AND PROPHYLAXIS (continued)

End-Points   Termination of seizure

Adults, total dose = no more than 300 mg

Children, total dose = 3 mg/kg

Paraldehyde (Paral)

Initial Dose   Adults: IM, 0.1–0.2 ml/kg (usually 5–10 ml); IV, 5 ml diluted 1:20 with normal saline, at a rate of 1 ml/min; per rectum, 4–8 ml delivered with normal saline flush; by nasogastric tube, 12 ml diluted with normal saline

Children: IM, 0.15 ml/kg; IV, 0.1–0.15 ml/kg diluted 1:20 with normal saline; per rectum, 0.3 ml/kg delivered with normal saline flush; by nasogastric tube, 0.3 ml/kg diluted with normal saline

Repeat Dose   Once in 20–30 minutes

End-Points   Termination of seizure

Total IM dose = 5–10 ml

Total IV dose = 0.3 ml/kg

Discussion

The general principles of drug action and therapy described in the section on convulsive status epilepticus hold true for seizures resulting from neurosurgical problems and prophylactic therapy.

Most significant head trauma is not isolated, and the search for other trauma must be exhaustive. Initial stabilization includes assessment of airway, breathing, and circulation. Cervical spine injury must always be seriously considered in patients with significant head trauma and should be assumed to be present until proved otherwise. Spinal immobilization is therefore essential. Intravenous access is important to allow the administration of drugs and intravenous fluids if needed for hemodynamic stabilization. Patients with significant trauma and who present with decreased level of consciousness or seizures should be treated for reversible causes of coma; these patients should receive naloxone, dextrose, and thiamine. In addition to routine screening laboratory tests, a urine toxicology screen should be performed on the trauma patient with altered levels of consciousness or seizures.

A patient with head trauma who develops seizures will experience an acute increase in intracranial pressure during the seizure that can precipitate herniation syndrome in the presence of an intracranial mass (such as an acute hematoma). Termination and prevention of seizure activity are therefore important aspects in the initial care of patients with head trauma. As with control of seizures from most causes, the rapidly acting benzodiazepines are the first-line drugs used to terminate seizures. A longer-acting anticonvulsant is administered to prevent seizure recurrence. Although the administration of a drug with sedating properties (such as diazepam) is not the optimal treatment in patients with head trauma, acute seizure control is essential and best achieved by rapidly acting benzodiazepines. Phenytoin is the long-acting anticonvulsant of choice to be used if treatment with diazepam has failed and for prevention of subsequent seizures. Phenobarbital is avoided because it is sedating and can obscure the findings of the mental status examination.

Patients with depressed skull and/or open skull fractures are frequently given prophylactic anticonvulsant therapy even if no seizures have occurred. This is especially important if the patient is to be transferred to another institution or to an area where close observation is not possible. The drug of choice for prophylaxis of seizures is phenytoin. It is effective in preventing the occurrence of seizures and has the advantage of not causing sedation, which could interfere with the ongoing neurologic evaluation of the patient. Likewise, patients who have recently undergone high-risk neurosurgical procedures and who require seizure prophylaxis also usually receive phenytoin.

SPECIFIC AGENTS

Diazepam (Valium)

Pharmacology

Chemical Structure

Diazepam (7-chloro-1,3-dihydro-1-methyl-5-phenyl-2H-1,4-benzodiazepin-2-one), like all benzodiazepines, is synthesized by substitutions into the benzophenone ring. It is poorly soluble in water and is supplied in 40% propylene glycol at a pH of 6.4 to 6.9.

Distribution

Diazepam is highly lipid-soluble and rapidly distributes from the blood to lipid stores. Detectable brain tissue levels are reached within 10 seconds after an intravenous dose. Serum levels are negligible 20 minutes after a single intravenous dose. Because of its lipid solubility, the total volume of distribution is 133 l/kg. It is 98% protein bound.

Elimination

Serum levels of diazepam rapidly decline and result in an effective distribution half-life of 20 to 30 minutes. Because of its lipid storage, the elimination half-life is about 51 hours. It is metabolized by the liver, and three active metabolites contribute to its effect. It is excreted in the urine as active and inactive drug.

Actions

Diazepam probably controls seizures by enhancing inhibition pathways of gamma-aminobutyric acid (GABA) activity to suppress the spread of abnormal electrical discharge. Effects are exerted at the limbic, thalamic, and hypothalamic levels.

Indications

Diazepam is used for acute control of status epilepticus or severe recurrent seizures of all types until precipitating causes can be corrected and a longer-acting anticonvulsant can be given. It is also used for control of symptoms of acute alcohol withdrawal states and delirium tremens, relief of anxiety states, and treatment of muscle spasticity.

Cautions

Renal failure—lower doses should be administered chronically to patients with renal insufficiency, while carefully monitoring for signs of toxicity.

Cardiac failure—diazepam may produce a transient cardiac depression and should be used cautiously in patients with cardiac dysfunction. Impaired metabolism may occur in patients with decreased liver blood flow due to cardiac failure, and, if diazepam is used in such patients, lower doses should be employed.

Hepatic failure—metabolism of the drug is impaired, and, if used at all, lower doses should be employed.

Pregnancy—Category D. Elimination half-life is prolonged, and volume of distribution is increased, so lower doses should be used. The drug crosses the placenta and can be measured in breast milk. Chronic use of oral diazepam during pregnancy is associated with increased risk of oral palate deformities.

Other—dose should be reduced in the elderly because of changes in elimination half-life and volume of distribution. It is contraindicated in acute narrow-angle glaucoma.

Onset and Duration of Action

Dosage

Adults and children >10 years, 2–5 mg IV, over at least 1 minute

Children <10 years, 0.3 mg/kg IV, no more than 1 mg/minute

The drug is compatible with any intravenous solution. If given too slowly, it interacts with plastic intravenous containers and administration sets, which may decrease the amount of drug delivered.

Limits

The serum concentration for seizure control is 0.2 to 1.0 μg/ml but is rarely measured in clinical practice. Adults may receive a total of 20 mg for acute control of seizures. Children younger than 5 years of age should not receive more than 3 to 5 mg; children younger than 10 years of age should receive 5 to 10 mg maximum.

Repeat Dosing

The onset of anticonvulsant activity occurs between 1 and 5 minutes, with a duration of 20 minutes. Repeated doses are usually needed; the drug can be given in the same dose every 5 to 10 minutes until effective, until dosing limits are reached, or until any signs of toxicity occur.

Toxicity

Drug Interactions

Very common

Any drug that is highly protein bound could increase the serum level and enhance the action of diazepam.

CNS depressants, narcotics, antidepressants, antihistamines, and psychotropics have an additive sedative effect with diazepam.

Cimetidine and disulfiram inhibit metabolism and enhance the action of diazepam.

Lower doses of phenytoin are needed because of decreased liver metabolism.

Diazepam reduces the renal clearance of digoxin and potentiates its activity.

Adverse Effects

Respiratory depression is a risk, especially in newborns, infants, in patients with preexisting pulmonary disease, or in the presence of other CNS depressant drugs. Hypotension (in part due to the vehicle propylene glycol) and bradycardia can occur. If the drug is delivered into small veins, thrombophlebitis can occur.

Treatment of Toxicity

No antidote for overdosage of diazepam is currently available in the United States, although a benzodiazepine antagonist is used in some European countries. Treatment of toxicity is therefore supportive. Ventilatory support should be initiated if respiratory depression or arrest occurs. Hypotension induced by diazepam will usually respond to fluid administration; if not, a vasopressor such as dopamine or norepinephrine should be administered. Symptomatic bradycardia associated with intravenous diazepam is responsive to atropine. Diazepam is poorly dialyzable. Physostigmine, 0.5 to 4.0 mg IV, may reverse CNS and respiratory depression, but the risks of this antidote must be weighed against the benefits of its use.

Lidocaine (Xylocaine)

Pharmacology

Chemical Structure

Lidocaine (acetamide-2-(diethylamino)-N-(2,6-dimethylphenyl) monohydrochloride) is an amide-type local anesthetic. The drug is water- and lipid-soluble and is supplied with and without epinephrine in commercial preparations of pH 5 to 7.

Distribution

Lidocaine has a volume of distribution of about 1 l/kg. It is initially distributed rapidly through the blood volume and is then taken up by adipose tissue. Because of the combination of its lipid solubility and its favorable un-ionized state, the drug freely crosses the blood–brain barrier. Lidocaine binds to plasma proteins in a dose-dependent fashion. At its therapeutic concentration of 1.5 to 5 μg/ml, it is between 60 to 80% protein bound. Its pKa is 8 to 9, so it is largely in the un-ionized state at physiologic pH.

Elimination

As the blood level of lidocaine falls, the resulting concentration gradient between the blood and adipose tissue pulls the drug from its lipid-binding sites back into the bloodstream; blood levels therefore can exhibit a biphasic pattern. Its serum half-life is 1 to 2 hours. Lidocaine is 90% metabolized in the liver to one major active metabolite, which may contribute to its effects. About 10% of the drug is excreted unchanged in the urine.

Actions

The anticonvulsant action of lidocaine is not well understood; it probably exerts its effects by stabilizing neuronal membranes by preventing calcium uptake or by blocking sodium–potassium exchange during the process of membrane polarization and repolarization.

Indications

Acute control of status epilepticus and severe recurrent seizures of all types unresponsive to other therapy; especially useful in treatment of seizures caused by acute brain lesions and drug-induced seizures.

Acute control of many ventricular arrhythmias

Local anesthetic agent

Cautions

Renal failure—doses should be reduced by half in the presence of renal failure.

Cardiac failure—the rate of elimination of lidocaine is dependent on liver blood flow. Caution should therefore be exercised when giving the drug to patients with poor perfusion states such as congestive heart failure (administer half the normal dose). Patients with ventricular escape rhythms should not receive the drug for seizure control.

Hepatic failure—reduced doses (half dose) should be given, if the drug is used at all, in patients with severe liver disease.

Pregnancy—Category B. The use of lidocaine in pregnancy is not well studied; animal studies do not report harmful effects during pregnancy. Lidocaine crosses the placenta and is secreted into breast milk.

Other—a reduced dose (half of normal) is recommended in elderly or debilitated patients.

Onset and Duration of Action

Dosage

Loading dose: adults, 1.5 to 2.0 mg/kg IV (50 mg/min); children, 0.5 to 1.0 mg/kg IV (20 mg/min)

Maintenance infusion: adults, 1 to 4 mg/min; children, 10 to 20 μg/kg/min

Limits

The therapeutic window for lidocaine's anticonvulsant activity is narrow; doses resulting in blood levels >5.0 μg/ml can irritate cortical tissue and precipitate seizure activity. Onset of anticonvulsant action occurs in 60 to 90 seconds, and it has a duration of action of 10 to 20 minutes. Adults should not receive more than 300 mg of lidocaine in 1 hour. If seizures persist in children, the loading dose may be repeated once.

Repeat Dosing

If seizure activity continues after the loading dose has been delivered, another dose of 0.5 to 1.0 mg/kg (to a total dose of 3 mg/kg) can be given within 2 to 5 minutes.

Toxicity

Drug Interactions

Not well studied

Lidocaine potentiates drug action of neuromuscular blocking agents and antidysrhythmics.

Lidocaine's actions are potentiated by beta-blockers and cimetidine.

Lidocaine's action is reduced by phenytoin.

Adverse Effects

Adverse effects of lidocaine are dose related and are rare unless the patient has compromised hepatic or cardiac function. Extremely high plasma levels can cause hypotension, arrhythmias, cardiac arrest, and motor nerve paralysis with resultant respiratory arrest. CNS effects ranging from blurred vision to seizures and coma can occur.

Treatment of Toxicity

When any signs of toxicity occur, the administration of lidocaine should be discontinued and resuscitation begun. Airway management followed by hemodynamic support should be initiated promptly. Vasopressors may be needed if hypotension occurs. If seizures occur, diazepam should be administered.

Lorazepam (Ativan)

Pharmacology

Chemical Structure

Lorazepam (7-chloro-5-(2-chlorophenyl)-1,3-dihydro-3-hydroxy-2-H-1,4-benzodiazepin-2-one) is synthesized by substitution into the benzophenone ring. It is insoluble in water and is prepared in propylene glycol, polyethylene glycol, and benzyl alcohol.

Distribution

Detectable brain tissue levels of lorazepam are attained rapidly following a single intravenous dose. It is 85 to 90% protein bound. It is not as extensively distributed in lipids as is diazepam. Its volume of distribution is 12.0 l/kg.

Elimination

The elimination half-life is 15.7 hours. Lorazepam is metabolized by the liver, and no active metabolites are produced. The drug is excreted in the urine in an inactive form.

Actions

Lorazepam probably suppresses the epileptogenic focus by enhancement of GABA-mediated inhibitor pathways; it probably does not abolish abnormal discharge from the focus.

Indications

Acute control of nonstatus and status epilepticus and of severe recurrent seizures of all types until a longer-acting anticonvulsant can be given.

Relief of anxiety states; used for sedation.

Cautions

Renal failure—if used at all, administer lowest effective dose to avoid toxicity from reduced clearance.

Cardiac failure—may produce a transient cardiac depression; lorazepam should be used cautiously in patients with cardiac dysfunction.

Hepatic failure—not recommended for use in severe liver disease because of increased elimination half-life; for mild disease, administer lowest effective dose.

Pregnancy—Category D. Elimination half-life and volume of distribution are increased, and, if used at all, lower doses should be administered. In animal studies, fetal reabsorption and fetal loss are seen with high doses. Fetal abnormalities in humans have been noted with all benzodiazepines if given chronically during the first trimester of pregnancy. Lorazepam crosses the placenta and is secreted in breast milk. Neonates lack the liver maturity to biotransform the drug completely to its inactive metabolite and may experience prolonged effects.

Other—reduced doses should be used in the elderly. It is contraindicated in acute narrow-angle glaucoma.

Onset and Duration of Action

Dosage

Adults, 4.0 mg IV over 2 minutes
Children, 1.5 mg IV over 2 minutes

The drug is compatible with all intravenous solutions. It should be diluted with an equal volume of solution for intravenous delivery.

Limits

The serum concentration for seizure control is 30 to 100 ng/ml but is rarely measured in clinical practice. Adults should probably receive no more than 8 mg acutely, and children should not be given more than 3 mg.

Repeat Dosing

The onset of action is 3 minutes, and peak anticonvulsant action occurs within 45 to 60 minutes. The initial dose can be repeated in 5 minutes if no effect is observed. Because of its relatively long duration of action (up to 4 hours) repeat dosing is rarely needed.

Toxicity

Drug Interactions

Not well studied
CNS depressants, narcotics, antidepressants, psychotropics, and antihistamines produce additive sedative effects with lorazepam.

Scopolamine produces additive sedative effects, hallucinations, and agitation.

Adverse Effects

Occasional respiratory, CNS, and cardiovascular depressant effects but fewer than with other benzodiazepines. Complications are usually seen in the elderly or debilitated patients.

Treatment of Toxicity

The drug is poorly dialyzable. Physostigmine, 0.5 to 4.0 mg, may reverse the depressant effects of the drug; the potential risks of its use must be weighed against its benefits. Patients experiencing toxicity should receive maximal supportive therapy, as outlined for diazepam.

Paraldehyde (Paral)

Pharmacology

Chemical Structure

Paraldehyde (2,4,6-trimethyl, 1,3,5-trioxane) is a polymer of acetaldehyde. On exposure to light, it decomposes and is further oxidized to acetic acid.

Distribution

Paraldehyde is water-soluble and somewhat lipid-soluble. It is rapidly absorbed from the gastrointestinal tract and from intramuscular injection sites. Its cerebrospinal fluid levels are 25 to 30% lower than its corresponding blood levels regardless of the route of administration. The volume of distribution is not established.

Elimination

The drug is 80% metabolized in the liver. Most unmetabolized drug is excreted through the lungs by exhalation; only trace amounts are excreted in the urine. Its biologic half-life is 7.5 hours.

Actions

The mechanism of the anticonvulsant activity of paraldehyde has not been defined. It may exert its action by causing an imbalance between inhibitory and facilitory mechanisms involved in spread of seizure activity.

Indications

Acute control of status epilepticus resistant to other interventions

Alcohol withdrawal seizures and other symptoms of alcohol withdrawal

(Paraldehyde may become of historical interest only; its manufacturer may remove it from the market because of economic reasons.)

Cautions

Renal failure—no alteration in dosing necessary

Cardiac failure—no alteration in dosing necessary

Hepatic failure—use cautiously if at all and in reduced doses in patients with liver disease.

Pregnancy—Category C. Use during pregnancy is not well studied; it crosses the placenta and appears in measurable quantities in the fetal circulation. Neonates delivered shortly after administration of paraldehyde to the mother have experienced respiratory depression.

Other—patients with bronchospastic disease or other pulmonary disease may be unable to excrete the drug as expected, with resulting prolonged drug activity.

Onset and Duration of Action

Dosing

Adults: oral dose by nasogastric tube = 12 ml of 10% solution, diluted with normal saline; IM dose = 5 to 10 ml; IV dose = 5 ml diluted with 100 ml normal saline administered at a rate of 1 ml/min; rectal dose = 4 to 8 ml, delivered with normal saline flush, or in mineral oil as a retention enema

Children: oral dose by nasogastric tube = 0.3 ml/kg; IM dose = 0.15 ml/kg, or 6

ml/m² body surface area; IV dose = 0.1 to 0.15 ml/kg diluted with normal saline and delivered slowly; rectal dose = 0.3 ml/kg, delivered with normal saline flush (a rough dose of 1 ml/year of age, not to exceed 5 ml, and followed by a saline flush, can also be used)

Paraldehyde is incompatible with plastics and should be administered using glass equipment. It is extremely irritating if high doses of undiluted drug are given intramuscularly or by rectum. Rectal administration results in erratic absorption and mucosal irritation. Intramuscular injections must be deep into large muscles or absorption will be erratic, and tissue irritation or necrosis can occur.

Limits

Therapeutic serum concentration is reported to be from 34 to 150 μg/ml; brain tissue levels reach maximum concentrations within 30 to 60 minutes after administration by any route. Its onset of action for its hypnotic effect occurs in about 15 minutes; its onset for seizure control occurs in less than 15 minutes; its hypnotic effect lasts about 8 hours. There is a very narrow therapeutic window between blood levels that terminate seizures and those that cause sedation.

Repeat Dosing

If the first dose fails to terminate seizure activity, one dose may be repeated in 20 to 30 minutes.

Toxicity

Drug Interactions

Paraldehyde potentiates actions of CNS depressants, alcohol, anesthetics, tricyclic antidepressants, and monoamine oxidase inhibitors.

Paraldehyde's actions are reduced by disulfiram (also produces antabuse-like reaction).

Adverse Effects

Pulmonary symptoms, edema, and hemorrhage have been noted following intravenous administration. Right-sided heart failure and CNS depression are also reported. Severe metabolic acidosis can occur and may result in renal dysfunction.

Treatment of Toxicity

Airway stabilization and hemodynamic support should be initiated. Bicarbonate should be administered in cases of severe metabolic acidosis; hemodialysis or peritoneal dialysis may be necessary to treat the severe acidosis and oliguric acute renal failure. Ventilatory assistance may enhance elimination by exhalation. Paraldehyde itself is too rapidly absorbed by all routes to be bound to activated charcoal. Although theoretically dialyzable, paraldehyde has not been detected in the dialysate after hemodialysis, and no antidote is available to reverse its adverse effects.

Phenobarbital (Luminal Sodium)

Pharmacology

Chemical Structure

Phenobarbital (5-ethyl-5-phenylbarbituric acid) is a substituted pyrimidine derivative of barbituric acid. It is a long-acting barbiturate. It is available in solution with propylene glycol at a pH of 8.5 to 10.5, and the parenteral form is its sodium salt.

Distribution

Phenobarbital has limited lipid solubility and penetrates the blood–brain barrier slowly. Its volume of distribution is 0.8 to 1.0 l/kg. From 20 to 60% of the drug is protein bound. The pKa of phenobarbital is 7.4; at physiologic pH, 50% of the drug is un-ionized. Very small shifts of serum pH will alter the degree of ionization and can markedly affect its distribution.

Elimination

The plasma half-life of phenobarbital averages about 90 hours (36 hours to 6 days) in adults. Its half-life is shorter in children. Phenobarbital stimulates enzyme induction of at least the cytochrome P-450 and UDP–glucuronyl transferase systems, both of which are involved in its metabolism. About 60% of the drug is hydroxylated in the liver to one major inactive and several minor active metabolites. The remaining drug is excreted unchanged in the urine.

Actions

Phenobarbital probably selectively suppresses the epileptogenic focus by enhancing GABA-induced inhibition or prolonging the polarized state of the membrane through calcium entry blockade. It depresses postsynaptic activity and decreases the electrical potentials generated during seizure activity to prevent the spread of seizures.

Indications

Prophylaxis for all types of seizures except absence seizures

Drug of choice for control of febrile, neonatal, and alcohol withdrawal seizures

Second-line drug used instead of or in addition to phenytoin for the treatment of status epilepticus that has not responded to first-line anticonvulsants

Instead of phenytoin in sensitive patients (i.e., cardiac conduction abnormalities)

Cautions

Renal failure—lower chronic doses may be necessary in patients with renal dysfunction.

Cardiac failure—may produce myocardial depression; lower doses should be given.

Hepatic failure—lower doses should be administered in the presence of liver dysfunction.

Pregnancy—safe use in pregnancy not established; has been associated with fetal abnormalities. It can reduce uterine contractions and should be avoided during labor.

Other—may increase potential for respiratory compromise in the presence of prior pulmonary insufficiency. It may cause confusion and acute delirium in the elderly.

Onset and Duration of Action

Dosage

Initial IV dose = 10 mg/kg, at no more than 60 mg/min for adults and 20 mg/min for children

The drug will precipitate in acidic solutions but can be delivered through commonly used intravenous fluids.

Limits

Maximum anticonvulsant effects are seen at 30 minutes; duration of action is 4 to 6 hours. Anticonvulsant effects are seen within 5 minutes; sedative effects are delayed. Adults should receive no more than 600 mg acutely or no more than 1.5 g over 24 hours. Children should receive no more than 400 mg for acute seizure control. Serum levels of 15 to 45 μg/ml are considered therapeutic for seizure control.

Repeat Dosing

The dose may be repeated once after 30 minutes, for a total dose of 20 mg/kg. Patients receiving a repeat dose or who have previously received diazepam are at increased risk for respiratory depression.

Toxicity

Drug Interactions

Very common

Phenobarbital potentiates action (additive effect or decreased metabolism) of CNS depressants, alcohol, antipsychotics, antihistamines, tricyclic antidepressants, and doxycycline.

Phenobarbital reduces action (enhanced metabolism) of anticoagulants, beta-blockers, corticosteroids, digitalis, estrogens, haloperidol, methyldopa, oral contraceptives, phenothiazines, phenytoin, and quinidine.

Phenobarbital action is decreased (increased metabolism) by rifampin and other drugs that stimulate liver enzymes.

Phenobarbital action is increased (decreased metabolism, reduced protein binding) by chloramphenicol, disulfiram, monoamine oxidase inhibitors, sulfonamides, oral antihyperglycemics, and valproic acid.

Adverse Effects

CNS and respiratory depression can occur but is unusual unless more than 500 mg has been given or other depressant drugs are also present. Myocardial depression has been reported. In the presence of hypercapnia, phenobarbital administration has been associated with increased sedation and circulatory collapse.

Treatment of Toxicity

There is no specific antidote for phenobarbital toxicity. Phenobarbital is dialyzable, and urinary excretion of the drug is enhanced if the urine is made alkaline. Orally administered activated charcoal will reduce the serum half-life of phenobarbital; repeated dosing of charcoal has been shown to enhance the elimination of the drug and shorten the duration of CNS and respiratory depression. Maximum supportive care (i.e., intubation, vasopressors) may be necessary for patients who have toxic effects.

Phenytoin (Dilantin)

Pharmacology

Chemical Structure

Phenytoin (5,5-diphenylhydantoin) is a hydantoin derivative, structurally related to the barbiturates. The parenteral form is the sodium salt, which is supplied in 40% propylene glycol and buffered to a pH of 12 (the drug will precipitate in storage at a pH of 11.5). Its sodium content is approximately 0.2 mEq (4.5 mg)/ml.

Distribution

Phenytoin is rapidly distributed through the blood volume after intravenous administration and is highly lipid-soluble, crossing the blood–brain barrier within 3 to 6 minutes. Peak brain/blood ratios are reached in 20 to 30 minutes. Its pKa is 8.03 to 8.33, so it is almost completely in an un-ionized state at physiologic pH. Its volume of distribution is 0.9 l/kg following an intravenous load. Phenytoin is extensively bound (approximately 95%) by serum proteins.

Elimination

Elimination half-life follows zero-order kinetics and increases with increasing dose, between 7 to 42 hours (average is about 22 hours for the sodium salt). Phenytoin undergoes hepatic degradation to one major and a few minor inactive metabolites. The oxidative systems involved in its metabolism can become saturated, so small increases in dosing can result in large increases in drug levels. Only 1% of the drug is excreted unchanged in the urine.

Actions

Phenytoin probably prevents the spread of seizure activity by stabilizing neuronal cell membranes through alteration of ionic transmembrane flux of sodium ions during the spread of nerve impulses and by activating inhibitory pathways extending to the cerebral cortex. It may inhibit the release of neurotransmitters at the presynaptic membrane of the epileptogenic focus and may alter the activity of membrane enzymes at the focus, thereby inhibiting the seizure focus itself.

Indications

Prophylaxis of all types of recurrent seizures, except petit mal seizures; usually given after acute control of seizures has been achieved

For acute control of frequent recurrent seizures or status epilepticus, when short-acting agents are unsuccessful in initial management

For treatment of cardiac dysrhythmias due to digitalis

Cautions

Renal failure—elimination is prolonged in the presence of uremia; doses should be lowered in patients with renal dysfunction. Clinical signs of toxicity should be monitored.

Cardiac failure—it has direct effects on cardiac ventricular automaticity and should not be used in patients with high-degree atrioventricular heart blocks, sinoatrial blocks, sinus bradycardia, or Adams-Stokes syndrome.

Hepatic failure—metabolism is prolonged; dosage should be lowered and adjustment directed by serum blood levels.

Pregnancy—the metabolism and/or protein binding of phenytoin changes during pregnancy; pregnant women who chronically receive phenytoin for seizure control may experience an increase in seizure frequency even at serum drug levels that were therapeutic prior to pregnancy. Phenytoin crosses the placenta, and many fetal abnormalities have been reported to be associated with its use. The risk of fetal abnormalities must be considered against the benefit of rapidly terminating maternal seizure activity, which in itself poses a serious risk of hypoxia to the fetus. Phenytoin is excreted in breast milk, and large amounts can be ingested by the nursing infant.

Onset and Duration of Action

Dosage

IV loading dose = 15 to 18 mg/kg at 50 mg/min for adults and 3 mg/kg/min for children

Maintenance dose = 100 mg IV or PO every 6 hours for adults and 5 mg/kg IV or PO bid or tid for children up to 60 kg

In debilitated adults, the delivery rate should be at no more than 50 mg/2 to 3 min. Administer by slow intravenous push or diluted in 30 to 50 ml of normal saline by a continuous infusion. The drug is incompatible with many other drugs and is best delivered if given in a separate line and flushed with normal saline. Constant cardiac monitoring and frequent assessment of blood pressure during drug loading are recommended. Phenytoin loading in a patient who may have previously taken the drug should be directed by serum drug levels.

Limits

The usual adult dose is 1000 to 1500 mg. If seizures do not terminate within 20 to 30 minutes after the intravenous loading dose, another intravenous bolus, to a total dose of 20 mg/kg, should be given. The maximum dose should not exceed 1.5 g IV/24 hours in adults or 20 mg/kg/24 hours in children. Serum level measurements report the total (protein-bound and unbound) drug levels; for most patients, therapeutic serum levels are between 10 to 20 μg/ml.

Repeat Dosing

If seizures do not terminate within 20 to 30 minutes after the intravenous load, another intravenous bolus, to a total dose of 20 mg/kg, should be given. The maximum dose should not exceed 1.5 g/24 hours IV in adults or 20 mg/kg/24 hours in children.

Toxicity

Drug Interactions

Very common

Increased activity of phenytoin is caused by inhibited metabolism or displacement from serum protein with alcohol, chloramphenicol, cimetidine, diazepam, disulfiram, trimethoprim, valproate, and salicylates.

Decreased activity of phenytoin is caused by increased metabolism, occurring in the presence of barbiturates, theophylline, calcium, and antacids.

Decreased activity of other drugs is caused by increased metabolism, occurring in the presence of corticosteroids, coumarin, digitoxin, oral contraceptives, doxycycline, and furosemide.

Adverse Effects

Adverse effects of phenytoin are dose related. In acute therapy, CNS clinical signs seen at serum levels of 20 to 25 μg/ml include ataxia, diplopia, and nystagmus; at 30 μg/ml, patients are lethargic; and at 50 μg/

ml, coma can occur. Hypotension, resulting either from the drug itself or from the large volume of propylene glycol delivered with a full load of phenytoin, is also reported during intravenous infusion and is not related to dosing.

Treatment of Toxicity

If the systolic blood pressure drops by 20 mmHg or more during intravenous infusion, the rate of infusion should be slowed. Intravenous fluid bolus, MAST garment inflation, or infusion of a vasopressor should be used if necessary for hemodynamic support. If any change in the cardiac rhythm occurs during administration of an intravenous loading dose, the infusion should be slowed or terminated. CNS toxic effects are usually transient; if airway patency is in question in a lethargic or comatose patient, the patient should be intubated. There is no antidote for phenytoin, and it is poorly dialyzable.

REFERENCES

Celesia GG: Prognosis in convulsive status epilepticus. in Delgrado-Escueta AV, Wasterlain CG, Treiman DM, et al (eds): Advances in Neurology, Vol 34. New York, Raven Press, 1983, pp 55–59.

Dailey RH: Grand mal (major motor) seizures. In Callaham ML (ed): Current Therapy in Emergency Medicine. Toronto, Becker, 1987, pp 292–295.

Delgrado-Escueta AV, Enrile-Bascal F: Combination therapy for status epilepticus: IV diazepam and phenytoin. In Delgrado-Escueta AV, Wasterlain CG, Treiman DM, et al (eds): Advances in Neurology, Vol 34. New York, Raven Press, 1983, pp 477–485.

Delgrado-Escueta AV, Wasterlain C, Treiman DM: Status epilepticus: Summary. In Delgrado-Escueta AV, Wasterlain CG, Treiman, DM et al (eds): Advances in Neurology, Vol 34. New York, Raven Press, 1983, pp 537–541.

Dodson WE: Epilepsy in children. In Edlich RF, Spiker DA (eds): Current Emergency Therapy, 3rd ed. Rockville, MD, Aspen, 1986, pp 424–430.

Eisner FR, Turnbull TL, Howes DS, et al: Efficacy of a "standard" seizure workup in the emergency department. Ann Emerg Med 15(1); 33–39, 1986.

Gangeness DE, White RD: Emergency Pharmacology. Bowie, MD, Prentice-Hall, 1985.

Glaser GH: Medical complications of status epilepticus. In Delgrado-Escueta AV, Wasterlain CG, Treiman DM, et al (eds): Advances in Neurology, Vol 34. New York, Raven Press, 1983, pp 395–398.

Goldberg MA, McIntyre HB: Barbituates in the treatment of status epilepticus. In Delgrado-Escueta AV, Wasterlain CG, Treiman DM, et al (eds): Advances in Neurology, Vol 34. New York, Raven Press, 1983, pp 499–503.

Homan RW, Walker JE: Clinical studies of lorazepam in status epilepticus. In Delgrado-Escueta AV, Wasterlain CG, Treiman DM, et al (eds): Advances in Neurology, Vol 34. New York, Raven Press, 1983, pp 493–498.

Janz P: Etiology of convulsive status epilepticus. In Delgrado-Escueta AV, Wasterlain CG, Treiman DM, et al (eds): Advances in Neurology, Vol 34. New York, Raven Press, 1983, pp 47–54.

Katsrup EK, Olin BR, Hunsaker LM (eds): Drug Facts and Comparisons. Philadelphia, JB Lippincott, 1986.

Loebl S, Spratto G, Heckheimer E: The Nurse's Drug Handbook. New York, John Wiley & Sons, 1983.

McEvoy GK (ed): American Hospital Drug Formulary Drug Information 1987. Bethesda, MD, ASHP Publishers, 1987.

Pincus JH: Status epilepticus. In Edlich RF, Spiker DA (eds): Current Emergency Therapy, 3rd ed. Rockville, MD, Aspen, 1986, pp 430–433.

Seyffart G: Paraldehyde. In Haddad LM, Winchester JF (eds): Clinical Management of Poisoning and Drug Overdose. Philadelphia, WB Saunders, 1983, pp 410–412.

Tomlanovich MC, Yee AS: Seizures. In Rosen P, Baker FJ, Barkin RM, et al (eds): Emergency Medicine: Concepts and Clinical Practice. St Louis, CV Mosby, 1988, pp 1751–1771.

Treiman DM: General principles of treatment: Responsive and intractable status epilepticus in adults. In Delgrado-Escueta AV, Wasterlain CG, Treiman DM, et al (eds): Advances in Neurology, Vol 34. New York, Raven Press, 1983, pp 377–384.

Volow MR: Pseudoseizures: An overview. South Med J 79(5):600–607, 1986.

Wilder BJ: Efficacy of phenytoin in treatment of status epilepticus. In Delgrado-Escueta AV, Wasterlain CG, Treiman DM, et al (eds): Advances in Neurology, Vol 34. New York, Raven Press, 1983, pp 441–451.

Wilder BJ, Bruni J: Seizure Disorders: A Pharmocologic Approach to Treatment. New York, Raven Press, 1981.

Wilder BJ, Leppik I, Ramsay RE: Protocols for emergency room treatment of epileptic patients. Neurology Viewpoints, New Jersey, Parke-Davis Co, 1987, pp 1–9.

Woodbury DM, Penry JK, Pippenger CE (eds): Antiepileptic Drugs, 2nd ed. New York, Raven Press, 1982.

CHAPTER 11

Antiarrhythmics

W. BRIAN GIBLER, M.D.

INTRODUCTION

Rapid interpretation and treatment of cardiac arrhythmias are fundamental skills of the acute care physician. Basic understanding of cardiac electrophysiology and arrhythmia pathogenesis is required to differentiate atrial from ventricular arrhythmias. This knowledge allows the selection of appropriate treatment. Cardiac arrhythmia pathogenesis is briefly discussed in this chapter. Primary emphasis is placed on therapeutic maneuvers and drugs used in the adult patient. If known, the mechanism of action of the drugs is addressed.

Pathogenesis of Cardiac Tachyarrhythmias and Bradyarrhythmias

Cardiac tachyarrhythmias result from aberrations in impulse initiation or conduction. An ectopic focus in the atrial or ventricular myocardium can generate ventricular rates greater than 200 beats per minute. The adult patient tolerates this poorly, often decompensating from decreased oxygen supply to the myocardium. Reduced cardiac output from inadequately filled ventricles may result in impaired cerebral perfusion or cessation of myocardial work. Emergent treatment is necessary to suppress this ectopic cardiac pacemaker and resume normal impulse initiation from the sinoatrial (SA) node.

Conduction abnormalities may result in reentry tachyarrhythmias, which are caused when closed loops of rapidly conducted impulses effectively prevent normal sinus triggering of the ventricles. Such reentry pathways may be due to anatomic accessory pathways or functional pathways secondary to electrophysiologic differences between adjacent myocardial tissue. Accessory atrioventricular (AV) pathways cause supraventricular arrhythmias associated with the Wolff-Parkinson-White syndrome. Myocardial infarction may be associated with functional reentry pathways that cause cardiac arrhythmias, including atrial and ventricular fibrillation.

Bradyarrhythmias may result from suppression of SA nodal impulse generation or from defects in the conduction of this impulse. Myocardial infarction may cause either difficulty. Many antiarrhythmics, such as digitalis and beta-adrenergic blockers, may also cause AV blockade. Profound block of this atrial-generated impulse can allow other myocardial conducting tissue to begin initiating impulse production, usually at or below the level of the AV node. Complete dissociation of the ventricular pacemaker from the SA node, usually at a rate less than 40 beats per minute, often requires electrical pacing or pharmacologic therapy. The agents used in this therapy are discussed in later sections of this chapter.

Types of Antiarrhythmics and Their Actions

The antiarrhythmic agents are classified by a system designed to group drugs by their electrophysiologic effects on human myocardium. The action potential responsible for impulse origination, repolarization, or conduction in myocardial cells may be altered. Perturbation of the sodium "fast channels" by Class I drugs, such as lidocaine, phenytoin, and procainamide, can affect depolarization, repolarization, or impulse conduction. The subclasses of Class I agents allow selection of the desired effect in the individual patient, since it is recognized that these drugs have different effects on action potential duration and the refractory period. Class II agents antagonize beta-adrenergic receptors, acting as antiarrhythmics by slowing SA nodal excitation and prolonging conduction through the AV node. Bretylium and amiodarone comprise the Class III antiarrhythmic drug group. These agents prolong the action potential duration and refractoriness of the myocardium. Class IV antiarrhythmic drugs include calcium channel blockers such as verapamil. Verapamil acts by antagonizing calcium "slow" channels, such as those found in the AV node, thus slowing antegrade conduction. Drugs such as digitalis and magnesium have antiarrhythmic properties; however, these agents do not have a separate group classification.

Rationale for Arrhythmia Treatment

Cardiac arrhythmias may compromise the patient by decreasing cardiac output or ultimately deteriorating into ventricular fibrillation or asystole. Healthy adults tolerate wide extremes of heart rate through physiologic compensation of the vascular system. Maintenance of blood pressure necessary to sustain brain, heart, and renal perfusion allows pulse variability from 40 to 160 beats per minute without tissue ischemia. Rates outside this range in the healthy patient may cause inadequate organ oxygenation with symptoms such as anginal chest pain or syncope. In the patient with preexisting vascular disease of the heart or other major organ systems, symptomatic bradycardia or tachycardia may occur within this "normal boundary." Unfortunately, prolongation of ischemia with arrhythmias often causes a spiraling phenomenon. Prolonged hypoxia of the myocardium, for example, will decrease cardiac output and worsen ischemia. This cycle may evolve into frank cardiac arrest. Some arrhythmias will spontaneously degenerate into ventricular fibrillation or asystole, causing immediate cessation of meaningful cardiac output. Either mechanism for arrhythmia-induced loss of cardiac output is lethal unless it is rapidly diagnosed and treatment is initiated immediately. The urgency for treatment in the various atrial and ventricular arrhythmias will be explored based on these concepts.

Complications of Treatment

Complications associated with arrhythmia therapy may result from misdiagnosis of the arrhythmia or side effects of the antiarrhythmic drug. The differentiation between wide-complex supraventricular tachycardia and ventricular tachycardia can be difficult. Treatment of ventricular tachycardia with calcium channel blockers has been associated with rapid deterioration of the patient and death. Atrial fibrillation in patients with Wolff-Parkinson-White syndrome treated with agents that block AV nodal conduction may actually accelerate ventricular conduction through the accessory pathway. This rapid ventricular response may not be tolerated or may degenerate into ventricular fibrillation.

The proarrhythmic effect of antiarrhythmic drugs is becoming recognized as a major hazard in their use. Digitalis has a narrow therapeutic "window," with toxicity reflected by cardiac arrhythmias. Agents such as quinidine may prolong the QT interval, resulting in torsades de pointes, a malignant ventricular tachycardia. Flecainide and encainide, two of the newer Class Ic oral agents, frequently cause proarrhythmic adverse effects, and initial therapy with these agents must be carefully monitored. Any therapeutic regimen for acute cardiac arrhythmias requires constant monitoring for adverse effects or proarrhythmic complications. The complications associated with each agent are discussed in detail later in this chapter.

CONDITIONS

Supraventricular Tachyarrhythmias

Reentry and *increased automaticity* are considered to be the primary mechanisms causing supraventricular tachycardia. Reentry pathways may be present in the atria or AV node or may bypass the AV node by connecting the atria to the ventricles directly or to the infranodal conduction system. Increased automaticity usually results from an ectopic atrial or junctional focus firing impulses at an increased rate. The actual conduction system of the heart is normal. *Triggered activity* is another mechanism proposed for supraventricular tachycardia. If threshold potential amplitude is achieved, depolarizations in atrial myocardium can generate a rapid sustained impulse that is conducted through the normal cardiac electrical circuit. Digitalis-induced supraventricular tachycardia may result from this triggered activity.

Increased automaticity and triggered activity can cause junctional tachycardia and multifocal atrial tachycardia. Digitalis toxicity may be present, or an underlying disease of the heart or lungs can manifest itself through these arrhythmias. The reentry phenomenon is associated with most clinically significant supraventricular tachyarrhythmias, including atrial fibrillation and flutter and reentrant (paroxysmal) supraventricular tachycardia. The preexcitation syndromes, including the Wolff-Parkinson-White and Lown-Ganong-Levine syndromes, are associated with large reentrant circuits that bypass all or part of the AV node. These disease processes are discussed individually in the following sections.

Junctional Tachycardia
Diagnosis

Junctional tachycardia (JT) is a narrow-complex tachycardia with a QRS width < 0.12 second originating at the junction of the atria and the AV node or immediately below the AV node at the proximal portion of the His bundle. These two areas contain pacemaker cells that function if the sinus mechanism is not perceived by these specialized myocardial cells. The SA node may function independently from this new pacemaker unit, causing AV dissociation. Although the QRS complexes are usually similar to those seen in sinus rhythm, a wide-complex tachycardia may result from a right or left bundle branch block. The ventricular rate usually ranges from 100 to 150 beats per minute and P waves are absent. Multiple cardiac abnormalities, including myocarditis, acute inferior wall myocardial infarction, and recent valvular surgery, are associated with JT. Digitalis toxicity can initiate JT and must be considered if this arrhythmia is present.

Indications for Treatment

Hemodynamic compromise is unusual with JT because the ventricular rate seldom exceeds 130 to 140 per minute. Therapy for this arrhythmia includes treating the underlying disease, if possible. In patients with digitalis toxicity, digitalis preparations should be discontinued and hypokalemia and other electrolyte disorders should be corrected. Administration of digoxin immune Fab fragments may be considered if more rapid elimination of digitalis is necessary. Fab fragments are the active portion of cleared digoxin antibodies, which selectively bind to free digoxin. (See Fig. 11-1 and box.)

Discussion

Correction of the underlying disease process should be attempted if possible. Because JT is commonly seen as a manifestation of digitalis toxicity, this possibility should be explored in any presentation of this arrhythmia. Digitalis preparations should be stopped and hypokalemia corrected by slowing infusing up to 30 mEq/hour of KCl, to a total of 40 to 80 mEq. Other electrolyte abnormalities should also be corrected. The use of digitalis Fab antibody fragments will rapidly lower free serum digoxin levels.

Multifocal Atrial Tachycardia
Diagnosis

Multifocal atrial tachycardia (MAT) is an irregular supraventricular tachycardia that has a rate ranging from 100 to 200 beats per minute and is caused by multiple premature atrial beats, demonstrating P waves of at least three different morphologies. The baseline is isoelectric; however, varying PR intervals are noted along with many nonconducted P waves. Usually the sinus mechanism is competing with two or more atrial ectopic impulse generators.

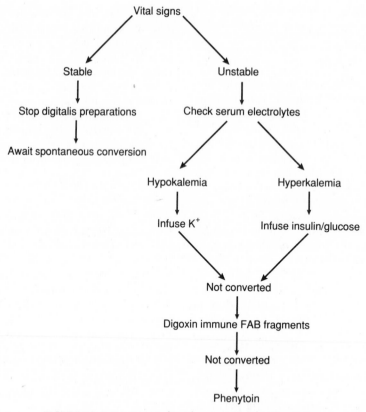

FIGURE 11–1. Treatment algorithm: junctional tachycardia.

DRUG TREATMENT: JUNCTIONAL TACHYCARDIA

First-Line Drug for Digitalis Toxicity
Digoxin Immune Fab Fragments

Dose	The amount of FAB fragments used should be in equimolar concentration to the suspected digoxin concentration present (see Table 11–1); initial small IV dose (1:100 dilution or 10 μg) to test for immediate hypersensitivity, then up to 20 vials (800 mg) given over 30 minutes; infuse through a 0.22-μm membrane filter. In the event of imminent cardiac arrest, bolus injection is given.
End-Points	Hypersensitivity reaction to antibody preparation
	Arrhythmia termination

Second-Line Drug
Phenytoin

Initial Dose	100 mg IV over 5 minutes
Repeat Dose	100 mg IV over 5 minutes until a full loading dose of 18 mg/kg is achieved
End-Points	Hypotension
	18 mg/kg loading dose
	Arrhythmia termination

TABLE 11–1. Estimated Dosages of Digoxin Immune Fab Fragments (Digibind) for Adults and Children

Approximate Digibind Dose for Reversal of a Single-Ingestion Digoxin Overdose

Number of Digoxin Tablets or Capsules Ingested°	Digibind Dose	
	(mg)	(No. Vials)
25	340	8.5
50	680	17
75	1000	25
100	1360	34
150	2000	50
200	2680	67

Adult Dose Estimate of Digibind (in No. of Vials) from Serum Digoxin Concentration

Patient Weight (kg)	Serum Digoxin Concentration (ng/ml)						
	1	2	4	8	12	16	20
40	0.5 v†	1 v	2 v	3 v	5 v	6 v	8 v
60	0.5 v	1 v	2 v	5 v	7 v	9 v	11 v
70	1 v	2 v	3 v	5 v	8 v	11 v	13 v
80	1 v	2 v	3 v	6 v	9 v	12 v	15 v
100	1 v	2 v	4 v	8 v	11 v	15 v	19 v

Infants and Children Dose Estimates of Digibind (in mg) from Serum Digoxin Concentration

Patient Weight (kg)	Serum Digoxin Concentration (ng/ml)						
	1	2	4	8	12	16	20
1	0.5‡ mg	1‡ mg	1.5† mg	3 mg	5 mg	6 mg	8 mg
3	1‡ mg	2‡ mg	5 mg	9 mg	13 mg	18 mg	22 mg
5	2‡ mg	4 mg	8 mg	15 mg	22 mg	30 mg	40 mg
10	4 mg	8 mg	15 mg	30 mg	40 mg	60 mg	80 mg
20	8 mg	15 mg	30 mg	60 mg	80 mg	120 mg	160 mg

(From Digibind package insert, Burroughs Wellcome Co., Research Triangle Park, NC.)
°0.25-mg tablets with 80% bioavailability.
†v = vials. One vial of Digibind = 40 mg of digoxin-specific Fab fragments.
‡Dilution of reconstituted vial to 1 mg/ml may be desirable.

Chronic obstructive pulmonary disease (COPD), theophylline toxicity, congestive heart failure, and sepsis are associated with this arrhythmia. Hemodynamic stability is initially not compromised, although a rapid ventricular rate may cause hypotension, particularly in patients with underlying pulmonary or cardiac disease.

Indications for Treatment

Hemodynamic instability with MAT may occur because the patient with pulmonary or cardiac disease may not tolerate an accelerated ventricular rate. Hypoxemia may exacerbate MAT or make it refractory to pharmacologic therapy and should be corrected. Underlying disease processes, including bronchospasm or congestive heart failure, should be treated.

A ventricular rate less than 100 beats per minute is defined as a wandering atrial pacemaker and does not require therapy. (See Fig. 11–2 and box.)

Discussion

Standard antiarrhythmics are ineffective in suppressing multiple atrial ectopic foci. The depression of AV nodal function with digitalis may result in toxicity, and this agent should be avoided. Reports describing verapamil combined with calcium gluconate therapy suggest that calcium channel blockage may effectively control ventricular rate in this supraventricular tachycardia. Magne-

DRUG TREATMENT: MULTIFOCAL ATRIAL TACHYCARDIA

First-Line Drug

Verapamil

Initial Dose	5–10 mg IV initially; may pretreat with calcium chloride, 1 g IV, if hypotension is a problem	
Repeat Dose	10 mg IV for a total of 20 mg or continuous IV infusion of 1–5 mg/hour	
End-Points	Hypotension	
	Total dose of 20 mg	
	Arrhythmia terminated	

Second-Line Drug

Magnesium Sulfate

Initial Dose	2 g IV over 10–20 minutes	
Repeat Dose	Infusion of 1–2 g/hour over 5 hours; maintain serum K^+ level > 4 mEq/liter	
End-Point	Arrhythmia terminated	

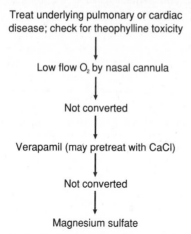

FIGURE 11–2. Treatment algorithm: multifocal atrial tachycardia.

sium sulfate offers an additional therapeutic agent as a general suppressor of atrial ectopy and should be considered with verapamil failure. Treatment of the underlying cardiac or pulmonary disorder, testing for theophylline toxicity, and correction of hypoxemia with oxygen therapy remain the primary therapeutic modalities in MAT.

Atrial Fibrillation
Diagnosis

Atrial fibrillation (AF) is one of the most frequently encountered supraventricular ar-

rhythmias. Multiple areas of atrial myocardium are depolarizing, repolarizing, and discharging repeatedly in a chaotic fashion, resulting in ineffectual atrial contractions. These foci are believed to represent multiple reentry circuits, giving an atrial electrical rate of greater than 400 beats per minute. With the loss of a coordinated atrial contraction, blood flow into the ventricles is impaired. The multiple electrical impulses from the fibrillating atria are not effectively transmitted to the ventricles because of the inherent refractory period of the AV node. Ventricular rates over 180 per minute are unusual in the healthy adult heart.

The electrocardiogram (ECG) in patients with AF will not demonstrate normal P waves. Instead, fibrillatory waves at a rate of 350 to 450 per minute will produce an irregular, nearly isoelectric baseline. QRS complexes will be irregularly irregular with rates up to 200 per minute. In patients with preexcitation syndromes, rates greater than 200 may occur. Accessory circuits may bypass the AV node, which normally prevents conduction at rates faster than 200 per minute.

Acute onset of AF is seen with acute myocardial infarction, alcohol intoxication ("holiday heart"), pulmonary embolism, pericarditis, and pneumonia. AF may also be chronic, developing in patients with hypertension, rheumatic mitral valve disease, ischemic heart disease, COPD, alcoholic cardio-myopathy, and thyrotoxicosis. It is important to differentiate acute from chronic AF as vascular stasis may result in thrombus formation within the chronically fibrillating atria. Electrical or chemical cardioversion can cause pulmonary or systemic embolization in patients with chronic AF. Anticoagulant therapy for two weeks prior to elective cardioversion is prudent in patients with chronic AF.

Indications for Treatment

Hemodynamic instability in acute or chronic AF is an indication for electrical cardioversion. Accelerating angina, congestive heart failure with pulmonary edema, or diminishing mentation from reduced cerebral perfusion demands rapid synchronized electrical cardioversion.

The acute onset of AF without decreased end-organ perfusion can be managed through pharmacologic therapy to decrease AV nodal conduction, slowing the ventricular rate. Treatment of the disease entity responsible for AF should be undertaken concurrently.

Cardioversion, either electrical or chemical, is unlikely to be successful in chronic AF, especially if the left atrium is dilated. If a patient with chronic AF presents with an acute rate acceleration that causes hemodynamic instability, electrical cardioversion may be attempted but will probably be unsuccessful. If cardioversion is initially successful but the patient quickly reverts to AF, further attempts at cardioversion will be fruitless, and the situation will require drug therapy for ventricular slowing. (See Fig. 11–3 and box.)

Discussion

Treatment of AF requires rapid intervention if the ventricular rate compromises cardiac output. All pharmacologic regimens described above are effective, and the decision to use a particular agent should reflect the urgency for reducing the ventricular rate and the underlying disease process, if any. Digitalization for reduction of ventricular response to atrial fibrillation is associated with a delay in onset of approximately 30 minutes. The serum potassium level should be determined after the first dose of digoxin to prevent the administration of additional digoxin to the patient with hypokalemia. Esmolol should not be given to patients with congestive heart failure, asthma, or COPD; it should be noted, however, that esmolol has demonstrated increased clinical safety when compared to longer-acting beta-blockers in patients with these conditions. Pretreatment with calcium gluconate may prevent hypotension associated with verapamil administration, while not altering AV nodal inhibition. Patients with AF should be questioned

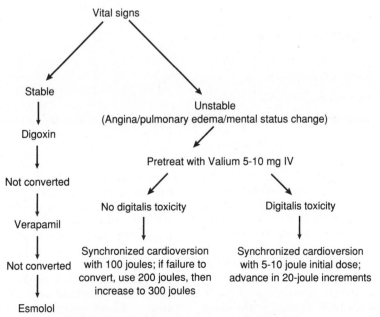

FIGURE 11–3. Treatment algorithm: atrial fibrillation.

DRUG TREATMENT: ATRIAL FIBRILLATION

If the patient is hemodynamically stable with an undesired rapid ventricular rate, all of the following are first-line agents; all modalities require that atropine, isoproterenol, and cardiac pacemaker equipment be nearby in the event of complete AV block.

First-Line Drugs

Digoxin

Initial Dose	Digoxin, 0.25–0.50 mg IV
Repeat Dose	0.25 mg IV given 30–60 minutes after initial dose. AV blockade may take 30 minutes or longer.
End-Points	Desired ventricular rate achieved
	Total of 1 mg given
	Development of complete AV blockade

Verapamil

Initial Dose	Verapamil, 5–10 mg IV given over 2–3 minutes; calcium gluconate, 1 g IV, can be used to pretreat or treat hypotension or complete heart block.
Repeat Dose	10 mg IV in 20–30 minutes
End-Points	20 mg total dose given
	Hypotension
	Development of complete AV blockade
	Desired ventricular rate achieved

Esmolol

Initial Dose	500 µg/kg loading dose over 1 minute, followed by a 4-minute infusion, starting with 50 µg/kg/min
Repeat Dose	Rate of infusion can be increased 50 µg/kg/min every 5 minutes, not to exceed 200 µg/kg/min. An additional loading dose of 500 µg/kg should be given with each increase in the infusion rate.
End-Points	Infusion rate of 200 µg/kg/min
	Hypotension
	Development of complete AV blockade
	Desired ventricular rate achieved

regarding possible accessory pathway disease, such as Wolff-Parkinson-White syndrome. AV nodal blockade in these patients may paradoxically accelerate ventricular rate as some fibrillatory impulses are transmitted in a competitive antegrade fashion through the AV node. AV nodal suppression with verapamil may result in chaotic rapid ventricular stimulation through the accessory pathway, sometimes resulting in ventricular fibrillation. These patients should receive synchronized electrical cardioversion. Acceleration of ventricular response to AF in any patient treated with drugs designed to slow AV conduction should alert the physician to the possibility of accessory pathway disease. The infusion of these agents should be stopped prior to cardioversion.

Chronic AF with a rapid ventricular rate, if previously treated with digitalis preparations, can be treated with digoxin until appropriate ventricular slowing occurs. Patients with chronic AF should receive anticoagulant therapy prior to cardioversion to prevent systemic or pulmonary embolization of atrial thrombi. Left atrial dilatation, however, is associated with likely degeneration of sinus rhythm into AF, and atrial enlargement should be investigated prior to attempted cardioversion.

Atrial Flutter

Diagnosis

Atrial reentry is the likely mechanism responsible for atrial flutter (AFL). Patients with acute myocardial infarction or recent cardiac surgery are prone to this atrial arrhythmia, which may cause hemodynamic impairment. Up to 10% of patients with acute myocardial infarction develop AFL, usually associated with a 2:1 AV block. As AFL generally has an atrial rate of 250 to 350 beats per minute, the ventricular response is often 150 per minute. In some cases, the presence of an accessory pathway or a short AV nodal refractory period will cause direct transmission of the atrial flutter rate to the ventricles. This 1:1 AV excitation is dangerous and may rapidly cause hemodynamic compromise. Rapid electrical cardioversion is indicated in these patients. AFL is not considered a chronic rhythm and usually degenerates into AF after several days.

The 12-lead ECG often demonstrates the classic "saw-tooth" morphology in the atrial waves, particularly visible in leads II, III, aVF, and V_1. The atrial rate will range from 250 to 350 beats per minute, with a ventricular rate of 150 per minute secondary to a 2:1 AV block. Carotid sinus massage may help diagnose this arrhythmia because it increases AV blockade of atrial impulse transmission, revealing the characteristic flutter waves hidden in the QRS complexes. Slowing of the ventricular rate with vagal maneuvers decreases the likelihood of an accessory pathway, since these techniques for increasing vagal tone do not affect accessory myocardial tissue.

Indications for Treatment

Hemodynamic compromise is an emergent indication for synchronized cardioversion of AFL. Patients with chest pain, altered mental status, pulmonary edema, or other evidence of end-organ ischemia are candidates for this regimen. A rapid ventricular rate not associated with end-organ hypoperfusion may be treated with pharmacologic agents that lengthen the AV nodal refractory period, slowing AV transmission of the atrial impulses. (See Fig. 11–4 and box.)

Discussion

Atrial flutter is sensitive to low-energy cardioversion. Synchronized cardioversion with

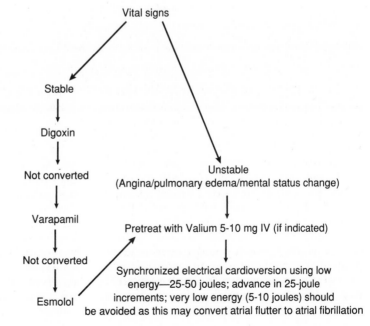

FIGURE 11–4. Treatment algorithm: atrial flutter.

DRUG TREATMENT: ATRIAL FLUTTER

First-Line Drugs

Digoxin

Initial Dose	Digoxin, 0.25–0.50 mg IV
Repeat Dose	0.25 mg IV given 30–60 minutes after initial dose. AV blockade may take 30 minutes or longer.
End-Points	Desired ventricular rate achieved
	Total of 1 mg given
	Development of complete AV blockade

Verapamil

Initial Dose	Verapamil, 5–10 mg IV given over 2–3 minutes; calcium gluconate, 1 g IV, can be used to pretreat or treat hypotension or complete heart block.
Repeat Dose	10 mg IV in 20–30 minutes
End-Points	20 mg total dose given
	Hypotension
	Development of complete AV blockade
	Desired ventricular rate achieved

Esmolol

Initial Dose	500 μg/kg loading dose over 1 minute, followed by a 4-minute infusion, starting with 50 μg/kg/min
Repeat Dose	Rate of infusion can be increased 50 μg/kg/min every 5 minutes, not to exceed 200 μg/kg/min. An additional loading dose of 500 μg/kg should be given with each increase in the infusion rate.
End-Points	Infusion rate of 200 μg/kg/min
	Hypotension
	Development of complete AV blockade
	Desired ventricular rate achieved

25 to 50 joules usually successfully terminates this arrhythmia. Hemodynamic instability should be treated in this fashion. Using very low energy cardioversion (5 to 10 joules) may only convert AFL to AF.

Verapamil and esmolol provide rapid AV nodal refractory period elongation, which slows the ventricular rate. Digoxin, although also effective, often requires at least 30 minutes to produce the desired effect, making this regimen less desirable for rapid ventricular slowing. Once AV nodal conduction is controlled, intravenous or oral procainamide or oral quinidine can be used to convert AFL to sinus rhythm.

Reentrant (Paroxysmal) Supraventricular Tachycardia

Diagnosis

In reentrant supraventricular tachycardia (PSVT), impulses from the atrial source are captured in a reentry circuit within the AV node. In some individuals, two parallel conduction pathways are present, one allowing faster impulse transmission than the other. Normally, these two pathways function together to transmit SA nodal impulses to the ventricles. An ectopic atrial impulse can be received by the AV node fast-conduction pathway while in a refractory period. As this impulse is transmitted along the slow-conduction pathway in an antegrade fashion, retrograde transmission of the impulse by the fast-conduction pathway results in the creation of a reentry circuit. Circular impulse production through this circuit continually travels down the bundle of His to fire the ventricles. The atria are depolarized repeatedly in a retrograde fashion, preventing normal SA nodal function.

The 12-lead ECG demonstrates a regular rhythm with a narrow QRS complex (<0.12 second). P waves from the retrograde depolarization of the atria may be hidden within or appear after the QRS complex. The ventricular rate usually ranges from 150 to 200 beats per minute. Aberrant conduction of these impulses due to a preexisting anatomic block or a rate-related functional block causes a wide-complex tachycardia. Distinguishing PSVT from ventricular tachycardia in these patients is nearly impossible. Wide QRS complex tachycardia will be considered in a separate section.

Indications for Treatment

Hemodynamic compromise with evidence of end-organ ischemia, such as angina, change in mental status, pulmonary edema, or hypotension, requires immediate synchronized cardioversion. If the patient is stable, increasing vagal tone through a variety of physical maneuvers may convert PSVT to sinus rhythm. Pharmacologic agents that decrease conduction through the AV node are used if vagal stimulation is ineffective in converting this arrhythmia. (See Fig. 11–5 and box.)

Discussion

PSVT is a supraventricular tachycardia that is readily treatable. Hemodynamic instability must be alleviated with electrical cardioversion. Although vagal maneuvers are routinely stressed as first-line management for PSVT, they are seldom effective alone. Combining pharmacologic AV nodal blockade using verapamil, adenosine, or esmolol

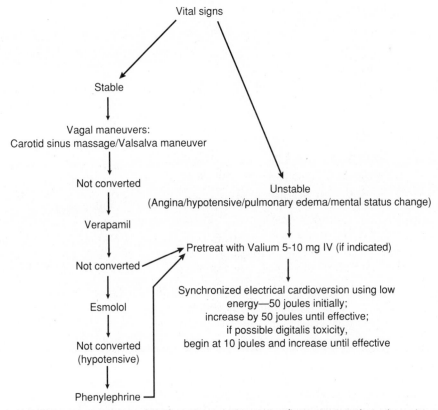

FIGURE 11–5. Treatment algorithm: reentrant (paroxysmal) supraventricular tachycardia.

DRUG TREATMENT: REENTRANT (PAROXYSMAL) SUPRAVENTRICULAR TACHYCARDIA

First-Line Drugs

Verapamil

Initial Dose	Verapamil, 5–10 mg IV given over 2–3 minutes; calcium gluconate, 1 g IV, can be used to pretreat or treat hypotension or complete heart block.
Repeat Dose	10 mg IV in 20–30 minutes
End-Points	20 mg total dose given
	Hypotension
	Development of complete AV blockade
	Desired ventricular rate achieved

Adenosine

Initial Dose	Adenosine, 6 mg IV given as a rapid 1- to 2-second bolus, followed by a saline flush of the IV line
Repeat Dose	If the initial 6-mg dose is not successful within 2 minutes, 12 mg should be given as a rapid 1- to 2-second bolus.
End-Points	18 mg total dose given
	Hypotension
	Development of complete AV blockade
	Arrhythmia termination

Esmolol

Initial Dose	500 μg/kg loading dose over 1 minute, followed by a 4-minute infusion, starting with 50 μg/kg/min
Repeat Dose	Rate of infusion can be increased 50 μg/kg/min every 5 minutes, not to exceed 200 μg/kg/min. An additional loading dose of 500 μg/kg should be given with each increase in the infusion rate.
End-Points	Infusion rate of 200 μg/kg/min
	Hypotension
	Development of complete AV blockade
	Desired ventricular rate achieved

Phenylephrine

Initial Dose	Mix 30–60 mg in 500 ml D_5W and infuse by IV drip, closely monitoring blood pressure; keep diastolic blood pressure < 130 mmHg; may combine with carotid sinus massage to increase effectiveness.
Repeat Dose	Infusion should be discontinued on termination of arrhythmia.
End-Points	Diastolic blood pressure > 130 mmHg
	Arrhythmia terminated

with vagal stimulation may increase the likelihood of conversion in PSVT.

Preexcitation Syndromes with Supraventricular Tachycardia

Diagnosis

This atrial arrhythmia group is perhaps the most interesting and challenging for the acute care physician. Preexcitation syndromes (PES) imply the existence of accessory myocardial conduction pathways connecting the atria to the infranodal conducting system or directly to the ventricles. The Wolff-Parkinson-White (WPW) syndrome activates the ventricular muscle mass directly from the atria through the Kent bundle. This myogenic connection bypasses the AV node and conducting system. A narrow QRS complex is most often seen in WPW because the AV node tends to have a shorter refractory period than does the accessory pathway, allowing normal conduction through the AV node. If the bypass connection has a shorter refractory period than does the AV node, however, more atrial impulses will be conducted through the Kent bundle, resulting in a wide QRS complex. James fibers, associated with the Lown-Ganong-Levine (LGL) syndrome, connect the atria directly to the infranodal conducting system. Some accessory myogenic pathways connect the AV node, His bundle, or bundle branches directly into the ventricle and are termed the *Mahaim bundles.* Through a reentrant mechanism using the accessory pathway and the normal AV nodal circuit, a narrow-complex or wide-complex tachycardia can be produced.

Electrocardiographic features of the WPW syndrome include a short PR interval (<0.12 second) with initial slurring of the QRS complex, resulting in a delta wave. The Kent bundle serves as an anatomic bypass of the AV node, allowing early depolarization of the ventricles with standard excitation through the AV node. In the LGL syndrome, the connection of the James fibers directly to the infranodal conducting system produces a short PR interval without the delta wave characteristic of the WPW syndrome. In SVT, reentrant ventricular excitation in the WPW syndrome, which occurs through the standard antegrade AV nodal conduction system, results in a narrow-complex tachycardia with a rate ranging from 150 to 200 beats per minute. Atrial excitation is accomplished

through retrograde conduction of ventricular depolarization by the accessory pathways. This occurs in 80% of cases of SVT associated with WPW. Retrograde depolarization of the atria through the AV node with antegrade excitation of the ventricles causes a wide-complex tachycardia. This is present in less than 5% of patients with WPW. Atrial fibrillation in patients with WPW allows rapid conduction of the fibrillatory waves through the Kent bundle, resulting in a wide QRS complex that is irregular on a 12-lead ECG. AV nodal blockade in patients with WPW and antegrade excitation of the ventricles through the Kent bundle may be disastrous, converting SVT into ventricular fibrillation. The hemodynamically stable patient presenting emergently should be questioned about a previous history of WPW or LGL, especially in the presence of a wide-complex tachycardia with AF. Wide-complex supraventricular tachycardia and its distinction from ventricular tachycardia are discussed in a later section.

Indications for Treatment

Synchronized cardioversion remains the appropriate treatment for hemodynamic instability associated with tachycardia resulting from PES, including wide-complex SVT. Complaints of angina, change in mental status, pulmonary edema, or hypotension should be promptly treated with electrical cardioversion. Stable patients may receive vagal maneuvers including carotid sinus massage or Valsalva maneuver. If vagal stimulation is unsuccessful, pharmacologic therapy is indicated, with verapamil as the drug of choice. (See Fig. 11–6 and boxes, Drug Treatment: Narrow-Complex Supraventricular Tachycardia and Drug Treatment: Atrial Fibrillation in Wolff-Parkinson-White Syndrome.)

Discussion

The treatment of PES SVT requires understanding the interaction of an accessory pathway with the normal AV node/His bundle conduction system. Treatment of reentrant SVT, particularly in the WPW syndrome, may be hazardous if the direction of the depolarization current is not known. Excitation of the ventricles through the AV nodal system represents antegrade conduction, which is represented by a narrow-complex QRS on the 12-lead ECG. Retrograde

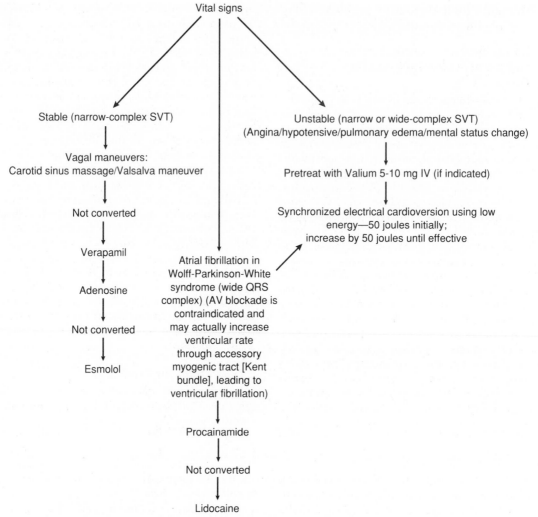

FIGURE 11–6. Treatment algorithm: preexcitation syndrome supraventricular tachycardia.

DRUG TREATMENT: NARROW-COMPLEX SUPRAVENTRICULAR TACHYCARDIA

First-Line Drugs

Verapamil

Initial Dose   Verapamil, 5–10 mg IV given over 2–3 minutes; calcium gluconate, 1 g IV, can be used to pretreat or treat hypotension or complete heart block.

Repeat Dose   10 mg IV in 20–30 minutes

End-Points   20 mg total dose given

Hypotension

Development of complete AV blockade

Arrhythmia terminated

DRUG TREATMENT: NARROW-COMPLEX SUPRAVENTRICULAR TACHYCARDIA *Continued*

Adenosine

Initial Dose	Adenosine, 6 mg IV given as a rapid 1- to 2-second bolus, followed by a saline flush of the IV line
Repeat Dose	If the initial 6-mg dose is not successful within 2 minutes, 12 mg should be given as a rapid 1- to 2-second bolus.
End-Points	18 mg total dose given
	Hypotension
	Development of complete AV blockade
	Arrhythmia termination

Esmolol

Initial Dose	500 μg/kg loading dose over 1 minute, followed by a 4-minute infusion, starting with 50 μg/kg/min
Repeat Dose	Rate of infusion can be increased 50 μg/kg/min every 5 minutes, not to exceed 200 μg/kg/min. An additional loading dose of 500 μg/kg should be given with each increase in the infusion rate.
End-Points	Infusion rate of 200 μg/kg/min
	Hypotension
	Development of complete AV blockade
	Arrhythmia terminated

DRUG TREATMENT: ATRIAL FIBRILLATION IN WOLFF-PARKINSON-WHITE SYNDROME (WIDE QRS COMPLEX)

First-Line Drug
Procainamide

Initial Dose	20 mg/min until arrhythmia is converted
Repeat Dose	Infusion, 1–4 mg/min, to prevent arrhythmia recurrence
End-Points	QRS duration is increased by 50% of original width
	Hypotension develops
	Total dose 1 g

Second-Line Drug
Lidocaine

Initial Dose	1 mg/kg initial bolus (75–100 mg)
Repeat Dose	Infusion may be given at 2–4 mg/min to prevent recurrence.
	Second bolus, 0.5–0.75 mg/kg, 15–20 minutes later
End-Points	Arrhythmia terminated
	Toxic effects such as seizures, central nervous system changes, AV heart block

conduction through the AV node implies antegrade excitation of the ventricles through the accessory Kent bundle, causing a wide-complex QRS. SVT in WPW with a regular-rate wide-complex QRS can be very difficult to distinguish from ventricular tachycardia and must be treated with extreme caution. AV nodal blockade with verapamil is not indicated. Similarly, atrial fibrillation in WPW may actually result in a hazardous increase in ventricular rate with inhibition of the AV node. This arrhythmia should be treated with procainamide or lidocaine to decrease conduction through the accessory pathway. This allows the native slower conduction rate of the AV nodal system to become the major conductor of atrial impulses to the ventricles.

Bradyarrhythmias

Sinus Bradycardia and Conduction System Blockade

Diagnosis

A decrease in the discharge rate of the SA node or difficulty in the transmission of impulses through the ventricular conduction system may be caused by pharmacologic agents or pathologic conditions. Beta-adrenergic antagonists such as propranolol, as well as digitalis and quinidine, can cause bradycardia of sufficient magnitude to hinder cardiac output. Pathologic conditions associated with bradycardia include SA or AV nodal injury or damage to the heart's conductive system from acute myocardial infarction, hypothyroidism, or carotid sinus hypersensitivity. As impulses conducted through the vagus nerve regulate the rate of SA node discharge, pharmacologic therapy is targeted at this site.

The ECG in sinus bradycardia demonstrates a normal P wave and PR interval and 1:1 atrial:ventricular conduction with a rate less than 60 per minute. If suppression of the AV node is sufficient to prevent ventricular depolarization by atrial impulses, or if a functional block of the distal conduction system exists, secondary pacemaker cells within the heart will begin to pace the heart. This pacemaker usually proceeds at a rate slower than that of the SA node. Junctional pacemakers within the AV node may excite the ventricles in the usual fashion, resulting in a narrow QRS complex. Distal conduction system pacemakers or actual ventricular myocardial cell rhythmic depolarization will cause a wide QRS complex regular bradycardic rhythm, usually at rates ranging from 40 to 50 beats per minute.

Indications for Treatment

Hemodynamic instability with bradycardia requires immediate intervention because decreasing cardiac output produces myocardial ischemia, worsening cardiac output further. Bradycardia in the setting of acute myocardial infarction, particularly with increasing AV block, may progress to electrical dissociation of the atria and ventricles. An external or transvenous pacemaker is necessary in complete heart block and should be considered in Mobitz Type II second-degree block secondary to acute myocardial infarction, even in asymptomatic patients. (See Fig. 11–7 and box.)

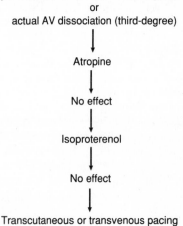

Sinus/junctional/ventricular bradycardia, hemodynamically unstable or advanced AV block (second-degree Type II)
or
actual AV dissociation (third-degree)

↓

Atropine

↓

No effect

↓

Isoproterenol

↓

No effect

↓

Transcutaneous or transvenous pacing

FIGURE 11–7. Treatment algorithm: bradycardia.

DRUG TREATMENT: BRADYCARDIA

First-Line Drug
Atropine

Initial Dose	0.5 mg IV
Repeat Dose	0.5 mg IV every 5 minutes
End-Points	Heart rate 60–80/min with adequate end-organ perfusion
	Total 2 mg

Second-Line Drug
Isoproterenol

Initial Dose	1 mg is added to 500 ml D_5W; this gives a concentration of 2 μg/ml; infuse at 2–20 μg/min to obtain a heart rate of 60–80/min.
Repeat Dose	Titrate rate of IV infusion to desired heart rate of 60–80/min.
End-Points	Infusion rate of 20 μg/min without desired change in heart rate
	Hypotension
	Development of cardiac arrhythmias

Discussion

Symptomatic bradycardia or progressive heart block must be treated aggressively to prevent worsening cardiac output from myocardial ischemia. Atropine produces vagolysis, which is effective in increasing heart rate if prolonged myocardial ischemia has not been present. Isoproterenol is a pure beta-adrenergic receptor stimulator; however, because of peripheral vasodilation, the use of this agent may not be appropriate in the presence of hypotension. Early intervention with transcutaneous pacing may be lifesaving in these conditions if pharmacologic therapy is not helpful. Transvenous pacing of the heart should be established as soon as feasible in the presence of Mobitz Type II second-degree heart block or complete AV dissociation. Hemodynamically unstable bradycardia of any type responsive only to transcutaneous pacing is another indication for transvenous pacing. Ideally, acceleration of the heart rate by means of drugs or electrical pacing should increase heart rate to a degree that will maximize cardiac output without causing excessive myocardial oxygen demand. Maintaining a heart rate of 60 to 80 beats per minute is optimal; however, a rate greater than 100 may worsen ischemia in an already compromised myocardium.

Wide-Complex Tachycardia
Diagnosis

The presentation of patients with wide QRS complex (W QRS C) tachycardia requires distinguishing ventricular tachycardia (VT) from supraventricular tachycardia (SVT) with aberrant conduction. Clinical information and a 12-lead ECG are essential to discriminate between these two arrhythmias. Both VT and SVT may be tolerated without evidence of hemodynamic compromise; therefore, patient stability should not be used as a criterion for diagnosis. VT tends to be associated with patient age greater than 35 years, male sex, and a history of myocardial infarction. Other factors increasing the likelihood of VT in W QRS C tachycardia are a history of valvular or congenital heart disease, coronary artery bypass grafting, and recent onset of angina pectoris or congestive heart failure. The patient should be questioned about previous cardiac illnesses, particularly Wolff-Parkinson-White syndrome, or other sources of recurrent SVT. Physical examination may demonstrate "cannon" A waves in the internal jugular veins (caused by AV dissociation with VT as the atria contract against a closed tricuspid valve), cardiomegaly with an S_3 gallop, or pulmonary edema.

TABLE 11–2. Guidelines for the Differential Diagnosis of a Wide QRS Tachycardia

Characteristic	Ventricular Tachycardia	Supraventricular Tachycardia Aberrant
AV dissociation	+	−
QRS width ≥ 0.14 sec	+	−
QRS extreme axis	+	−
QRS morphology		
Right bundle-branch block V_1	*(ECG waveforms)*	*(ECG waveforms)*
Right bundle-branch block V_6	*(ECG waveforms)*	*(ECG waveform)*
Left bundle-branch block	*(ECG waveform)*	*(ECG waveform)*
Fusions, captures	+	−
Concordant pattern	+	−

Graner K: Surmounting clinical hurdles in supraventricular tachyarrhythmias. Emerg Med Rep (Suppl) 9(7):49, 1988.

The 12-lead ECG is helpful in differentiating VT from SVT. Carotid sinus massage may precipitate a transient AV block, possibly terminating reentrant SVT or slowing the tachycardia sufficiently to distinguish P wave morphology. QRS width greater than 140 msec, left axis deviation, slight variation in R-R intervals, and AV dissociation are typical findings with VT. Morphologic characteristics of the QRS wave in SVT and VT are given in Table 11–2. It is important to determine the presence of a regular rate, since atrial fibrillation with aberrant conduction may have an irregular rate and a W QRS C tachycardia.

Indications for Treatment

Synchronized cardioversion is the treatment of choice for hemodynamic instability associated with W QRS C tachycardia. Complaints of angina, change in mental status, pulmonary edema, or hypotension should be promptly treated with electrical cardioversion. Stable patients may receive pharmacologic therapy, with procainamide and lidocaine indicated. Because of the possibility that W QRS C tachycardia is ventricular tachycardia with a pulse, prompt treatment is recommended. Verapamil is contraindicated in this setting because degeneration of ventricular arrhythmias is associated with this drug. (See Fig. 11–8 and box.)

Discussion

Care must be taken with W QRS C tachycardia not to assume the rhythm displayed is SVT with aberrant conduction. Treatment of W QRS C tachycardia with drugs used for SVT may be hazardous, resulting in hypotension, or lethal if associated with ventricular fibrillation. A safer approach is to assume the arrhythmia to be malignant if a diagnosis of SVT is not obtained from the history, physical examination, or ECG. Synchronized cardioversion should be rapidly provided with W QRS C tachycardia and unstable vital signs or end-organ ischemia. VT may be accelerated or converted to ventricular fibrillation with verapamil. The mechanism for verapamil-associated ventricular fibrillation in patients with VT is unclear. It has been postulated that hypotension with reflex autonomic release of catecholamines and heart rate acceleration induces ventricular fibrillation. Wolff-Parkinson-White syndrome, in the presence of atrial fibrillation, may cause a W QRS C tachycardia. AV nodal blockade by verapamil in patients having antegrade conduction through the accessory pathway can produce an accelerated ventricular rate or may degenerate to ventricular fibrillation. Synchronized cardioversion is indicated in the unstable patient with Wolff-Parkinson-White syndrome and atrial fibrillation. Using procainamide to slow conduction through the accessory tract is appropriate in the stable patient. Lidocaine may be used as a second-line agent if procainamide treatment is unsuccessful.

Digitalis Toxicity Arrhythmias
Diagnosis

Digitalis toxicity was described over 200 years ago by Dr. William Withering and re-

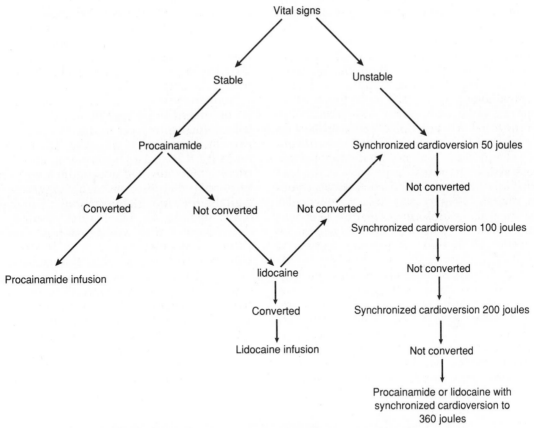

FIGURE 11–8. Treatment algorithm: wide QRS complex tachycardia.

DRUG TREATMENT: WIDE QRS COMPLEX TACHYCARDIA

First-Line Drug
Procainamide

Initial Dose	20 mg/min until arrhythmia is converted
Repeat Dose	1–4 mg/min infusion to prevent arrhythmia recurrence
End-Points	QRS duration increased by 50% of original width
	Hypotension
	Total dose 1 g

Second-Line Drug
Lidocaine

Initial Dose	1 mg/kg initial bolus (75–100 mg)
Repeat Dose	Additional bolus every 5 minutes (0.5–0.75 mg/kg) to maximum total dose ≤3 mg/kg
	Infusion may be given at 2–4 mg/min to prevent recurrence.
End-Points	Arrhythmia terminated
	Toxic effects such as seizures, CNS changes, AV heart block
	Maximum IV bolus dose ≤3 mg/kg

mains a challenging management problem today. Digitalis toxicity causes atrial and ventricular arrhythmias mediated by the autonomic nervous system. The digitalis effect seen in the atrial myocardium, the SA node, and the AV node is antiadrenergic and parasympathomimetic. Atrial arrhythmias may include atrial tachycardia with block, nonparoxysmal AV junctional tachycardia with or without block, atrial fibrillation with ventricular ectopy, and nonconducted premature atrial complexes. Stimulation of the His-Purkinje fibers and ventricular myocardium in digitalis toxicity can induce ventricular tachycardia, multiform premature ventricular complexes, and bigeminal or trigeminal ventricular rhythms. A primary feature of digitalis toxicity is the simultaneous occurrence of depressed impulse conduction with increased atrial and ventricular ectopy or automaticity. Although a normal therapeutic level of digoxin is 0.5 to 1.9 ng/ml, toxic arrhythmias may occur within this range. Digitalis-induced arrhythmias increase in frequency as the serum digoxin level rises. Digitalis binds to and inhibits sarcolemmal membrane NaK-ATPase and increases the calcium available to contractile elements of the cardiac muscle. Transient delayed afterdepolarizations may give rise to "triggered arrhythmias," which appear to be due to intracellular calcium excess.

Nonparoxysmal AV junctional tachycardia is considered to be specific for digitalis toxicity, representing up to one-half of all arrhythmias induced by this drug. The rate can range from 70 to 140 beats per minute. Ventricular bigeminy and nonconducted premature atrial complexes are highly suggestive of digitalis toxicity. Manifestations of digitalis effect include AV block (first, second, or third degree) with associated bradycardia. Often this toxic effect is reversed with atropine, since it is mediated by the parasympathetic nervous system. Atrial tachycardia with AV block is frequently detected. The atrial rate ranges from 150 to 250 per minute with a 2:1 atrial:ventricular rate. This arrhythmia is associated with a high mortality and requires rapid treatment. Ventricular ectopy in digitalis toxicity is worrisome and can evolve into ventricular tachycardia, ventric-

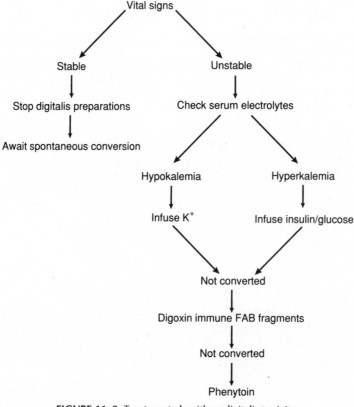

FIGURE 11–9. Treatment algorithm: digitalis toxicity.

ular fibrillation, and death. Patients with atrial fibrillation may have digitalis toxicity with complete AV block and junctional escape at 45 to 55 beats per minute. Nonparoxysmal AV junctional tachycardia may also be evident in atrial fibrillation and digitalis toxicity.

Indications for Treatment

Patients with presumed massive digitalis overdose need rapid therapy with digoxin immune Fab fragments in addition to other antiarrhythmic therapy (see Drug Treatment: Digitalis Toxicity, for details). In patients with benign atrial arrhythmias or low-grade AV block, cessation of digitalis therapy and correction of hypokalemia will likely be sufficient intervention. Rapid atrial tachycardia with increasing AV blockade, ventricular ectopy, or total AV dissociation must be treated aggressively. If rapid response to pharmacologic therapy with antiarrhythmics

is not detected, digoxin immune Fab fragments should be used. Ventricular tachycardia or atrial fibrillation with a rapid ventricular rate in an unstable patient will require synchronized electrical cardioversion. Lower energy is required to convert digitalis-induced arrhythmias than non–digitalis-induced myocardial arrhythmias. (See Figs. 11–9 to 11–12 and box.)

Discussion

Treatment of digitalis toxicity arrhythmias requires familiarity with a variety of treatment modalities. Initially, elevation of serum potassium increases the sodium–potassium pump activity, which decreases intracellular calcium concentration. Toxic levels of digitalis may be associated with hyperkalemia; therefore, treatment with potassium supplementation should be withheld in suspected overdose until the serum potassium level is determined. Rapid administration of digoxin

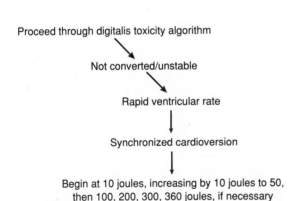

FIGURE 11–10. Treatment algorithm: atrial fibrillation with digitalis intoxication.

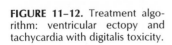

FIGURE 11–11. Treatment algorithm: bradycardia with digitalis toxicity.

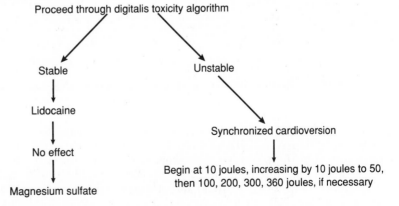

FIGURE 11–12. Treatment algorithm: ventricular ectopy and tachycardia with digitalis toxicity.

DRUG TREATMENT: DIGITALIS TOXICITY

First-Line Drugs

Digoxin Immune Fab Fragments

Dose	The amount of Fab fragments used should be in equimolar concentration to the suspected digoxin concentration present (see Table 11–1); initial small IV dose (1:100 dilution or 10 μg) to test for immediate hypersensitivity, then up to 20 vials (800 mg) given over 30 minutes; infuse through a 0.22-μm membrane filter. In the event of imminent cardiac arrest, bolus injection is given.
End-Points	Hypersensitivity reaction to antibody preparation
	Arrhythmia termination

Phenytoin

Initial Dose	100 mg IV over 5 minutes
Repeat Dose	100 mg IV over 5 minutes until a full loading dose of 18 mg/kg is achieved
End-Points	Hypotension
	18 mg/kg loading dose
	Arrhythmia termination

Second-Line Drugs

Magnesium Sulfate

Initial Dose	2 g IV over 10–20 minutes
Repeat Dose	Infusion of 1–2 g/hour over 5 hours. Maintain serum K^+ level > 4 mEq/liter.
End-Point	Arrhythmia terminated

Lidocaine

Initial Dose	1 mg/kg initial bolus (75–100 mg)
Repeat Dose	Additional bolus every 5 minutes (0.5–0.75 mg/kg) to maximum total dose $\leq$3 mg/kg
	Infusion may be given at 2–4 mg/min to prevent recurrence.
End-Points	Arrhythmia terminated
	Toxic effects such as seizures, central nervous system changes, AV heart block
	Maximum IV bolus dose $\leq$3 mg/kg

Atropine

Initial Dose	0.5 mg IV
Repeat Dose	Give 0.5 mg IV every 5 minutes.
End-Points	Heart rate 60–80/min with end-organ perfusion
	Total 2 mg

immune Fab fragments is clearly the most important therapy for digitalis toxicity that has evolved in the past ten years. This therapy should be employed in cases of life-threatening ventricular or atrial arrhythmias and prophylactically in massive overdosage of digitalis. Delayed serum sickness is a potential complication of treatment with digoxin immune Fab fragments.

Phenytoin reduces the automaticity and afterdepolarizations seen in digitalis toxicity. AV nodal blockade may also be reversed using this agent. The major side effect, hypotension, may preclude its use or limit its effectiveness.

In the presence of digitalis toxicity, the energy necessary to cardiovert the heart is greatly reduced. Fatal ventricular arrhythmias may result from overzealous cardioversion of atrial arrhythmias. Lower energy should also be used for ventricular arrhythmias.

Bradycardia with hypotension, chest pain, and change in mental status associated with SA and AV nodal conduction delay may be reversed by atropine. If atropine is ineffective, atrial pacing through low-energy atrial catheter pacing should be instituted. The digitalis-toxic ventricular myocardium may be stimulated to ventricular fibrillation by misplacement of an atrial pacing wire.

The use of lidocaine and magnesium sulfate should be reserved for refractory cases of ventricular ectopy and tachycardia. While lidocaine decreases delayed afterdepolarizations and inhibits automaticity, it may suppress an ectopic focus that is acting as the only ventricular pacemaker. This can result in ventricular asystole. Magnesium has been shown to be effective in suppressing ventricular arrhythmias and has also been used for AV junctional tachycardia.

Premature Ventricular Contractions

Diagnosis

Premature ventricular contractions (PVCs) are extrasystoles originating from ventricular myocardium. Chronic antiarrhythmic therapy for the individual with frequent or multifocal PVCs is probably not indicated routinely. No clear evidence exists that suppression of PVCs or nonsustained ventricular tachycardia (VT) reduces mortality in patients without underlying cardiac disease. Patients with sustained VT or survivors of sudden cardiac death will likely benefit from antiarrhythmic therapy when the therapy is guided by electrophysiologic testing. Implantation of automatic defibrillators will further lower the risk of mortality in these patients.

Congestive cardiomyopathies, hypokalemia, digitalis toxicity, hypoxemia, and sympathomimetic drugs such as cocaine or amphetamine may cause PVCs. Treatment of the underlying disorder will often preclude the need for specific antiarrhythmic therapy.

On the 12-lead ECG, PVCs are single wide-complex QRS beats without preceding P waves. PVCs may join as couplets, or three PVCs may occur in succession, indicating nonsustained VT. Multiple areas in the ventricle may fire in a disjointed fashion, resulting in differences in QRS morphology.

Indications for Treatment

The acute phase of myocardial infarction is frequently associated with PVCs. In the first 48 hours after infarction, antiarrhythmics are considered beneficial in the presence of PVCs. The American Heart Association recommends prophylactic treatment of "warning arrhythmias," including frequent (more than 6/min) PVCs, coupled PVCs or runs of VT, multifocal PVCs, or PVCs that fall on the T wave of the preceding complex (R-on-T phenomenon). Use of lidocaine to prevent ventricular fibrillation in all patients with acute myocardial infarction is controversial and determined by physician preference. Patients with sustained ectopy after 72 hours are at increased risk of mortality. (See Fig. 11–13 and box.)

Discussion

Lidocaine is the most frequently used agent for prophylaxis of PVCs and is quite effective. Bretylium and procainamide should be considered second-line agents for PVC suppression after a careful analysis of the risk-versus-benefit ratio. Treatment of underlying electrolyte abnormalities, hypoxemia, or drug toxicity may successfully treat PVCs.

FIGURE 11–13. Treatment algorithm: premature ventricular contractions.

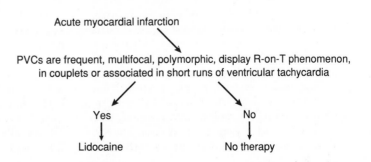

DRUG TREATMENT: PREMATURE VENTRICULAR CONTRACTIONS

First-Line Drug
Lidocaine

Initial Dose	1 mg/kg initial bolus (75–100 mg)
Repeat Dose	Additional bolus every 5 minutes (0.5–0.75 mg/kg) to maximum total dose ≤3 mg/kg
	Infusion may be given at 2–4 mg/min to prevent recurrence.
End-Points	Arrhythmia terminated
	Toxic effects such as seizures, central nervous system changes, AV heart block
	Maximum IV bolus dose ≤3 mg/kg

Second-Line Drugs
Bretylium

Initial Dose	5 mg/kg IV over 5–10 minutes
Repeat Dose	10 mg/kg IV over 10–20 minutes; may repeat once
	If arrhythmia terminated, may give infusion at 2 mg/min
End-Points	Arrhythmia terminated
	Postural hypotension
	Nausea, vomiting
	Maximum bolus dose ≤25 mg/kg

Procainamide

Initial Dose	20 mg/min until arrhythmia terminated
Repeat Dose	Infusion of 1–4 mg/min to prevent recurrence
End-Points	QRS duration increased by 50% of original width
	Hypotension
	Total dose 1 g
	Arrhythmia terminated

Ventricular Tachycardia
Diagnosis

Ventricular tachycardia (VT) is a wide-complex tachycardia that originates below the His bundle bifurcation. Although sometimes associated with hemodynamic stability, VT should be considered potentially lethal and requires rapid diagnosis and therapy. This tachyarrhythmia may be self-terminating or sustained. Degeneration into ventricular fibrillation should be anticipated if cardioversion is not successful in treating sustained VT. This arrhythmia is often associated with underlying heart disease, particularly ischemia. Drug toxicity, including tri-cyclic antidepressant overdose and digitalis toxicity, may cause VT (therapy for each is discussed in other sections). Congestive or hypertrophic cardiomyopathy and mitral valve prolapse are also associated with VT.

The ECG demonstrates at least three consecutive wide QRS complexes with a rate greater than 100 beats per minute. The QRS axis and morphology remain similar in the usual cases of VT. Complex VT, characterized by polarity reversal of the QRS axis, is termed torsades de pointes and is described in a later section in this chapter. Although VT usually has a rate ranging from 150 to 200 beats per minute, the distinction between accelerated idioventricular rhythm and VT often blurs at rates between 100 and 150. Treatment of ventricular rates greater than 100 with standard agents used to treat VT is prudent.

A 12-lead ECG should be obtained prior to pharmacologic intervention in the stable patient. In sustained common VT, long bursts of coupled wide QRS complexes are noted at rates from 100 to 250 per minute. The QRS morphology usually varies little between complexes, which occur at a regular rate with a nearly identical axis from complex to complex. In the unstable patient, a rhythm strip obtained before electrical cardioversion may provide helpful information should the arrhythmia recur. Once cardioversion is performed, the 12-lead ECG may depict underlying ischemia or infarction.

Indications for Treatment

Sustained VT in the unstable patient requires immediate electrical cardioversion. Synchronized cardioversion may not be effective because a definite QRS complex is sometimes unrecognized by the cardioversion instrument. If immediate synchronized cardioversion does not occur, unsynchronized cardioversion with equivalent energy should be used. VT in the stable patient should be treated aggressively with pharmacologic agents, since rapid deterioration of this rhythm to ventricular fibrillation is possible. (See Figs. 11–14 and 11–15 and box.)

DRUG TREATMENT: VENTRICULAR TACHYCARDIA

First-Line Drug

Lidocaine

Initial Dose	1 mg/kg initial bolus (75–100 mg)
Repeat Dose	Additional bolus every 5 minutes (0.5–0.75 mg/kg) to maximum total dose $\leq$3 mg/kg
	Infusion may be given at 2–4 mg/min to prevent recurrence.
End-Points	Arrhythmia terminated
	Toxic effects such as seizures, central nervous system changes, AV heart block
	Maximum IV bolus dose $\leq$3 mg/kg

Second-Line Drugs

Procainamide

Initial Dose	20 mg/min until arrhythmia is converted
Repeat Dose	Infusion of 1–4 mg/min to prevent arrhythmia recurrence
End-Points	QRS duration increased by 50% of original width
	Hypotension develops
	Total dose 1 g
	Arrhythmia terminated

Bretylium

Initial Dose	5 mg/kg IV bolus
Repeat Dose	10 mg/kg IV bolus in 10–20 minutes; may repeat once
	If arrhythmia is terminated, may infuse at 2 mg/min
End-Points	Arrhythmia terminated
	Postural hypotension
	Nausea and vomiting
	Maximum bolus dose $\leq$25 mg/kg

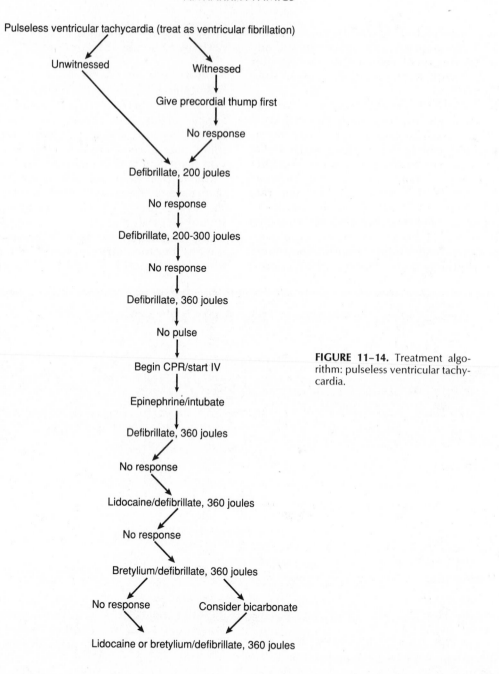

FIGURE 11–14. Treatment algorithm: pulseless ventricular tachycardia.

Discussion

The recommendations for VT therapy given here are adapted from the American Heart Association guidelines and represent a distillation of current research in advanced cardiac life support. Variations from this regimen for treatment of individual patient situations may be necessary, particularly in the use of sodium bicarbonate in prolonged arrest times. Measurement of arterial blood gases may prove helpful to individualize therapy. The treatment of torsades de pointes and the treatment of arrhythmias induced by tricyclic antidepressant overdose do not follow these common VT guidelines and are discussed in the following sections.

Torsades de Pointes Ventricular Tachycardia

Diagnosis

Torsades de pointes (TdP) is a unique form of VT first described by Dessertenne in 1966. In this arrhythmia, the polarity of the wide QRS complex appears to spiral around

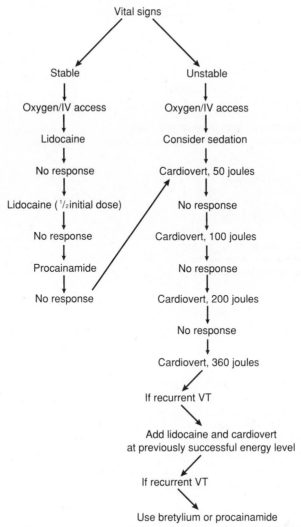

FIGURE 11-15. Treatment algorithm: sustained ventricular tachycardia with a pulse. (Adapted from the Textbook of Advanced Cardiac Life Support. Dallas, American Heart Association, 1987.)

the ECG baseline. This results in apparent reversals of the QRS polarity that are distinctive for TdP. This form of VT is associated with prolongation of the QT interval and does not respond to conventional antiarrhythmic therapy. TdP is also seen as a proarrhythmic effect of antiarrhythmic drugs that prolong the QT interval, such as quinidine, procainamide, disopyramide, encainide, flecainide, and sotalol. Other drugs, such as the psychotropic agents lithium carbonate, tricyclic antidepressants, and thioridazine, may cause TdP. Hypomagnesemia, hypokalemia, and hypocalcemia all increase the QT interval, increasing the likelihood of TdP development. Prolongation of the QT interval also occurs as a congenital disorder

that may result in sudden death, presumably due to TdP. TdP originates in a small area of ventricular myocardium and is likely caused by triggered automaticity.

TdP is identified on the ECG by the undulating sinusoidal twisting of a wide-complex tachycardia around the ECG baseline. Although often it may last for only short runs of 5 to 15 seconds, it may rapidly degenerate into ventricular fibrillation. Between runs of TdP, a prolonged QT interval is often seen on the standard 12-lead ECG.

Indications for Treatment

Recurrent or sustained TdP, an unusual form of VT, must be treated in order to prevent degeneration into ventricular fibrilla-

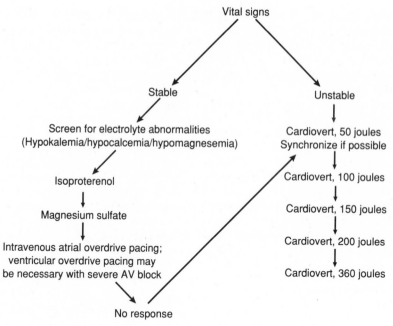

FIGURE 11–16. Treatment algorithm: torsades de pointes (TdP).

tion. In cases of TdP caused by drug overdose, the drug causing the arrhythmia should be removed by gastric lavage if possible, and activated charcoal should be given. Treatment of tricyclic antidepressant overdose is discussed later in this chapter. (See Fig. 11–16 and box.)

Discussion

TdP is an interesting variant of VT that requires different therapeutic intervention. Lidocaine is ineffective in treating TdP. Class I antiarrhythmic agents such as procainamide and quinidine prolong the QT interval and are absolutely contraindicated. Removal of

---

DRUG TREATMENT: TORSADES DE POINTES (TdP)

First-Line Drugs

Isoproterenol

Initial Dose	1 mg is added to 500 ml D_5W, which gives a concentration of 2 $\mu g/ml$; infuse at 2–20 $\mu g/min$ to increase heart rate to 100–120/min and shorten the QT interval.
Repeat Dose	Titrate IV infusion to desired heart rate.
End-Points	Infusion rate of 20 $\mu g/min$ without desired change in heart rate
	Hypotension
	Development of cardiac arrhythmias

Magnesium Sulfate

Initial Dose	2 g IV over 10–20 minutes
Repeat Dose	Infusion of 1 g/hour if successful; maintain serum K^+ level > 4 mEq/liter
End-Points	Arrhythmia terminated

offending agents from the gastrointestinal tract using activated charcoal should be attempted in overdose. Electrolyte abnormalities, particularly hypokalemia, hypocalcemia, and hypomagnesemia, should be sought and corrected if present.

Isoproterenol and atrial overdrive pacing are the mainstay of therapy for TdP. Recent reports indicate magnesium sulfate may effectively treat TdP resistant to standard therapy. The mechanism for magnesium abolition of TdP is unclear; however, magnesium is a known cofactor of ATPase. It acts to transport potassium into cells while extruding sodium. The preservation of intracellular potassium has been postulated to contribute to electrical stabilization.

Tricyclic Antidepressant Arrhythmias
Diagnosis

Tricyclic antidepressant (TCA) overdose is commonly encountered, and the arrhythmias associated with TCA toxicity can be fatal. Toxicity associated with TCA overdose results in multiple cardiac effects, including cholinergic blockade, increased serum catecholamine levels through inhibition of uptake of these neural transmitters, and direct myocardial cell inhibition of the fast sodium channel. The anticholinergic effects of TCA may cause tachycardia, which is often the first sign of impending cardiac dysfunction. Elevated catecholamine levels can increase ventricular arrhythmias and contribute to sinus tachycardia. Inhibition of the myocardial sodium fast current slows phase 0 depolarization, prolonging the QRS complex and the QT interval. Elevated TCA levels, like the Class Ia antiarrhythmics quinidine and procainamide, decrease the automaticity of atrial pacemaker tissue, often resulting in a ventricular escape rhythm. The newer Class Ic agents, including encainide and flecainide, have similar toxic effects.

Hypotension is also a major feature of TCA overdose and is probably caused by decreased contractility with impaired cardiac output. Acidemia may occur in TCA overdose secondary to combined hypotension and hypoventilation. Hyperthermia may result from increased muscle tone combined with impaired heat dissipation from cholinergic blockade. Confusion, agitation, seizures, and coma are frequent central nervous system manifestations of TCA overdose.

The ECG will confirm the tachycardia associated with TCA toxicity. The QRS complex may become prolonged to greater than 0.12 second, and the QT interval may increase as well. This slurring of the QRS complex portends the actual VT seen in TCA toxicity. Both common VT and torsades de pointes may be associated with TCA overdose, and resistance to treatment is frequently observed.

Indications for Treatment

TCA toxicity may initially be manifested by sinus tachycardia alone. Although this condition does not require treatment, any QRS prolongation greater than 0.12 second indicates the need for sodium bicarbonate therapy. Arrhythmias associated with TCA toxicity, especially ventricular arrhythmias, should be considered malignant and require therapy. Hypotension should be aggressively treated as well. If overdose is the cause of TCA toxicity, gastric lavage and the use of activated charcoal are indicated. (See Fig. 11–17 and box.)

DRUG TREATMENT: TRICYCLIC ANTIDEPRESSANT CARDIAC TOXICITY

First-Line Drugs
Sodium Bicarbonate (NaHCO₃)

Initial Dose	1 mEq/kg IV push
Repeat Dose	0.5 mEq/kg IV push
End-Points	Serum pH greater than 7.50
	Arrhythmia terminated

Chart continued on following page

DRUG TREATMENT: TRICYCLIC ANTIDEPRESSANT CARDIAC TOXICITY *Continued*

Lidocaine

Initial Dose	1 mg/kg initial bolus (75–100 mg)
Repeat Dose	Additional bolus every 5 minutes (0.5–0.75 mg/kg) to maximum total dose ≤3 mg/kg
	Infusion may be given at 2–4 mg/min to prevent recurrence.
End-Points	Arrhythmia terminated
	Toxic effects such as seizures, central nervous system changes, AV heart block
	Maximum IV bolus dose ≤3 mg/kg

Normal Saline

Initial Dose	500 ml (add 1.0 mEq/kg sodium bicarbonate to 1000 ml normal saline)
Repeat Dose	250-ml bolus as necessary
End-Points	Excessive serum alkalization
	Pulmonary edema or fluid overload

Second-Line Drugs
Phenytoin

Initial Dose	100 mg IV over 5 minutes
Repeat Dose	100 mg IV over 5 minutes until a full loading dose of 18 mg/kg is achieved
End-Points	Hypotension
	18 mg/kg loading dose
	Arrhythmia termination

Norepinephrine Bitartrate

Initial Dose	Infusion through central venous catheter at 2–12 µg/min
Repeat Dose	Titrate IV infusion to desired blood pressure.
End-Points	Desired pressure obtained
	Maximum 12–15 µg/min dosage
	Severe peripheral vasoconstriction without central venous pressure maintenance

Dobutamine

Initial Dose	2.5–20 µg/kg/min IV infusion
Repeat Dose	Continue infusion necessary to maintain adequate pressure.
End-Points	Tachycardia
	Arrhythmia generation
	Desired blood pressure maintenance
	Maximal dose ≤20 µg/kg/min

Discussion

TCA cardiac toxicity is treated initially with alkalization using hypertonic sodium bicarbonate. Animal studies have demonstrated that this agent has beneficial effects by increasing extracellular sodium and the serum pH. The improvement in phase 0 depolarization appears to be the primary effect

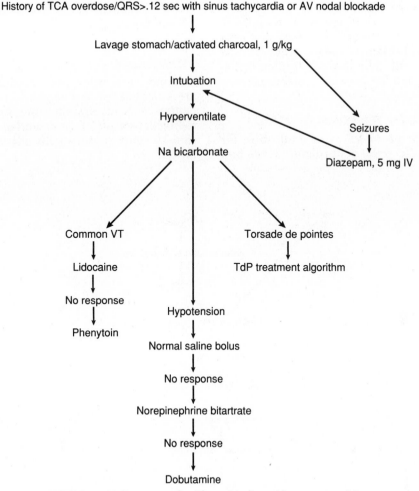

FIGURE 11–17. Treatment algorithm: tricyclic antidepressant toxicity.

of increased extracellular sodium. Elevating serum pH increases the protein binding of the TCA, presumably decreasing the availability of free drug to block fast sodium channels.

Lidocaine, a Class Ib antiarrhythmic drug, does not depress myocardial conduction or contractility, making it a good first-line agent for rapid treatment of ventricular arrhythmias. Because lidocaine does not mimic Class Ia antiarrhythmic agents such as quinidine and procainamide, prolongation of the QT interval does not occur. Phenytoin, another Class Ib agent, appears to improve conduction through specialized conductive tissues of the heart and increases phase 0 depolarization. The use of phenytoin for treatment of TCA toxicity is controversial, and therefore it should only be considered a second-line drug. Physostigmine may be hazardous when given to patients with TCA toxicity

and is not recommended for use in this setting.

Ventricular Fibrillation
Diagnosis

Ventricular fibrillation (VF) is a terminal arrhythmia. Fibrillating ventricles have no effective cardiac output, and electrical defibrillation is required to prevent death. The reentry mechanism is postulated as the cause of VF. There are many known causes of VF, including electrolyte abnormalities, hypoxemia, acidosis, and electrical injuries. Myocardial ischemia and infarction are the most frequent causes. VF results in sudden death if not reversed rapidly.

On the 12-lead ECG, VF is recognized as disorganized waveforms of varying amplitude. The QRS complex is not identifiable. Multiple areas of the ventricle depolarize and repolarize simultaneously; therefore, cardiac mechanical function is minimized. Coarse VF is represented by relatively high-amplitude fibrillatory waves, whereas fine VF is represented by low-amplitude fibrillatory waves and may even be misinterpreted as asystole.

Indication for Treatment

The presence of VF is an indication for treatment. Electrical defibrillation is the first line and mainstay of treatment. (See Fig. 11–18 and box.)

Discussion

Rapid recognition and termination of VF are essential for a successful outcome with central nervous system resuscitation. Early defibrillation of VF is essential for conversion to sinus rhythm with effective cardiac output.

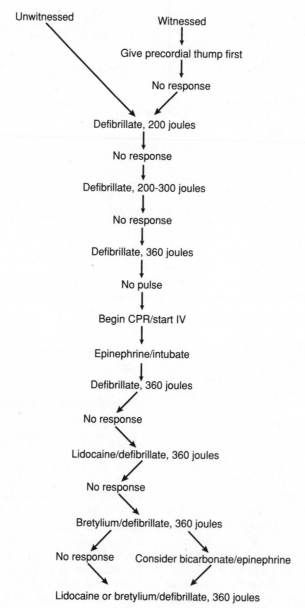

FIGURE 11–18. Treatment algorithm: ventricular fibrillation. (Adapted from the Textbook of Advanced Cardiac Life Support. Dallas, American Heart Association, 1987.)

DRUG TREATMENT: VENTRICULAR FIBRILLATION

First-Line Drugs

Epinephrine

Initial Dose	0.5–1.0 mg IV push (1:10,000 concentration)
Repeat Dose	0.5–1.0 mg IV every 5 minutes
End-Points	Return of pulse with rhythm
	Severe arrhythmia generation

Lidocaine

Initial Dose	1 mg/kg initial bolus (75–100 mg)
Repeat Dose	Additional bolus every 5 minutes (0.5–0.75 mg/kg) to maximum total dose ≤3 mg/kg
	Infusion may be given at 2–4 mg/min to prevent recurrence.
End-Points	Arrhythmia terminated
	Toxic effects such as seizures, central nervous system changes, AV heart block
	Maximum IV bolus dose ≤3 mg/kg

Second-Line Drugs

Bretylium

Initial Dose	5 mg/kg IV bolus
Repeat Dose	10 mg/kg IV bolus in 10–20 minutes; may repeat once
	If arrhythmia is terminated, may infuse at 2 mg/min
End-Points	Arrhythmia terminated
	Postural hypotension
	Nausea and vomiting
	Maximum bolus dose ≤25 mg/kg

Sodium Bicarbonate (NaHCO₃)

Initial Dose	1 mEq/kg IV push
Repeat Dose	0.5 mEq/kg IV push
End-Points	Alkalotic pH
	Arrhythmia terminated

SPECIFIC AGENTS

Adenosine (Adenocard)

Pharmacology

Distribution

Adenosine is a purine nucleoside found in every body cell. Within the intravascular volume, adenosine is eliminated quite rapidly with a half-life of 10 seconds through erythrocyte and vascular endothelial cell uptake.

Elimination

Adenosine is rapidly eliminated through erythrocyte and vascular endothelial cell uptake. Adenosine undergoes metabolism to adenosine monophosphate (AMP) and inosine.

Cardiovascular Actions

Adenosine exerts its primary antiarrhythmic activity through slowing of AV conduction time, which can terminate supraventricular arrhythmias through interruption of reentry pathways. Dilation of peripheral arteries may cause hypotension at high dosages.

Indications

Adenosine is indicated for reentrant (paroxysmal) supraventricular tachycardia and narrow-complex supraventricular tachycardia associated with accessory bypass tracts such as in Wolff-Parkinson-White and Lown-Ganong-Levine syndromes. Currently, *no* indication is given for the use of adenosine for wide QRS complex tachycardias, although experimental work is under way in this area.

Cautions

Cardiovascular—in patients with second- or third-degree heart block, complete heart block, including asystole, may result with the use of adenosine, except in the presence of a functioning artificial pacemaker. In patients with sick sinus syndrome, a functioning pacemaker is necessary prior to adenosine use in these patients. In patients with atrial flutter, atrial fibrillation, or ventricular tachycardia, adenosine is not effective in converting these arrhythmias to sinus rhythm.

Hepatic or renal failure—no effect on adenosine elimination, which is removed from circulation by vascular endothelial cells and erythrocytes.

Pregnancy—Category C. No studies have been performed on pregnant women. Risk versus benefit must be weighed, although it must be understood that adenosine is a naturally occurring substance in the body. Breast milk contamination with adenosine is unlikely, but no information is available in this area.

Children—not recommended because experience is limited

Onset and Duration of Action

Dosage

Initial dose, 6 mg given as a rapid IV bolus over 1 to 2 seconds

Limit

Maximum dosage, 18 mg

Repeat Dosing

If no effect is seen within 2 minutes after the initial 6-mg bolus, a second rapid IV bolus of 12 mg should be administered.

Toxicity

Drug Interactions

Adenosine is potentiated by dipyridamole, a blocker of nucleoside transport. Smaller doses of adenosine are therefore appropriate in this setting. Methylxanthines such as caffeine and theophylline antagonize adenosine. Larger doses of adenosine may be required in the patient using these drugs.

Carbamazepine has been reported to increase the likelihood of high-degree AV nodal blockade with adenosine.

Specific Adverse Effects

Facial flushing (18%), chest pain or pressure (7%), headache (2%), and hypotension (<1%) are the primary side effects of adenosine. Transient bradycardia, varying degrees of AV block, and premature ventricular contractions may be seen on arrhythmia conversion. Shortness of breath and asthma exacerbation may occur in some patients, but these side effects are quite transient because of the short half-life of adenosine. Dizziness and nausea have also been reported.

Treatment of Toxicity

Because the half-life of adenosine is less than 10 seconds, adverse effects are usually self-limited. Patients should be treated individually if symptoms persist beyond several minutes after bolus infusion of adenosine.

Atropine

Pharmacology

Distribution

Atropine disappears rapidly from the blood and is distributed throughout the entire body, including the central nervous system.

Elimination

The drug is excreted in the urine within 12 hours, up to one-half unchanged.

Actions

Central nervous system—restlessness, irritability, disorientation, delirium, hallucinations

Eye—mydriasis and cycloplegia

Respiratory tract—dries secretions and acts as a bronchodilator

Cardiovascular—causes tachycardia through vagolytic action; accelerates the SA nodal pacemaker and increases AV nodal conduction time through decreasing vagal influence on the heart; may cause cutaneous flushing through dilatation of surface vessels

Gastrointestinal tract—reduces salivary and gastric acid secretion; decreases gastrointestinal motility

Skin—inhibits sweating

Indications

Atropine is indicated for symptomatic bradycardia in patients with myocardial infarction, digitalis toxicity, and other causes of increased vagal tone.

Cautions

Renal failure—reduced dosage necessary because the kidneys are primary organs for drug elimination

Heart failure—no dose adjustment necessary, but increasing tachycardia may worsen myocardial ischemia

Hepatic failure—no dose adjustment necessary

Pregnancy—Category B. Risk versus benefit must be weighed; atropine is found in bodily secretions, including breast milk.

Onset and Duration of Action

Dosage

Initial dose, 0.5 to 1.0 mg IV
Children, 0.01 to 0.03 mg/kg

Limit

Maximum parasympatholytic dose, 2.0 mg

Repeat Dosing

Effect may be seen up to 12 hours.

Toxicity

Drug Interactions

No specific antiarrhythmic interaction

Specific Adverse Effects

Inappropriate tachycardia in patients treated for symptomatic bradycardia is a potential adverse effect. In patients with atropine toxicity, tachycardia is associated with palpitations, dry mouth, flushing, reduced heat dissipation, blurred vision, decreased gastrointestinal peristalsis, ataxia, restlessness, hallucinations, and delirium. Coma and death may occur in severe intoxication.

Treatment of Toxicity

Significant anticholinergic toxicity can be treated with physostigmine, 1 to 2 mg IV given over 3 to 5 minutes. This can be repeated in 20 minutes if no effect is seen. Physostigmine, an acetylcholinesterase inhibitor, increases the availability of acetylcholine at the cholinergic neuroreceptor.

Bretylium (Bretylol)

Pharmacology

Elimination

Excreted entirely in the urine, unchanged
Half-life = 8 hours

Cardiovascular Actions

When bretylium is taken up by the presynaptic nerve terminal, a transient release of norepinephrine is observed, which may cause hypertension. The drug increases the action potential duration and effective refractory period of myocardium without changing the heart rate. It also increases the ventricular fibrillation threshold. An increase in pacemaker spontaneous firing may be seen, with an increase in ventricular conduction velocity. After initial hypertension, postural hypotension is observed.

Indications

Bretylium is indicated for ventricular tachycardia and ventricular fibrillation.

Cautions

Renal failure—reduced dosage necessary because the kidneys are primary organs for drug elimination; increased dosage interval also necessary

Heart failure—with a fixed cardiac output, severe hypotension possible with the fall in vascular resistance noted with peripheral adrenergic blockade

Hepatic failure—no dose adjustment necessary

Pregnancy—risk versus benefit must be weighed because bretylium is most frequently used in life-threatening situations; safety has not been established in human pregnancy. It is not known whether bretylium is excreted in breast milk.

Children—safety and efficacy have not been established.

Onset and Duration of Action

Dosage

Initial dose is 5.0 mg/kg IV given over 5 to 10 minutes for premature ventricular contractions or given as a bolus for ventricular fibrillation. In ventricular fibrillation, a second dose of 10 mg/kg is given prior to defibrillation.

Limit

Maximum loading dose is 20 mg/kg.

Repeat Dosing

Dose may be repeated in 20 minutes if no effect and again in 1 to 2 hours. Maintenance dose is given as a constant infusion of 1 to 4 mg/min.

Toxicity

Drug Interactions

The release of norepinephrine by bretylium may result in worsening of digitalis-induced arrhythmias. Bretylium should not be used in this setting.

Specific Adverse Effects

Postural hypotension is frequently seen, and supine hypotension may be observed in up to 50% of patients. Bradyarrhythmias may be seen at loading doses greater than 20 mg/kg. Vomiting is common after intravenous bolus injection.

Treatment of Toxicity

Hypotension, caused by vasodilation from adrenergic blockade, should be treated with dopamine or norepinephrine infusion to increase blood pressure.

Digoxin (Lanoxin)

Pharmacology

Distribution

After drug administration, a 6- to 8-hour distribution phase is observed with most of the drug found in the tissues. Approximately 20 to 25% of plasma digoxin is bound to protein. Dialysis does not effectively remove the drug because most of the drug is found in the tissue, not circulating in the blood.

Elimination

From 50 to 70% of the dose is excreted unchanged in the urine following first-order kinetics. In patients with normal renal function, the half-life is 1 to 2 days. In anuric patients, the half-life is prolonged to 4 to 6 days.

Cardiovascular Actions

Inotropic action of the drug increases cardiac output, decreasing evidence of congestive heart failure such as pulmonary venous congestion, dyspnea, pedal edema, and orthopnea. Digoxin increases vagal tone, decreasing activity of the SA and AV nodes and acting as a negative chronotrope. It also decreases conduction velocity through the AV node.

Indications

Digitalis is indicated for the treatment of atrial fibrillation and flutter, although its onset of action is slower than agents such as verapamil and esmolol. It is also used as a second-line agent for paroxysmal supraventricular tachycardia. This drug is a mainstay for the chronic treatment of congestive heart failure.

Cautions

Renal failure—reduced dosage necessary because the kidneys are primary organ for drug elimination. Because of the drug's prolonged half-life, a longer period of time is necessary to achieve steady state in the patient with renal disease.

Electrolyte abnormalities—hypokalemia and hypomagnesemia are associated with increased digitalis toxicity. Serum levels of potassium and magnesium should be monitored and normal to high-normal levels of these serum electrolytes should be maintained.

Heart failure—no dose adjustment necessary

Hepatic failure—no dose adjustment necessary

Pregnancy—Category C. Risk versus benefit must be weighed; studies involving pregnant women have not been performed. Breast milk concentrations are the same as serum concentrations. This amount of drug in the breast milk should have no pharmacologic effect on the nursing infant.

Onset and Duration of Action

Dosage

Initial dose is 0.25 to 0.50 mg IV.

Limit

Maximum initial digitalizing dose is 1.0 mg IV.

Repeat Dosing

In 30 to 60 minutes, an additional 0.25-mg dose is given to a maximum dose of 1.0 mg. An initial dose of 600 to 1000 μg (0.6 to 1.0 mg) is necessary to achieve 8 to 15 μg/kg peak body stores, necessary for control of atrial arrhythmias in a 70-kg patient. A 6- to 10-μg/kg digitalization dose should be used in the patient with renal insufficiency.

Children

Half the digitalizing dose should be given initially and the remainder over 24 hours as clinically indicated.

Age	Digitalizing Dose (μg/kg)
Premature	15–25
Full term	20–30
1–24 months	30–50
2–5 years	25–35
5–10 years	15–30
>10 years	8–12

Toxicity

Drug Interactions

Diuretics and corticosteroids can decrease serum potassium levels, resulting in significant arrhythmias with digitalis use. Rapid calcium infusion may also acutely lower the serum potassium level, causing arrhythmias. Succinylcholine may cause sudden extrusion of myocardial intracellular potassium, resulting in cardiac arrhythmias.

Specific Adverse Effects

Digitalis has a significant proarrhythmic action when toxic serum levels are achieved. Premature ventricular contractions including bigeminy and trigeminy, ventricular tachycardia, AV dissociation, accelerated junctional rhythm, and atrial tachycardia with block are frequently seen with digitalis toxicity. Non-cardiac adverse effects include anorexia, nausea and vomiting, visual disturbances (yellow-green vision), headache, and psychosis.

Treatment of Toxicity

Digitalis should be discontinued. Serum potassium and magnesium levels should be maintained at the upper limits of normal. Potassium salts, magnesium sulfate, phenytoin, and lidocaine may all be used to treat digitalis toxic rhythms (see Drug Treatment: Digitalis Toxicity, earlier). Digoxin immune Fab fragments should be used early in a clinically significant overdose of digitalis.

Esmolol (Brevibloc)

Pharmacology

$$CH_3O_2CCH_2CH_2 - \text{〈benzene ring〉} - OCH_2CHOHCH_2NHCH(CH_3)_2 \cdot HCl$$

Distribution

Esmolol has a rapid distribution half-life of approximately 2 minutes. Using the appropriate loading dose, steady-state blood levels can be achieved in 5 minutes. Without a loading dose, steady-state blood levels will be reached in 30 minutes.

Elimination

Esmolol is metabolized by red blood cell cytosol esterase and has an elimination half-life of 9 minutes. Elimination is not dependent on blood flow through the liver or kidneys.

Actions

Cardiovascular—beta-adrenergic blocking agent that is relatively cardioselective, acting primarily on $beta_1$-receptors. A decrease in sinus rate is seen with a decreased conduction of the AV node and a prolonged refractoriness. Decreased blood pressure often accompanies beta-adrenergic blockade.

Respiratory tract—mild $beta_2$-receptor blockade may worsen asthma and cause bronchoconstriction.

Indications

Esmolol is indicated for supraventricular tachycardias, including atrial fibrillation and flutter, paroxysmal supraventricular tachycardia, and hypertensive emergencies. Wide QRS complex tachycardias or atrial fibrillation in patients with accessory pathway disease, such as Wolff-Parkinson-White syndrome, should *not* be treated with this agent.

Cautions

General—infusion concentrations greater than 10 mg/ml are associated with an increased risk of venous irritation and thrombophlebitis.

Renal failure—the acid metabolite of esmolol is excreted unchanged in the urine. Patients with renal insufficiency should be treated with caution.

Heart failure—should be used with caution, since esmolol and all beta-adrenergic blocking drugs are negative inotropic agents. Early indications suggest esmolol can be given safely in some patients with left ventricular failure, because of its ultra-short half-life.

Hepatic failure—no dose adjustment necessary

Pregnancy—Category C. Risk versus benefit must be weighed; no teratogenicity has been demonstrated in rat studies. It is not known whether esmolol is excreted in breast milk.

Children—adequate experience is not available.

Onset and Duration of Action

Dosage

Initial dose is 500 µg/kg given over 1 minute; this is followed by a 4-minute infusion started with 50 µg/kg/min.

Limit

Maximum infusion dose is 200 µg/kg/min.

Repeat Dosing

A loading dose of 500 µg/kg is repeated every 5 minutes, with an increase in infusion dose by 50 µg/kg/min. Most patients respond to 100 µg/kg/min.

Toxicity

Drug Interactions

Use with other agents that cause AV nodal blockade may result in complete AV dissociation. Use with catecholamine-depleting drugs such as reserpine may cause significant bradycardia or hypotension.

Specific Adverse Effects

Dose-related hypotension occurred in 20 to 50% of patients given esmolol in early clinical trials. This hypotension usually resolved within 30 minutes after the infusion was discontinued. Because of esmolol's brief half-life and cardioselectivity, bronchospasm may occur less frequently than with the longer-acting beta-adrenergic agents. This agent should be used cautiously in the presence of congestive heart failure because it is a negative inotrope.

Treatment of Toxicity

Discontinue infusion. Adverse effects resolve quickly because of the short 9-minute half-life.

Isoproterenol (Isuprel)

Pharmacology

Elimination

Isoproterenol is metabolized primarily in the liver and other tissues by catechol-o-methyl transferase. Its half-life is less than 10 minutes.

Actions

Respiratory tract—acts as a bronchodilator due to beta-adrenergic stimulation
Cardiovascular—tachycardia and increased cardiac output; decrease in peripheral vascular resistance caused by vasodilation of peripheral and coronary arteries. Isoproterenol increases venous return to the heart, increasing cardiac output through this mechanism.
Gastrointestinal tract—decreases gastrointestinal motility and tone

Indications

Isoproterenol is useful in complete heart block and symptomatic bradycardia unresponsive to anticholinergic blockade.

It is also used for torsades de pointes ventricular tachycardia for increasing the ventricular rate and decreasing the QT interval.

Cautions

General—reduced dosage necessary for coronary insufficiency, diabetes, or hyperthyroidism
Renal failure—no dose adjustment necessary

Heart failure—no dose adjustment necessary; however, increasing tachycardia may worsen myocardial ischemia.
Hepatic failure—reduced dosage necessary because drug is metabolized by the liver
Pregnancy—Category C. Risk versus benefit must be weighed; no teratogenic potential is known. It is not known whether isoproterenol is excreted in breast milk.

Onset and Duration of Action

Dosage

Dilute 1 mg isoproterenol in 500 ml diluent for a final concentration of 1:500,000. The infusion rate is 0.5 to 5.0 μg/min (0.25 to 2.5 ml/min) for the initial dose. Titrate cardiac rate to 110 beats/min. Heart rates greater than 130 beats/min are associated with ventricular arrhythmias.

Limit

Maximum infusion rate is 30 μg/min.

Children: initial infusion 0.1 μg/kg/min; maximum infusion < 1.0 μg/kg/min

Toxicity

Drug Interactions

Isoproterenol should not be used in tachycardia associated with digitalis toxicity. Because of potential additive arrhythmogenic effect, epinephrine and isoproterenol should not be used simultaneously.

Specific Adverse Effects

Facial flushing, palpitations, mild tremors, headache, and nervousness are potential adverse effects of isoproterenol.

Treatment of Toxicity

Stop infusion of isoproterenol.

Lidocaine (Xylocaine)

Pharmacology

Distribution

Oral lidocaine is subject to extensive first-pass hepatic metabolism, making it unsuitable as an oral agent. About 50% of the drug is bound to albumin in the bloodstream after intravenous administration. Distribution is rapid, with apparent volume of distribution of 1 liter per kilogram. The effective half-life is approximately 2 hours.

Elimination

Minimal amounts of lidocaine are excreted in the urine. Primary metabolism occurs through the liver, with the clearance of lidocaine directly proportional to hepatic blood flow.

Cardiovascular Actions

Lidocaine depresses depolarization slightly and slows conduction. Repolarization is shortened, with a corresponding decrease in action potential duration. Abnormal automaticity of Purkinje cells is decreased. Reentrant ventricular arrhythmias are often abolished.

Indications

Lidocaine is indicated for intravenous treatment of ventricular arrhythmias, particularly those associated with acute myocardial infarction.

Cautions

General—lidocaine is potentially associated with the development of malignant hyperthermia. Use in patients with sinus bradycardia or incomplete heart block may result in ventricular arrhythmias or complete heart block.

Renal failure—metabolite accumulation may be observed in patients with renal failure. Less than 10% of a dose is excreted unchanged by the kidneys.

Heart failure—associated with decreased hepatic blood flow, it decreases lidocaine metabolism.

Hepatic failure—significant reduction in liver metabolism results in the rapid accumulation of lidocaine and metabolites. Extreme caution must be used in these patients.

Pregnancy—Category B. Risk versus benefit must be weighed; no evidence of teratogenicity. It is not known whether lidocaine is excreted in breast milk.

Onset and Duration of Action

Dosage

Initial dose is 1.0 mg/kg IV.

Limit

Maximum dose is 3 mg/kg or 300 mg total initially.

Repeat Dosing

After initial bolus, a second bolus of 0.5 mg/kg can be given in 8 to 10 minutes and repeated until desired effect is seen or 3 mg/kg has been infused. After the arrhythmia is abolished, constant infusion of 1 to 4 mg/min should be given as maintenance therapy as follows:

Bolus	Maintenance
1 mg/kg	2 mg/min
1–2 mg/kg	3 mg/min
2–3 mg/kg	4 mg/min

Children: loading dose 1 mg/kg; infusion 20 to 50 μg/kg/min

Toxicity

Drug Interactions

Lidocaine should be used with caution in digitalis toxicity accompanied by AV block. Beta-adrenergic blocking agents may reduce hepatic blood flow, decreasing lidocaine metabolism.

Specific Adverse Effects

In patients with severely compromised cardiac function, bradycardia or hypotension may occur with lidocaine usage. This may cause cardiac arrest. Signs and symptoms of central nervous system toxicity associated with lidocaine use includes euphoria, nausea, confusion, tremors, twitching, seizures, respiratory depression, and possible respiratory arrest. Allergic reaction to lidocaine may occur.

Treatment of Toxicity

Discontinue lidocaine. Convulsions due to lidocaine may be treated with benzodiazepines (diazepam, 5 mg IV). The use of short-acting barbiturates such as pentobarbital (100 mg IV given at 50 mg/min) may also be effective.

Magnesium Sulfate

Pharmacology

MgSO$_4$

Elimination

Excreted in the urine. The renal threshold for magnesium is slightly greater than the upper limit of normal for serum magnesium. It is unusual for patients with normal renal function to develop hypermagnesemia. The initial dose of magnesium is rapidly cleared because of slow equilibration of serum magnesium levels with the intracellular stores.

Cardiovascular Actions

Through magnesium sulfate's effect of stabilization of the transmembrane potassium gradient, the PR interval is prolonged primarily through direct AV nodal effect. The SA nodal conduction time is prolonged, as is the effective AV nodal refractory period.

Indications

Magnesium sulfate is indicated for digitalis toxic arrhythmias, torsades de pointes ventricular tachycardia, and multifocal atrial tachycardia.

Cautions

Renal failure—hypermagnesemia may result because of impaired renal excretion of magnesium. Serum creatinine and magnesium levels must be carefully monitored during therapy.

Heart failure—no dose adjustment necessary

Hepatic failure—no dose adjustment necessary

Pregnancy—risk versus benefit must be weighed; seizures associated with eclampsia of pregnancy are an indication for magnesium therapy. Magnesium readily crosses the placenta and may cause hypotension and respiratory depression in the neonate. Problems associated with breast feeding have not been documented.

Onset and Duration of Action

Dosage

A dose of 2 g of 10% magnesium sulfate solution is given intravenously over 10 to 20 minutes. It may be given more rapidly in torsades de pointes therapy, but magnesium will be rapidly cleared because the renal threshold is only slightly greater than the upper limit of normal concentration for serum magnesium.

Limit

Maximum dose is 2.0 g.

Repeat Dosing

Continuous infusion of 1 to 2 g/hour may be given. Magnesium serum level should be maintained between 4 and 5 mEq/liter.

Toxicity

Drug Interactions

No specific antiarrhythmic interaction is known.

Specific Adverse Effects

Hypermagnesemia results in muscle weakness, hypotension, sedation, and confusion. Deep tendon reflexes are decreased as magnesium serum levels exceed 4 mEq/liter, and disappear at 6 mEq/liter. Respiratory paralysis may occur as serum levels approach 10 mEq/liter.

Treatment of Toxicity

The magnesium infusion should be stopped. Intravenous calcium salt infusion with 1 g calcium chloride given intravenously may offer temporary reversal of the effects of hypermagnesemia. Hemodialysis is indicated with significant respiratory paralysis, since magnesium is readily dialyzable.

Phenytoin (Dilantin)

Pharmacology

Distribution

After intravenous administration, phenytoin is rapidly distributed to the tissues.

About 90% of plasma phenytoin is bound to albumin.

Elimination

Hepatic hydroxylation metabolizes this drug, which has an effective half-life of 24 hours. Hepatic blood flow changes do not greatly influence this degradation. The microsomal enzyme system responsible for phenytoin metabolism may become saturated in the therapeutic range, resulting in unexpected toxicity secondary to this zero-order kinetics.

Actions

Central nervous system—membrane stabilization, increasing seizure threshold
Cardiovascular—phenytoin can reverse experimental SA nodal block caused by digitalis. Also, it is effective in decreasing abnormal automaticity due to digitalis-induced delayed afterdepolarizations in Purkinje fibers. Some shortening of the QT interval can also occur.

Indications

Phenytoin is considered the drug of choice for arrhythmias of digitalis toxicity or prolonged QT syndromes. It is a second-line agent for arrhythmias induced by tricyclic antidepressants. Phenytoin is not approved by the Food and Drug Administration for either indication.

Cautions

Renal failure—protein binding is decreased in uremia, in hyperbilirubinemia, and in late pregnancy, potentially causing toxicity despite "therapeutic" levels.
Hepatic failure—caution must be used because this drug is eliminated through liver metabolism.
Cardiac failure—no dose adjustment necessary
Pregnancy—risk versus benefit must be weighed. It is unclear whether phenytoin is teratogenic when administered to pregnant women. Phenytoin exposure of the fetus prior to delivery may cause hemorrhage in the neonate. Vitamin K should be given to the exposed neonate after birth. Phenytoin is excreted in the breast milk and should not be given to nursing mothers.

Onset and Duration of Action

Dosage

Phenytoin, 15 to 18 mg/kg, should be infused at a rate of 20 to 50 mg/min intravenously; in children, the dosage is 1 to 3 mg/kg/min. The serum phenytoin level should not exceed 20 μg/ml; therapeutic levels range from 10 to 20 μg/ml. Infusion should cease if (1) therapeutic effect is observed; (2) toxicity is noted; or (3) 18 mg/kg has been infused.

Limit

Maximum dose is usually 18 mg/kg.

Repeat Dosing

Further doses of phenytoin should not exceed the 20 μg/ml serum level.

Toxicity

Drug Interactions

Drugs such as dicumarol, isoniazid, diazepam, cimetidine, and trazodone may increase serum phenytoin levels. Phenytoin serum levels may be reduced by carbamazepine and reserpine. Chronic alcohol abuse can also decrease phenytoin levels. Phenobarbital and valproic acid may either increase or decrease serum levels of phenytoin.

Specific Adverse Effects

Signs and symptoms of central nervous system toxicity from phenytoin include nystagmus, ataxia, confusion, and decreased coordination. Cardiovascular toxicity may be manifested by hypotension, decreased contractility, and ventricular fibrillation.

Treatment of Toxicity

Supportive care is essential because no specific therapy exists. Hemodialysis is not indicated since phenytoin is primarily protein bound.

Procainamide (Pronestyl)

Pharmacology

Distribution

Intravenous procainamide infusion can produce therapeutic levels within minutes, with 15 to 20% reversibly bound to plasma proteins. The apparent volume of distribution is 2 liters per kilogram weight, with binding in the heart, kidney, liver, and lung. The drug is dialyzable.

Elimination

Procainamide elimination follows first-order kinetics, with over half the drug excreted unchanged in the urine. In addition, the hepatic enzyme N-acetyltransferase metabolizes the remaining procainamide, producing N-acetylprocainamide (NAPA), which also has antiarrhythmic action. The half-life of procainamide is 3 to 6 hours.

Cardiovascular Actions

Procainamide slows conduction throughout the heart, making it particularly effective against reentrant arrhythmias. Myocardial excitability is reduced in the atria, ventricles, and His-Purkinje system. Ectopic pacemaker activity is also suppressed. Contractility of ischemic myocardium may be decreased, resulting in a decreased cardiac output.

Indications

Procainamide is indicated in the treatment of premature ventricular contractions and ventricular tachycardia. It is especially useful in the treatment of wide QRS complex tachycardias, since supraventricular tachyarrhythmias with aberrancy are difficult to distinguish from ventricular tachycardia.

Cautions

Renal failure—reduced dosage is necessary because the kidneys eliminate over half the procainamide dose.

Heart failure—impaired hepatic and renal blood flow can effectively reduce elimination, resulting in toxic accumulation of procainamide. Preexisting AV nodal blockade can be increased with procainamide.

Hepatic failure—dose reduction is necessary because acetylation of procainamide will be reduced, resulting in drug accumulation.

Pregnancy—Category C. Risk versus benefit must be weighed; teratogenicity studies in humans have not been performed. Procainamide is excreted in breast milk and should not be used in nursing mothers.

Children—safety and effectiveness have not been established.

Onset and Duration of Action

Dosage

Initial dose is 50 mg every 5 minutes until (1) the arrhythmia is suppressed, (2) the QRS complex is widened by 50% of the original width, (3) hypotension develops, or (4) 1 g of the drug has been injected. A therapeutic range for procainamide (procainamide plus NAPA) of 4 to 8 μg/ml should be maintained. Toxicity is usually encountered at levels greater than 16 μg/ml.

Limit

Maximum dose is 1 g.

Repeat Dosing

A maintenance infusion of 1 to 4 mg/min can be used once the arrhythmia is successfully abolished.

Toxicity

Drug Interactions

Anticholinergic drugs such as atropine used simultaneously with procainamide may cause additive vagolytic effects on AV nodal conduction. Neuromuscular blocking agents such as succinylcholine may require a reduced dose because of the effect of procainamide on acetylcholine release.

Specific Adverse Effects

Hypotension, bradycardia, and QRS prolongation are the primary cardiovascular adverse effects. A lupus erythematosus–like syndrome may accompany long-term procainamide use but is not associated with the emergent use of the drug for arrhythmia suppression.

Treatment of Toxicity

Discontinue infusion. Supportive measures are indicated if toxicity is observed. Pressor agents can be instituted if necessary. Serum procainamide and NAPA levels should be followed.

Verapamil (Calan or Isoptin)

Pharmacology

Distribution

After intravenous infusion, verapamil has a rapid early distribution phase. The drug disappears from the plasma following first-order kinetics. Nearly 90% of verapamil is bound to plasma proteins.

Elimination

Extensive metabolism occurs in the liver, and over 12 metabolites of verapamil have been identified. Seventy percent of the administered dose is excreted in the urine and approximately 16% is excreted in the feces. Less than 5% is excreted in the urine unchanged. The elimination half-life is approximately 3 hours.

Cardiovascular Actions

Verapamil exerts a primary antiarrhythmic effect through the blockade of calcium slow channels in the AV node. Some associated inhibition of calcium-mediated excitation–contraction coupling occurs, resulting in a negative inotropic effect. Dilatation of the coronary and peripheral arteries is an additional effect.

Indications

Verapamil is indicated for use in paroxysmal supraventricular tachycardias resulting from reentrant mechanisms or narrow-complex tachycardias associated with accessory bypass tracts (Wolff-Parkinson-White and Lown-Ganong-Levine syndromes) and MAT. It is also indicated for use in atrial fibrillation or flutter *not* associated with accessory tract syndromes. Verapamil is contraindicated in wide QRS complex tachycardias because aberrant conduction of supraventricular impulses often cannot be distinguished from ventricular tachycardia.

Cautions

Renal failure—prolonged duration of action may occur because kidneys are major elimination organs for this drug.

Heart failure—negative inotropic effect of verapamil may worsen failure. Renal and hepatic perfusion may be impaired, slowing elimination.

Hepatic failure—substantial elimination occurs through hepatic metabolism. Repeated dosing may cause accumulation of verapamil and should be avoided if possible.

Cardiovascular—patients with simultaneous presence of drugs that slow AV conduction, such as beta-blockers or digitalis, may develop an additive effect with profound AV blockade. Bradycardia or periods of asystole in sick sinus syndrome may be worsened by verapamil infusion.

Pregnancy—Category C. Risk versus benefit must be weighed; teratogenicity studies have not been performed in humans. Verapamil is excreted in breast milk and should not be used in nursing mothers.

Onset and Duration of Action

Dosage

Initial dose is 5 to 10 mg IV. May pretreat with calcium, 1 g IV, if hypotension is a problem.

Limit

Maximum dose is 20 mg.

Repeat Dosing

If no effect is seen after the initial 5- to 10-mg dose, an additional 10-mg dose should be given in 20 minutes. An IV infusion of 1 to 5 mg/hour may be used.

Children

Age	Initial Dose
<12 months	0.1–0.2 mg/kg
1-15 years	0.1–0.3 mg/kg

Toxicity

Drug Interactions

Use of verapamil with digitalis requires careful monitoring for increasing AV nodal block or bradycardia. Use with beta-adrenergic blocking agents is not recommended because of potential additive effects. Verapamil may potentiate the effect of neuromuscular blocking agents; therefore, lowering the dose of either or both agents is indicated.

Specific Adverse Effects

Hypotension, severe bradycardia, and tachycardia are potential adverse cardiovascular effects of verapamil. Some dizziness and headaches have also been reported.

Treatment of Toxicity

Hypotension can be treated with calcium chloride, 1 g IV. If ineffective, dopamine may be infused at an initial rate of 5 to 10 μg/kg/min. Intravenous fluids should also be helpful. Bradycardia or asystole may be treated with calcium chloride infusion or with an isoproterenol drip, titrated for effect starting at 2 to 10 μg/min. Rapid ventricular rate and ventricular fibrillation secondary to accessory pathway conduction in Wolff-Parkinson-White or Lown-Ganong-Levine syndromes require electrical cardioversion.

REFERENCES

Adenosine

Bush A, Busst CM, Clarke B, Barnes PJ: Effect of infused adenosine on cardiac output and systemic resistance in normal subjects. Br J Clin Pharmacol 27:165–171, 1989.

DiMarco JP, Sellers TD, Lerman BB, et al: Diagnostic and therapeutic use of adenosine in patients with supraventricular tachyarrhythmias. J Am Coll Cardiol 6:417–425, 1985.

Garratt C, Linker N, Griffith M, et al: Comparison of adenosine and verapamil for termination of paroxysmal junctional tachycardia. Am J Cardiol 64:1310–1316, 1989.

Griffith MJ, Garratt CJ, Ward DE, Camm AJ: The effects of adenosine on sinus node reentrant tachycardia. Clin Cardiol 12:409–411, 1989.

Griffith MJ, Ward DE, Linker NJ, Camm AJ: Adenosine in the diagnosis of broad complex tachycardia. Lancet 1:672–675, 1988.

Lin C-I, Tao P-L, Chang Y-F, Chiang BN: Pacemaker activity is modulated by tissue levels of cyclic adenosine 3′,5′-monophosphate in human atrial fibers. Int J Cardiol 25:39–46, 1989.

Moro C, Lorio N, Nunez A, et al: Dose related efficacy of adenosine triphosphate in spontaneous supraventricular tachyarrhythmias. Int J Cardiol 25:207–212, 1989.

Rankin, AC, Oldroyd KG, Chong E, et al: Value and limitations of adenosine in the diagnosis and treatment of narrow and broad complex tachycardias. Br Heart J 62:195–203, 1989.

Rinne C, Sharma AD, Klein GJ, et al: Comparative effects of adenosine triphosphate on accessory pathway and atrioventricular nodal conduction. Am Heart J 115:1042–1047, 1988.

Amiodarone

Greenspon AJ, Volosin KJ, Greenberg RM: Amiodarone therapy: Role of early and late electrophysiologic studies. J Am Coll Cardiol 11:117–123, 1988.

Heger JJ, Prystowsky EN, Jackman WM, et al: Amiodarone: Clinical efficacy and electrophysiology during long-term therapy for recurrent ventricular tachycardia or ventricular fibrillation. N Engl J Med 305:539–545, 1981.

Kato R, Venkatesh N, Kamiya K, et al: Electrophysiologic effects of desethylamiodarone, an active metabolite of amiodarone: Comparison with amiodarone during chronic administration in rabbits. Am Heart J 115:351–359, 1988.

Klein RC, Machell C, Rushforth N, Standefur J: Efficacy of intravenous amiodarone as short-term treatment for refractory ventricular tachycardia. Am Heart J 115:96–101, 1988.

Robinson KC, McKenna WJ, Krikler DM: Amiodarone: Current perspectives from Europe. Heart Lung 16:636–639, 1987.

Saksena S, Rothbart ST, Shah Y, Cappello G: Clinical efficacy and electropharmacology of continuous intravenous amiodarone infusion and chronic oral amiodarone in refractory ventricular tachycardia. Am J Cardiol 54:347–352, 1984.

Atrial Fibrillation and Flutter

Blumlein SL, Armstrong R, Haywood LJ: Atrial flutter associated with acute myocardial infarction. West J Med 135:97–103, 1981.

Fenster PE, Comess KA, Marsh R, et al: Conversion of atrial fibrillation to sinus rhythm by acute intravenous procainamide infusion. Am Heart J 106:501–504, 1983.

Waxman HL, Myerburg RJ, Appel R, Sung RJ: Verapamil for control of ventricular rate in paroxysmal supraventricular tachycardia and atrial fibrillation or flutter: A double-blind randomized cross-over study. Ann Intern Med 94:1–6, 1981.

Atropine

Cooper MJ, Abinader EG: Atropine-induced ventricular fibrillation: Case report and review of the literature. Am Heart J 97:225–228, 1979.

Greenberg MI, Mayeda DV, Chrzanowski R, et al: Endotracheal administration of atropine sulfate. Ann Emerg Med 11:546–548, 1982.

Prete MR, Hannan CJ, Burkle FM: Plasma atropine concentrations via intravenous, endotracheal, and intraosseous administration. Am J Emerg Med 5:101–104, 1987.

Stueven HA, Tonsfeldt DJ, Thompson BM, et al: Atropine in asystole: Human studies (Part 2). Ann Emerg Med 13:815–817, 1984.

Bretylium

Dronen SC: Antifibrillatory drugs: The case for bretylium tosylate (Part 2). Ann Emerg Med 13:805–807, 1984.

Euler DE, Scanlon PJ: Mechanism of the effect of bretylium on the ventricular fibrillation threshold in dogs. Am J Cardiol 55:1396–1401, 1985.

Euler DE, Zeman TW, Walleck ME, Scanlon PJ: Deleterious effects of bretylium on hemodynamic recovery from ventricular fibrillation. Am Heart J 112:25–31, 1986.

Haynes RE, Chinn TL, Copass MK, Cobb LA: Comparison of bretylium tosylate and lidocaine in management of out of hospital ventricular fibrillation: A randomized clinical trial. Am J Cardiol 48:353–356, 1981.

Olson DW, Thompson BM, Darin JC, Milbrath MH: A randomized comparison study of bretylium tosylate and lidocaine in resuscitation of patients from out-of-hospital ventricular fibrillation in a paramedic system (Part 2). Ann Emerg Med 13:807–810, 1984.

Digoxin and Digitalis Toxicity

Bhatia SJS: Digitalis toxicity—turning over a new leaf? West J Med 145:74–82, 1986.

Mann DL, Maisel AS, Atwood JE, et al: Absence of cardioversion ventricular arrhythmias in patients with therapeutic digoxin levels. J Am Coll Cardiol 5:882–888, 1985.

Mogensen L: Digitalis-two hundred years. Acta Med Scand 220:97–100, 1986.

Ordog GJ, Benaron S, Bhasin V: Serum digoxin levels and mortality in 5,100 patients. Ann Emerg Med 16:32–39, 1987.

Schwartz JS, Bache RJ: Effect of ouabain on large coronary artery diameter. J Cardiovasc Pharmacol 11:608–613, 1988.

Sharma VK, Pottick LA, Banerjee SP: Ouabain stimulation of noradrenaline transport in guinea pig heart. Nature 286:817–819, 1980.

Springer M, Olson KR, Feaster W: Acute massive digoxin overdose: Survival without use of digitalis-specific antibodies. Am J Emerg Med 4:364–368, 1986.

Smith TW: Digitalis: Mechanism of action and clinical use. N Engl J Med 318:358–365, 1988.

Smith TW, Butler VP, Haber E, et al: Treatment of life-threatening digitalis intoxication with digoxin-specific Fab antibody fragments—experience in 26 cases. N Engl J Med 307:1357–1362, 1982.

General—Antiarrhythmic Therapy

Adams PC, Campbell RWF, Julian DG: The clinical pharmacology of antiarrhythmic drugs. In Conti CR (ed): Cardiac Drug Therapy. Cardiovascular Clinics. Philadelphia, FA Davis, 1984.

American Heart Association. Textbook of Advanced Cardiac Life Support. Dallas, American Heart Association, 1987.

Batsford WP: Are ambient and induced ventricular arrhythmias related phenomena? J Am Coll Cardiol 10:105–106, 1987.

Bigger JT: Methodology for clinical trials with antiarrhythmic drugs to prevent cardiac death: U.S. experience. Cardiology 74(Suppl 2): 40–56, 1987.

Bolton EC: Dysrhythmias in emergency medicine. In Rosen P, Baker FJ, Barkin RM, et al (eds): Concepts and Clinical Practice. St Louis, CV Mosby, 1988.

Drugs for cardiac arrhythmias. Med Lett 28:111–116, 1986.

Echt DS, Mason JW: Management of serious cardiac arrhythmias with drugs. In Conti CR (ed): Cardiac Drug Therapy. Cardiovascular Clinics. Philadelphia, FA Davis, 1984.

Graboys TB, Lown B, Podrid PJ, DeSilva R: Long-term survival of patients with malignant ventricular arrhythmia treated with antiarrhythmic drugs. Am J Cardiol 50:437–443, 1982.

Gettes LS, McAllister RG: Electrophysiology and clinical pharmacology of antiarrhythmic drugs. In Eliot RS, Saenz A, Forker AD (eds): Cardiac Emergencies. Mt Kisco, NY, Futura, 1982, pp 241–279.

Harken AH, Honigman B, VanWay CW: Cardiac dysrhythmias in the acute setting: Pathophysiology or anyone can understand cardiac dysrhythmias. J Emerg Med 5:123–128, 1987.

Hong RA, Bhandari AK, McKay CR, et al: Life-threatening ventricular tachycardia and fibrillation induced by painless myocardial ischemia during exercise testing. JAMA 257:1937–1940, 1987.

Johnson RA, Haber E, Austen WG (eds): The Practice of Cardiology. Boston, Little, Brown Co, 1980.

Kessler KM, Kissane B, Cassidy J, et al: Dynamic variability of binding of antiarrhythmic drugs during the evolution of acute myocardial infarction. Circulation 70:472–478, 1984.

Kron J, Kudenchuk PJ, Murphy ES: Ventricular fibrillation survivors in whom tachyarrhythmia cannot be induced: Outcome related to selected therapy. PACE 10:1291–1300, 1987.

Liem LB, Franz MR: A review of new antiarrhythmic drugs. Topics in Emergency Medicine, October 23–35, 1986.

Marcus FI, Ruskin JN, Surawicz B: Arrhythmias. J Am Coll Cardiol 10:66A–72A, 1987.

Morganroth J: Differential utility of antiarrhythmic agents. Cardiology 74(Suppl 2):57–66, 1987.

Nakamura M, Suyama A: Ventricular tachycardia: Variation with underlying heart disease. Cardiology Board Review 4:99–104, 1987.

Ruskin JN, DiMarco JP, Garan H: Out-of-hospital cardiac arrest: Electrophysiologic observations and selection of long-term antiarrhythmic therapy. N Engl J Med 303:607–613, 1980.

Roberts R, Husain A, Ambos HD, et al: Relation between infarct size and ventricular arrhythmia. Br Heart J 37:1169–1175, 1975.

Siddoway LA, Roden DM, Woosley RL: Clinical pharmacology of old and new antiarrhythmic drugs. In Josephson ME (ed): Sudden Cardiac Death. Cardiovasc Clin 15:199–233, 1985.

Stapczynski JS: Update on the emergent treatment of arrhythmias. In Overton DT (ed): Selected Topics on Emergency Cardiology. Emerg Med Clin North Am 6:267–288, 1988.

Stapczynski JS: Update on antiarrhythmic drugs in emergency medicine. In Overton DT (ed): Selected Topics on Emergency Cardiology. Emerg Med Clin North Am 6:289–315, 1988.

Surawicz B: Prognosis of ventricular arrhythmias in relation to sudden cardiac death: Therapeutic implications. J Am Coll Cardiol 10:435–447, 1987.

Swerdlow CD, Bardy GH, McAnulty J, et al: Determinants of induced sustained arrhythmias in survivors of out-of-hospital ventricular fibrillation. Circulation 76:1053–1060, 1987.

Vlay SC: Catecholamine-sensitive ventricular tachycardia. Am Heart J 114:455–461, 1987.

Waller TJ, Kay HR, Spielman SR, et al: Reduction in sudden death and total mortality by antiarrhythmic therapy evaluation by electrophysiologic drug testing: Criteria of efficacy in patients with sustained ventricular tachyarrhythmia. J Am Coll Cardiol 10:83–89, 1987.

Watanabe Y, Dreifus LS, Likoff W, et al: Electrophysiologic antagonism and synergism of potassium and antiarrhythmic agents. Am J Cardiol 11:702–710, 1963.

Woosley RL, Wood AJJ, Roden DM: Drug therapy: Encainide. N Engl J Med 318:1107–1115, 1988.

Isoproterenol

Andrieu J-L, Vial C, Font B, et al: Effects of isoproterenol on the metabolism of normal and ischemic heart. Arch Int Pharmacodyn 244:255–269, 1980.

Cuccurullo F, Mezzetti A, Lapenna D, et al: Mechanism of isoproterenol-induced angina pectoris in patients with obstructive hypertrophic cardiomyopathy and normal coronary arteries. Am J Cardiol 60:667–673, 1987.

Lupi-Herrera E, Sandoval J, Seoane M, et al: The role of isoproterenol in the preoperative evaluation of high-pressure, high-resistance ventricular septal defect. Chest 81:42–46, 1982.

Makdessi SA, Andrieu J-L, Herilier H, Fancon G: Effect of isoproterenol on the metabolism of myocardial fatty acids. J Mol Cell Cardiol 19:141–149, 1987.

Reddy CP, Gettes LS: Use of isoproterenol as an aid to electric induction of chronic recurrent ventricular tachycardia. Am J Cardiol 44:705–713, 1979.

Lidocaine

Carruth JE, Silverman ME: Ventricular fibrillation complicating acute myocardial infarction: Reasons against the routine use of lidocaine. Am Heart J 104:545–550, 1982.

Koster RW, Dunning AJ: Intramuscular lidocaine for prevention of lethal arrhythmias in the prehospitalization phase of acute myocardial infarction. N Engl J Med 313:1105–1110, 1985.

Lown B: Lidocaine to prevent ventricular fibrillation: Easy does it. N Engl J Med 313:1154–1156, 1985.

Nattel S, Elharrar V, Zipes DP, Bailey JC: pH-dependent electrophysiological effects of quinidine and lidocaine on canine cardiac Purkinje fibers. Circ Res 48:55–61, 1981.

Waller ES: Pharmacokinetic principles of lidocaine dosing in relation to disease state. J Clin Pharmacol 21:181–194, 1981.

Magnesium Sulfate

Cohen L, Kitzes R: Magnesium sulfate and digitalis-toxic arrhythmias. JAMA 249:2808–2810, 1983.

Reisdorff EJ, Clark MR, Walters BL: Acute digitalis poisoning: The role of intravenous magnesium sulfate. J Emerg Med 4:463–469, 1986.

Multifocal Atrial Tachycardia

Iseri LT, Fairshter RD, Hardemann JL, Brodsky MA: Magnesium and potassium therapy in multifocal atrial tachycardia. Am Heart J 110:789–794, 1985.

Iseri L, Fairshter R, Hardemann JL, Brodsky MA: Magnesium therapy in multifocal atrial tachycardia (abstr). Circulation 70(Suppl II):II-444, 1984.

Levine JH, Michael JR, Guarnieri T: Treatment of multifocal atrial tachycardia with verapamil. N Engl J Med 312:21–25, 1985.

Salerno DM, Anderson B, Sharkey PJ, Iber C: Intravenous verapamil for treatment of multifocal atrial tachycardia with and without calcium pretreatment. Ann Intern Med 107:623–628, 1987.

Paroxysmal Supraventricular Tachycardia

Denes P, Delon W, Dhingra RC: Demonstration of dual A-V nodal pathways in patients with paroxysmal supraventricular tachycardia. Circulation 48:549–555, 1973.

Grauer K, Karkal SS: Surmounting clinical hurdles in supraventricular tachyarrhythmias. Emerg Med Rep 9:49–56, 1988.

Marinchak RA, Friehling TD, Kowey PR: A clinician's approach to diagnosing supraventricular tachycardia. J Crit Illness 3:39–70, 1988.

Rosen KM, Mehta A, Miller RA: Demonstration of dual atrioventricular nodal pathways in man. Am J Cardiol 33:291–294, 1974.

Singh BN: Intravenous calcium and verapamil—when the combination may be indicated. Int J Cardiol 4:281–284, 1983.

Weiss AT, Lewis BS, Halon DA, et al: The use of calcium with verapamil in the management of supraventricular tachyarrhythmias. Int J Cardiol 4:275–280, 1983.

Phenytoin

Garson A, Kugler JD, Gillette PC, et al: Control of late postoperative ventricular arrhythmias with phenytoin in young patients. Am J Cardiol 46:290–294, 1980.

Karey REW, Blackman MS, Sondheimer HM: Phenytoin therapy for ventricular arrhythmias occurring late after surgery for congenital heart disease. Am Heart J 104:794–798, 1982.

Tsuchioka Y, Yamaoka K, Hashimoto M, et al: Electrophysiologic effects of diphenylhydantoin in patients with sinus node dysfunction. Jpn Heart J 27:159–165, 1986.

Preexcitation Syndromes

Feld GK, Nademanee K, Stevenson W, et al: Clinical and electrophysiologic effects of amiodarone in patients with atrial fibrillation complicating the Wolff-Parkinson-White syndrome. Am Heart J 115:102–107, 1988.

Gallagher JJ: Localization of accessory atrioventricular pathways: What's the "gold standard"? Pace 10:583–584, 1987.

Gulamhusein S, Ko P, Carruthers SG, Klein GJ: Acceleration of the ventricular response during atrial fibrillation in the Wolff-Parkinson-White syndrome after verapamil. Circulation 65:348–354, 1982.

Moraday F, DiCarlo LA, Baerman JM, DeBuitleir M: Effect of propranolol on ventricular rate during atrial fibrillation in the Wolff-Parkinson-White syndrome. PACE 10:492–496, 1987.

Premature Ventricular Contractions

Abdalla ISH, Prineas RJ, Neaton JD, et al: Relation between ventricular premature complexes and sudden cardiac death in apparently healthy men. Am J Cardiol 60:1036–1042, 1987.

Proarrhythmic Effect on Antiarrhythmic Drugs

Creamer JE, Nathan AW, Camm AJ: The proarrhythmic effects of antiarrhythmic drugs. Am Heart J 14:397–406, 1987.

Nuyaard TW, Sellers TD, Cook TS, Dimarco JP: Adverse reactions to antiarrhythmic drugs during therapy for ventricular arrhythmias. JAMA 256:55–57, 1986.

Ruskin JN, McGovern B, Garan H, et al: Antiarrhythmic drugs: A possible cause of out-of-hospital cardiac arrest. N Engl J Med 309:1302–1306, 1983.

Torres V, Flowers D, Somberg JC: The arrhythmogenicity of antiarrhythmic agents. Am Heart J 109:1090–1097, 1985.

Procainamide

Boucher M, Dubray C, Paire M, Duchene-Marullaz P: Comparative effects of procainamide and its N-acetylated metabolite in conscious dogs with atrioventricular block: Plasma concentration–response relationship. J Cardiovasc Pharmacol 10:562–567, 1987.

Dutty CE, Swiryn S, Bauernfeind RA, et al: Inducible sustained ventricular tachycardia refractory to individual class I drugs: Effect of adding a second class I drug. Am Heart J 106:450–458, 1983.

Greenspan AM, Horowitz LN, Spielman SR, Josephson ME: Large dose procainamide therapy for ventricular tachyarrhythmia. Am J Cardiol 46:453–462, 1980.

Olshansky B, Okumura K, Hess PG, et al: Use of procainamide with rapid atrial pacing for successful conversion of atrial flutter to sinus rhythm. J Am Coll Cardiol 11:359–364, 1988.

Roden DM, Reele SB, Higgins SB, et al: Antiarrhythmic efficacy, pharmacokinetics and safety of N-acetylprocainamide in human subjects: Comparison with procainamide. Am J Cardiol 46:463–468, 1980.

Winkle RA, Jaillon P, Kates RE, Peters F: Clinical pharmacology and antiarrhythmic efficacy of N-acetylprocainamide. Am J Cardiol 47:123–130, 1981.

Propranolol

Baber NS, Wainwright Evans D, Howitt G, et al: Multicentre postinfarction trial of propranolol in 49 hospitals in the United Kingdom, Italy, and Yugoslavia: Br Heart J 44:96–100, 1980.

B-Blocker Heart Attack Trial Research Group: A randomized trial of propranolol in patients with acute myocardial infarction: 1. Mortality results. JAMA 247:1707–1714, 1982.

Khurmi NS, O'Hara MJ, Bowles MJ, Raftery EB: Effect of diltiazem and propranolol on myocardial ischaemia during unrestricted daily life in patients with effort-induced chronic stable angina pectoris. Eur J Clin Pharmacol 32:443–447, 1987.

Peduzzi P, Hultgren H, Thomsen J, Detre K: Ten-year effect of medical and surgical therapy on quality of life: Veterans Administration cooperative sutdy of coronary artery surgery. Am J Cardiol 59:1017–1023, 1987.

Thadini U, Parker JO: Propranolol in angina pectoris: Comparison of therapy given two to four times daily. Am J Cardiol 46:117–123, 1980.

Thompson DS, Naqri N, Juul SM, et al: Effects of propranolol on myocardial oxygen consumption, substrate extraction, and haemodynamics in hypertrophic obstructive cardiomyopathy. Br Heart J 44:488–498, 1980.

Torsades de Pointes

Abildskov JA: Adrenergic effects on the QT interval of the electrocardiogram. Am Heart J 92:210–216, 1976.

Burgess KR, Jefferis RW, Stevenson IF: Fatal thioridazine cardiotoxicity. Med J Aust 2:177–178, 1979.

Chadda K, Ballas M, Bodenheimer MM: Efficacy of magnesium replacement in patients with hypomagnesemia and cardiac arrhythmia (abstr). Circulation 70(Suppl):II-444, 1989.

Hollister LE, Kosek JC: Sudden death during treatment with phenothiazine derivatives. JAMA 192:1035–1038, 1965.

Kemper AJ, Dunlap R, Pietro DA: Thioridazine-induced torsades de pointes: Successful therapy with isoproterenol. JAMA 249:2931–2934, 1983.

Krikler DM, Curry PVL: Torsades de pointes, an atypical ventricular tachycardia. Br Heart J 38:117–120, 1976.

Kulick DL, Hong R, Ryzen E, et al: Electrophysiologic effects of intravenous magnesium in patients with normal conduction systems and no clinical evidence of significant cardiac disease. Am Heart J 115:373, 1988.

Martinez R: Torsades de pointes: Atypical rhythm, atypical treatment. Ann Emerg Med 16:878–884, 1987.

Moss AJ: Prolonged QT-interval syndromes. JAMA 256:2985–2987, 1986.

Smith WM, Gallagher JJ: "Les torsades de pointes": An unusual ventricular arrhythmia. Ann Intern Med 93:578–584, 1980.

Tzivoni D, Keren A, Cohen AM, et al: Magnesium therapy for torsades de pointes. Am J Cardiol 53:528–530, 1984.

Tricyclic Antidepressant–Induced Arrhythmias

Frommer DA, Kulig KW, Marx JA, Rumack P: Tricyclic antidepressant overdose: A review. JAMA 257:521–526, 1987.

Molly DW, Penner SB, Rabson J, Hall KW: Use of sodium bicarbonate to treat tricyclic antidepressant-induced arrhythmias in a patient with alkalosis. Can Med Assoc J 130:1457–1459, 1984.

Nattel S, Keable H, Sasyniuk BI: Experimental amitriptyline intoxication: Electrophysiologic manifestations and management. J Cardiovasc Pharmacol 6:83–89, 1984.

Nattel S, Mittleman M: Treatment of ventricular tachyarrhythmias resulting from amitriptyline toxicity in dogs. J Pharmacol Exp Ther 231:430–435, 1984.

Pentel PR, Benowitz NL: Tricyclic antidepressant poisoning: Management of arrhythmias. Med Toxicol 1:101–121, 1986.

Pentel PR, Benowitz NL: Efficacy and mechanisms of action of sodium bicarbonate in the treatment of desipramine toxicity in rats. J Pharmacol Exp Ther 230:12–19, 1984.

Pentel PR, Goldsmith SR, Salerno DM, et al: Effect of hypertonic sodium bicarbonate on encainide overdose. Am J Cardiol 57:878–880, 1986.

Sasyniuk BI, Jhamandas V: Mechanism of reversal of toxic effects of amitriptyline on cardiac Purkinje fibers by sodium bicarbonate. J Pharmacol Exp Ther 231:387–394, 1984.

Sasyniuk BI, Jhamandas V, Valois M: Experimental amitriptyline intoxication: Treatment of cardiac toxicity with sodium bicarbonate. Ann Emerg Med 15:1052–1059, 1986.

Weld FM, Bigger JT: Electrophysiological effects of imipramine on ovine cardiac Purkinje and ventricular muscle fibers. Circ Res 46:167–175, 1980.

Verapamil

Buxton AE, Waxman HL, Macklinski FE, Josephson ME: Electropharmacology of nonsustained ventricular tachycardia: Effects of class I antiarrhythmic agents, verapamil and propranolol. Am J Cardiol 53:738–744, 1984.

Pariser R, Kluger J: Verapamil responsive ventricular tachycardia. Conn Med 50:612–614, 1986.

Porter CJ, Gillette PC, Garson A, et al: Effects of verapamil on supraventricular tachycardia in children. Am J Cardiol 48:487–491, 1981.

Przyklenk K, Kloner RA: Effect of verapamil on post-ischemic "stunned" myocardium: Importance of the timing of treatment. J Am Coll Cardiol 11:614–623, 1988.

Schwartz JB, Keefe D, Kates RE, et al: Acute and chronic pharmacodynamic interaction of verapamil and digoxin in atrial fibrillation. Circulation 65:1163–1170, 1982.

Sternbach G, Eliastam M: Verapamil in the treatment of ventricular tachycardia. Am J Emerg Med 3:536–540, 1985.

Sung RJ, Elser B, McAllister RG: Intravenous verapamil for termination of re-entrant supraventricular tachycardias. Ann Intern Med 93:682–689, 1980.

Woelfel A, Foster JR, McAllister RG, et al: Efficacy of verapamil in exercise-induced ventricular tachycardia. Am J Cardiol 56:292–297, 1985.

Wide-Complex Tachycardia

Baerman JM, Morady F, DiCarlo LA, de Buitleir M: Differentiation of ventricular tachycardia from supraventricular tachycardia with aberration: Value of the clinical history. Ann Emerg Med 16:40–43, 1987.

Nguyen NX, Yang P-T, Huycke E, Sung RJ: Verapamil and ventricular tachyarrhythmias. PACE 10:571–578, 1987.

Stewart RB, Bardy GH, Greene HL: Wide-complex tachycardia: Misdiagnosis and outcome after emergent therapy. Ann Intern Med 104:766–771, 1986.

Wellens HJJ, Bar FWHM, Lie KI: The value of the electrocardiogram in the differential diagnosis of a tachycardia with a widened QRS complex. Am J Med 64:27–33, 1978.

CHAPTER 12

Antihypertensives

MICHAEL S. JASTREMSKI, M.D.

INTRODUCTION

Simply defined, hypertension is an elevation of the blood pressure above normal. However, additional factors, such as the degree of blood pressure elevation, the clinical status of the patient, associated conditions, and the presence or absence of secondary complications, affect decisions concerning the need for and type and timing of antihypertensive therapy. Thus, a brief definition of the problem is necessary before the specifics of emergency therapy for hypertension can be discussed.

CONDITIONS

Asymptomatic Hypertension

Diagnosis

The 1988 report of the Joint National Committee on Detection, Evaluation, and Treatment of High Blood Pressure provides a broad consensus on the categorization of hypertension. Hypertension in adults (age > 18 years) may be categorized by the following guidelines:

Diastolic Blood Pressure (DBP)*
(mmHg)

<85	Normal
85–89	High normal
90–104	Mild hypertension
105–114	Moderate hypertension
≥115	Severe hypertension

Systolic Blood Pressure (SBP)*†
(mmHg)

<140	Normal
140–159	Borderline isolated systolic hypertension
>160	Systolic hypertension

*Average of two determinations at different times during the visit.
†When diastolic pressure is normal.

Hypertension is unusual in children and is almost always associated with some underlying pathologic state. Thus, a very careful evaluation for the causes of secondary hypertension is mandatory in children. The approach to the immediate treatment of hypertension in children, however, is the same as for adults. The Joint National Committee on High Blood Pressure suggests the following upper limits of normal pressure in children:

Age (Years)	Blood Pressure (mmHg)
14–18	<135/90
10–14	<125/85
6–10	<120/80
<6	<110/75

Indications for Treatment

The emergency department and other outpatient settings should function as a detection point for asymptomatic hypertensive patients. Every patient presenting in an emergency or outpatient setting should have an accurate and properly obtained blood pressure recorded. However, this may cause the physician the dilemma of deciding how to act on the finding of incidental hypertension in an otherwise asymptomatic individual. The physician must first decide if he or she should initiate antihypertensive treatment or refer the patient for follow-up before starting treatment. The 1988 report of the Joint National Committee on High Blood Pressure recommends that the blood pressure be averaged on two or more visits before a patient is assigned the diagnosis of hypertension. This is because there may be considerable lability of the blood pressure, with transient elevations occurring during exertion or stress (i.e., as a result of coming to the emergency department to have a laceration sutured). The Committee has recommended that follow-up of asymptomatic patients be obtained according to the following schedule:

Initial Blood Pressure (mmHg)	Follow-Up
A. DBP <85 or SBP <140	Within 2 years
B. DBP 85–89	Within 1 year
C. DBP 90–104 or SBP 140–199	Within 2 months
D. DBP 105–114 or SBP >200	Within 2 weeks
E. DBP ≥ 115	Immediate

We interpret these guidelines to imply that asymptomatic individuals with a DBP ≥ 115 mmHg should be started on the initial treatment step (see box, Stepped Care Approach to Drug Therapy) immediately and referred for follow-up evaluation in 24 to 48 hours. Although the Joint Committee report does not recommend treatment for the other categories (A to D, above) until a second confirmatory blood pressure measurement, we feel that some patients in category D should be started on treatment at the initial visit. Specifically, it is prudent and safe to start step-1 therapy (see below) for middle-aged patients with other cardiovascular risk factors, especially smoking, abnormal renal function, or a family history of cerebrovascular events. A prescription for a small starter quantity of an antihypertensive medication may help motivate the asymptomatic, high-risk patient to seek follow-up care.

STEPPED CARE APPROACH TO DRUG THERAPY: ASYMPTOMATIC HYPERTENSION

Step 1 Thiazide-type diuretic
or
Beta-blocker
or
Calcium channel blocker
or
ACE* inhibitor

Step 2 Second drug of different class
or
Increase dose of first drug
or
Discontinue first drug and substitute another drug

Step 3 Third drug of different class
or
Substitute second drug
or
Calcium channel blocker

Step 4 Third or fourth drug
and
Reevaluate

*ACE, angiotensin converting enzyme

Discussion

This stepped care outlines a graduated approach to the drug therapy of asymptomatic hypertension and is adapted from the 1988 report of the Joint National Committee on Detection, Evaluation and Treatment of High Blood Pressure. In this approach, the patient is started on small doses of a single drug, and the dose of that drug is increased or additional drugs are added until the desired blood pressure is achieved, side effects become intolerable, or the maximum dose of a drug is reached. A multiple synergistic drug regimen that allows lower doses of each individual drug may cause fewer side effects than immediately prescribing the maximum dosage of a single agent. Several months should be allowed at each step, and the reasons for lack of responsiveness (e.g., noncompliance, excess salt or weight gain, competing drugs, unrecognized secondary hypertension) should be investigated before proceeding to the next treatment step.

Symptomatic Hypertension

Diagnosis

Symptomatic hypertensive patients who require prompt treatment are commonly classified into two subsets: hypertensive emergencies and hypertensive urgencies (Table 12–1). Hypertensive emergencies mandate control of the blood pressure within an hour or less. It is the associated complications and *not* the level of blood pressure elevation that represent the danger in these situations. Hypertensive urgencies require blood pressure control within 24 hours or less because of the high risk of progression to one of the hypertensive emergencies. Accelerated or malignant hypertension is defined as a grossly elevated blood pressure in association with fundoscopic finding of grade III (accelerated) or grade IV (malignant) retinopathy. Table 12–1 possibly overclassifies conditions into the hypertensive emergency category, and clinical judgment must be applied when deciding how rapidly to lower the blood pressure in a given patient. However, it is much better to institute therapy too soon rather than too late.

Indications for Treatment

See Table 12–1 and boxes, Drug Treatment: Hypertensive Emergencies and Drug Treatment: Hypertensive Urgencies.

TABLE 12–1. Classification of Hypertensive Emergencies and Urgencies

Hypertensive Emergencies
Hypertensive encephalopathy
Aortic dissection
Eclampsia
Hypertension with acute myocardial ischemia or pulmonary edema
Cerebral hemorrhage
Pheochromocytoma crisis
Sympathomimetic drug overdose
Monoamide oxidase inhibitor–tyramine interaction
Rebound from abrupt cessation of antihypertensive medication (e.g., clonidine)
Perioperative hypertension

Hypertensive Urgencies
Accelerated or malignant hypertension
Diastolic pressure >130 mmHg
Hypertension associated with rapidly deteriorating renal function
Intractable nasal hemorrhage

Discussion: Hypertensive Emergencies

The drug treatment of hypertensive emergencies outlined in the box represents my preferred sequential approach to this problem based on personal experience and review of the literature. This algorithmic approach has not been tested in a prospective, controlled clinical trial. Most patients with hypertensive emergencies will need admission to an intensive care unit, but treatment must begin immediately in the emergency department. An arterial line is necessary for constant monitoring of the blood pressure (I usually use a 20-gauge 2-inch catheter in the radial artery of the nondominant wrist) and should be inserted as soon as feasible *after* treatment has begun.

It is important to remember that patients with chronic hypertension have their autoregulation curve for cerebral blood flow shifted upward; they may develop hypoperfusion and cerebral ischemia at higher pressures than would a normal individual. Therefore, it is prudent to aim for an initial blood pressure reduction of 25 to 30% of the patient's pretreatment blood pressure, with care being taken to avoid abrupt falls below a systolic pressure of 150 to 160 mmHg and a diastolic pressure of 100 mmHg. If this level of pressure reduction does not abolish the hypertensive complication, the blood pressure should be cautiously lowered further. If this level of blood pressure reduction is associated with evidence of hypoperfusion, such as a decreasing urine output or al-

DRUG TREATMENT: HYPERTENSIVE EMERGENCIES

First-Line Drug
Sodium Nitroprusside

Initial Dose	0.5 μg/kg/min by continuous IV infusion (1 ml of a solution of 50 mg sodium nitroprusside in 250 ml D$_5$W contains 200 μg). *Add a beta-blocker if aortic dissection is present.*
Repeat Dose	Increase infusion rate by 0.1–0.5 μg/kg/min every 5 minutes.
End-Point	Higher of systolic blood pressure no lower than 160 mmHg and diastolic blood pressure no lower than 100 mmHg, or 25% reduction in starting blood pressure with relief of signs and symptoms of clinical problem and no evidence of hypoperfusion; in aortic dissection, systolic blood pressure of 100–110 mmHg or signs of cerebral hypoperfusion

Second-Line Drug
Diazoxide

Initial Dose	1–3 mg/kg IV bolus (maximum bolus 150 mg) every 5 minutes to maximum total dose of 600 mg
Alternate Dosing Regimen	IV infusion of 15 mg/min (1 ml of solution containing 300 mg diazoxide in 20 ml) for 20 to 30 minutes; must pretreat with 0.02 mg/kg propranolol IV
End-Point	Higher of systolic blood pressure no lower than 160 mmHg and diastolic blood pressure no lower than 100 mmHg, or 25% reduction in starting blood pressure with relief of signs and symptoms of clinical problem and no evidence of hypoperfusion

SPECIAL CIRCUMSTANCES

Eclampsia (See Chap. 23)

First-Line Drug
Hydralazine

Initial Dose	5 mg IV bolus
Repeat Dose	5–10 mg IV bolus at 15- to 20-minute intervals
End-Point	Diastolic pressure 90–100 mmHg

Pheochromocytoma or Monoamide Oxidase Inhibitor Crisis

First-Line Drug
Sodium Nitroprusside

Initial Dose	0.5 μg/kg/min by continuous IV infusion (1 ml of a solution of 50 mg sodium nitroprusside in 250 ml D$_5$W contains 200 μg)
Repeat Dose	Increase infusion rate by 0.1–0.5 μg/kg/min every 5 minutes.
End-Point	Higher of systolic blood pressure no lower than 160 mmHg and diastolic blood pressure no lower than 100 mmHg, or 25% reduction in starting blood pressure with relief of signs and symptoms of clinical problem and no evidence of hypoperfusion

Chart continued on following page

DRUG TREATMENT: HYPERTENSIVE EMERGENCIES *Continued*

Second-Line Drug

Phentolamine

Initial Dose	Continuous IV infusion of 0.1 to 2 mg/min
Alternate Dosing Regimen	Repeated 5-mg IV boluses
End-Point	25% reduction from starting blood pressure. In patients with a pheochromocytoma, add a beta-blocker at this time when alpha blockade is ensured.

Clonidine Withdrawal

First-Line Drug

Clonidine

Initial Dose	0.2 mg orally
Repeat Dose	0.1 mg every hour to maximum of 0.8 mg
End-Point	Higher of systolic blood pressure no lower than 160 mmHg and diastolic blood pressure no lower than 100 mmHg, or 25% reduction in starting blood pressure with relief of signs and symptoms of clinical problem and no evidence of hypoperfusion

Second-Line Drug

Sodium Nitroprusside

Initial Dose	0.5 μg/kg/min by continuous IV infusion (1 ml of a solution of 50 mg sodium nitroprusside in 250 ml D_5W contains 200 μg)
Repeat Dose	Increase infusion rate by 0.1–0.5 μg/kg/min every 5 minutes.
End-Point	Higher of systolic blood pressure no lower than 160 mmHg and diastolic blood pressure no lower than 100 mmHg, or 25% reduction in starting blood pressure with relief of signs and symptoms of clinical problem and no evidence of hypoperfusion

Third-Line Drug

Diazoxide

Initial Dose	IV infusion of 7.5 mg/min for 20–30 minutes (0.5 ml of a solution containing 300 mg diazoxide in 20 ml)
Alternate Dosing Regimen	50-mg IV boluses every 5 minutes until desired blood pressure reduction or maximum dose of 600 mg
End-Point	25% reduction in starting blood pressure

terations in neurologic function, the blood pressure should be allowed to rise to a systolic pressure of 160 to 180 mmHg with a diastolic pressure of approximately 120 mmHg. The exception to this end-point is acute aortic dissection. In this condition, the blood pressure is lowered to a systolic of 100 to 110 mmHg unless vital organ perfusion is compromised.

Sodium nitroprusside, given by titrated intravenous infusion, is the preferred drug for the immediate control of most hypertensive emergencies. It is rapid acting, with the maximal response to each dosage increase apparent in minutes. Therefore, after starting at 0.5 μg/kg/min, the infusion rate should be increased by 0.1 to 0.5 μg/kg/min every 5 minutes until the desired reduction in blood

DRUG TREATMENT: HYPERTENSIVE URGENCIES

First-Line Drug

Nifedipine

Initial Dose	10 mg sublingually
Repeat Dose	10 mg sublingually or orally in 1–2 hours and then every 6 hours
End-Point	25–30% reduction from the starting blood pressure without evidence of hypoperfusion

Second-Line Drug

Sodium Nitroprusside

Initial Dose	0.1–0.2 µg/kg/min by continuous IV infusion (1.0 ml of a solution of 50 mg sodium nitroprusside in 250 ml D$_5$W contains 200 µg)
Repeat Dose	Increase by 0.1 µg/kg/min every 10–15 minutes.
End-Point	25–30% reduction from the starting blood pressure without evidence of hypoperfusion

Third-Line Drug

Diazoxide

Initial Dose	50 mg IV bolus every 5 minutes to maximum of 600 mg
Alternate Dosing Regimen	IV infusion of 7.5 mg/min (0.5 ml of a solution of 300 mg diazoxide in 20 ml) for 20–30 minutes
End-Point	25–30% reduction from the starting blood pressure without evidence of hypoperfusion

Fourth-Line Drug

Labetalol

Initial Dose	20 mg IV bolus
Repeat Dose	40 mg IV bolus every 10 minutes to maximum of 300 mg
End-Point	25–30% reduction from the starting blood pressure without evidence of hypoperfusion

pressure is achieved. Each dosage increase should be smaller as the targeted blood pressure is approached. Considerable individual variation exists in the response to sodium nitroprusside, so the effective level may range from as little as 0.1 to 0.2 µg/kg/min up to 8 or 10 µg/kg/min. The other favorable pharmacokinetic characteristic of sodium nitroprusside is its very short effective half-life. Thus, if sodium nitroprusside causes an excessive decrease in the blood pressure, the intravenous drip can be stopped, and the blood pressure will come back up in a few minutes, at which time the drip is restarted at a dose lower than the one that produced the low pressure.

Diazoxide is an accepted alternative to intravenous sodium nitroprusside for the management of hypertensive emergencies. Diazoxide is usually not the first-choice drug because its pharmacokinetics do not allow for the minute-to-minute fine tuning of the blood pressure that is possible with sodium nitroprusside. The current dosing approach of using a 15-mg/min infusion over 20 to 30 minutes or a 50- to 150-mg bolus every 5 minutes until the desired blood pressure is achieved is less likely to produce hypotension than the original approach of giving a single 300-mg rapid IV bolus, which is no longer recommended. However, diazoxide may still produce excessive lowering of the blood pressure that is more difficult to reverse than that caused by sodium nitroprusside. In addition, diazoxide should not be used in patients with acute aortic dissection, myocardial ischemia, or pulmonary edema.

Some suggestions have appeared in the literature that sublingual nifedipine, intravenous labetalol, or oral clonidine might be used in hypertensive emergencies. Their use has been reported in small case series consisting mostly of patients with hypertensive urgencies rather than hypertensive emergencies. It is the opinion of this author that these regimens have not been proved and do not offer any advantage in the management of hypertensive emergencies.

The flow sheet for managing hypertensive emergencies suggests some variation in the initial management based on the etiology of the hypertension. Eclampsia is clearly a special circumstance that should be quite easy to diagnose. Hydralazine is the drug of choice for blood pressure control in this setting, along with magnesium sulfate to control the neuromuscular irritability (see Chap. 23 for a more complete discussion). The definitive management of eclampsia in pregnancy is delivery of the baby. In the unusual case of eclampsia that does not respond to hydralazine, sodium nitroprusside may be tried. The hypertensive emergencies created by a pheochromocytoma, clonidine withdrawal, or monoamide oxidase inhibitor–tyramine interaction are best treated with phentolamine. However, these conditions will also respond well to sodium nitroprusside, which may be more readily available than phentolamine, so it is not a problem if their etiology is not immediately identified. Clonidine withdrawal can also be managed with oral clonidine loading.

Oral drug therapy for long-term definitive control of the blood pressure should be started as soon as the blood pressure has been stabilized at the targeted level for several hours with parenteral therapy. Multiple drug therapy is begun at the outset in these patients because of the seriousness of the problem. A useful drug combination is hydralazine and propranolol or labetalol. Captopril may be used instead of hydralazine. Captopril is favored for use in patients with renal failure because it selectively increases renal blood flow. Some clinicians may choose to use a calcium blocker such as nifedipine in the initial oral drug regimen, especially in patients with coexisting angina. However,

the role and utility of calcium blockers in the management of hypertension have not been clearly elucidated, and they are not yet approved by the Food and Drug Administration for this purpose. Minoxidil may be valuable in refractory cases, particularly if the patient has renal disease. Patients who have developed a hypertensive emergency because of noncompliance with drug therapy may be restarted on an oral regimen known to have been effective previously in controlling their blood pressure.

As the oral medications begin to exert their effect, the parenteral medication is progressively tapered to maintain the desired blood pressure. Sodium nitroprusside pharmacokinetics coupled with continuous intra-arterial blood pressure monitoring in an intensive care unit allow a smooth transition from parenteral to oral therapy.

Discussion: Hypertensive Urgencies

Hypertensive urgencies do not require quite as immediate control of the blood pressure as do hypertensive emergencies, but they do require initiation of treatment in the emergency department before admission to the inpatient ward. Many clinicians manage hypertensive urgencies using an approach identical to that for hypertensive emergencies. Therapy is started with intravenous sodium nitroprusside or diazoxide, an intra-arterial monitoring line is inserted, and the patient is admitted to an intensive care unit; after the blood pressure is brought under control with the parenteral drug regimen, the patient is switched to multiple drug oral therapy for long-term management. In contrast to hypertensive emergencies where the major problem is a complication of hypertension rather than the degree of blood pressure elevation, in hypertensive urgencies the problem is the degree of blood pressure elevation and the prevention of complications. The clinician needs to be concerned about both complications resulting from the hypertension and complications resulting from excessive lowering of the blood pressure. Therefore, in hypertensive urgencies, it is prudent to aim for a 25 to 30% reduction in the blood pressure at a gradual rate over 12 to 24 hours to minimize the possibility of overshoot hypotension. If using sodium nitroprusside, start at 0.1 to 0.2 μg/kg/min, wait 10 or 15 minutes at each dosing level, and increase the dose by only 0.1 μg/kg/min at a time. If using diazoxide, administer 50-

mg boluses or a drip of only 7.5 to 10 mg/ min.

Nifedipine, given orally or sublingually, is an attractive alternative to sodium nitroprusside or diazoxide for managing hypertensive urgencies and is now my first choice when treating this problem. In a recent prospective trial, oral nifedipine compared favorably with intravenous nitroprusside in terms of blood pressure control and morbidity. Nifedipine is advantageous because it is simpler and easier to use and may resolve the problem quickly, obviating the need for intensive care unit admission; however, these patients generally still require inpatient admission for institution of a long-term management regimen. Nifedipine is given as a 10-mg oral dose, repeated in 1 to 2 hours and then at 6-hour intervals until the desired reduction of blood pressure is achieved or a total dose of 60 mg has been administered. A more rapid initial effect can be achieved if the initial dose is administered intraorally in liquid form. The majority of patients in the clinical trial responded to 20 mg of nifedipine, and no nifedipine-treated patients had hypotension requiring treatment. Nifedipine has not yet been approved by the Federal Drug Administration for this use.

The combined alpha- and beta-blocker labetalol also shows some promise for use in hypertensive urgencies; however, it probably offers no advantages over sodium nitroprusside, diazoxide, or nifedipine and has a much smaller experience base than these drugs. Labetalol can be given as an intravenous infusion at a rate of 2 mg/min or by intermittent intravenous boluses given over 2 minutes. If the intravenous bolus technique is used, the first dose is 20 mg, and subsequent boluses of 40 to 80 mg are given every 10 minutes until the targeted blood pressure is reached or a maximum dose of 300 mg has been given. In one controlled study using the intravenous bolus technique, there was no hypotension but also no response in 2 of 17 patients. Because of its beta-blocking effect, labetalol is less likely to cause reflex tachycardia but more likely to cause bradyarrhythmias or heart failure. In my opinion, labetalol requires the same intensive care unit monitoring as does sodium nitroprusside or diazoxide, has a greater potential for side effects, and offers no advantage over more proven approaches to this problem.

Once the blood pressure has been stabilized at the desired level for several hours by the acute regimen, multiple drug oral therapy is started in a fashion identical to that described for hypertensive emergencies.

SPECIFIC AGENTS

Detailed information concerning the various drugs used for the treatment of hypertension is provided in this section. The drugs are grouped by their mechanism of action. Table 12-2 provides a summary of the important features of each drug.

Adrenergic Inhibitors

Alpha-Blockers

The peripherally acting alpha-blocking drugs lower blood pressure by modulation of catecholamine stimulation of the sympathetic nerves serving the vasculature. Catecholamines, such as epinephrine and norepinephrine, stimulate postsynaptic alpha$_1$-receptors, causing vasoconstriction and hypertension. Alpha$_1$-receptor blockade opposes this effect and lowers blood pressure. Stimulation of presynaptic alpha$_2$-receptors inhibits norepinephrine release from sympathetic neurons and thus lowers blood pressure. Therefore, alpha$_2$-receptor blockade can increase vascular tone and blood pressure. In addition, the increased norepinephrine release produced by alpha$_2$ blockade leads to beta-receptor stimulation, which can cause dysrhythmias and angina.

Phenoxybenzamine (Dibenzyline)

Pharmacology

Haloarylamine
Blocks both alpha$_1$- and alpha$_2$-receptors with alpha$_1$ effect predominant

Kinetics (Oral Formulation Only)

Onset	Variable
Peak	Variable
Duration	Variable
Half-life	12 hours to up to a week

Metabolism

Molecular conversion to reactive caronium ion
Renal excretion

Text continued on page 208

TABLE 12–2. Summary of Features of Antihypertensive Drugs

Drug	Route	How Supplied	Starting Dose	Onset of Action	Maintenance Dose
Adrenergic Inhibitors					
Alpha-Blockers					
Phenoxybenzamine	PO	10-mg capsules	10 mg bid	Variable	10–100 mg bid
Phentolamine	IV	5-mg/ml	5-mg IV bolus	Minutes	IV infusion, 0.2–0.5 mg/min
Prazosin	PO	1-, 2-, 5-mg capsules	1 mg bid or tid	30 min	6–20 mg in divided doses
Beta-Blockers°					
Propranolol	IV	1 mg/ml	1 mg	Minutes	Repeated 1–2 mg boluses as needed
	PO	10-, 20-, 40-, 60-, 80-, 90-mg tablets	40 mg bid	Days to weeks	120–480 mg daily in divided doses
Esmolol	IV	2.5 g/10 ml	500 μg/kg	Immediate	100–200 μg/kg/min
Alpha- and Beta-Blocker					
Labetalol	IV	5 mg/ml	20 mg over 2 min	5 min	40–80 mg bolus q 5 min until desired blood pressure or maximum 300 mg
	PO	100-, 200-, 300-mg tablets	200 mg	2 hours	400–1200 mg in divided doses
Central Adrenergic Inhibitors					
Clonidine	PO	0.1-, 0.2-, 0.3-mg tablets	0.1 mg	30–60 min	0.2–1.0 mg in divided doses
	Transdermal	0.1-, 0.2-, 0.3-mg qd systems	TTS-1†	30–60 min	TTS-1 to TTS-3 weekly
Guanabenz	PO	4-, 8-, 16-mg tablets	4 mg	60 min	8–32 mg in divided doses
Guanfacine	PO	1-mg tablets	1 mg	60 min	1–3 mg daily
Methyldopa	IV	250 mg/5 ml	250 mg/30–60 min	4–6 hours	250–2000 mg
	PO	125-, 250-, 500-mg tablets	250 mg	4–6 hours	500–2000 mg in divided doses
Peripheral Adrenergic Antagonists					
Guanethidine	PO	10-, 25-mg tablets	10 mg	Days	10–100 mg qd
Reserpine	PO	0.1-, 0.25-mg tablets	0.05 mg	Days	0.05–0.25 qd

Adverse Effects	Interactions	Use in Pregnancy	Use in Nursing Mother
Hypotension Tachycardia	Exaggerated hypotensive response to vasodilating agents	Category C	Avoid
Hypotension Tachycardia	Exaggerated hypotensive response to vasodilating agents	Category C	No data; avoid
Syncope	Reduce dose of prazosin when adding other antihypertensives Nonsteroidals decrease effect	Category C	No infant toxicity reported; small quantities in breast milk
Hypotension/cardiac failure Bronchospasm Bradycardia	Increases theophylline toxicity Barbiturates decrease effect Cimetidine increases effect Severe vasoconstriction with ergot alkaloids Additive adverse cardiac effects with calcium channel blockers Decreased effect of oral hypoglycemics Prolonged hypoglycemia with insulin and oral hypoglycemics Salicylates decrease antihypertensive effect	Category C	Appears in breast milk
Same as propranolol	Increases digoxin levels	Category C	No data
Cardiac failure Rapid hypotension Bradycardia Branchospasm	Cimetidine increases bioavailability Blunts bronchodilator effects of beta-agonist bronchodilators Tremor with tricyclics Synergistic hypotension with halothane	Category C	Appears in breast milk
Severe rebound hypertension	Tricyclics reduce clonidine effect Hypertension with beta-blockers	Category C	High concentrations in breast milk
Sedation	Increased effect of CNS depressants	Category C	No data
Rebound hypertension		Category B	No data
Hemolytic anemia Orthostatic hypotension Sedation Hepatitis	Hypertension with beta-blockers Hypotension with anesthetics Oral contraceptives decrease effect Additive effect on conduction with digoxin	Category C	Appears in breast milk
Postural hypotension Bronchospasm Cardiac failure	*Do not use with MAO inhibitors* Hypotensive effect reduced by amphetamines, ephedrine, methylphenicate, tricyclic antidepressants, phenothiazides, and oral contraceptives	Category C	Appears in breast milk
Depression Postural hypotension	Hypotension with barbituates and general anesthetics Arrhythmias when used with digitalis or quinidine Do not use with MAO inhibitors Hypertension with sympathomimetics Tricyclic antidepressants decrease hypotensive action	Category D	Appears in breast milk

Table continued on following page

TABLE 12–2. Summary of Features of Antihypertensive Drugs *Continued*

Drug	Route	How Supplied	Starting Dose	Onset of Action	Maintenance Dose
Angiotensin Converting Enzyme Inhibitors					
Captopril	PO	12.5-, 25-, 50-, 100-mg tablets	25 mg	60–90 min	25–50 mg bid or tid
Enalapril	PO	5-, 10-, 20-mg tablets	5 mg	1 hour	10–40 mg qd or bid Reduce dose in renal failure
Enalaprilat	IV	1.25 mg/ml	1.25 mg (0.625 mg with diuretic)	15 min	1.25 mg q 6 hours
Calcium Blockers					
Nifedipine	PO	10-, 20-mg capsules	10 mg	15–30 min	Repeat q 1–2 hours until desired blood pressure achieved, then 10–30 mg q 6 hours
	Sublingual		10 mg	5–10 min	
Diuretics°					
Furosemide	IV	10 mg/ml	20–40 mg	30–60 min	20–200 mg q 2–6 hours
	PO	20-, 40-, 80-, mg tablets, 10 mg/ml oral solution	40 mg	Hours	80–240 mg daily in 2 divided doses
Vasodilators					
Diazoxide	IV	300 mg/20 ml ampule	1–3 mg/kg q 5 min or 15 mg/min × 20–30 min	1–5 min	May repeat initial dose q 4–24 hours if needed
Hydralazine	IV	20 mg/ml ampule	10–20 mg	10–30 min	Repeat as needed q 2–4 hours
	IM		10–20 mg	10–80 min	
	PO	10-, 25-, 50-, 100-mg tablets	5 mg	1–2 hours	40–300 mg in divided doses
Minoxidil	PO	2.5-, 10-mg tablets	5 mg	30 min–2 hours	10–40 mg qd or bid
Sodium nitroprusside	IV	50-mg vial	0.5 μg/kg/min	Seconds	0.25–10.0 μg/kg/min
Trimethaphan	IV	500 mg/10 ml ampule	0.5 mg/min continuous infusion	1–5 min	0.3–6 mg/min infusion

°There are many drugs in this class, but they all have similar effects. Major differences exist in duration of action, which is important therapeutically.
†TTS = transdermal therapeutic system.

Adverse Effects	Interactions	Use in Pregnancy	Use in Nursing Mother

Hypotension
Renal failure
Neutropenia
Angioedema
	Exaggerated hypotensive effect
	  with diuretics
	Hyperkalemia with potassium-
	  sparing diuretics
	Increased risk of renal failure with
	  diuretics
	Neuropathy with cimetidine
	Hypoglycemia with insulin and
	  oral hypoglycemics
		Category C	Low level in breast milk

Same as captopril	Same as captopril	Category C	Appears in breast milk
Same as captopril	Same as captopril	Category C	Avoid; no data

Hypotension
Heart failure
	Additive adverse effects on
	  contractility and AV conduction
	  with beta-blockers
	Increases digoxin levels
	Increases coumadin effect
	Cimetidine and ranitidine
	  increase nifedipine levels
	Decreased quinidine effect
	Severe hypotension with prazosin
		Category C	No data

Hypokalemia
Hypovolemia
Aplastic anemia
Pancreatitis
	Phenytoin decreases diuretic
	  effect
	Increases digoxin toxicity
	Enhances lithium toxicity
	Increases salicylate level
	Indomethacin blocks diuretic
	  effect
	Enhances cephalosporin
	  nephrotoxicity
	Enhances aminoglycoside
	  nephrotoxicity and ototoxicity
	Increases quinidine absorption
	Increases propranolol effect
	Enhanced neuromuscular
	  blockade
		Category C	Avoid; may cause infant
			thrombocytopenia

Rapid hypotension
Hyperglycemia
Cardiac failure
	Increases coumadin effect
	Severe hypotension with beta-
	  blockers, nitrates, vasodilators,
	  narcotics
	Decreases phenytoin effect
		Category C	No data

Tachycardia
Postural hypotension
Lupus syndrome
	Do not use with MAO inhibitors or
	  diazoxide
	Increases effect of propranolol
	  and metoprolol
	Decreases digoxin effect
	Nonsteroidals decrease
	  hydralazine's effect
		Category B
		Drug of choice
		  in
		  pregnancy
			No data

Cardiac failure Tachycardia Rapid hypotension Pericardial effusion	Do not use with guanethidine or diazoxide	Category D	Appears in breast milk
Rapid hypotension Cyanide toxicity Vomiting	Decreased digoxin effect	Category C	No data

Respiratory arrest
Rapid hypotension
Pupillary dilation
	Hypotensive effect enhanced by
	  diuretics, anesthetics, and other
	  antihypertensives
		Category D	No data

> *Note:* The variable kinetics of phenoxybenzamine are due to a combination of erratic absorption and the active molecule being a metabolite of the orally administered prodrug.

Indications

Pheochromocytoma (for chronic blood pressure control, *not* during crisis)

Dosage

Needs careful individual titration
Initial—10 mg twice daily
Additional—increase each dose by 10 mg after several days until desired control of blood pressure is achieved.

Cautions

Dosage adjustments—reduce dose in hepatic or renal failure.
Use in pregnancy—Category C. Although this drug is mutagenic in some models, the risk of maternal and fetal mortality from pheochromocytoma far outweighs the mutation risk.
Use in lactation—no data
Use in childhood—no data

Toxicity

Side Effects

Common: hypotension, tachycardia, miosis, nasal congestion, inhibition of ejaculation, fatigue, sedation
Uncommon: convulsions, nausea and vomiting
Dangerous: convulsions, hypotension

Treatment of Acute Toxicity

Stop drug.
For hypotension, elevate patient's legs; give fluid bolus and norepinephrine (*not* epinephrine) infusion, 0.1 to 0.5 μg/kg/min.
For convulsion, give intravenous diazepam.

Interactions

Enhanced hypotensive effect with other vasodilating drugs (e.g., beta-blockers, opiates, alcohol)
Urinary incontinence with methyldopa

Phentolamine (Regitine)

Pharmacology

2-substituted imidazoline
Alpha-blocker with predominant alpha$_1$ effect

Kinetics (IV Administration Only)

Onset	0.5–1 minute
Peak	0.5–1 minute
Duration	10–20 minutes
Half-life	15 minutes

Metabolism

Unclear—10% urinary excretion

Indications

Acute pheochromocytoma crisis
Treatment of vasoconstrictor extravasation
Monoamide oxidase inhibitor–tyramine reaction

Dosage (IV or IM)

Initial—5-mg bolus
Maintenance—continuous IV infusion of 0.2 to 0.5 mg/min

Cautions

Dosage adjustments in organ failure—none
Use in pregnancy—Category C; avoid.
Use in lactation—no data
Use in childhood—yes; bolus dose, 1 mg

Hemodynamic Effects

Heart rate	Increased
Afterload	No change
Cardiac output	Decreased
Renal blood flow	Increased or no change
Cerebral blood flow	No change

Toxicity

Side Effects

Common: hypotension, tachycardia, abdominal pain, nausea and vomiting, diarrhea
Dangerous: myocardial infarction, stroke, ischemic dysrhythmias

Treatment of Acute Toxicity

Stop drug.
Volume infusion

Norepinephrine (*not* epinephrine) infusion at 0.1 to 0.5 μg/kg/hour

Antiarrhythmics

Interactions

Hypotension enhanced by other vasodilating agents and hypovolemia (diuretics)

Prazosin (Minipress)

Pharmacology

Quinazoline derivative

Alpha$_1$-receptor blocker

Affects both arteries and veins

Phosphodiesterase inhibition yields bronchodilatation.

Kinetics

Onset	30 minutes
Peak	2–3 hours
Duration	8 hours
Half-life	2–3 hours

Metabolism

Hepatic demethylation and conjugation, then biliary excretion

Indication

Chronic blood pressure control, especially with coexisting renal dysfunction or congestive heart failure

Contraindications

Not useful for acute management of hypertensive urgencies or emergencies

Dosage

Initial—1 mg at bedtime

Maintenance—6 to 20 mg daily in two or three divided doses (achieved by increasing daily dose by 1 or 2 mg every few days until the desired level of blood pressure is achieved)

Effect enhanced by addition of diuretic therapy

Cautions

Dose adjustments in organ failure—none

Use in pregnancy—Category C

Use in lactation—excreted in breast milk, avoid.

Use in childhood—no data

Beware: "First-dose syncope" may occur with prazosin. This is due to hypotension, usually postural, resulting from alpha-induced venous dilation. It occurs 30 to 90 minutes after the first dose (incidence is increased if 2 mg or more used) or after large increases in dose. Concomitant diuretic use increases the risk of this complication.

Hemodynamic Effects

Heart rate	No change or increased
Preload	Decreased
Afterload	Decreased
Cardiac output	No change
Renal blood flow	No change
Cerebral blood flow	No change

Toxicity

Side Effects

Common: dizziness, drowsiness, headache, lassitude, palpitations, nausea

Uncommon: vomiting, diarrhea, constipation, edema, rash, blurred vision, nasal congestion, dry mouth, paresthesias, tinnitus, incontinence, priapism

Dangerous: syncope due to hypotension

Treatment of Acute Toxicity

Supine position, legs elevated

Volume infusion

Vasopressor

Decrease dose of drug.

Interactions

Increased hypotensive effect with beta-blockers, diazoxide, nifedipine, diuretics, verapamil

Nonsteroidal anti-inflammatory agents decrease prazosin effect.

Beta-Blockers

The beta-blockers have limited utility in the management of hypertensive urgencies and emergencies. Their role in these situations is primarily as adjunctive therapy to block the reflex tachycardia induced by vasodilating drugs. A beta-blocker is specifically indicated in hypertension associated with aortic dissection to reduce the force of cardiac contraction. Beta-blockers are also used in hypertension associated with myocardial ischemia because of their favorable effects on myocardial oxygen supply–demand balance. A large number or oral beta-blockers are now available that differ in their selectivity for the beta$_1$ cardiac receptors and duration of action. The oral agents are a mainstay in the stepped-care management of chronic hypertension but are not useful in hypertensive crises and so will not be discussed here.

Esmolol (Brevibloc)

Pharmacology

($\pm$)-Methyl   p-[2-hydroxy-3-(isopropyl-amino)propoxy]hydrocinnamate hydrochloride
Cardioselective beta$_1$-receptor antagonist
No intrinsic sympathomimetic activity

Kinetics (IV Loading Bolus)

Onset	Immediate
Peak	5 minutes
Duration	20 minutes
Half-life	9 minutes

Metabolism

Hydrolysis by circulating esterases

Indications

Supraventricular tachycardia
Hypertension (especially in the postoperative period)

Contraindications

Sinus bradycardia
Hypotension
Heart block greater than first-degree
Congestive heart failure

Dosage

(*Note:* Dilute before infusion by adding 5 g (2 ampules) of esmolol to 480 ml D$_5$W to yield concentration of 10 mg/ml.)
500 μg/kg loading dose over 1 minute, followed by a 4-minute infusion of 50 μg/kg/min
If no response, repeat loading dose and increase infusion by 50 μg/kg/min. This may be repeated twice more to achieve maximum recommended infusion rate of 200 μg/kg/min.
When desired therapeutic effect is achieved, continue maintenance infu-

sion at dose that was effective (esmolol infusions have been well tolerated for 24 to 48 hours).

Cautions

Dose adjustments in organ failure—none
Use in pregnancy—Category C; avoid.
Use in lactation—no data
Use in childhood—no clinical experience

Hemodynamic Effects

Heart rate	Decreased
Preload	Increased
Afterload	Decreased
Cardiac output	Decreased
Renal blood flow	Decreased
Cerebral blood flow	Decreased

Toxicity

Side Effects

(Current clinical experience is limited, so complete side effect profile may not yet be apparent.)
Common: hypotension (usually transient and asymptomatic), diaphoresis, dizziness, somnolence, nausea, inflammation at infusion site (incidence increases with increasing duration of infusion), headache
Uncommon: bronchospasm (drug seems to be safe to use in patients with reactive airway disease), bradycardia, myocardial depression
Dangerous: bradycardia, hypotension, heart failure

Treatment of Acute Toxicity

Stop infusion.
For bradycardia, give atropine, isoproterenol; use external pacer.
For hypotension, give dopamine or dobutamine infusion.
For bronchospasm, provide inhalation treatment with metaproterenol (Alupent) or albuterol.

Interactions

Additive effect with catecholamine-depleting drugs (reserpine)
Increases digoxin levels
Slightly increases duration of succinylcholine effect
Morphine increases esmolol steady-state levels.

Propranolol (Inderal)

Pharmacology

1-(isopropylamino)-3-(1-naphthyloxy)-2-propanol hydrochloride
Nonselective beta-adrenergic blocker
No intrinsic sympathomimetic activity
Strong membrane-stabilizing activity
Antihypertensive effect produced by combination of cardiac, central nervous system, and humoral actions

Kinetics

	IV Bolus	Oral
Onset	1 minute	30–60 minutes
Peak	5–10 minutes	60–90 minutes
Duration	4 hours	8–12 hours
Half-life	4–6 hours	4–6 hours

Metabolism

Hepatic

Indications

Aortic dissection (to decrease aortic shearing forces)
Control of tachycardia induced by other antihypertensives
Chronic blood pressure control
Angina
Antiarrhythmic
Following myocardial infarction
Migraine prophylaxis
Essential tremor
Hypertrophic subaortic stenosis

Contraindications

Bronchospasm
Heart block greater than first-degree
Acute cardiac failure

Dosage (IV for Acute Situations)

Initial—1-mg bolus over 1 minute
Repeat—1-mg bolus over 1 minute every 5 minutes until targeted heart rate is achieved
Maintenance—1 to 2 mg/hour by continuous fusion

Cautions

Reduce dose of maintenance infusion if cardiac, hepatic, or renal failure
Use in pregnancy—Category C
Use in lactation—avoid; excreted in breast milk
Use in childhood—no data on intravenous use

Hemodynamic Effects

Heart rate	Decreased
Preload	Increased
Afterload	Increased
Cardiac output	Decreased
Renal blood flow	Decreased
Cerebral blood flow	Decreased

Toxicity

Side Effects

Common: bronchospasm, bradyarrhythmias, heart failure, gastrointestinal disturbances, depression, malaise, vivid dreams
Uncommon: Raynaud's arterial insufficiency, renal failure, catatonia, agranulocytosis, thrombocytopenia purpura, impotence, hypoglycemia, rash
Dangerous: bronchospasm, bradyarrhythmias, heart failure, agranulocytosis, thrombocytopenia purpura, renal failure, severe depression, hypoglycemia

Treatment of Acute Toxicity

Stop drug.
Glucagon, 0.05 mg/kg/bolus, then infusion of 2 to 5 mg/hour
Epinephrine infusion
Electrical pacemaker

Interactions

Propranolol effect enhanced by calcium blockers, cimetidine and ranitidine, oral contraceptives, cyclopropane, diazoxide, disopyramide, furosemide, haloperidol, hydralazine, neuromuscular blockers, chlorpromazine
Propranolol effect decreased by antacids, barbiturates, cholestyramine, nonsteroidal anti-inflammatory drugs, rifampin, salicylates, sympathomimetic amines
Hypertension with clonidine, methyldopa, phenformin, sympathomimetic amines
Propranolol increases toxicity from warfarin, diazepam, calcium blockers, lidocaine, narcotics, oral hypoglycemics, insulin, theophylline, thiazide diuretics (hyperglycemia).
Propranolol decreases effect of bronchodilators, oral hypoglycemics, thyroid hormones.
Gangrene with ergot alkaloids

Alpha- and Beta-Blocker
Labetalol (Normodyne, Trandate)

Pharmacology

5-[1-hydroxy-2-[(1-methyl-3-phenylpro-
pyl)amino]ethyl] salicylamide monohydrochloride

Selective, competitive alpha$_1$-blocker
Nonselective, competitive beta-blocker
Alpha-to-beta blockade ratio 1:7 after in-
travenous administration
Has some beta$_2$ agonist activity

Kinetics (IV Route)

Onset	5 minutes
Peak	10 minutes
Duration	3–6 hours
Half-life	5–6 hours

Metabolism

Hepatic conjugation to inactive glucu-
ronides
Renal excretion of both metabolites and
unaltered drug

Indications

Labetalol is a second-line drug for treatment of hypertensive urgencies. As an intravenous agent that blocks both alpha$_1$- and
beta-receptors, it seems an attractive drug
for the rapid management of severe hypertension. It has been used successfully in severe hypertension alone or in association
with dissecting aortic aneurysm, left ventricular failure, acute myocardial infarction, or
hypertensive encephalopathy. However, the
experience base with this drug is small, and
it has yet to be proved to be better than more
traditional regimens. Although labetalol has
not been specifically studied as an anti-angi-
nal agent, its beta-blocking properties appear to be advantageous in hypertensive patients with myocardial ischemia. The
combined alpha- and beta-blocking properties of labetalol seem to be ideal for managing patients with pheochromocytoma; however, some patients with this condition
experience paradoxical hypertension when
given labetalol. This presumably occurs because labetalol is a more active beta-blocker
than an alpha-blocker. The oral administration of labetalol for acute hypertensive problems has been of only variable success and is
not recommended.

Contraindications

Bradyarrhythmias/heart block greater than
first degree
Bronchospasm
Cardiac failure
Hepatic failure

Dosage

Only intravenous administration is suitable
for acute hypertensive problems. Switch to
oral labetalol after blood pressure has been
controlled by intravenous drug.

Alternative 1: Continuous Titrated Infusion

Prepare solution containing 200 mg labetalol in 200 ml solution by adding 40 ml
labetalol solution to 160 ml of intravenous fluid (i.e., D$_5$W).
Start administration at 2 ml (2 mg)/min
and adjust rate to desired blood pressure. Usual range for desired response is
0.5 to 4 mg/min.
Stop infusion when targeted blood pressure is achieved.
This technique results in the least hypotension but is most labor intensive, requiring intensive care unit admission
and intra-arterial pressure monitoring.

Alternative 2: Multiple Miniboluses

Initial IV bolus—20 mg over 2 minutes
Repeat IV boluses—40 to 80 mg every 5
minutes until desired reduction in blood
pressure or maximum dose of 300 mg
has been administered

The minibolus approach causes less hypotension than the large single bolus technique
but is not always successful in lowering the
blood pressure. This technique usually produces a satisfactory decrease in blood pressure in 30 to 60 minutes, which will be sustained without further treatment for 5 to 6
hours. Thus, patients managed with the
minibolus technique who achieve satisfactory blood pressure control in the emergency department may not need admission
to an intensive care unit.

Alternative 3: Single Bolus

Administer 1 to 2 mg/kg as a 10-minute IV
infusion.
Not recommended because it may cause
severe hypotension

Oral Maintenance Therapy

Begin when diastolic blood pressure has increased 10 mmHg above the minimum pressure achieved with intravenous loading.
Initial dose—200 mg
Range—200 to 1200 mg bid

Cautions

Dose adjustment in organ failure—none
Use in pregnancy—Category C
Use in lactation—no; excreted in breast milk
Use in childhood—no data

Hemodynamic Effects

Heart rate	Little change
Preload	Little change
Afterload	Decreased
Cardiac output	Little change
Renal blood flow	Little change
Cerebral blood flow	No data

Toxicity

Side Effects

Common: dizziness, fatigue, nausea, postural hypotension, tingling of skin
Uncommon: vomiting, numbness, taste distortion, headache, jaundice, pruritus
Dangerous: bradyarrhythmias, cardiac failure, bronchospasm, severe hypotension

Treatment of Acute Toxicity

Stop labetalol.
Bradycardia—atropine, epinephrine, and pacemaker
Hypotension—supine position with legs elevated, norepinephrine infusion 0.1 to 0.5 μg/kg/min
Cardiac failure—dopamine or dobutamine infusion, digitalization, diuretic
Bronchospasm—beta$_2$ agonist by inhalation
Seizures—diazepam intravenously

Interactions

Labetalol effect enhanced by other antihypertensives, diuretics, anesthetic agents (especially halothane), cimetidine, nitroglycerin
Tremor when used with tricyclic antidepressants

Labetalol decreases effect of beta-agonist bronchodilators.

Central Adrenergic Inhibitors

The drugs in this class of antihypertensives are alpha$_2$-receptor agonists that act on vasomotor centers in the brain to cause a decrease in afferent sympathetic outflow with a resultant lowering of vascular tone and pressure. Clonidine is the only drug in this class that is currently recommended for acute hypertensive problems. Drugs of this class should not be used in combination because they all have the same site of action and, in high doses, can increase blood pressure by causing a direct alpha-stimulating effect on the peripheral vasculature.

Clonidine (Catapres)

Pharmacology

Imidazoline derivative
Centrally acting alpha$_2$-receptor stimulator
Decreases sympathetic activity and plasma epinephrine, norepinephrine, and renin levels

Kinetics (Oral Dose Only)

Onset	30–60 minutes
Peak	2–4 hours
Duration	6–8 hours
Half-life	8–12 hours

Metabolism

Renal excretion of unchanged compound

Indications

Step-2 adrenergic inhibitor
First-line agent for clonidine withdrawal hypertensive crisis

Dosage

Acute Hypertension due to Clonidine Withdrawal

Initial dose—0.2 mg orally
Repeat dose—0.1 mg every hour until targeted blood pressure achieved or maximum dose of 0.8 mg used

Chronic Therapy

Initial—0.1 mg bid
Maintenance—0.1 to 0.4 mg bid

Transdermal system available for once weekly dosing schedule

Cautions

Reduce dose in renal failure and in the elderly.
Use in pregnancy—avoid; Category C
Use in lactation—avoid; excreted in breast milk
Use in childhood—unknown

Toxicity

Side Effects

Common: dry mouth, drowsiness/sedation, nightmares
Uncommon: contact dermatitis (transdermal system), angioneurotic edema, postural hypotension, seizures, diarrhea
Dangerous: congestive heart failure, bradyarrhythmias, coma, seizures

Treatment of Acute Toxicity

Stop drug and consider gastric emptying.
Ventilatory support
Hypotension—Trendelenburg position, volume infusion, dopamine infusion
Bradycardia with hemodynamic compromise—atropine, pacemaker
Seizure—diazepam intravenously

Beware: **Life-threatening rebound hypertension due to sympathetic hyperactivity may develop with abrupt cessation of clonidine therapy. Treat with intravenous phentolamine and reinstitution of oral clonidine. Do *not* treat with beta-blockers.**

Interactions

Effect enhanced by diuretics
Effect diminished by tricyclic antidepressants, beta-blockers
Additive sedative effect with methyldopa, alcohol, barbiturates, other sedatives
Hypertension with beta-blockers

Guanabenz (Wytensin) and Guanfacine (Tenex)

Guanabenz and guanfacine are two recently introduced centrally active alpha$_2$-adrenergic agonists that have actions similar to clonidine. Both are given orally for chronic blood pressure control and have no role in the management of hypertensive emergen-

cies or urgencies. Their major advantage over clonidine seems to be that their sudden cessation is less often followed by severe rebound hypertension.

Methyldopa (Aldomet)

Methyldopa is one of the older antihypertensives that was used for acute hypertensive problems in the past, but it has now been replaced by more reliable and rapidly acting agents. Although it is available for intravenous administration, its prolonged onset of action (2 to 6 hours) and erratic effectiveness make it unsuitable for rapid control of life-threatening hypertension. The antihypertensive effect of methyldopa is primarily due to its metabolism to alpha-methyl-norepinephrine, which then stimulates central nervous system inhibiting neurons. The long latent period before methyldopa's hypotensive effect begins is the result of this need for metabolism to produce the active compound. The main value of methyldopa is as an oral agent for chronic blood pressure control, although some clinicians may use intravenous methyldopa to maintain blood pressure control in a patient whose hypertension is chronically controlled with oral methyldopa but who has a short-term interruption of bowel function.

Peripheral Adrenergic Antagonists

The peripheral adrenergic antagonists guanethidine and reserpine have been part of the antihypertensive armamentarium for many years. However, they have now been surplanted by more effective, less toxic agents and have no role in the emergency department management of acute hypertension and only a limited role in the management of chronic hypertension refractory to other therapy.

Angiotensin-Converting Enzyme Inhibitors

Angiotensin-converting enzyme inhibitors are now widely used as step-1 agents for asymptomatic hypertension. They have a high success rate of chronic blood pressure control and cause few side effects. There are reports describing the successful management of hypertensive emergencies with both oral and sublingual captopril; enalaprilat is available in an intravenous formulation that might be considered for use in hypertensive emergencies, but it has not been tested in a comparison trial with proven agents. However, it is my opinion that there is not enough data to recommend any use of the angiotensin-converting enzyme inhibitors in acute hypertensive emergencies or urgencies.

Captopril (Capoten)

Pharmacology

Competitive inhibitor of angiotension-converting enzyme

Blocks production of the potent vasoconstrictor angiotensin II

Increases concentration of the vasodilators bradykinin and prostaglandin E_2

Decreases aldosterone release and, thus, sodium and water retention

Kinetics

	Oral	Sublingual
Onset	30 minutes	5 minutes
Peak	60–90 minutes	15 minutes
Duration	8 hours	8 hours
Half-life	2–3 hours	2–3 hours

Metabolism

Renal excretion
50% unchanged drug
50% disulfide metabolites

Indications

Chronic control of hypertension
Heart failure

Captopril is not recommended for acute hypertensive emergencies or urgencies.

Contraindications

Prior hypersensitivity
Agranulocytosis

Dosage

Initial—25 mg two or three times daily
Titration—increase each dose by 25 mg every 2 weeks until adequate blood pressure or maximum of 150-mg dose reached. Add thiazide diuretic if no response at 50 mg tid dose before further increase in captopril.

Cautions

Reduce dose in cardiac and renal failure.
Use in pregnancy—no; crosses placenta; increases fetal malformations and stillbirths in animals; Category C
Use in lactation—no; excreted in breast milk
Use in childhood—yes; reduce dose proportionate to weight

Hemodynamic Effects

Heart rate	Little change
Preload	Decreased
Afterload	Decreased
Cardiac output	Little change
Renal blood flow	Increased
Cerebral blood flow	No change

Toxicity

Side Effects

Common: first-dose hypotension (especially if patient is receiving diuretics or other vasodilators), pruritus, rash, altered taste perception

Uncommon: angioedema, flushing, tachycardia, postural hypotension, hyperkalemia, proteinuria

Dangerous: agranulocytosis, renal failure, first-dose hypotension

Treatment of Acute Toxicity

Supine position
Volume infusion
Vasopressor

Interactions

Captopril effect enhanced by diuretics, vasodilators (nitrates, calcium channel blockers, other antihypertensives), beta-blockers, anesthetics

Hyperkalemia with potassium supplements, spironolactone, triamterene, amiloride

Captopril effect decreased by food, antacids, aspirin, naloxone, nonsteroidal anti-inflammatory drugs

Higher incidence or renal failure with furosemide, thiazides

Neuropathies with cimetidine

Stevens-Johnson syndrome with allopurinol

Captopril enhances hypoglycemic effect of both insulin and oral hypoglycemics

Enalaprilat (Vasotec)
Pharmacology

Active metabolite of orally administered
  prodrug enalapril
Competitive inhibitor of angiotensin$_1$-con-
  verting enzyme
Blocks production of the potent vasoconstrictor angiotensin II
Increases concentration of the vasodilators
  bradykinin and prostaglandin E$_2$
Decreases aldosterone release and, thus,
  sodium and water retention

Kinetics (IV Administration)

Onset	15 minutes
Peak	1–4 hours
Duration	6 hours
Half-life	11 hours

Metabolism

Renal elimination of unchanged drug

Indications

Intravenous—short-term maintenance of
  blood pressure control in patients receiving oral ACE inhibitors and who
  have bowel dysfunction
Oral—chronic control of hypertension

Note: **Intravenous enalaprilat cannot
be recommended for management of
acute hypertensive emergencies because appropriate controlled studies
are lacking. It may have a role in this
setting in the future as more data become available.**

Contraindications

Hypersensitivity
Agranulocytosis

Dosage

Initial—1.25 mg given as a 5-minute IV
  bolus. Repeat in 1 hour if desired blood
  pressure reduction is not achieved.
Maintenance—1.25 mg IV over 5 minutes
  every 6 hours

Cautions

Reduce dose to 0.625 mg if the patient is
  also receiving diuretics or if in renal failure with a serum creatinine level >3
  mg/dl.

Use in pregnancy—Category C; avoid.
Use in lactation—found in breast milk;
  avoid.
Use in childhood—no data

Hemodynamic Effects

(Little data; assumed to be the same as
  captopril)

Heart rate	Little change
Preload	Decreased
Afterload	Decreased
Cardiac output	Little change
Renal blood flow	Increased
Cerebral blood flow	No change

Toxicity

Side Effects

(New drug, so side effect profile not fully
  developed yet)
Common: hypotension, headache, nausea
Uncommon: syncope, angioedema, fatigue, fever, rash, constipation, palpita-
  tion, pancreatitis, hepatitis, depression,
  fatigue/somnolence, insomnia, hyperkalemia, and syndrome of fever, myalgia,
  and arthralgia with increased erythrocyte sedimentation rate
Dangerous: hypotension with stroke or
  myocardial infarction, renal failure,
  bone marrow suppression

Treatment of Acute Toxicity

Stop drug.
Supine position
Volume infusion
Vasopressor

Interactions

(Limited usage to date, so all interactions
  probably not yet recognized)
Enalaprilat effect enhanced by diuretics
Hyperkalemia with potassium, spironolactone, triamterene
Enhances hypoglycemia of oral hypoglycemics

Calcium Blocker

Nifedipine (Procardia, Adalat)
Pharmacology

3,5-Pyridinedicarboxylic acid, 1,4-dihy-
  dro-2,6-dimethyl-4-(2-nitrophenyl)-di-
  methyl ester

Inhibits transmembrane influx of calcium ions via slow channels into cardiac and smooth muscle

Lowers blood pressure by lessening contractile state of vascular smooth muscle

Kinetics

	Sublingual	Oral and Rectal
Onset	5–10 minutes	15–30 minutes
Peak	20–30 minutes	30–60 minutes
Duration	4–6 hours	4–6 hours
Half-life	2 hours	2 hours

Metabolism

Renal elimination of inactive metabolites

> *Note:* Biting the nifedipine capsule before swallowing it gives an earlier onset of action for the oral route.

Indications

First-line drug for hypertensive urgencies (*Note:* Nifedipine is not yet approved by the Food and Drug Administration for use as an antihypertensive.)
Angina

Contraindication

Known hypersensitivity

Dosage

Initial—10 mg orally (Puncture capsule and squeeze in mouth or have patient bite the capsule and swallow.)
Repeat—10 mg orally in 1 to 2 hours, depending on blood pressure response, and then 10 to 30 mg every 6 hours
Expect each 10 mg of nifedipine to produce a 25% reduction in the predose systolic, diastolic, and mean blood pressures.

Cautions

Dose reduction in organ failure—none
Use in pregnancy—Category C; avoid
Use in lactation—no data
Use in childhood—no data

Hemodynamic Effects

Heart rate	Increased
Preload	Decreased
Afterload	Decreased
Cardiac output	Small increase
Renal blood flow	Little change
Cerebral blood flow	Increased

Toxicity

Side Effects

Common: tachycardia, nausea, headache, fluid retention, paresthesias, flushing, muscle cramps, fatigue, dizziness
Uncommon: hypotension, pruritus/dermatitis, sexual dysfunction
Dangerous: hypotension-induced myocardial infarction, renal failure, increased intracranial pressure if preexisting cerebral edema (not yet reported, but theoretical risk)

Treatment of Acute Toxicity

Stop drug and consider gastric emptying.
Supine position
Volume infusion
Calcium chloride, 1 g IV
Glucagon, 0.05 mg/kg IV bolus, then 2 to 5 mg/hour IV infusion
Norepinephrine IV infusion, 0.1 to 0.5 μg/kg/min

Interactions

Nifedipine effects increased by beta-blockers, cimetidine/ranitidine, prazosin
Nifedipine increases toxicity of coumadin, digoxin, phenytoin, theophylline.
Quinidine effect decreased by nifedipine

Diuretics

Diuretic agents have a limited role in the emergency management of most hypertensive urgencies and emergencies. In fact, they are contraindicated in most of these patients because the pathophysiologic events lending to an acute hypertensive event actually produce and are further accelerated by hypovolemia. Therefore, a diuretic should be included in the initial therapeutic approach only in those patients who have hypertension and pulmonary edema. The diuretics do play an important role in the chronic control of asymptomatic hypertension, either as a single agent or as adjunctive therapy to counteract the fluid-retaining side effect of many of the other antihypertensive drugs. In the unusual acutely hypertensive patient who needs diuretic therapy, my choice is intravenous furosemide.

Furosemide
Pharmacology

4-Chloro-n-furfuryl-5-sulfamoylanthranilic acid

Mechanism of Action

Inhibits reabsorption of sodium and chloride in loop of Henle and proximal and distal tubules

Kinetics (IV)

Onset	5 minutes
Peak	10–30 minutes
Duration	2 hours
Half-life	1 hour

Metabolism

35% hepatic metabolism to glucuronide
65% renal excretion
95% protein-bound

Indications

Diuresis
Intracranial hypertension
Increased intraocular pressure
Hypertension
Hypercalcemia

Contraindication

Anuria

Dosage

Initial—20 to 40 mg IV bolus over 1 to 2 minutes
Repeat—every 2 hours. Increase dose if no or minimal response to initial dose.

Cautions

Increase dose in renal failure to 100 to 200 mg IV bolus.
Use in pregnancy—no; Category C
Use in lactation—no; appears in breast milk
Use in childhood—yes; dose, 1 mg/kg initial to maximum of 6 mg/kg

Toxicity

Side Effects

Common: hypokalemia, hypomagnesemia, hyperuricemia, hyponatremia, hypochloremic alkalosis, hypocalcemia, hyperglycemia, gastrointestinal upset, rash/pruritus, headache, dizziness (may be postural), paresthesias

Uncommon: pancreatitis, deafness, marrow suppression, exacerbation of lupus erythematosus, cholestatic jaundice
Dangerous: hypokalemia, pancreatitis, aplastic anemia, hypovolemia

Treatment of Acute Toxicity

Stop drug.
Normalize intravascular volume.
Correct electrolyte imbalances.

Note: Patients who are allergic to sulfonamides may also have serious allergic reactions to furosemide.

Interactions

Increases digoxin toxicity
Increases lithium toxicity
Increases salicylate toxicity
Enhances neuromuscular blockade of succinylcholine
Increases nephrotoxicity and ototoxicity of aminoglycosides
Increases nephrotoxicity of cephalosporins
Increases captopril-induced renal failure
Vasomotor instability with cloral hydrate
Nonsteroidal anti-inflammatory drugs decrease furosemide effects.
Phenytoin decreases furosemide effects.
Furosemide decreases theophylline effects.

Vasodilators

Diazoxide (Hyperstat)
Pharmacology

Benzothiadiazine
Direct-acting arteriolar dilator

Kinetics (IV Infusion Only)

Onset	1–2 minutes
Peak	2–5 minutes
Duration	4–12 hours
Half-life	28 ± 8 hours

Metabolism

90% albumin-bound
Renal elimination

Indications

Hypertensive emergencies and urgencies

> *Note:* Diazoxide is best avoided in acute myocardial infarction, aortic dissection, and pheochromocytoma.

Dosage

1 to 3 mg/kg IV bolus (150-mg maximum bolus) every 5 minutes until desired blood pressure achieved or total dose of 600 mg administered

Alternate regimen: pretreat with 0.020 mg/kg propranolol IV; infuse diazoxide at rate of 15 mg/min for 20 to 30 minutes.

Cautions

Dose adjustments in organ failure—none
Use in pregnancy—Category C; crosses placenta and has caused neonatal hyperglycemia and thrombocytopenia; inhibits uterine contractions and may arrest labor
Use in lactation—no data; best avoided
Use in childhood—yes

Hemodynamic Effects

Heart rate	Increased
Preload	Increased
Afterload	Decreased
Cardiac output	Increased
Renal blood flow	Increased
Cerebral blood flow	Decreased

Toxicity

Side Effects

Common: reflex tachycardia, fluid retention, nausea and vomiting, hyperglycemia
Uncommon: pancreatitis, rash, pain in injected vein, choking sensation, parotid swelling, diarrhea
Dangerous: shock, myocardial ischemia, cerebral ischemia, hyperglycemia

Treatment of Acute Toxicity

Hypotension—stop drug; Trendelenburg position; volume infusion; vasopressor
Hyperglycemia—insulin

Interactions

Enhances coumadin effect
Diazoxide effect increased by diuretics, sympatholytics, nitrates
Decreases phenytoin effect

Hydralazine (Apresoline)
Pharmacology

1-Hydrazinophthalazine
Direct-acting arteriolar dilator (no venous effect)

Kinetics (IV Infusion)

Onset	10–30 minutes
Peak	2 hours
Duration	6–12 hours
Half-life	6 hours

Metabolism

10% hepatic
90% renal excretion

Indications

First-line drug for eclampsia
Step-3 or -4 therapy for asymptomatic hypertension

> *Note:* Do not use in the treatment of aortic dissection. Hydralazine is best avoided in patients with ischemic heart disease.

Dosage

10 to 20 mg IV drip over 20 minutes, repeated every 6 hours

Cautions

Dose adjustments in organ failure—dosing interval increased to 8 hours in severe renal failure
Use in pregnancy—drug of choice; Category C
Use in lactation—no data; avoid if possible.
Use in childhood—yes; dose is 1.7 to 3.5 mg/kg daily in four divided doses.

Hemodynamic Effects

Heart rate—pronounced reflex tachycardia
Preload—increased due to sodium and water retention
Afterload—decreased
Cardiac output—increased
Renal blood flow—increased
Cerebral blood flow—increased

Toxicity

> *Note:* Coadminister beta-blocker with hydralazine, except in eclampsia, to prevent reflex tachycardia.

Side Effects

Common: headache, dizziness, nausea, anorexia, palpitations, nasal congestion, fluid retention, diarrhea
Uncommon: conjunctivitis, rash, tremor, paresthesias, depression
Dangerous: myocardial ischemia, hepatitis, lupus syndrome, bone marrow suppression, glomerulonephritis, polyneuritis

Treatment of Acute Toxicity

Stop drug.
Supine position
Volume infusion
Vasopressor if hypotension
Beta-blocker for tachycardia

Interactions

Decreases digoxin effect
Increases propranolol and metoprolol effects
Nonsteroidal anti-inflammatory drugs decrease hydralazine effect.

Minoxidil (Loniten)
Pharmacology

2,4-pyridiminediamine, 6-[1-piperidinyl]-3-oxide
Direct-acting arteriolar dilator (no venous dilation)

Kinetics (Oral Formulation Only)

Bioavailability	90%
Onset	30 minutes
Peak	2–3 hours
Duration	12 hours
Half-life	4.2 hours

Metabolism

90% hepatic conjugation
10% renal excretion

Indication

Hypertension refractory to maximum doses of a diuretic and two other agents

We do not recommend minoxidil for the initial management of hypertensive urgencies or emergencies.

Contraindication

Pheochromocytoma

Dosage

Initial—5 mg once daily
Increase by 5 to 10 mg daily until desired blood pressure achieved
Usual effective dose range is 10 to 40 mg daily given once or twice
Maximum—100 mg total daily dose

Cautions

Reduce dose in renal failure and childhood.
Use in pregnancy—Category C; do not use.
Use in lactation—do not use.
Use in childhood—yes, at reduced dose

Hemodynamic Effects

Heart rate	Increased
Preload	Increased
Afterload	Decreased
Cardiac output	Increased
Renal blood flow	Increased
Cerebral blood flow	Increased

Toxicity

> *Note:* A beta-blocker and a diuretic must be coadministered with minoxidil.

Side Effects

Common: hypertrichosis, fluid retention, tachycardia
Uncommon: nausea, breast tenderness, coarsening of facial features, rash
Dangerous: hypotension, pericardial tamponade, congestive heart failure

Treatment of Acute Toxicity

Hypotension—stop drug, volume infusion, dopamine, echocardiogram to look for tamponade
Congestive heart failure—diuresis

Interactions

Profound hypotension with guanethidine and diazoxide

Sodium Nitroprusside (Nipride)
Pharmacology

Disodium pentacyanonitrosylferrate (2)—
dihydrate
Acts directly on vasodilating receptor of
vascular smooth muscle
Affects both arteries and veins

Kinetics (IV Infusion Only)

Onset—0.5 to 5 minutes
Peak—0.5 to 5 minutes
Duration—1 to 10 minutes after infusion
discontinued
Half-life—nitroprusside, minutes; thiocy-
anate, 1 week
Tachyphylaxis—no

Metabolism

1. Rapid nonenzymatic breakdown by hemoglobin to cyanide
2. Hepatic conversion of cyanide to thiocyanate
3. Renal excretion of thiocyanate

Indications

Drug of choice for rapid, acute blood pressure control in hypertensive emergencies
Hypotensive anesthesia

Dosage

Initial—0.5 μg/kg/min
Maximum—10 μg/kg/min
Average effective dose—3 μg/kg/min

Cautions

Dose adjustments in organ failure—none,
but cyanide and thiocyanate toxicity
more likely with prolonged use in hepatic and renal failure
Use in pregnancy—yes, for short-term use
if absolutely necessary; Category C
Use in lactation—do not use.
Use in childhood—yes; dose as above

Note: Protect sodium nitroprusside solution from light with opaque covering.
Discard solution after 24 hours or if
discolored. Beware of hypotension at
previously good infusion rate when
hanging a new bottle.

Hemodynamic Effects

Heart rate	Increased or no change
Preload	Decreased
Afterload	Decreased
Cardiac output	Increased or no change
Renal blood flow	Increased unless excessive decrease in blood pressure
Cerebral blood flow	Increased

Toxicity
Side Effects

Common: hypotension, vomiting, headache, diaphoresis, apprehension
Uncommon: rash, bradycardia, methemo-
globinuria, increased intracranial pressure, cyanide or thiocyanate toxicity
Dangerous: hypotension (if uncorrected),
cyanide or thiocyanate toxicity, increased intracranial pressure

Interactions

Effect enhanced by other antihypertensives and anesthetic agents
Increases renal excretion of digoxin; decreases digoxin effect

Trimethaphan (Arfonad)
Pharmacology

Thiophanium derivative
Vasodilation due to ganglionic blockade
Also blocks parasympathetic ganglia
Causes histamine release

Kinetics (IV Infusion Only)

Onset	1 minute
Peak	2–5 minutes
Duration	10 minutes

Metabolism

Renal excretion

Indications

Hypotensive anesthesia
Aortic dissection

Dosage

Start continuous intravenous infusion at
0.5 mg/min and increase by 0.5 mg/min
at 5-minute intervals until desired blood
pressure is achieved.
Maximum dose 6 mg/min
Tachyphylaxis common after several days

Cautions

Dose adjustments in organ failure—none,
  but titrate carefully
Use in pregnancy—no; Category D
Use in lactation—do not use.
Use in childhood—do not use.

Note: **Coadminister beta-blocker with
trimethaphan when treating aortic dissection.**

Hemodynamic Effects

Heart rate	Decreased
Preload	Decreased
Afterload	Decreased
Cardiac output	Decreased
Renal blood flow	Decreased
Cerebral blood flow	No change

Toxicity

Side Effects

Common: constipation, urinary hesitancy,
  mydriasis, loss of ocular accommodation, dry mouth
Uncommon: paralytic ileus, urinary retention, glaucoma
Dangerous: respiratory arrest (especially
  with high doses), syncope, myocardial
  ischemia, ileus, urinary retention

Treatment of Acute Toxicity

Stop drug.
Ventilatory support
Vasopressor (phenylephrine or norepi-
  nephrine) for hypotension

Interaction

Severe hypotension with other antihypertensives and diuretics

REFERENCES

Alpert MA, Bauer JH: Hypertensive emergencies: Recognition and pathogenesis. Cardiovasc Rev Rep
6:407, 1985.
Alpert MA, Bauer JH: Control of severe hypertension
with minoxidil. Arch Intern Med 142:2099, 1982.
Bauer JH, Alpert MA: Rapid reduction of severe hypertension with minoxidil. J Cardiovasc Pharmacol
2:5189, 1980.

Benfield P, Sorkin EM: Esmolol: A preliminary review
of its pharmacodynamic and pharmacokinetic properties and therapeutic efficacy. Drugs 33:392, 1987.
Bertez O, Conen D, Radu EW, et al: Nifedipine in hypertensive emergencies. Br Med J 286:19, 1983.
Biollaz J, Waeber B, Brunner MR: Hypertensive crisis
treated with orally administered captopril. Eur J Clin
Pharmacol 25:145, 1983.
Cohen IM, Katz MA: Oral clonidine loading for rapid
control of hypertension. Clin Pharmacol Ther 24:11,
1978.
Cohn JN, Burke LP: Nitroprusside. Ann Intern Med
91:752, 1979.
Cressman MD, Vidt DG, Gifford RW, et al: Intravenous
labetalol in the management of severe hypertension
and hypertensive emergencies. Am Heart J 107:980,
1984.
Dinsdale HB: Hypertensive encephalopathy. Curr Concepts Cerebrovasc Dis Stroke 17:5, 1982.
DiPette DJ, Ferrapo JC, Evans PR, Martin M: Enalaprilat, an intravenous angiotensin converting enzyme inhibitor, in hypertensive crises. Clin Pharmacol Ther
38:199, 1985.
Esmolol—a short-acting IV beta blocker. Medical Letter 29:57, 1987.
Ferlinz J: Nifedipine in myocardial ischemia, systemic
hypertension, and other cardiovascular disorders.
Ann Intern Med 105:714, 1986.
Franklin C, Nightingale S, Mamdani B: A randomized
comparison of nifedipine and sodium nitroprusside in
severe hypertension. Chest 90:500, 1986.
Frishman WH, Weinberg P, Peled HB, et al: Calcium
entry blockers for the treatment of severe hypertension and hypertensive crisis. Am J Med 77:35, 1984.
Garrett BN, Kaplan NM: Efficacy of slow infusion of di-
azoxide in the treatment of severe hypertension without organ hypoperfusion. Am Heart J 103:390, 1982.
Hayes JM: Prazosin in severe hypertension: Effect on
blood pressure, plasma renin activity and in hypertensive emergencies. Med J Aust 2:30, 1977.
Houston MC: Hypertensive urgencies and emergencies:
Pathophysiology, clinical aspects and treatment. In
Chernow B, Shoemaker WC (eds): Critical Care: State
of the Art, Vol. 7. Fullerton, Society of Critical Care
Medicine, 1986, pp 151–246.
Huymans FT, Thien TA, Koene RA: Combined intrave-
nous administration of diazoxide and beta blocking
agents in acute treatment of severe hypertension or
hypertensive crisis. Am Heart J 103:395, 1982.
Kincaid-Smith P: Malignant hypertension. Cardiovasc
Rev Rep 1:42, 1980.
Koch-Weser J: Diazoxide. N Engl J Med 244:1271,
1976.
The 1988 Report of the Joint National Committee on
Detection, Evaluation and Treatment of High Blood
Pressure. Arch Intern Med 148:1023, 1988.
Ogilvie RI, Nadeau JH, Sitar DS: Diazoxide concentration response relation in hypertension. Hypertension
4:167, 1982.
Ram CVS, Hyman D: Hypertensive crises. J Intensive
Care Med 2:151, 1987.
Rosei EA, Brown JJ, Lever AF, et al: Treatment of
phaeochromocytoma and of clonidine withdrawal hy-
pertension with labetalol. Br J Clin Pharmacol
20:237, 1981.
Rumbozdt Z, Bagatin J, Vidoril A: Diazoxide vs. labetalol: A crossover comparison of short term effects in
hypertension. Int J Clin Pharmacol Res 3:47, 1983.

Spitalewitz S, Porush JG, Oquagha C: Use of oral clonidine for rapid titration of blood pressure in severe hypertension. Chest 83:404, 1983.

Strandgaurd S, Paulson OB: Cerebral autoregulation. Stroke 15:413, 1984.

Stumpe KO, Kolloch R, Overlack A: Captopril and enalapril: Evaluation of therapeutic efficacy and safety. Pract Cardiol 10:111, 1984.

Tinker JH, Michenfelder JD: Sodium nitroprusside: Pharmacology, toxicology and therapeutics. Anesthesiology 45:340, 1976.

Vasoactive Agents

CHARLES E. SAUNDERS, M.D.

INTRODUCTION

Vasopressors, inotropic agents, and vasodilators are drugs that are commonly used to increase cardiac output or systemic blood pressure in low cardiac output states, hypotension, and shock from a variety of causes. Agents discussed in this chapter are listed in Table 13–1. Vasopressors are agents that usually cause arterial vasoconstriction by stimulation of alpha-adrenergic receptors. Inotropic agents act on the myocardium, either directly or through beta$_1$-adrenergic receptors, to increase the strength of myocardial contraction (contractility). Vasodilators influence cardiac function by reducing preload with venous dilation or reducing afterload by arterial dilation. Most agents of either group mediate their effects on various effector organs depending on the type and number of receptors present and the affinity of the agent for the receptors. Table 13–2 summarizes the distribution and action of adrenergic receptors in the body. The choice of agent depends on the physiologic effect desired, which, in turn, depends on the pathophysiologic derangement present.

Hypotension

Hypotension has diverse causes, but can be expressed physiologically by the relationship between three variables:

$$BP = CO \times SVR$$
$$BP = \text{blood pressure}$$
$$CO = \text{cardiac output}$$
$$SVR = \text{systemic vascular resistance}$$

More precisely, the correct expression includes an adjustment for central venous pressure (CVP) and a conversion constant:

$$MAP - CVP = (CO \times SVR)/80$$
$$MAP = \text{mean arterial pressure}$$

Cardiac output is the product of two variables, heart rate (HR) and stroke volume (SV). Therefore, total expression for mean arterial pressure is the following:

$$MAP = CVP + (HR \times SV \times SVR)/80$$

Clearly, blood pressure is affected by several variables. Hypotension may be caused by decreases in systemic vascular resistance,

TABLE 13–1. Vasoactive Agents Discussed
in this Chapter

Amrinone
Digoxin
Dobutamine
Dopamine
Epinephrine
Glucagon
Isoproterenol
Levarterenol (norepinephrine)
Metaraminol
Methoxamine
Nitroglycerin
Nitroprusside
Phenylephrine
Vasopressin

Spitalewitz S, Porush JG, Oquagha C: Use of oral cloni-dine for rapid titration of blood pressure in severe hy-pertension. Chest 83:404, 1983.

Strandgaurd S, Paulson OB: Cerebral autoregulation. Stroke 15:413, 1984.

Stumpe KO, Kolloch R, Overlack A: Captopril and ena-lapril: Evaluation of therapeutic efficacy and safety. Pract Cardiol 10:111, 1984.

Tinker JH, Michenfelder JD: Sodium nitroprusside: Pharmacology, toxicology and therapeutics. Anesthe-siology 45:340, 1976.

CHAPTER 13

Vasoactive Agents

CHARLES E. SAUNDERS, M.D.

INTRODUCTION

Vasopressors, inotropic agents, and vasodilators are drugs that are commonly used to increase cardiac output or systemic blood pressure in low cardiac output states, hypotension, and shock from a variety of causes. Agents discussed in this chapter are listed in Table 13–1. Vasopressors are agents that usually cause arterial vasoconstriction by stimulation of alpha-adrenergic receptors. Inotropic agents act on the myocardium, either directly or through beta$_1$-adrenergic receptors, to increase the strength of myocardial contraction (contractility). Vasodilators influence cardiac function by reducing preload with venous dilation or reducing afterload by arterial dilation. Most agents of either group mediate their effects on various effector organs depending on the type and number of receptors present and the affinity of the agent for the receptors. Table 13–2 summarizes the distribution and action of adrenergic receptors in the body. The choice of agent depends on the physiologic effect desired, which, in turn, depends on the pathophysiologic derangement present.

Hypotension

Hypotension has diverse causes, but can be expressed physiologically by the relationship between three variables:

$$BP = CO \times SVR$$
$$BP = \text{blood pressure}$$
$$CO = \text{cardiac output}$$
$$SVR = \text{systemic vascular resistance}$$

More precisely, the correct expression includes an adjustment for central venous pressure (CVP) and a conversion constant:

$$MAP - CVP = (CO \times SVR)/80$$
$$MAP = \text{mean arterial pressure}$$

Cardiac output is the product of two variables, heart rate (HR) and stroke volume (SV). Therefore, total expression for mean arterial pressure is the following:

$$MAP = CVP + (HR \times SV \times SVR)/80$$

Clearly, blood pressure is affected by several variables. Hypotension may be caused by decreases in systemic vascular resistance,

TABLE 13–1. Vasoactive Agents Discussed in this Chapter

Amrinone
Digoxin
Dobutamine
Dopamine
Epinephrine
Glucagon
Isoproterenol
Levarterenol (norepinephrine)
Metaraminol
Methoxamine
Nitroglycerin
Nitroprusside
Phenylephrine
Vasopressin

TABLE 13–4. Differential Features of Various Shock States°

	Hypovolemic	Cardiogenic	Distributive	Anaphylactic

Clinical features	Cool, clammy skin
	± Trauma
	± Vomiting
	± Diarrhea
		Cool, clammy skin
		Rales, gallop,
		    jugular venous
		    distention
		± Dysrhythmia
		± Murmur
			Warm skin
			± Fever
			± Neurologic abnormality
				Warm skin
				± Wheezing
				± Urticaria
				± Angioedema

Laboratory
    findings
	± Anemia
	± Hyper- or
	    hyponatremia
		ECG abnormal
		↑ Cardiac
		    enzymes
			± X-ray infiltrate
			± Pyuria
			± Cultures
				PEFR or FEV$_1$
				    diminished

SVR	Increased	Increased	Decreased	Decreased

CO	Decreased	Decreased	Increased	Normal,
				    increased,
				    or decreased

PWP	Decreased	Increased	Normal to
			    decreased
				Normal to
				    decreased

SvO$_2$	<30 mmHg	<30 mmHg	35–50 mmHg	35–40 mmHg

°Common findings are listed (exceptions occur). ± = present in some cases; SVR = systemic vascular resistance; CO = cardiac output; PWP = pulmonary wedge pressure; SvO$_2$ = mixed venous oxygen saturation; PEFR = peak expiratory flow rate; FEV$_1$ = forced expiratory volume in 1 second.

panied by systemic and pulmonary venous engorgement due to compensatory mechanisms that result in sodium retention through the renin-angiotensin axis and water retention through increased antidiuretic hormone secretion. CHF may be due to acute or chronic left ventricular disease, mechanical failure of the heart valves, abnormal heart rhythms that reduce pump efficiency, or systemic conditions of markedly increased demand that exceed the normal performance capacity of the heart. The latter group includes such conditions as beriberi, thyrotoxicosis, Paget's disease of bone, arteriovenous shunts, and extreme anemia and will not be included in this discussion.

Clinical symptoms and signs vary somewhat, reflecting the etiology. Low cardiac output produces fatigue, weakness, oliguria, and somnolence. Pulmonary vascular congestion produces dyspnea on exertion, orthopnea, and paroxysmal nocturnal dyspnea. Systemic vascular congestion produces edema, ascites, hepatic congestion, and nocturia.

On examination, the pulse may be abnormal in certain conditions. A pulsus alternans may occur with severe left ventricular failure, *pulsus parvus et tardus* (upstroke weak and slow) may occur with aortic stenosis, a dicrotic notch may also be palpated with aortic stenosis, and a Corrigan's (water hammer) pulse may be seen with aortic insufficiency. Blood pressure may be low, normal, or elevated. If elevated, it may be due to underly-

ing hypertension or to activation of the renin-angiotensin axis and high circulating catecholamine levels. Jugular venous distention may be present, the precordium may exhibit a sustained and laterally displaced left ventricular impulse ("heave") or parasternal right ventricular "lift," and auscultation may reveal an S$_3$ gallop. Other abnormal cardiac sounds, such as murmurs, an S$_4$ gallop, an opening snap, or an accentuated P$_2$ component, may be heard associated with various etiologies. The lungs may contain bibasilar rales, the liver edge may be palpably enlarged, ascites may be present, and pedal edema may be noted.

Laboratory data help confirm the diagnosis of CHF and suggest its etiology. The chest x-ray film usually reveals an enlarged cardiac silhouette with variably abnormal contours, depending on the etiology. Pulmonary vascular congestion may be present in varying degrees from interstitial and septal edema, to pleural effusions, to frank pulmonary edema. The latter is recognized by the characteristic "bat-wing" pattern of perihilar infiltrates. The electrocardiogram may show a left or right ventricular strain pattern or other features reflective of the etiology, such as acute or chronic ischemic changes, left ventricular hypertrophy, or P-pulmonale. The electrocardiogram, however, may be normal. Blood chemistries may be normal or may show mild to moderate hyponatremia. Arterial blood gases may show mild to marked hypoxemia if pulmonary edema is

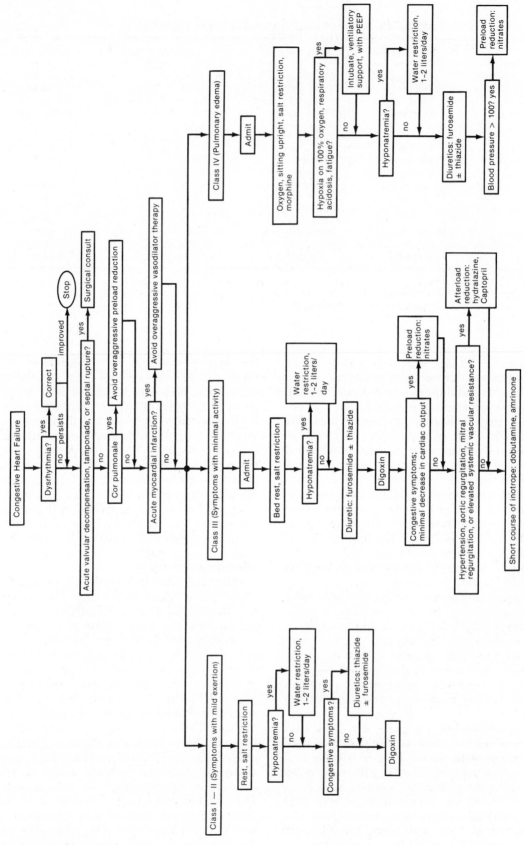

FIGURE 13–2. Treatment algorithm: congestive heart failure.

present and a respiratory alkalosis progressing to respiratory acidosis in preterminal cases.

Invasive hemodynamic data, if available, are the most revealing. The central venous pressure is elevated, as are the right atrial and pulmonary artery pressures. If left ventricular failure is present, the pulmonary wedge pressure is also elevated. Cardiac output is reduced as is stroke work index. Mixed venous oxygen saturation is low, and the oxygen extraction ratio is high.

Indications for Treatment

Vasodilator therapy is often the most effective treatment for CHF in that it improves the abnormal physiology while decreasing myocardial oxygen needs. The emergency use of vasopressors and inotropic agents in CHF is limited and must be seen in the context of other modes of treatment and in consideration of the underlying causes (Fig. 13–2). Vasopressors have little place in the treatment of CHF because systemic vascular resistance is already elevated as a result of high levels of circulating catecholamines. Also, in CHF, the relationship between afterload and stroke work index is an inverse one. Increases in afterload from the use of vasopressor agents may cause further deterioration in myocardial performance and increase myocardial oxygen demand.

Inotropic agents may, however, be employed in some cases. Patients with chronic CHF may present to the emergency department with acute decompensation due to a variety of factors, including worsening of the underlying condition, dietary indiscretion, or noncompliance with medications. If the patient is already on an oral form of digoxin and has been noncompliant, the drug may be continued along with other modes of therapy such as salt restriction, bed rest, additional diuresis, vasodilator therapy, or other measures as necessary. If digoxin has not been previously instituted, it may be beneficial over the long run and may be begun in the emergency department provided there are no contraindications. This is especially true if CHF is due to hypertensive, ischemic, chronic valvular, or congenital heart disease. Dixogin is less effective if CHF is due to myocarditis, congestive cardiomyopathy, and high-output states, and probably ineffective if due to cor pulmonale (unless left ventricular dysfunction is present), mitral stenosis, or obstructive causes. (See boxes, Drug Treatment: Vasoactive Drugs in Acute Heart Failure with Normotension; Drug Treatment: Vasoactive Drugs in Acute Congestive Heart Failure with Hypotension; and Drug Treatment: Vasoactive Support in Acute Congestive Heart Failure with Hypertension.)

DRUG TREATMENT: VASOACTIVE DRUGS IN ACUTE HEART FAILURE WITH NORMOTENSION

First-Line Drug

Dobutamine

Initial Dose	2.5 µg/kg/min constant IV infusion
Repeat Dose	Titrate dose to clinical response up to 15 µg/kg/min. Occasionally, higher doses may be effective.
End-Points	Optimization of cardiac output, pulmonary wedge pressure, urine output
	Arrhythmias

AND

Nitroglycerin

Initial Dose	20 µg/min constant IV infusion
Repeat Dose	Titrate to clinical response up to 400 µg/min.
End-Points	Optimization of cardiac output, pulmonary wedge pressure, and urine output
	Hypotension

Chart continued on following page

DRUG TREATMENT: VASOACTIVE DRUGS IN ACUTE HEART FAILURE WITH NORMOTENSION Continued

Second-Line Drug

Amrinone

Initial Dose	0.75 mg/kg IV loading dose over 2–3 minutes
Repeat Dose	5 µg/kg/min–10 µg/kg/min constant IV infusion; may repeat loading dose after 30 minutes
End-Points	<10 mg/kg/day total dose
	Optimization of cardiac output, wedge pressure, urine output
	Hypotension
	Thrombocytopenia

DRUG TREATMENT: VASOACTIVE DRUGS IN ACUTE CONGESTIVE HEART FAILURE WITH HYPOTENSION

First-Line Drug

Dopamine

Initial Dose	5.0 µg/kg/min constant IV infusion
Repeat Dose	Titrate dose up to 20 µg/kg/min
End-Points	Optimization of cardiac output, wedge pressure, urine output
	Arrhythmias
	Decreased urine output

DRUG TREATMENT: VASOACTIVE SUPPORT IN ACUTE CONGESTIVE HEART FAILURE WITH HYPERTENSION

First-Line Drug

Nitroprusside

Initial Dose	5 µg/min constant IV infusion
Repeat Dose	Titrate to desired effect by increasing 10 µg/min q 5 minutes.
End-Points	Normalized blood pressure
	Improved hemodynamics
	Relief of symptoms
	Hypotension

Discussion

Severe exacerbations of chronic CHF or new-onset CHF usually require hospitalization. If pulmonary edema is present, the first priority of treatment is oxygen and ventilation. The patient is placed in an upright position and morphine and diuretics are administered. Vasodilators may be employed acutely in the form of intravenous nitroglycerin or nitroprusside (especially if hypertension is present). Long-acting inotropic agents, such as digoxin, are of little acute benefit unless rapid atrial fibrillation is present and control of atrioventricular nodal conduction is required to slow the ventricular rate. In conditions of reduced myocardial contractility or myocardial disease, short-term intravenous inotropic support may be necessary. In cases where mentation is diminished, oliguria is present, reduced cardiac output has resulted in extreme weakness, or shock is present, inotropic agents may be indicated. Occasionally, in the presence of severe chronic CHF, a short course (e.g., 1 to 2 days) of an intravenous inotropic agent, such as dobutamine or amrinone, may result in hemodynamic improvement that may transiently improve the patient's functional class. It should be emphasized, however, that the benefits from intravenous inotropic agents are short term and may not alter the long-term disease course. Also, mitral stenosis, cor pulmonale, high-output failure, and obstructive etiologies (e.g., tamponade) benefit little from inotropic support.

The parenteral agent of choice for acute inotropic support of CHF (in the absence of cardiogenic shock and hypotension) is dobutamine. Dobutamine is a selective beta$_1$-adrenergic agonist that increases cardiac output primarily through increasing stroke volume with little chronotropic effect. It reduces pulmonary wedge pressure but has little effect on systemic vascular resistance and hence does not elevate blood pressure. For this reason, it is ideally suited for the treatment of CHF associated with adequate systemic blood pressure, especially if the pulmonary wedge pressure is elevated. Coadministration of intravenous nitroglycerin relieves pulmonary congestion by causing venous dilation and may relieve angina if present. If hypertension is present, afterload reduction with a vasodilator, such as sodium nitroprusside, should be the first modality employed.

If hypotension is present, dopamine is more effective than dobutamine at raising blood pressure due to greater alpha-adrenergic stimulation. At low doses, dopamine stimulates dopaminergic receptors in the kidney, resulting in increased renal blood flow, but at higher doses, alpha and beta$_1$ effects are dominant. Thus, dopamine is the agent of choice for CHF associated with hypotension. Increases in blood pressure, however, result in greater stroke work and, hence, greater myocardial oxygen consumption. This may result in ischemia if coronary artery disease is present. In cases where renal blood flow is diminished and sodium retention is present, low-dose infusions will increase renal blood flow and sodium excretion. Dopamine does not reduce pulmonary wedge pressure, however, and may not improve pulmonary congestion.

Isoproterenol should not be used because of the marked tachycardia it produces and because of the possible hypotension that may be induced from its beta$_2$-mediated vasodilation.

Amrinone, a newly released inotropic agent that acts independently of the adrenergic receptors, increases cardiac output without an increase in heart rate. It also reduces systemic vascular resistance and pulmonary wedge pressure, making it an attractive inotropic agent with both preload- and afterload-reducing capacity. It is occasionally used in patients with refractory CHF when a trial of vasodilators or dobutamine has failed to produce hemodynamic improvement. Because amrinone is a vasodilator as well as an inotropic agent, it does not increase blood pressure but rather may reduce it slightly. It is therefore not useful for CHF with hypotension or cardiogenic shock. Also, there are toxicities associated with its use and experience is still limited.

In all cases, the use of these agents is intended to be short term and should be accompanied by hemodynamic monitoring in an intensive care setting. Adequate filling pressures are necessary to optimize the results from inotropic agents.

Cardiogenic Shock

Diagnosis

Cardiogenic shock results from failure of the heart to pump blood in an amount sufficient to meet the body's needs. This results in inadequate cellular perfusion and oxygen delivery to tissues. Although most discussions of cardiogenic shock focus on failure of the left ventricular myocardium following myocardial infarction (MI), a diversity of etiologies may result in pump failure. These may be mechanical, with acute valvular dysfunction or septal rupture; obstructive, with valvular stenosis, tamponade, or pulmonary emboli; due to arrhythmias; or conditions of "high-output" failure (Table 13–5).

In most cases the diagnosis is suggested by the history. Crushing substernal chest pain with radiation down the left arm or into the neck or jaw should suggest an acute MI, especially with history of angina or known ischemic disease. A history of heart murmur, rheumatic fever as a child, or congenital heart disease may be a clue to valvular dysfunction. Pericardial tamponade is suggested by a history of pericardial effusion (chronic renal failure, ascites, cancer, tuberculosis, connective tissue disease). Conditions associated with high-output failure, such as thyrotoxicosis, Paget's disease of bone, recently acquired arteriovenous shunts, or severe malnutrition, may be present but are less common causes. A massive pulmonary embolus may be suggested by sudden shock in the setting of obesity, deep venous thrombois, or recent leg or pelvic trauma or surgery.

Physical signs of cardiogenic shock include cool, mottled, moist skin; acral cyanosis; extreme weakness; diminished mentation; and oliguria. The systolic blood pressure is usually less than 90 mmHg. A narrow pulse pressure and pulsus paradoxus may be demonstrated if pericardial tamponade is pres-

ent. Jugular venous distention is often present, and hepatomegaly may also be present, especially in the presence of chronic right heart failure. Dyspnea may be noted if pulmonary edema is present. In such cases rales or wheezes may be audible. Cardiac auscultatory signs differ depending on the etiology, but an S_3 gallop, heart murmurs, or a pericardial friction rub may suggest the cause.

Although the electrocardiogram (ECG) may be nonspecific, it may show changes indicative of the underlying etiology. Acute myocardial infarction is indicated by ST segment elevations, "hyperacute" T waves, T wave inversions, or Q waves. Pericarditis may appear as diffuse ST segment elevations with T wave flattening or inversions; large effusions may exhibit electrical alternans. Acute pulmonary emboli may show signs of acute right heart strain, right axis deviation, and nonspecific T wave abnormalities. Cardiogenic shock due to a dysrhythmia is evident from the ECG (e.g., a tachydysrhythmia or bradydysrhythmia).

Acute hemodynamic data are most revealing. Most commonly, in cardiogenic shock due to acute left ventricular failure, the cardiac index is below normal, the systemic vascular resistance is elevated, and the pulmonary wedge pressure is elevated (Table 13–6). Also, the heart rate is increased, central venous pressure and right atrial pressure (RAP) are elevated, stroke volume and stroke work index are reduced, and the mixed venous oxygen saturation is low. If other causes of cardiogenic shock are present, some differences in these variables may be observed. Cardiac tamponade will result in an equalization of diastolic pressures with an accentuated x-descent in the RAP tracing ("square-root sign"); a massive pulmonary embolus will usually be associated with high central venous and pulmonary artery pressures and a low pulmonary wedge pressure; mitral regurgitation (e.g., due to papillary muscle dysfunction) will result in transmitted v waves in the pulmonary wedge pressure trace; and a ruptured ventricular septum will produce very high right ventricular pressures with a step up in oxygen saturation of mixed venous blood when a right atrial sample is compared to a pulmonary artery sample.

Indications for Treatment

Cardiogenic shock is a life-threatening condition and must be treated immediately.

TABLE 13–5. Etiologies of Cardiogenic Shock

Myocardial disease
  Myocardial infarction
  Myocarditis
  Cardiomyopathy
Valvular disease
  Ruptured chordae tendineae
  Acute papillary muscle dysfunction
  Acute aortic insufficiency
  Prosthetic valve dysfunction
  Ruptured intraventricular septum
Dysrhythmia
  Ventricular tachycardia
  Supraventricular tachycardia
  Atrial fibrillation/flutter
  Heart block
Drugs or toxins that alter cardiac function

TABLE 13–6. Clinical Features of Cardiogenic Shock of Various Etiologies

Etiology	Cardiac Index	Stroke Volume	Central Venous Pressure	Pulmonary Wedge Pressure	Other
Left ventricular dysfunction	L	L	H	H	Normal RAP, PAP
Cardiac tamponade	L	L	H	H	High RAP = RVDP = PADP = PWP
Mitral valve dysfunction	L	L	H	H	V waves on PWP trace
High output failure	H	H	N/H	N/H	Fever, thyrotoxicosis, etc.
Septal rupture	L	L	H	L	Increased RVSP, SvO₂
Right ventricular infarction	L	L	H	N	High RVDP, low RVSP, low PAP

L = low; N = normal; H = high; PADP = pulmonary artery diastolic pressure; RVDP = right ventricular diastolic pressure; RVSP = right ventricular systolic pressure; PAP = pulmonary artery systolic pressure; RAP = right atrial systolic pressure; PWP = pulmonary wedge pressure; SvO_2 = mixed venous oxygen saturation.

Approximately 15% of acute myocardial infarctions are complicated by cardiogenic shock, and the mortality approaches 85%. Treatment differs depending on the cause. Rhythm disorders should be corrected immediately by cardioversion (tachydysrhythmias) or pacing (bradydysrhythmias) (Fig. 13–3). When pericardial tamponade, ventricular septum or free-wall rupture, or acute valvular dysfunction has occurred, the treatment is surgical. Oxygen should be administered and intensive care monitoring begun. In pericardial tamponade and massive pulmonary embolus, temporary improvement occurs with rapid volume expansion using crystalloid solution. Aspiration of pericardial fluid may also produce temporary improvement. As soon as possible, invasive monitoring should be initiated with continuous measurement of arterial pressure, central venous pressure, and pulmonary artery pressure, and with periodic measurement of pulmonary wedge pressure, cardiac output, mixed venous oxygen saturation, and arterial blood gases.

In the vast majority of cases, cardiogenic shock is due to left ventricular dysfunction from acute myocardial infarction. The objective is to restore perfusion without placing the myocardium in further jeopardy by increasing oxygen demand. If pulmonary edema is present, diuresis with intravenous furosemide may improve oxygenation and reduce edema; occasionally with extreme hypoxia or hypercapnia, endotracheal intubation is necessary. Most patients with early cardiogenic shock are functionally volume contracted. The poorly compliant left ventricle functions best with pulmonary wedge pressure around 18 mmHg (above 20 mmHg, pulmonary edema occurs). For this reason, pulmonary wedge pressure monitoring with a balloon-tipped catheter to accurately guide volume therapy is important. If the pulmonary wedge pressure is below this range, careful volume expansion should be beneficial. If shock is still present, parenteral inotropic agents should be employed.

Because systemic vascular resistance is maximally elevated due to high circulating catecholamine levels, vasopressor agents are not indicated. Increases in afterload result in greater myocardial oxygen demand. There is an abnormal inverse relationship between stroke work and afterload in the failing heart. Further attempts to increase afterload may cause deterioration of stroke work index. Inotropic agents may be useful over the short term. (See box.)

Discussion

The agent of choice in cardiogenic shock with hypotension is dopamine. At low doses (e.g., below 3 to 5 µg/kg/min) dopaminergic effects dominate and increases in renal blood flow and sodium excretion occur. However, at these doses blood pressure and systemic perfusion may not improve, and, in fact, blood pressure may decrease due to vasodilation. Above 3 to 5 µg/kg/min, beta₁-adrenergic effects are dominant, leading to increases in cardiac output with a modest increase in heart rate and no change in pulmonary wedge pressure or systemic vascular resistance. At higher doses, alpha-adrenergic effects are prominent and systemic vascular resistance increases. Dopamine should be begun at 5 µg/kg/min and increased slowly to achieve improvement in perfusion and blood pressure. High doses and marked increases

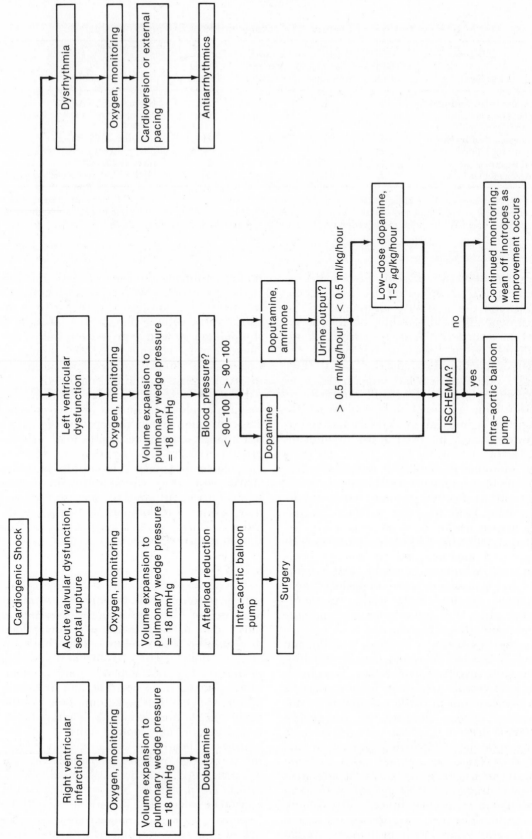

FIGURE 13–3. Treatment algorithm: cardiogenic shock.

DRUG TREATMENT: INOTROPIC SUPPORT IN CARDIOGENIC SHOCK

First-Line Drug

Dopamine

Initial Dose	5.0 µg/kg/min constant IV infusion
Repeat Dose	Titrate dose up to 20 µg/kg/min.
End-Points	Optimization of cardiac output, pulmonary wedge pressure, urine output
	Arrhythmias
	Decreased urine output

Second-Line Drug

Dobutamine

Initial Dose:	2.5 µg/kg/min constant IV infusion
Repeat Dose	Titrate dose to clinical response up to 15 µg/kg/min. Occasionally, higher doses may be effective.
End-Points	Optimization of cardiac output, pulmonary wedge pressure, urine output
	Arrhythmias

in systemic vascular resistance should be avoided.

Dobutamine has advantages in that it has little alpha-adrenergic or chronotropic effects and it reduces pulmonary wedge pressure. Because it has little effect on blood pressure, its use in cardiogenic shock is limited to cases where blood pressure is adequate. The combination of dobutamine and dopamine, however, is useful and may result in higher systemic pressure and cardiac output than with either agent alone.

Amrinone, a recently released inotropic agent, acts independently of the adrenergic receptors. Experience with it is limited. Amrinone increases cardiac output but decreases systemic vascular resistance and pulmonary wedge pressure, with usually a modest decrease in blood pressure. For this reason, it is not beneficial in cardiogenic shock.

Isoproterenol should not be used in cardiogenic shock. It may actually decrease blood pressure through its beta$_2$-adrenergic receptor stimulation and resulting vasodilation and decreased systemic and coronary perfusion pressures. In addition, it causes tachycardia, which further increases myocardial oxygen demand, and may lead to worsening ischemia or ventricular arrhythmias.

Intra-aortic balloon counterpulsation (IABP) may be used as an adjunctive measure in cases of cardiogenic shock associated with ongoing ischemia. Improvements in diastolic blood pressure and coronary filling occur and will lessen or alleviate ischemia. IABP should be reserved for candidates who are likely to survive or have an operable lesion.

Patients on parenteral inotropic agents or vasopressors should undergo continuous monitoring of hemodynamic variables with an indwelling arterial line and a pulmonary artery catheter, with intermittent assessment of preload (e.g., pulmonary wedge pressure or central venous pressure), cardiac output, and other indices of perfusion, such as urine output and mixed venous oxygen saturation, in an intensive care setting.

Septic Shock

Diagnosis

Septic shock is a form of distributive shock. It is characterized by maldistribution and shunting of pulmonary and systemic blood flow. The presence of infection produces a variety of metabolic and systemic reactions, including activation of the complement cascade and platelet activation. Early in septic shock, fever is typically present, although hypothermia may occur. Patients may exhibit confusion, weakness, tachycardia, hyperpnea, and oliguria. The skin is warm, and blood pressure may be normal or slightly decreased. Later, cool, moist skin and hypotension develop as cardiac output begins to decline.

Hemodynamically, septic shock is a dynamic process. Early in its course, a hyperdynamic state predominates, with increased cardiac output and low systemic vascular resistance, stroke volume, stroke work index, oxygen consumption (VO_2), and arterial and mixed venous oxygen content (CaO_2 and CvO_2). As it progresses, cardiac output falls below normal and is associated with elevated systemic vascular resistance. Urine output ceases, intrapulmonic shunting occurs, and hypoxia develops, initially accompanied by respiratory alkalosis and later by increasing metabolic acidosis. Adult respiratory distress

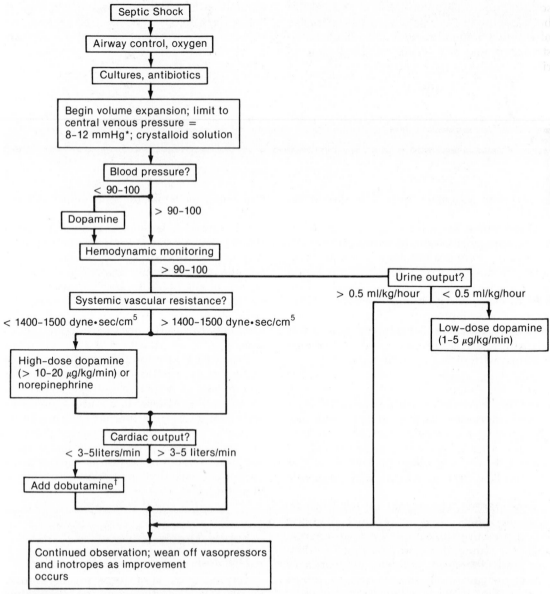

FIGURE 13–4. Treatment algorithm: septic shock. (*Limit central venous pressure to 8 to 12 mmHg or pulmonary pressure to 12 to 15 mmHg to prevent pulmonary edema due to increased capillary permeability. †Dobutamine plus low-dose dopamine is useful in low cardiac output states with adequate blood pressure but poor renal perfusion.)

syndrome (ARDS), multiple organ system failure, and disseminated intravascular coagulation are common.

Other features of the illness depend on the focus of infection. There may be signs of pneumonia, meningitis, peritonitis, or cutaneous infection. On the other hand, the focus may be occult with no specific findings.

Indications for Treatment

In most cases of septic shock, blood volume is mildly to moderately diminished and volume replacement is necessary. This is accomplished by infusing balanced crystalloid solution rapidly until an optimal preload has been achieved (pulmonary wedge pressure of 12 to 15 mmHg) in order to maximize stroke volume (Fig. 13–4). Capillary integrity is compromised in septic shock, and larger volumes may precipitate pulmonary edema. For this reason, it is desirable to guide volume expansion with some measure of filling pressure such as central venous pressure or, preferably, pulmonary wedge pressure. Colloid infusions may pass quickly into the interstitium and increase the accumulation of interstitial edema and should probably be avoided.

Oxygen should be provided to correct hypoxia, and antibiotics should be instituted promptly as indicated by the anticipated source of infection. Although high-dose corticosteroids have been used for septic shock in the past, recent studies have failed to demonstrate a benefit from their use. If blood pressure does not respond to volume infusion, vasopressor and inotropic support is necessary to maintain a mean arterial pressure greater than 60 mmHg.

DRUG TREATMENT: SEPTIC SHOCK WITH DECREASED SYSTEMIC VASCULAR RESISTANCE

First-Line Drug
Dopamine
Initial Dose	5.0 μg/kg/min constant IV infusion
Repeat Dose	Titrate dose up to 20 μg/kg/min.
End-Points	Optimization of cardiac output, pulmonary wedge pressure, urine output
	Arrhythmias
	Decreased urine output

Second-Line Drugs
Norepinephrine
Initial Dose	8–12 μg IV loading dose
Repeat Dose	Titrate constant IV infusion starting at 2 μg/min.
End-Points	Adequate blood pressure and perfusion
	Cardiac arrhythmias
	Decreased urine output

OR

Phenylephrine
Initial Dose	100–180 μg/min constant IV infusion to elevate blood pressure
Repeat Dose	After blood pressure elevated, continuous IV infusion at 40 μg/min and titrate
End-Points	Adequate blood pressure and perfusion
	Decreased urine output

DRUG TREATMENT: SEPTIC SHOCK WITH INCREASED SYSTEMIC VASCULAR RESISTANCE

First-Line Drugs

Dopamine

Initial Dose	5 μg/kg/min constant IV infusion
Repeat Dose	Titrate to 10 μg/kg/min or higher.
End-Points	Adequate cardiac output and pulmonary wedge pressure
	Adequate urine output

PLUS

Dobutamine

Initial Dose	2.5 μg/kg/min constant IV infusion
Repeat Dose	Titrate dose to clinical response up to 15 μg/kg/min. Occasionally, higher doses may be effective.
End-Points	Optimization of cardiac output, pulmonary wedge pressure, urine output
	Arrhythmias

Discussion

The parenteral agent of choice in early hyperdynamic shock is dopamine. Its alpha-adrenergic agonist effects increase systemic vascular resistance and raise the blood pressure. Its dopaminergic effects on the kidney increase renal blood flow. In later stages of shock, cardiac output is augmented through its beta$_1$-mediated inotropic effects. Dopamine should be started at a low dose (5 μg/kg/min) and titrated to the desired effect.

Other agents have a potential role depending on the hemodynamic derangement present. If severe hypotension is present with markedly reduced systemic vascular resistance (e.g., blood pressure <60 to 70 mmHg), the use of norepinephrine or other alpha-adrenergic agonists (e.g., metaraminol, phenylephrine, or methoxamine) will effectively raise blood pressure by causing vasoconstriction. Caution should be exercised with prolonged use. Very high systemic vascular resistance may result in hypoperfusion of the renal bed and other tissues whose arterial blood supply is mediated by alpha-adrenergic receptors, leading to renal shutdown and ischemia of digits. Late in the course of septic shock, as systemic vascular resistance increases and cardiac output declines, this scenario is common.

Shock with depressed myocardial function and increasing systemic vascular resistance may benefit from the combination of dopamine and dobutamine. Dobutamine, through its beta$_1$-agonist activity, increases cardiac output without increasing systemic vascular resistance, while low dose dopamine augments renal blood flow.

All patients should be intensively monitored with continuous determinations of blood pressure and heart rate and frequent determinations of pulmonary wedge pressure or central venous pressure, mixed venous oxygen saturation, cardiac output, urine output, and arterial blood gases.

Spinal Shock

Diagnosis

Neurogenic shock is a form of distributive shock resulting from loss of vasomotor tone. Reduced sympathetic stimulation of vascular smooth muscle in arterioles results in decreased systemic vascular resistance and hypotension. Cardiac contractility and heart rate, also under sympathetic control, fail to compensate. Venodilation occurs as well and results in expansion of the venous capacitance system, creating a relative volume deficit. This produces diminished venous return to the heart and a reduction in stroke volume and, hence, cardiac output.

Loss of vasomotor tone may occur from many mechanisms, including brain or spinal cord injury, anesthesia, or drugs that inhibit the formation or transmission of neural impulses that mediate vascular tone. Exposure to noxious stimuli may produce a transient interruption of vascular sympathetic tone and an increase in parasympathetic tone manifested commonly as "fainting."

Clinically, neurogenic shock is characterized by hypotension, with warm, dry, flushed skin reflecting vasodilation. The absence of tachycardia suggests the loss of appropriate sympathetic responses. Other signs present may reflect the underlying etiology, such as unconsciousness or a neurologic deficit, signs of drug ingestion, or acute trauma. Vagal episodes may, in addition, be accompanied by nausea, vomiting, salivation, or diarrhea.

Hemodynamic signs include reduced systemic vascular resistance, usually with reduced cardiac output reflecting diminished venous return, which is confirmed by finding a low central venous pressure and pulmonary wedge pressure. Heart rate is normal or low, as is stroke volume.

Indications for Treatment

Initial treatment of spinal shock should be to support the airway, provide oxygen, and assist ventilation as needed (Fig. 13–5). If the spinal shock is trauma-induced, associated injuries should be sought and treated. Because the primary hemodynamic impairment in spinal shock is diminished systemic vascular resistance and venodilation, treatment is aimed at restoring vascular tone using vasopressor agents. Venodilation expands the vascular pool and results in diminished venous return; thus left ventricular filling pressure is frequently low. Therefore, the first step is to optimize left ventricular filling pressure by careful volume expansion using crystalloid solutions. A gradual rise in arterial pressure will occur. However, because overhydration may result in increasing cerebral edema if head injury is present, monitoring of central venous pressure or pulmonary wedge pressure and maintaining them at near normal levels is desirable. In transient vasomotor fainting episodes, volume expansion alone may be sufficient.

In more severe cases that fail to respond to volume expansion, and in those cases of head injury where excessive volume expansion is to be avoided, vasopressor agents such as phenylephrine will raise arterial pressure. (See box.)

Discussion

These drugs are given as a continuous intravenous infusion and titrated to the desired effect. Hemodynamic monitoring is required. During the administration of spinal anesthesia, injections of phenylephrine (subcutaneous, intramuscular, or intravenous) may be employed as a prophylactic measure.

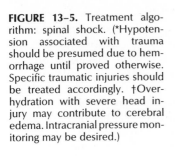

FIGURE 13–5. Treatment algorithm: spinal shock. (*Hypotension associated with trauma should be presumed due to hemorrhage until proved otherwise. Specific traumatic injuries should be treated accordingly. †Overhydration with severe head injury may contribute to cerebral edema. Intracranial pressure monitoring may be desired.)

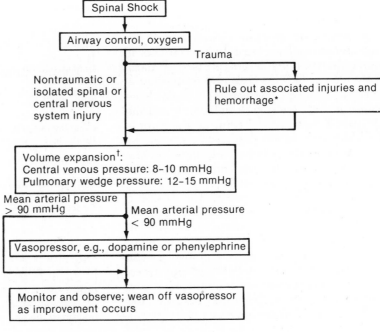

DRUG TREATMENT: SPINAL SHOCK

First-Line Drug

Dopamine

Initial Dose	10 μg/kg/min constant IV infusion
Repeat Dose	Titrate to maximal dose of 20/μg/kg/min.
End-Points	Adequate blood pressure and perfusion
	Decreased urine output

OR

Phenylephrine

Initial Dose	100–180 μg/min constant infusion to elevate blood pressure
Repeat Dose	After blood pressure elevated, continuous infusion at 40 μg/min and titrate
End-Points	Adequate blood pressure and perfusion
	Decreased urine output

It is important to remember, however, that hypotension accompanying acute head injury, especially in the presence of multiple injuries, should be presumed due to hypovolemia until proved otherwise and treated initially with volume expansion. Also, overzealous use of alpha-agonist agents may elevate blood pressure at the expense of organ perfusion.

Anaphylactic Shock

Diagnosis

Anaphylactic shock is a syndrome of cardiovascular collapse resulting from the action of humoral mediators released primarily from mast cells when exposed to an inciting antigen. Primary mediators include histamine, leukotrienes, prostaglandins, platelet activating factor, kallikrein, and serotonin. In addition, the effects of secondary mediators, such as the products of platelets, neutrophils, and eosinophils, and of complement activation may contribute.

Cardiovascular collapse is the result of several parallel processes (Table 13–7). Most commonly, vasodilation occurs with increased vascular permeability and a resultant decrease in plasma volume. Hemoconcentration may occur, along with reductions in central venous pressure and pulmonary wedge pressure. Early on, there may be an endogenous catecholamine response to vasodila-

tion, and tachycardia and increased cardiac output may occur transiently. When anaphylactic shock is fully developed, however, stroke volume and cardiac output are decreased, partly due to reduced plasma volume and partly to direct cardiac effects. Cardiac effects include dysrhythmias and depressed myocardial contractility, resulting from diverse factors, including acidosis, hyp-

TABLE 13–7. Pathophysiology of Anaphylactic Shock

Mediators of Anaphylaxis
Histamine
Leukotrienes
Prostaglandins
Platelet activating factor
Kallikrein
Serotonin
Complement
Products of platelets, neutrophils, eosinophils

Mechanisms of Shock
Vasodilation
Vascular permeability, loss of plasma volume
Depressed myocardial contractility
   Mediator effect
   Acidosis
   Hypoxia
   Ischemia
Dysrhythmias
Pulmonary hypertension

(Adapted from Perkin RM, Nick NG: Mechanisms and management of anaphylactic shock not responding to traditional therapy. Ann Allerg 54:202–207, 1985.)

oxemia, myocardial ischemia, and the direct effects of mediators and exogenous drugs. Further contributing to the deteriorating cardiac output is the frequent finding of pulmonary hypertension, which may be the result of pulmonary vasoconstriction or microvascular plugging by aggregates of platelets and neutrophils.

Clinically, angioedema and urticaria are almost universal, occurring early and involving lips, periorbital area, hands, feet, and genitalia. Upper airway obstruction with laryngeal edema is common, as is bronchospasm. Patients may complain of a choking sensation, coughing, or wheezing. Diaphoresis may occur, as well as pupillary dilation, flushing, dizziness, and gastrointestinal upset. In more severe cases, syncope occurs, accompanied by hypotension and dysrhythmias (sinus tachycardia, supraventricular dysrhythmias, intraventricular conduction delays). Extreme cases may manifest coma, seizures, and death.

Indications for Treatment

Supportive measures should be instituted promptly, including airway control, oxygen, and intravenous access. (See Fig. 13–6 and box.)

DRUG TREATMENT: ANAPHYLACTIC SHOCK

First-Line Drugs
Epinephrine

Initial Dose	0.1 mg (1 ml of 1:10,000 solution) IV over 2–3 minutes
Repeat Dose	0.1 mg every 5 minutes or constant IV infusion from 1–5 μg/min and titrate
End-Points	Adequate blood pressure and perfusion
	Cardiac arrhythmias
	Myocardial ischemia

Second-Line Drugs
Dopamine

Initial Dose	5 μg/kg/min constant IV infusion
Repeat Dose	Titrate to 10 μg/kg/min or higher.
End-Points	Adequate cardiac output and pulmonary wedge pressure
	Adequate urine output

Third-Line Drugs
Norepinephrine

Initial Dose	8–12 μg loading dose
Repeat Dose	Titrate constant IV infusion starting at 2 μg/min.
End-Points	Adequate blood pressure and perfusion
	Cardiac arrhythmias

OR

Phenylephrine

Initial Dose	100–180 μg/min constant IV infusion to elevate blood pressure
Repeat Dose	After blood pressure elevated, continuous infusion at 40 μg/min and titrate
End-Points	Adequate blood pressure and perfusion

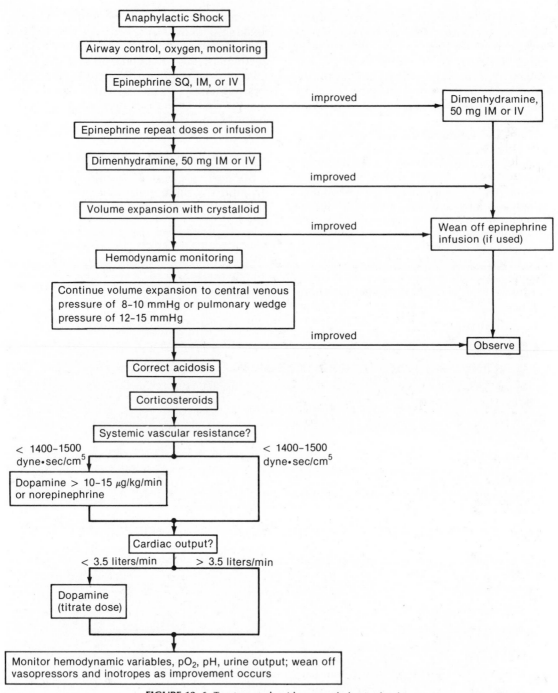

FIGURE 13–6. Treatment algorithm: anaphylactic shock.

Discussion

Pharmacologic treatment is indicated when hypotension is present along with signs of decreased end-organ perfusion, such as myocardial ischemia, alteration in mental status, and oliguria. Cases of marginal hypo-tension (systolic blood pressure 90 to 110 mmHg) may be initially managed with rapid intravenous crystalloid infusion or colloid infusion. Because of increased capillary permeability and the propensity for the development of pulmonary edema, indicators of left ventricular filling should be monitored and fluid administration restricted when the central venous pressure rises to 12 mmHg or the pulmonary wedge pressure rises to 15 mmHg.

Shock from Beta-Blockers

Diagnosis
Beta-blocker overdose is seldom a diagnostic dilemma. Patients exhibit signs of beta blockade with bradycardia, hypotension, prolongation of the QRS complex, atrioventricular nodal block, and heart failure. Bronchospasm may be prominent, and diffuse wheezing may be heard. Lethargy occurs, and seizures have been reported. Specific blood levels of the agent are elevated. Hemodynamically, heart rate and cardiac output are reduced and systemic vascular resistance is elevated due to unimpeded compensatory alpha-receptor stimulation. Characteristic of shock from beta blockade, no beneficial response occurs to the administration of inotropic or chronotropic agents that exert their action through the beta receptor.

Indications for Treatment
Initial treatment of beta-blocker overdose requires evacuation of the stomach with careful protection of the airway. If bronchospasm is present, inhaled beta agonists should be administered, and, if necessary, endotracheal intubation should be performed and assisted ventilation provided. (See treatment of bronchospasm in Chapter 18.) If hypotension is present, careful volume expansion is indicated to obtain optimal filling pressures. When volume is adequate but symptomatic hypotension persists, pharmacologic treatment is indicated. (See Fig. 13–7 and box.)

DRUG TREATMENT: SHOCK FROM BETA-BLOCKER OVERDOSE

Bradycardia

First-Line Drug
Atropine

Initial Dose	0.5 mg IV
Repeat Dose	0.5–1.0 mg IV
End-Points	Total dose of 3 mg
	Resolution of bradycardia

Second-Line Drug
Isoproterenol

Initial Dose	0.05 mg loading dose IV
Repeat Dose	Constant IV infusion beginning at 5 μg/min and titrate upward
End-Points	Resolution of bradycardia
	Excessive hypotension (add vasopressor)

Third-Line Drug
Glucagon

Initial Dose	5–10 mg IV
Repeat Dose	5 mg IV q 15–30 minutes or IV infusion starting at 1.0 mg/hour and titrate
End-Points	Adequate blood pressure and perfusion

Chart continued on following page

DRUG TREATMENT: SHOCK FROM BETA-BLOCKER OVERDOSE
Continued
Hypotension

First-Line Drug
Glucagon

Initial Dose	5–10 mg IV
Repeat Dose	5 mg IV q 15–30 minutes or IV infusion starting at 1.0 mg/hour and titrate
End-Points	Adequate blood pressure and perfusion
	5 mg/hour

Second-Line Drugs
Dobutamine

Initial Dose	2.5 μg/kg/min constant IV infusion
Repeat Dose	Titrate dose to clincial response up to 15 μg/kg/min. Occasionally, higher doses may be effective.
End-Points	Optimization of cardiac output, pulmonary wedge pressure, urine output
	Arrhythmias

OR

Dopamine

Initial Dose	5 μg/kg/min constant IV infusion
Repeat Dose	Titrate dose up to 20 μg/kg/min.
End-Points	Optimization of cardiac output, pulmonary wedge pressure, urine output
	Arrhythmias
	Decreased urine output

Discussion

Bradycardia should be treated with atropine, 0.5 to 1 mg, which may be repeated every 5 to 10 minutes to a total dosage of 3 mg. If atropine is ineffective, an isoproterenol infusion should be administered or an external pacer applied. Because beta-blockers are competitive antagonists of the beta receptors, high doses of isoproterenol may be required to overcome beta blockade. The presence of hypotension is also an indication for inotropic and chronotropic support. An isoproterenol infusion should be begun with dopamine added if cardiac output fails to rise or hypotension persists. Although volume deficits are not a hemodynamic consequence of beta-blocker overdose, inotropic agents will have limited effectiveness in the presence of a volume deficit. Thus, optimal filling pressures should be restored promptly by the infusion of crystalloid solutions.

Frequently, beta agonists exert little or no effect in overdoses with beta-blockers. However, agents that exert an inotropic effect independent of the beta receptor may be of dramatic benefit. Digitalis should not be used because its inhibition of atrioventricular nodal conduction may be potentiated by beta blockade leading to a high-grade atrioventricular block. Glucagon, however, has been shown to be effective at increasing cardiac output and reducing peripheral resistance in cases of beta-blocker overdose. It exerts an inotropic and chronotropic effect through a mechanism independent of beta receptors. Although its effects are not of long duration (e.g., 15 to 30 minutes), it has little toxicity and may be repeated as often as necessary. A glucagon infusion may be administered.

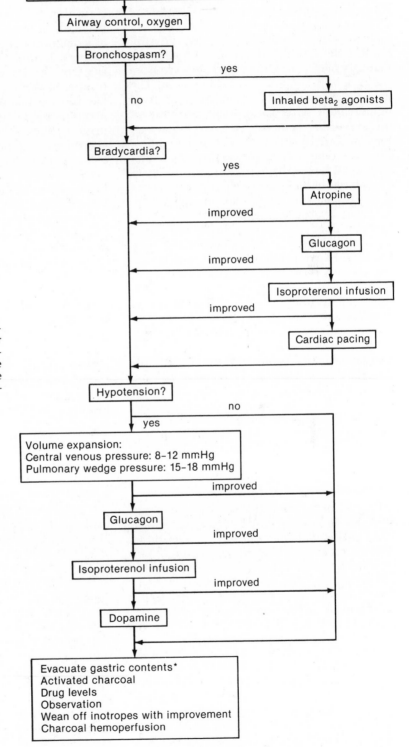

FIGURE 13–7. Treatment algorithm: shock from beta-blocker overdose. (*Evacuate gastric contents as soon as possible; may be done simultaneously with above measures. Emergency hemodynamic support has priority.)

Gastrointestinal Hemorrhage

Diagnosis

Gastrointestinal (GI) hemorrhage occurs when disruption of the mucosal lining of the GI tract extends into a blood vessel. The site may be at any point from the pharynx (including the nose) to the anus, although the majority of serious GI hemorrhages are from the esophagus, stomach, or duodenum. The majority of minor GI hemorrhages are from hemorrhoids. After appropriate resuscitative measures have been initiated and blood sent for complete blood count, a coagulation profile, and type and crossmatch, a good first step in GI hemorrhage treatment is to localize the site of bleeding to an upper (pharynx through small intestine) or lower (colon) site. A history or observation of hematemesis confirms an upper GI source. Bright red blood from the rectum is usually associated with lower GI bleeding but may sometimes be observed with very brisk upper GI bleeding. A nasogastric tube should be passed to confirm the diagnosis of upper GI bleeding and to be used for gastric lavage.

The next step is to more specifically localize the site of bleeding, which can usually be accomplished by endoscopy—anoscopy followed by sigmoidoscopy or colonoscopy for lower GI bleeding, upper endoscopy for upper GI bleeding. In some patients, particularly if they are bleeding from an unusual site (e.g., Meckel's diverticulum), angiography or a tagged red cell nuclear scan may be necessary to localize the bleeding site.

Indications for Treatment

Except for minor anal bleeding from hemorrhoids or fissures, all GI hemorrhages will need treatment. The mainstay of therapy is restoration of an adequate circulating blood volume by transfusion and control of the bleeding site. The need for resuscitation, hospitalization, and the specifics of therapy will depend on the degree of hemorrhage, the patient's overall health, and the site of bleeding.

Upper GI hemorrhage from esophageal or gastric varices is both a challenging and unique management problem; it is the only type of GI bleeding in which a vasoactive drug may be beneficial as adjunctive therapy. Esophageal varices result from an increase in portal venous pressure, usually as a result of advanced cirrhosis. These patients typically present with the various clinical signs of cirrhosis and a history of previous GI bleeding. It is important to remember that approximately a third of upper GI bleeding episodes in patients with cirrhosis will not be from varices. Therefore, early endoscopy is particularly important in these patients, both as a diagnostic tool and as the means for providing sclerotherapy if the site of bleeding is a varix. Endoscopic sclerotherapy is the treatment of choice for bleeding varices and has been a major advance in the management of bleeding esophageal varices from prior days of the Sengstaken-Blakemore tube and emergency portocaval shunt surgery.

Vasopressin has an adjunctive role in the management of bleeding esophageal varices. Vasopressin is an arterial constrictor that lowers portal and, thus, variceal pressure by reducing mesenteric arterial blood flow. A vasopressin infusion may be used to control or reduce variceal bleeding until sclerotherapy can be performed and is used by many endoscopists following sclerotherapy to reduce the incidence of rebleeding, especially in the first 24 hours.

Vasopressin is also occasionally given by direct intra-arterial infusion to control arterial bleeding sites at other locations in the gastrointestinal tract. This requires arteriography for catheter placement and is a specialized technique utilized by interventional radiologists. (See box.)

Discussion

Vasopressin should not be considered definitive therapy for GI hemorrhage, especially for variceal hemorrhage, because no well-designed clinical trial has shown that its use significantly affects outcome. However, vasopressin does clearly reduce the rate of blood loss from bleeding varices and thus is a useful agent to buy time until definitive treatment with endoscopic sclerotherapy or portocaval shunting can be accomplished. Sclerotherapy is technically easier when there is less active bleeding and thus is facilitated by the prior initiation of vasopressin.

The usual maximal and starting dose is 0.4 unit/min given by continuous intravenous infusion. If possible, the infusion should be given via a central vein because extravasation causes a severe skin slough if vasopressin leaks into the tissues. One series has recently reported a better outcome with very high-dose (1.0 to 1.5 units/min) vasopressin infusion compared to standard doses. In this series, all patients also received a portosys-

---

DRUG TREATMENT: GASTROINTESTINAL HEMORRHAGE

First-Line Drugs

Vasopressin

Initial Dose	Continous IV infusion of 0.4 unit/min
Repeat Dose	If bleeding is controlled, continue for 24 hours and then taper by decreasing by 0.1 unit q 12 hours.
	If bleeding persists, increase dose to maximum of 1.0 unit/min and consider alternative therapy.
End-Points	Control of bleeding
	Toxicity
	Maximum dose of 1 unit/min

PLUS

Nitroglycerin

Initial Dose	200 μg/min by continuous IV infusion
Repeat Dose	May increase infusion to 400 μg/min if evidence of coronary ischemia
End-Points	Control of bleeding
	Hypotension

---

temic shunt. There were more adverse events in the group receiving high-dose vasopressin. Based on this report, we would recommend increasing the dose of vasopressin to a maximum of 1.0 unit/min if bleeding persists. Continued bleeding on this dose of vasopressin calls for sclerotherapy or, if this has failed or is not available, placement of a Sengstaken-Blakemore tube and consideration of surgical intervention.

The major toxicity of vasopressin results from its arterial constricting action in the coronary and mesenteric vessels. Myocardial ischemia, infarction, and arrhythmias may result from the use of vasopressin in patients with coronary artery disease. Mesenteric vasoconstriction may result in bowel infarction. The simultaneous administration of nitroglycerin with vasopressin blocks vasopressin's adverse effects on coronary perfusion and also has some additive effect in lowering portal pressure. Nitroglycerin is best given to these acutely ill and unstable patients by a continuous intravenous infusion starting at 200 μg/min (100 μg/min if the patient is hypotensive) and titrated based on clinical response. The nitroglycerin is increased if the patient has chest pain, arrhythmias, or electrocardiographic changes and

decreased if the patient becomes hypotensive.

SPECIFIC AGENTS

Amrinone (Inocor)

Pharmacology

The volume of distribution is 1.2 liters/kg. Amrinone is 10 to 49% protein bound and has a distribution-phase half-life of approximately 4.6 minutes. The terminal elimination half-life is approximately 3.6 hours in normal individuals and 5.8 hours in the presence of congestive heart failure. Following the distribution phase, elimination follows first-order kinetics. The primary route of elimination is the urine.

Actions

Amrinone has positive inotropic and vasodilatory effects independent of beta receptors or Na^+/K^+-ATPase (Table 13–8). Its effects are mediated through direct inhibition of myocardial cyclic nucleotide phosphodiesterase. A dose-related increase in cardiac output occurs, primarily as a result of in-

TABLE 13–8. Comparison of the Effects of Inotropic Agents

Agent	Clinical Effect				Receptor Stimulation		
	HR	**BP**	**SVR**	**CO**	*Alpha*	*Beta₁*	*Beta₂*
Amrinone	N	N	D	I			
Digoxin	D	N	D	I			
Dobutamine	N/I	N/I	N/D	I	0/+	+++	0/+
Dopamine	I	I	I	I	0/+++	+++	+
Epinephrine	I	I	I	I	+++	+++	+++
Glucagon	I	I	D	I			
Isoproterenol	I	D	D	I	0	+++	+++
Levarterenol (norepinephrine)	D	I	I	D	+++	++	++
Metaraminol	D	I	I	D	++	0/+	0/+
Methoxamine	D	I	I	D	+++	0	0
Phenylephrine	D	I	I	D	+++	0	0

I = increases; D = decreases; N = no or minimal effect; HR = heart rate; BP = blood pressure; SVR = systemic vascular resistance; CO = cardiac output; 0 = no effect; + = positive effect or stimulating; ++ and +++ = stronger effect.

creased cardiac contractility. There is a dose-related decrease in pulmonary wedge pressure, right atrial pressure, and systemic vascular resistance. Heart rate and blood pressure are unchanged.

Indications

Amrinone is indicated for short-term treatment of congestive heart failure in a closely monitored setting. It is reserved for patients who have not responded adequately to conventional inotropic agents.

Cautions

Renal failure—careful monitoring of the hemodynamic effects of amrinone is necessary in patients with diminished renal perfusion because plasma concentrations of the drug may increase.

Cardiac failure—although the elimination half-life is prolonged in patients with congestive heart failure, the dosage is generally titrated to its desired effect. It may require a lower rate of infusion to maintain a therapeutic plasma concentration (approximately 0.5 to 7 μg/ml).

Hepatic failure—patients with reduced hepatic perfusion may experience higher plasma levels of amrinone. Therefore, it is necessary to monitor the hemodynamic effects closely in these patients.

Use in pregnancy—Category C. There are conflicting reports of teratogenic effects to the fetus at high doses in a rabbit model, but the drug has not been studied well in pregnant humans.

Use in childhood—safety and effectiveness not established

Onset and Duration of Action

Dosage

Amrinone should be initiated with a 0.75 mg/kg IV bolus given over 2 to 3 minutes, followed by an IV infusion at 5 to 10 μg/kg/min. A repeat bolus may be given 30 minutes after the first. The peak effect occurs within 10 minutes after the bolus injection and lasts 30 minutes to 2 hours. The therapeutic range of plasma concentrations over which a dose-related effect can be observed is between 0.5 and 7 μg/ml.

Limits

The maximum daily dose should not exceed 10 mg/day (bolus plus infusion).

Repeat Dosing

Because of the rapid distribution phase of amrinone, a second bolus may be repeated 30 minutes after the first.

Toxicity

Drug Interactions

Experience with amrinone is limited, and no drug interactions have been reported with the exception of one episode of excessive hypotension when used with disopyramide (Norpace).

Specific Adverse Effects

Amrinone may cause supraventricular and ventricular dysrhythmias, although it is not arrhythmogenic *per se.* In combination with other agents, in high-risk patients, and at high doses, the likelihood of dysrhythmias is increased. Like other inotropic agents, it should not be used in patients with ventricular outflow obstruction (e.g., aortic or pulmonic valve stenosis or hypertrophic subaortic stenosis) because it may increase the obstruction gradient. Nonimmune thrombocytopenia may occur due to direct platelet damage, but drops in platelet counts below 70,000/ml are uncommon, and the effect is reversible after cessation of the drug. Other effects include gastrointestinal upset in 2.4% of patients and hepatocellular injury at high doses (9 to 32 mg/kg/day).

Treatment of Toxicity

If the above-mentioned adverse reactions develop, the drug should be discontinued. Mild decreases in platelet counts or elevations in transaminase levels may respond to a reduction of the daily dose. The decision to discontinue amrinone will depend on whether the risks from mild hepatic injury or thrombocytopenia outweigh the potential benefits of continuing therapy.

Digoxin (Lanoxin)

See Chapter 11, Antiarrhythmics.

Dobutamine (Dobutrex)

Pharmacology

The half-life of dobutamine is 2 minutes. The drug is widely distributed. It is metabolized in the liver to inactive conjugates and excreted in the urine.

Actions

Dobutamine stimulates beta$_1$ receptors in the heart to exert a positive inotropic response. Unlike dopamine, it does not stimulate the release of endogenous norepinephrine, nor does it have an effect on dopaminergic receptors. It produces an increase in cardiac output primarily through an increase in stroke volume. Heart rate is minimally affected. At doses below 15 µg/kg/min, systemic vascular resistance may decline slightly, although at high doses or with concomitant beta blockade, it may rise slightly. Blood pressure is usually unchanged, and pulmonary wedge pressure declines. Dobutamine also enhances atrioventricular nodal conduction.

Indications

Dobutamine is indicated for short-term inotropic support of patients with depressed cardiac contractility. It should be used in a monitored setting. It is ideally suited for patients with depressed cardiac function without hypotension, especially those with congestive heart failure and elevated pulmonary wedge pressure.

Cautions

Renal failure—because dobutamine is metabolized to an inactive form by the liver, alterations in renal function do not markedly affect the action of dobutamine.

Cardiac failure—dobutamine's primary use is in cardiac failure. In extremely low flow states, elimination may be reduced. Because the infusion is titrated to the desired effect, a reduction in infusion rate may be necessary.

Hepatic failure—because dobutamine is inactivated in the liver, a reduction in infusion rate may be necessary in the presence of hepatic failure.

Use in pregnancy—Category C. Animal studies have not shown dobutamine to be teratogenic. Its effects in pregnant humans, however, are unknown. It should be used during pregnancy only if the benefits to its use outweigh the potential risks.

Use in childhood—may be used in children

Onset and Duration of Action

Dosage

After intravenous injection of dobutamine, the onset of action is 1 to 2 minutes, with a peak effect obtained in less than 10 minutes. The usual dosage ranges between 2.5 and 10 µg/kg/min, titrated to the desired effect. Occasionally higher doses may be needed. Because the half-life is short (2 minutes), reductions in the rate of infusion are followed within minutes by a decrease in dobutamine's effects.

Limits

There are no dosage limits. If toxicity occurs, the infusion rates should be reduced or the drug discontinued.

Repeat Dosing

Dobutamine is administered by continuous intravenous infusion.

Toxicity

Drug Interactions

There are no significant known drug interactions. Dobutamine may be combined with certain other agents, such as nitroprusside, to enhance hemodynamic effects.

Specific Adverse Effects

In a small percentage of patients (5 to 10%), a marked increase in heart rate and blood pressure may be observed, which responds promptly to reduction in the rate of infusion. Because atrioventricular nodal conduction is enhanced by dobutamine, patients with atrial fibrillation may experience an accelerated ventricular response when the drug is administered. Approximately 5% of patients may experience increased ventricular ectopy, but dobutamine appears to be less arrhythmogenic than dopamine or isoproterenol.

Other uncommon adverse effects include nausea, palpitations, shortness of breath, exacerbations of angina, and occasional allergic reactions.

Treatment of Toxicity

Increases in heart rate, blood pressure, or ventricular ectopy will respond to reduction of the rate of dobutamine infusion. Hypersensitivity reactions require discontinuation of the drug.

Dopamine (Intropin)

Pharmacology

Dopamine's half-life is 2 minutes. It is metabolized in the liver and excreted in the urine. Also metabolized by monoamine oxidase (MAO) and catecholamine-o-methyl transferase (COMT).

Actions

Dopamine is a positive inotropic agent that exerts its effect by stimulating beta$_1$ receptors. It can stimulate the release of epinephrine from presynaptic neurons and increases cardiac output through an increase in myocardial contractility. Systolic blood pressure is elevated, and heart rate may be slightly elevated. Systemic vascular resistance is not affected at low doses, but at high doses (e.g., above $10/\mu g/kg/min$), it rises due to dopamine's mild alpha-agonist properties. Pulmonary wedge pressure is minimally to slightly increased.

Dopamine stimulates "dopaminergic" receptors in the kidney to reduce renal vascular resistance when administered at low doses (e.g., 2 to 5 $\mu g/kg/min$). This results in an increase in renal blood flow and sodium excretion.

Indications

Dopamine is indicated in patients with reduced cardiac output and shock of diverse origin. It is particularly useful when renal hypoperfusion or oliguria is present. Hypovolemia must first be corrected for dopamine to be most effective.

Cautions

Renal failure—dopamine is metabolized in the liver to an inactive metabolite. Alterations in renal function do not markedly affect its action.

Cardiac failure—dopamine is useful in the treatment of cardiac failure due to reduced myocardial contractility. However, in the presence of obstructions to cardiac outflow (e.g., aortic or pulmonic valvular stenosis or hypertrophic subaortic stenosis), cardiac output may decrease with dopamine administration because of worsening of the outflow gradient.

Hepatic failure—because dopamine is metabolized in the liver, use of the drug in patients with liver failure may require reduction in the rate of infusion.

Use in pregnancy—Category C. No teratogenic effects from dopamine have been observed in laboratory animals, although a rat model showed reduced survival of offspring and a tendency toward cataract formation in the survivors. Sufficient studies involving pregnant humans are lacking. Therefore, dopamine should be used in pregnant women only if the benefits outweigh the potential risks.

Use in childhood—may be used in children

Use in vaso-occlusive disease—patients with Raynaud's disease, diabetic endarteritis, Buerger's disease, or other occlusive vascular disease may experience vasospasm with dopamine infusion, especially at high doses.

Onset and Duration of Action

Dosage

The dosage of dopamine depends on the desired effect. In patients with oliguria complicating congestive heart failure or sepsis, for example, dopamine at low dose (2 to 5 μg/kg/min) allows the dopaminergic effects to predominate with little beta$_1$- or alpha-receptor stimulation. If an increase in cardiac output is desired, the dosage may be increased. Above 5 μg/kg/min, beta$_1$ stimulation increases in a dose-related fashion, and increases in cardiac output and blood pressure may be observed. At doses above 10 to 20 μg/kg/min, alpha-receptor stimulation increases markedly and systemic vascular resistance rises. The latter effect may be particularly desirable, for example, in septic shock associated with hypotension and reduced systemic vascular resistance.

The onset of action is rapid, within 1 to 2 minutes, and will fall as abruptly with discontinuance of the infusion. In most cases, infusions may be initiated at 2 to 5 μg/kg/min and titrated upward to their desired effect, with adjustment made in increments of 2 to 5 μg/kg/min every 5 to 10 minutes.

Limits

Most patients require infusion rates of less than 20 μg/kg/min; however, dosages up to 50 μg/kg/min are occasionally used. At high doses, vasoconstriction of vascular beds is common and oliguria may occur.

Repeat Dosing

Dopamine is administered as a continuous intravenous infusion.

Toxicity

Drug Interactions

Because dopamine is a substrate for MAO, inhibitors of this enzyme may potentiate its action. In such cases, dopamine should be initiated at one-tenth the normal dose.

Specific Adverse Reactions

Most adverse reactions are related to the pharmacologic effects of the drug and include tachycardia, palpitations, exacerbation of angina, shortness of breath, nausea, vomiting, and headache. Ventricular ectopy may occur. Vasoconstriction may lead to necrosis of distal appendages and renal failure. If dopamine is extravasated subcutaneously, skin necrosis is likely to occur. For this reason, dopamine should be infused into a large vein by a secure intravenous catheter.

Treatment of Toxicity

Dose-related toxicities such as tachycardia, palpitations, and episodes of angina may be treated by reducing the rate of infusion or discontinuing the drug. The risk of discontinuing the agent must be weighed against the potential benefit of continuing it. If subcutaneous extravasation occurs, the area should be infiltrated as soon as possible with 5 to 10 mg of phentolamine (diluted to 10 to 15 ml with saline). This may limit the extent of the necrosis that may occur.

Epinephrine (Adrenalin, Sus-Phrine, Asthmanefrin, Micronefrin, Vaponefrin)

Pharmacology

Chemical Structure

Racemic epinephrine contains both the active ($-$) and inactive ($+$) isomers of epinephrine. Epinephrine suspension contains epinephrine, ascorbic acid, thioglycolic acid, phenol, and glycerin.

Distribution

Epinephrine is slowly absorbed from subcutaneous injection and more rapidly absorbed with intramuscular injection. Inhaled epinephrine has limited systemic absorption in conventional doses.

Elimination

Epinephrine is metabolized in sympathetic nerve endings, liver, and other tissues. Very little is excreted unchanged in the urine.

Actions

Bronchial—will relax bronchial smooth muscle and constrict bronchial arterioles
Cardiovascular—in low doses may elevate systolic and decrease diastolic pressure; in higher doses will increase both; will increase inotropy and chronotropy in the heart

Indications

Bronchial asthma
Reversible bronchospasm with acute or chronic airway disease
Croup
Anaphylaxis
Cardiac arrest
Low cardiac output (selected cases)

Cautions

Renal failure—no dosage adjustment necessary
Cardiac failure—will increase myocardial oxygen consumption and demand. This may precipitate arrhythmias. Epinephrine treatment for bronchospasm is contraindicated in heart failure or patients with suspected coronary artery disease.
Hepatic failure—no dosage adjustment necessary
Use in pregnancy—Category C; has been shown to be teratogenic in animals in large doses; may slow labor. Epinephrine is excreted in the breast milk and should not be used for treatment of asthma in nursing mothers.
Other—epinephrine treatment for asthma is contraindicated in patients known or suspected to have coronary artery disease or pheochromocytoma.
Use in childhood—may be used

Onset and Duration of Action

Dosage

Subcutaneous: epinephrine 1:1000, 0.2 to 0.5 ml (children, 0.01 ml/kg, up to 0.5 ml)
Epinephrine suspension: 0.2 ml (0.005 ml/kg in children, up to 0.2 ml)
Inhalation: epinephrine 1% or racemic epinephrine 2.25%, 0.5 ml in 4 ml saline
Intravenous: epinephrine 1:10,000 solution, 1.0 ml every 2 to 3 minutes (children, 0.02 ml/kg)

Onset of action is within minutes with subcutaneous or inhaled epinephrine. The duration of action of subcutaneous epinephrine 1:1000 and inhaled epinephrine is 2 to 3 hours. Epinephrine suspension will be active for 4 to 6 hours.

Limits

Determined by development of toxicity or clinical improvement

Repeat Dosing

Subcutaneous aqueous epinephrine: may repeat initial dose in 30 to 60 minutes if toxicity not present. Thereafter, repeat doses given every 3 to 4 hours.
Subcutaneous epinephrine suspension: every 6 hours
Inhalation epinephrine: repeat in 30 minutes if toxicity absent; thereafter every 2 to 4 hours

Toxicity

Drug interactions

Adrenergic blockers, haloperidol, labetalol, loxapine, phenothiazines, prazosin, thioxanthenes, vasodilators—may cause decreased blood pressure and tachycardia
Anesthetics—may increase arrhythmias
Antidiabetics—may increase serum glucose
Beta-adrenergic blockers—may increase blood pressure and decrease heart rate
Digitalis glycosides—may increase arrhythmias
Ergot alkaloids—May increase vasoconstriction
Guanethidine—may increase blood pressure
Maprotiline, nomifensine—may increase arrhythmias, blood pressure, and heart rate
Sympathomimetics, xanthines—may increase toxic side effects

Specific Adverse Effects

Anxiety, headaches, fear, and palpitations are most common. More worrisome side effects are chest pain, hypertension, arrhythmias, nausea, vomiting, seizures, pounding heartbeat, and severe anxiety.

Treatment of Toxicity

Reduction in dosage or discontinuation of drug is the treatment. Pressor effects may be treated with vasodilators, but prolonged hypotension may result. Arrhythmias may be treated with beta-adrenergic blockers, but caution should be used because hypertension may occur.

Glucagon

Pharmacology

Glucagon is a hormone manufactured in pancreatic islet cells. It binds to specific cell-surface receptors in target organs and stimulates adenylate cyclase to increase levels of intracellular cyclic adenosine monophosphate. Other effects include relaxation of smooth muscle in the stomach and bowel and stimulation of gluconeogenesis. It has positive inotropic and chronotropic effects on the heart independent of the beta-adrenergic receptors. Glucagon appears to be less arrhythmogenic than catecholamines. Its half-life is 3 to 6 minutes.

Indications

Acute hypoglycemic reactions in order to raise blood glucose concentrations

Diagnostic aid in certain gastrointestinal radiographic procedures

Effective inotropic and chronotropic agent, particularly in cases of beta-blocker overdose or calcium-blocker overdose

Cautions

Renal failure—no alterations in the dosage are required in patients with renal failure.

Hepatic failure—no alterations in the dosage are required in patients with hepatic failure. In advanced hepatic failure, gluconeogenesis may be impaired and the hyperglycemic response to glucagon may be less marked.

Cardiac failure—no alterations in the dosage are required in patients with cardiac failure. However, patients with advanced cardiac failure who continue to be stimulated by catecholamines may exhibit resistance to the inotropic action of glucagon.

Use in pregnancy—Category B. There are no known adverse effects of glucagon to the fetus. However, because data in pregnant humans are lacking, glucagon should be used during pregnancy only if the risks are outweighed by the potential benefits.

Use in childhood—may be used

Onset and Duration of Action

Dosage

The dosage of glucagon is 0.5 to 2 mg subcutaneously, intramuscularly, or intravenously. It is supplied as a lyophilized powder and must be reconstituted for use. Glucagon has been administered in experimental settings to cardiac patients for its inotropic effect in the form of a continuous infusion at dosages ranging from 0.5 to 16 mg/hour with few side effects.

Limits

Limits to the use of glucagon have not been established. It should not be administered, however, in a concentration greater than 1 mg/ml.

Repeat Dosing

Because of its short half-life and low toxicity, glucagon may be repeated as often as necessary. Usually, it is recommended every 10 to 25 minutes.

Toxicity

Drug Interactions

No significant drug interactions are known.

Specific Adverse Effects

Glucagon has very little toxicity. In rats, the LD_{50} was determined to be 300 mg/kg. In experimental settings where high doses of glucagon were administered by continuous infusion, nausea, vomiting, and hypokalemia were noted.

Treatment of Toxicity

There have been no reported cases of glucagon overdose. Hypokalemia occurring with glucagon infusion may be treated with supplemental potassium.

Isoproterenol (Isuprel)

See Chapter 11, Antiarrhythmics.

Levarterenol (Levophed)

Pharmacology

Levarterenol (norepinephrine) is a potent agonist of alpha and $beta_1$ receptors with little $beta_2$-receptor stimulation in comparison with epinephrine. It produces marked elevations in both systolic and diastolic blood pressure as a result of an increase in systemic vascular resistance. In hypotensive individuals, cardiac output is increased, but as blood pressure rises, reflex bradycardia predominates and stroke volume and cardiac output are usually reduced. $Beta_1$-mediated coronary dilation results in increased coronary blood flow. Splanchnic and hepatic blood flow and, at high doses, renal blood flow are reduced.

Indications

Levarterenol is indicated in the treatment of hypotensive or shock states, especially those in which elevating systemic vascular resistance would be of benefit, for example, in septic, neurogenic, or anaphylactic shock.

Cautions

Renal failure—adjustments in dosage are not necessary in renal failure *per se.* However, raising renal vascular resistance with levarterenol may itself cause a deterioration in renal function.

Cardiac failure—adjustments in dosage are not necessary in cardiac failure. Although increasing systemic and diastolic arterial pressures and increasing coronary blood flow may improve the failing heart if hypotension is present, cardiac work may also be increased if blood pressure elevations are too great, leading to greater myocardial oxygen consumption.

Hepatic failure—adjustments in dosage are not necessary in hepatic failure.

Use in pregnancy—Category C. Data on the safety of levarterenol to the human fetus are lacking. Therefore, it should be used during pregnancy only if the risks are outweighed by the potential benefits of its use.

Use in childhood—may be used

Occlusive vascular disease—individuals with occlusive vascular diseases such as Raynaud's disease, Buerger's disease, atherosclerosis, angina, and diabetic arteritis should receive levarterenol with caution because they may be more sensitive to the effects of alpha-adrenergic stimulation.

Onset and Duration of Action

Dosage

Levarterenol is usually given as a continuous intravenous infusion, beginning at a rate of 2.0 to 4.0 μg/min and titrated to the desired response. A test dose is recommended before beginning the infusion. Some individuals with coronary spasm may be hypersensitive to alpha-receptor stimulation and will experience angina at small doses. The onset of action is rapid (1 to 2 minutes), as is the termination of effect once the drug is stopped.

Limits

Administration of levarterenol is limited by the signs of toxicity or adverse reactions.

Repeat Dosing

Levarterenol is given as a continuous infusion.

Toxicity

Drug Interactions

Levarterenol used in combination with other sympathomimetic agents or vasopressors may have an additive effect. It should also be used with extreme caution in combination with MAO inhibitors because marked hypertension may occur.

Specific Adverse Reactions

Severe hypertension, reflex bradycardia, restlessness, anxiety, angina, and ventricular dysrhythmias may occur as with other sympathomimetic agents. If levarterenol is accidentally extravasated during intravenous infusion, skin necrosis and sloughing may occur. Also, prolonged use in shock states may cause tissue injury from hypoperfusion secondary to vasoconstriction. Ischemic digits and renal failure may occur.

Treatment of Toxicity

Most adverse consequences of levarterenol administration will abate with reduction in dosage or discontinuation of the drug. Extravasation must be treated promptly with the local infiltration of an alpha-receptor blocking agent. Phentolamine (5 to 10 mg in 10 to 15 ml of 0.9% saline) should be infiltrated in the area as soon as possible. To minimize the occurrence of extravasation-induced skin necrosis, levarterenol should always be administered into a large vein.

Metaraminol (Aramine)

Pharmacology

Distribution and elimination of metaraminol are not completely known. Following intravenous injection, it has a rapid onset of action (1 to 2 minutes), and the effects persist for 20 to 90 minutes. It stimulates alpha and beta$_1$ receptors, similarly to levarterenol, but is less potent and is longer acting. It causes an increase in systemic vascular resistance, which results in a rise in both systolic and diastolic pressure, usually with a reflex bradycardia. If the reflex mechanism is blocked by atropine, or if the drug is used in hypotensive states, there is also a marked increase in cardiac output through a direct inotropic effect. However, in normal individuals the cardiac output is unchanged or slightly decreased. Renal, central nervous system, splanchnic, and limb blood flows are reduced, but coronary blood flow is increased.

Indications

Metaraminol is indicated in conditions of shock associated with low systemic vascular resistance, such as neurogenic or spinal shock or anaphylaxis, and as an adjunct in the treatment of septic shock. In most cases of hypovolemic or cardiogenic shock, systemic vascular resistance is already high and further increases are unnecessary.

Metaraminol is also used in the treatment of supraventricular tachycardia. The reflex bradycardia that attends its administration may often cause conversion.

Cautions

Renal failure—no alterations in dosage are required in the presence of renal failure. However, because renal blood flow is diminished with the administration of metaraminol, care must be taken with its use in the presence of already diminished renal function, as complete renal shutdown may occur.

Cardiac failure—no alterations in dosage are necessary with cardiac failure.

Hepatic failure—there is one report of a death with metaraminol from ventricular arrhythmia in a patient with cirrhosis. It should be used with caution in patients with cirrhosis.

Use in pregnancy—insufficient data exist to recommend it as safe for use during pregnancy. It should therefore be used only if the risks are outweighed by the potential benefits to its use.

Use in childhood—safety and effectiveness not established

Occlusive vascular disease—individuals with occlusive vascular diseases such as Raynaud's disease, Buerger's disease, atherosclerosis, angina, or diabetic arteritis should receive metaraminol with caution as they may be more sensitive to the effects of alpha-receptor stimulation.

Onset and Duration of Action

Dosage

Given subcutaneously or intramuscularly, the dose is 2 to 10 mg. The onset of action is 5 to 20 minutes, and the duration is 20 to 90 minutes.

Metaraminol is given as an intravenous infusion by mixing 15 to 100 mg in 500 ml saline or 5% dextrose in water, starting at 30 ml/hour and titrating to the desired blood pressure response.

Limits

The dosage is limited only by signs of toxicity.

Repeat Dosing

Metaraminol is usually given as a continuous intravenous infusion. Repeat dosing should be guided by blood pressure response.

Toxicity

Drug Interactions

Metaraminol should be used with caution in patients taking MAO inhibitors because its effects may be more accentuated. The concomitant use of other sympathomimentic agents or vasopressors may have an additive effect.

Specific Adverse Effects

As with levarterenol, severe hypertension, reflex bradycardia, restlessness, anxiety, angina, and ventricular dysrhythmias may occur. If metaraminol is accidentally extravasated during intravenous infusion, skin necrosis and sloughing may occur. Also, prolonged use in shock states may cause tissue injury from hypoperfusion secondary to vasoconstriction. Ischemic digits and renal failure may occur.

Treatment of Toxicity

Most adverse consequences of metaraminol administration will abate with reduction in dosage or discontinuation of the drug. To minimize the occurrence of extravasation-induced skin necrosis, metaraminol should always be administered into a large vein.

Methoxamine (Vasoxyl)

Pharmacology

Methoxamine is a relatively pure alpha-receptor agonist. It produces an increase in systemic vascular resistance, which results in a rise in both systolic and diastolic blood pressure, usually attended by a reflex bradycardia that is blocked by atropine. There is no inotropic or chronotropic effect. Renal, central nervous system, splanchnic, and limb blood flows are reduced, and coronary blood flow is usually unchanged.

Indications

Acute hypotensive states characterized by reduced systemic vascular resistance, such as neurogenic and spinal shock

Treatment or prevention of hypotension associated with spinal anesthesia

Cautions

Renal failure—because methoxamine is administered in a dosage that is titrated to the desired clinical effect, no alterations in dosage are required in the presence of renal failure. As with all vasopressors, however, because renal blood flow is reduced with its use, care must be taken in giving it to individuals with renal insufficiency as renal shutdown may occur.

Cardiac failure—no alteration in dosage is necessary in the presence of cardiac failure. As with all vasopressors, it should be used with caution in individuals who have angina because they may experience myocardial ischemia.

Hepatic failure—no alteration in dosage is necessary in the presence of hepatic failure.

Use in pregnancy—insufficient data exist to recommend it as safe for use during pregnancy. It may reduce blood flow to the fetus and cause fetal bradycardia. It should therefore be used only if the risks are outweighed by the potential benefits to its use.

Use in childhood—safety and effectiveness not established

Occlusive vascular disease—individuals with occlusive vascular diseases, such as Raynaud's disease, Buerger's disease, atherosclerosis, angina, or diabetic arteritis, should receive methoxamine with caution, as they may be more sensitive to the effects of alpha stimulation.

Onset and Duration of Action

Dosage

The intramuscular dose is 10 to 15 mg given shortly before or simultaneously with the administration of spinal anesthesia. The peak effect occurs in 15 to 20 minutes, and the duration of action is 90 minutes. Intravenously, it may be given as a 3- to 5-mg bolus or, for supraventricular tachycardia, 10 mg over 3 to 5 minutes. With intravenous administration, the onset of action is 0.5 to 2 minutes and the duration of action is 10 to 15 minutes.

Limits

The use of the drug is limited to the above dosage guidelines and by signs of toxicity such as markedly elevated blood pressure.

Repeat Dosing

Doses may be repeated as often as necessary depending on the desired blood pressure response.

Toxicity

Drug Interactions

The effects of methoxamine may be potentiated by MAO inhibitors, tricyclic antidepressants, vasopressin, ergot alkaloids, ergonovine, or methylergonovine. Concomitant use of the drug with other sympathomimetic agents may have an additive effect.

Specific Adverse Effects

Adverse effects are excessive blood pressure elevations, nausea, vomiting, headache, anxiety, and ventricular ectopic beats. As with other vasopressor agents, angina, vaso-occlusive phenomena, and skin necrosis and sloughing (if extravasated) are a risk with its use.

Treatment of Toxicity

Excessive elevation in blood pressure may be treated with an alpha-receptor blocking agent (e.g., phentolamine) or vasodilator (e.g., nitroprusside). Excessive reflex bradycardia may be treated with atropine.

Nitroglycerin (Tridil, Nitro-Bid IV, Nitrostat)

Pharmacology

Nitroglycerin is the organic nitrate 1,2,3-propranetriol trinitrate. It is a directly acting smooth muscle relaxant. Its action is independent of innervation but can be antagonized by other drugs that cause smooth muscle contraction, such as norepinephrine or acetylcholine. Thus, the net effect of nitroglycerin depends on the concentration of these antagonist compounds.

Nitroglycerin dilates both veins and arteries, although the venous effects predominate at lower doses. The resultant effects on the determinants of cardiac performance include a reduction in preload (central venous pressure and pulmonary wedge pressure) and afterload. The output of a failing heart usually increases with nitroglycerin therapy, whereas there is usually little change in the output of a normal heart. Nitroglycerin causes some decrease in blood pressure, but unless this is excessive, coronary perfusion pressure is maintained and the myocardial oxygen supply–demand balance is improved because of a concomitant reduction in oxygen demand and nitroglycerin-induced coronary vasodilation.

Nitroglycerin causes a fall in portal venous pressure due to a direct vasodilating effect in these vessels.

Nitroglycerin has a half-life of 1 to 4 minutes due to rapid metabolism. The effects of a given dose are seen almost immediately and disappear within minutes of stopping the infusion.

Indications

Myocardial ischemia
Congestive heart failure
Bleeding esophageal varices
Perioperative hypertension
Hypotensive anesthesia

Contraindications

Hypovolemia
Cardiac tamponade
Increased intracranial pressure
Hypersensitivity to nitrates

Cautions

Renal failure—may be used
Hepatic failure—use cautiously because the liver is the principal organ for nitroglycerin metabolism.
Cardiac failure—may be used
Use in pregnancy—Category C; no data, so use only if clearly indicated.
Use in childhood—safety in children not established

Nitroglycerin is readily, but variably, absorbed by plastics. It should only be mixed and stored in glass bottles and given through the administration set supplied with the drug. Nitroglycerin administration should be controlled by a volumetric infusion pump.

Onset and Duration of Action

Dosage

The same dosing regimen can be used for all clinical settings. A continuous intravenous infusion is started at 5 μg/min and rapidly titrated by increments of 10 μg/min every 3 to 5 minutes, until the desired end-point is reached or hypotension occurs. The dose may be further titrated to the maximum of 400 μg/min if there is clinical evidence of coronary ischemia or ongoing congestive heart failure. When nitroglycerin is used as adjunctive therapy in the treatment of bleeding esophageal varices, the targeted end-point should be an infusion rate of 200 μg/min, unless hypotension occurs at a lower dose.

Limits

There is great variation in responsiveness to nitroglycerin so the dose must be titrated based on objective physiologic measurements.

Repeat Dosing

Nitroglycerin should be given as a continuous intravenous infusion in acute situations.

Toxicity

Drug Interactions

Additive hypotension with other vasodilators, calcium blockers, and ethanol
Tricyclic antidepressants decrease nitroglycerin effect.
Nitroglycerin decreases heparin effect with a potential for a marked increase in prothrombin time with discontinuation of the nitroglycerin.

Specific Adverse Reactions

Hypotension with the potential for cerebral, cardiac, renal, and hepatic hypoperfusion is the most serious side effect of nitroglycerin.

Headache is common with nitroglycerin administration. Rash, nausea, vomiting, flushing, and restlessness are uncommon side effects.

The vehicle for intravenous nitroglycerin contains ethanol. Patients receiving high doses of intravenous nitroglycerin for prolonged periods may become intoxicated. This should be considered when it is used in patients with alcoholic liver disease.

Treatment of Toxicity

Reduce or discontinue drip
Trendelenburg position
Volume infusion
Vasopressor if no response to above measures

Nitroprusside (Nipride)

See Chapter 12, Antihypertensives.

Phenylephrine (Neo-Synephrine)

Pharmacology

The distribution and elimination of phenylephrine are not completely known. Following intravenous injection, an effect is observed within 1 minute and persists for 15 to 20 minutes. It is metabolized primarily in the liver and intestine by MAO.

Actions

Phenylephrine is a potent alpha-receptor agonist with almost no effect on the beta receptor. It produces an increase in systemic vascular resistance, which results in a rise in systolic and diastolic blood pressure. Cardiac output remains unchanged or is slightly reduced. A reflex bradycardia occurs, which is blocked by atropine. Vasoconstriction occurs in most vascular beds, and renal, limb, and splanchnic blood flows are reduced, although coronary blood flow is increased. Pulmonary vascular resistance increases, and pulmonary artery pressure is raised.

Indications

Phenylephrine is indicated in hypotensive states associated with reduced systemic vascular resistance, including spinal and neurogenic shock, and during induction of anesthesia. It may be useful as an adjunct in the treatment of shock due to sepsis and anaphylaxis. It has also been used to treat supraventricular tachycardia. When administered, reflex bradycardia may cause the rhythm to convert.

Cautions

Renal failure—because phenylephrine is administered in a dosage that is titrated to the desired clinical effect, no alterations in dosage are required in the presence of renal failure. As with all vasopressors, however, because renal blood flow is reduced with its use, care must be taken in giving it to individuals with renal insufficiency because renal shutdown may occur.

Cardiac failure—no alteration in dosage is necessary in the presence of cardiac failure. As with all vasopressors, it should be used with caution in individuals who have angina because they may experience myocardial ischemia.

Hepatic failure—no alteration in dosage is necessary in the presence of hepatic failure.

Use in pregnancy—Category C. Insufficient data exist to recommend it as safe for use during pregnancy. It may reduce blood flow to the fetus and cause fetal bradycardia. It should therefore be used only if the risks are outweighed by the potential benefits to its use.

Use in childhood—may be used intramuscularly or subcutaneously at a dose of 0.5 to 1 mg per 25 lb.

Occlusive vascular disease—individuals with occlusive vascular diseases, such as Raynaud's disease, Buerger's disease, atherosclerosis, angina, or diabetic arteritis, should receive phenylephrine with caution because they may be more sensitive to the effects of alpha stimulation.

Onset and Duration of Action

Dosage

Subcutaneously or intramuscularly, 1 to 10 mg (usual dose, 2 to 5 mg) may be given. The duration of action is 1 to 2 hours. It may also be given as an intravenous bolus injection at a dosage of 0.5 mg. This will elevate the blood pressure for about 15 minutes. A continuous intravenous infusion may be given by mixing 10 mg in 500 ml of saline or 5% dextrose in water starting at 40 μg/min and titrating to the desired effect. The usual dose range is 40 to 180 μg/min. The onset of action will be within minutes.

Limits

The use of the drug is limited by the clinical response and by signs of toxicity.

Repeat Dosing

Intravenous injections should not be repeated more often than every 15 minutes.

Toxicity

Drug Interactions

Phenylephrine should be used with extreme caution in individuals taking MAO inhibitors, tricyclic antidepressants, or other vasopressors because they may markedly potentiate its action.

Specific Adverse Effects

Extreme hypertension, reflex bradycardia, headache, agitation, and rarely arrhythmias may occur. As with other vasopressor agents, angina, vaso-occlusive phenomena, and skin necrosis and sloughing (if extravasated) are a risk with its use.

Treatment of Toxicity

Excessive elevation in blood pressure may be treated with an alpha-receptor blocking agent (e.g., phentolamine) or vasodilator (e.g., nitroprusside). Excessive reflex bradycardia may be treated with atropine.

Vasopressin (Pitressin)

Pharmacology

Vasopressin is an octapeptide hormone produced by the posterior pituitary gland. It causes contraction of all elements of the vascular bed and also of the bowel by a direct stimulation of the smooth muscle constrictors. Vasopressin produces an antidiuretic effect by stimulating increased reabsorption of water by the renal tubules.

The plasma half-life of vasopressin is 10 to 20 minutes due to its rapid metabolism in the liver and kidneys. Thus, vasopressor activity ceases shortly after discontinuation of an intravenous infusion. When given by the subcutaneous or intramuscular route to treat diabetes insipidus, the antidiuretic effect lasts from 2 to 8 hours.

Indications

Bleeding esophageal varices
Diabetes insipidus

Cautions

Renal failure—use with caution because vasopressin may aggravate fluid retention.

Hepatic failure—may be used without dosage adjustment

Cardiac failure—use with great caution because vasopressin causes both fluid retention and coronary artery constriction with the potential of myocardial ischemia.

Use in pregnancy—Category C. No data exist concerning vasopressin's effects on the fetus. Since it is a naturally occurring hormone and since hemorrhagic shock is detrimental to the fetus, its use in a pregnant patient with bleeding esophageal varices would seem warranted.

Use in childhood—may be used

Onset and Duration of Action

Dosage

For bleeding esophageal varices, vasopressin is given as a continuous intravenous infusion, starting at a rate of 0.4 unit/min. If bleeding persists, the rate may be increased to 1.0 unit/min.

Limits

1.0 unit/min
Toxicity, especially signs of myocardial ischemia

Repeat Dosing

Vasopressin is given as a continuous infusion.

Toxicity

Drug Interactions

Vasopressin's antidiuretic effect is increased by carbamazepine, chlorpropamide, clofibrate, fluorocortisone, and tricyclic antidepressants.

Vasopressin's antidiuretic action is inhibited by demeclocycline, norepinephrine, lithium, heparin, and ethanol.

Vasopressin's vasoconstricting effect is enhanced by ganglionic blocking drugs.

Specific Adverse Reactions

Cardiac: Vasopressin increases afterload, directly decreases cardiac contractility, decreases coronary blood flow, and causes water retention. All of these effects are potentially detrimental to cardiac performance. Vasopressin may induce congestive heart failure, myocardial infarction, and dangerous dysrhythmias and should be used with great care in patients with known cardiac disease.

A reflex bradycardia is common with vasopressin infusion.

Anaphylaxis has occurred after vasopressin injection.

Gastrointestinal: vasopressin stimulates the smooth muscle of the bowel, producing cramps, vomiting, and diarrhea. Mesenteric ischemia and bowel infarction may result from its vasoconstricting action.

Renal: vasopressin causes increased tubular resorption of water with the potential for congestive heart failure or water intoxication.

Vasopressin causes skin necrosis if extravasation occurs; administer by central line.

Treatment of Toxicity

Coadminister nitroglycerin.
Discontinue infusion.
Antiarrhythmics

REFERENCES

Abraham E, Shoemaker WC, Bland RD, Cobo JC: Sequential cardiorespiratory patterns in septic shock. Crit Care Med 11:799, 1983.

Austen WG, Sokol DM, DeSanctis RW, et al: Surgical treatment of papillary muscle rupture complicating myocardial infarction. N Engl J Med 278:1137–1141, 1968.

Barach EM, Nowak RM, Lee TG, Tomlanovich MC: Epinephrine for treatment of anaphylactic shock. JAMA 251:2118–2122, 1984.

Benotti J, Grossman W, Braunwald E, et al: Hemodynamic assessment of amrinone: A new inotropic agent. N Engl J Med 299:1373–1377, 1978.

Billhardt RA, Stuart RW: Cardiogenic and hypovolemic shock. Med Clin North Am 4:853–876, 1986.

Bone RC, Fisher CJ, Clemmer TP, et al: A controlled trial of high-dose methylprednisolone in the treatment of severe sepsis and septic shock. N Engl J Med 317:653–658, 1987.

Bouzoukis JK: Shock. Primary Care 13:193–205, 1986.

Boxer M, Greenberger PA, Patterson R: Clinical summary and course of idiopathic anaphylaxis in 73 patients. Arch Intern Med 147:269–272, 1987.

Cohn JA: Nitrates for congestive heart failure. Am J Cardiol 56:19A–23A, 1985.

Cohn JN, Guiha NH, Broder MI, et al: Right ventricular infarction: Clinical and hemodynamic features. Am J Cardiol 33:209–214, 1974.

De La Cal MA, Miravelles E, Pascual T, et al: Dose-related hemodynamic and renal effects of dopamine in septic shock. Crit Care Med 12:22–25, 1984.

Dolan EJ, Tator CH: The treatment of hypotension due to acute experimental spinal cord compression injury. Surg Neurol 13:380–384, 1980.

Farah AE: Glucagon and the circulation. Pharmacol Rev 35:181–217, 1983.

Forrester JS, Diamond G, Chatterjee K, et al: Medical therapy of acute myocardial infarction by application of hemodynamic subsets: Parts I and II. N Engl J Med 295:1363–1365, 1404–1413, 1976.

Franciosa JA: Current indications for vasodilator therapy for left ventricular failure. Compr Ther 11:39–46, 1985.

Francis GS, Sharma B, Hodges M: Comparative hemodynamic effects of dopamine and dobutamine in patients with acute cardiogenic circulatory collapse. Am Heart J 103:995–1000, 1982.

Friedman WF, George BL: Treatment of congestive heart failure by altering loading conditions of the heart. J Pediatr 5:697–706, 1985.

Gascho JA, Martins JB, Marrus ML, et al: Effects of volume expansion and vasodilators in acute pericardial tamponade. Am J Physiol 240:H49–52, 1981.

Genton R, Jaffe AS: Management of congestive heart failure in patients with acute myocardial infarction. JAMA 256:2556–2560, 1986.

Goldberger M, Tabak SW, Shah PK: Clinical experience with intra-aortic balloon counterpulsation in 112 consecutive patients. Am Heart J 111:497–502, 1986.

Goodman LS, Gilman A: The Pharmacological Basis of Therapeutics, 7th ed. New York, Macmillan, 1985.

Gunnar RM, Loeb HS: Shock in acute myocardial infarction: Evolution of physiologic therapy. J Am Coll Cardiol 1:154–163, 1983.

Gunnar RM, Loeb HS, Pietras RJ, et al: Ineffectiveness of isoproterenol in the treatment of shock due to acute myocardial infarction. JAMA 202:1124–1128, 1967.

Gunnar RM, Loeb HS, Winslow EJ, et al: Hemodynamic measurements in bacteremia and septic shock in man. J Infect Dis 128:295–298, 1973.

Guntheroth WG, Jacky JP, Kawabori I, et al: Left ventricular performance in enotoxin shock in dogs. Am J Physiol 242:H172–176, 1982.

Hall-Boyer K, Zaloga GP, Chernow B: Glucagon: Hormone or therapeutic agent? Crit Care Med 12:584–589, 1984.

Herbert P, Tinker J: Inotropic drugs in acute circulatory failure. Intensive Care Med 6:101–111, 1980.

Hess ML, Hastillo A, Greenfield LJ: Spectrum of cardiovascular function during gram-negative sepsis. Prog Cardiovasc Dis 23:279–298, 1981.

Hill NS, Antiman EM, Green LH, Alpert JS: Intravenous nitroglycerin. Chest 179:69, 1981.

Houston MC, Thompson WL, Robertson D: Shock: Diagnosis and management. Arch Intern Med 144:1433–1439, 1984.

Illingworth RN: Glucagon for beta-blocker poisoning. Practitioner 223:683–685, 1979.

Iqbal MZ, Liebson PR: Counterpulsation and dobutamine: Their use in treatment of shock due to right ventricular infarction. Arch Intern Med 141:247–249, 1981.

Karakusis PH: Considerations in the therapy of septic shock. Med Clin North Am 70:933–944, 1986.

Kosinski EJ, Maldinzak GS: Glucagon and isoproterenol in reversing propranolol toxicity. Arch Intern Med 132:840–843, 1973.

Krausz MM, Perel A, Eimerl D, Cotev S: Cardiopulmonary effects of volume loading in patients in septic shock. Ann Surg 10:429–434, 1976.

Kubo SH, Fox SC, Prida XE, Cody RJ: Combined hemodynamic effects of nifedipine and nitroglycerin in congestive heart failure. Am Heart J 110:1032–1034, 1985.

Laks H, Rosenkranz E, Buckberg G: Surgical treatment of cardiogenic shock after myocardial infarction. Circulation 74 (Suppl III):11–16, 1986.

Lehr CV, Heban PT, Huss P, et al: Comparative systemic and regional hemodynamic effects of dopamine and dobutamine in patients with cardiomyopathic heart failure. Circulation 58:466–475, 1978.

Lorell B, Leinbach RC, Pohost GM, et al: Right ventricular infarction: Clinical diagnosis and differentiation from cardiac tamponade and pericardial constriction. Am J Cardiol 43:465–471, 1979.

Lucchesi BR: Cardiac actions of glucagon. Circ Res 22:777–787, 1968.

Luce JM: Pathogenesis and management of septic shock. Chest 91:883–888, 1987.

Mancini D, Thierry L, Sonnenblick E: Intravenous use of amrinone for the treatment of the failing heart. Am J Cardiol 56:8B–15B, 1985.

Moss J, Fahmy NR, Sunder N, et al: Hormonal and hemodynamic profile of an anaphylactic reaction in man. Circulation 63:210–213, 1981.

Oertel T, Loehr MM: Bee-sting anaphylaxis: The use of medical antishock trousers. Ann Emerg Med 13:459, 1984.

Packer M, Lee WH, Yushak M, Medina N: Comparison of captopril and enalapril in patients with severe chronic heart failure. N Engl J Med 315:847–853, 1986.

Packer M, Medina N, Yshak M: Hemodynamic and clinical limitations of long-term inotropic therapy with amrinone on patients with severe chronic heart failure. Circulation 70:1038–1047, 1984.

Packman MI, Rackow EL: Optimum left heart filling pressure during fluid resuscitation of patients with hypovolemic and septic shock. Crit Care Med 11:165–169, 1983.

Parker MM, Parillo JE: Septic shock: Hemodynamics and pathogenesis. JAMA 250:3324–3327, 1983.

Perkin RM, Anas NG: Mechanisms and management of anaphylactic shock not responding to traditional therapy. Ann Allergy 54:202–208, 1985.

Regnier B, Safran D, Carlet J, Teisseire B: Comparative hemodynamic effects of dopamine and dobutamine in septic shock. Intensive Care Med 5:115–120, 1979.

Richard C, Ricone JL, Rimailho A, et al: Combined hemodynamic effects of dopamine and dobutamine in cardiogenic shock. Circulation 67:620–626, 1983.

Salzberg M., Gallagher E.: Propranolol overdose. Ann Emerg Med 9:26–27, 1980.

Scholtz H: Inotropic drugs in the treatment of heart failure. Hosp Pract 19:57–71, 1984.

Shatney CH: Pathophysiology and treatment of circulatory shock. In Zschoche DA: Comprehensive Review of Critical Care. St Louis, CV Mosby, 1986.

Shoemaker WC: Circulatory mechanisms of shock and their mediators. Crit Care Med 15:787–794, 1987.

Shoemaker WC: Pathophysiology and therapy of shock syndromes. In Shoemaker WC, Thompson WL, Holbrook PR (eds): Textbook of Critical Care. Philadelphia, WB Saunders, 1984.

Sirinek KR, Levine BA: High dose vasopressin for acute variceal hemorrhage: Clinical advantages without adverse effects. Arch Surg 123:876–80, 1988.

Soderlund C: Vasopressin and glypressin in upper gastrointestinal bleeding. Scand J Gastroenterol (Suppl) 137:50–55, 1987.

Sonnenblick EH, Frishman WH, LeJemtel TH: Dobutamine: A new synthetic cardioactive sympathetic amine. N Engl J Med 300:17–22, 1979.

Tsai YT, Lay CS, Lai KH, et al: Controlled trial of vasopressin plus nitroglycerin vs vasopressin alone in the treatment of bleeding esophageal varices. Hepatology 6:406–409, 1986.

Vincent JL, Linden P, Domb M, et al: Dopamine compared with dobutamine in experimental septic shock. Anesth Analg 66:565–571, 1987.

Wallace CM, Tator CH: Successful improvement of blood pressure, cardiac output, and spinal cord blood flow after experimental spinal cord injury. Neurosurgery 20:710–715, 1987.

Wasserman, SI.: The heart in anaphylaxis. J Allergy Clin Immunol 77:663–666, 1986.

Weinstein RS: Recognition and management of poisoning with beta-adrenergic blocking agents. Ann Emerg Med 13:1123–1131, 1984.

Weinstein RS, Cole S, Knaster HB, Dahlbert T: Beta blocker overdose with propranolol and atenolol. Ann Emerg Med 14:161–163, 1985.

Westaby D, Gimson A, Hayes PC, Williams R: Hemodynamic response to intravenous vasopressin and nitroglycerin in portal hypertension. Gut 29:372–377, 1988.

Zaloga GP, Delacey W, Holmboe E, Chernow B: Glucagon reversal of hypotension in a case of anaphylactoid shock. Ann Intern Med 105:65–66, 1986.

Zimmerman JJ, Dietrich KA: Current perspective on septic shock. *Pediatr Clin North Am* 34:131–163, 1987.

CHAPTER 14

Emetics and Antiemetics

CLIFTON A. SHEETS, M.D.

INTRODUCTION

Nausea is a universally experienced dysphoric sensation that defies exact definition. It is believed to be mediated by the same neurogenic pathways as vomiting and is frequently accompanied by autonomic symptoms such as tachycardia and perspiration. Nausea is typically a precursor to vomiting; however, it may be absent if the cause of vomiting is increased intracranial pressure.

Vomiting is the vagally mediated forceful expulsion of gastric contents (and sometimes small bowel contents) through the mouth. Vomiting represents a complex coordinated sequence of events and is mediated by somatic rather than autonomic pathways. Vomiting begins with a deep inspiration followed by forceful downward contraction of the diaphragm. The soft palate simultaneously closes to protect the nasopharynx. A quick and forceful contraction of the abdominal muscles results in a rapid increase in intra-abdominal and intrathoracic pressure. Following the pressure gradient, gastric contents are expelled through the mouth. Segmental contractions of the small bowel cause reflux of proximal duodenal and jejunal contents into the stomach. Successful vomiting requires net positive pressures in both the abdomen and thorax.

Retching occurs when intra-abdominal pressures are positive but intrathoracic pressures remain negative. Regurgitation results from intraluminal pressure or gravitational differences and differs from true vomiting in that it does not involve forceful contraction of respiratory or abdominal muscles.

Sensory information mediating vomiting is processed in the medulla oblongata. This processing zone is referred to as the vomiting center (VC) and is the final common neuroanatomic pathway of the vomiting process. The VC is rich in histamine receptors and muscarinic cholinergic receptors. At least part of the antiemetic effect of antihistamines is the result of their activity at the level of the VC.

Sensory stimulation of the VC arrives through vagal, vestibular, corticobulbar, and chemoreceptor trigger zone (CTZ) afferent pathways. Stimulation of vagal (bowel distention, direct gastrointestinal irritants) and corticobulbar afferents (sight, smell, taste) result in increased activity in the VC.

The CTZ, located on the surface of the area postrema of the fourth ventricle and rich in dopamine receptors, is the site of action of many emetics and antiemetics. Ablation of the CTZ eliminates the emetic effect of many drugs, motion sickness, uremia, and radiation sickness. Antidopaminergic preparations such as the phenothiazines exert their antiemetic properties by inhibition of the CTZ.

Vestibular contributions to nausea and vomiting deserve special note. Motion sickness results from atypical vestibular stimulation. Rhythmic movements such as occur in a sea voyage cause abnormal motion of the endolymph in the semicircular canal. The ensuing noxious stimulation of the vestibular portion of the eighth cranial nerve results in activation of the VC. Vertigo from any cause will produce nausea and vomiting through similar pathways. The vestibular center, like the VC, is rich in muscarinic, cholinergic, and histamine receptors. Drugs used in the treatment of motion sickness and vertigo typically possess anticholinergic and antihistaminic properties.

CONDITIONS

Gastric Emptying

Diagnosis and Indications for Treatment

Currently, there are a few absolute indications for the use of emetic drugs. The sole remaining clinical arena for emetic use is in the management of acute poisoning and overdose. Emetic use in poisoning is often dependent on time of ingestion of the poison, dose and content of the ingestion, and toxicology of the poison. Despite these clinical variables, reasonable guidelines for emetic usage can be outlined that allow for flexibility and clinical judgment.

The induction of emesis is indicated when (1) a toxic ingestion is suspected; (2) the time since ingestion is reasonably short (generally less than 1 hour), and (3) no contraindications to use of emetics exist. Emesis induction is contraindicated (1) in corrosive, alkali, and some acid ingestions; (2) in the presence of altered mental status, airway control problems, or diminished gag reflexes; (3) following petroleum distillate ingestions; (4) in the presence of seizures; and (5) if the patient is less than 6 months of age.

When the need for emetic use is questionable, contact with a poison control center or other toxicologic source is recommended.

The algorithm in Figure 14–1 provides a decision tree for emetic management of the poisoned patient. (See box.)

Discussion

Syrup of ipecac is the only emetic in widespread use in the United States today. Copper sulfate, salt solutions, and apomorphine have been abandoned because of morbidity and mortality associated with their use.

Ipecac is highly effective in inducing emesis. In over 95% of patients, vomiting will occur within 30 minutes following a single dose. Repeat dosing, though rarely needed, increases the efficacy to nearly 100%. In drug recovery studies, the amount of drug removed with ipecac-induced emesis decreases rapidly as time after ingestion increases. Only about one-third of the total amount can be reliably recovered at 1 hour following ingestion. Studies comparing ipecac with lavage have generally demonstrated superior results with ipecac regardless of the time of administration. Lavage may be more beneficial when gastric emptying has been delayed (e.g., cyclic antidepressant overdose) or when concretions form in the stomach (e.g., aspirin overdose). Ipecac is routinely administered with water or other beverage. Administration of carbonated beverages has no clinical benefit over the use of water. Cold water and warm water are equally effective. Milk administration delays onset of vomiting. Administration of fluids before or after ipecac is equally effective.

DRUG TREATMENT: EMETICS

First-Line Agent

Syrup of Ipecac

Initial Dose	Age 6–12 months: 10 ml
	Age 1–5 years: 15 ml
	Age above 5 years: 30 ml
	Follow with 100–300 ml water.
Repeat Dose	Once if no vomiting after 30 minutes
End-Point	Vomiting

USE OF EMETICS

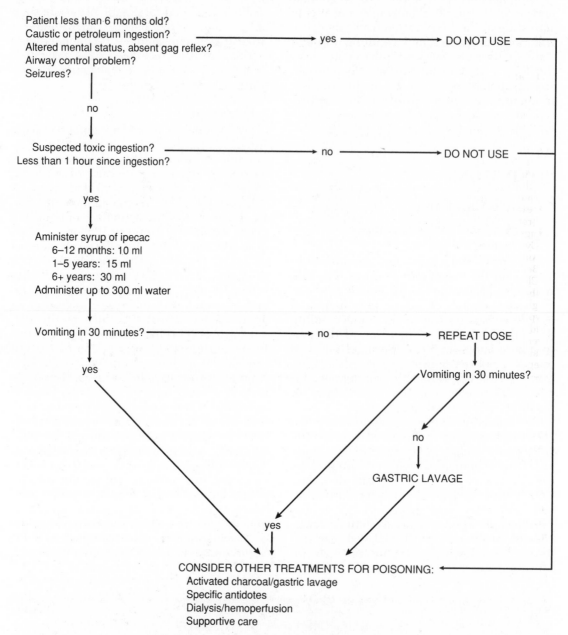

FIGURE 14–1. Treatment algorithm: the poisoned patient.

Vomiting

Diagnosis

The causes of nausea and vomiting are legion (Table 14–1). Nausea and vomiting are symptoms of disease and not disease processes themselves. The emergency evaluation of nausea and vomiting should always include an attempt to identify the underlying etiology and rule out life-threatening causes.

Acute vomiting is arbitrarily classified as vomiting of 48 hours' duration or less. Intractable vomiting is repeated vomiting over a prolonged time period (>48 hours) and often results in fluid and electrolyte imbalances. Anticipatory vomiting is common in cancer chemotherapy patients and occurs prior to the administration of the chemotherapeutic agent. Anticipatory vomiting results from corticobulbar influences on the VC and

TABLE 14–1. Causes of Vomiting

Anesthetics	**Miscellaneous Causes**
Halothane	Increased intracranial pressure
Cycloproprane	Radiation sickness
Medications	Pharyngeal stimulation
Opiates	Unpleasant sights, smells, tastes
Antibiotics	Glaucoma (acute)
Erythromycin	Erotic vomiting
Antineoplastics	**Psychogenic Causes**
Cisplatin	Bulimia/self-administered ipecac
Dacarbazine	Anorexia nervosa
Mustine	Malingering
Cyclophosphamide	**Gastrointestinal Disorders**
Mitomycin C	Peritonitis/appendicitis
Endocrine medications	Hepatitis
Bromocriptine	Pancreatitis
Cardiac drugs	Obstruction
Digoxin	Pseudo-obstruction
Levodopa	Decreased motility
Bretylium	Alcohol
Drugs decreasing gastrointestinal motility	Postsurgical
Cyclic antidepressants	Diabetic gastroparesis
Anticholinergics	Direct gastrointestinal irritants
Beta agonists	Enterotoxin
Clonidine	Alcohol
Metabolic Disorders	Copper sulfate
High fever	**Cardiac Causes**
Hypoglycemia	Acute myocardial infarction
Addisonian crisis	Congestive heart failure
Uremia	
Diabetic ketoacidosis	
Pregnancy/hyperemesis gravidarum	

can usually be managed with mild sedation. Vomiting as a form of erotic arousal has been reported and usually occurs in women.

Psychogenic vomiting is only diagnosed in cases with a prolonged history of vomiting (>6 months) when all organic causes of vomiting have been eliminated. It is commonly seen when there is a family history of vomiting, a childhood parental loss, or a sense of entrapment in a hostile relationship.

As a general rule, vomiting that is the result of viral gastroenteritis or psychogenic vomiting is closely related to meals. In contrast, vomiting from gastric outlet disorders or obstruction is typically delayed 2 to 3 hours following meals.

Acute nausea and vomiting are commonly related to toxins, drugs, infections, acute obstructions, or pain and may represent the largest category of patients seen emergently. Persistent vomiting is seen with pregnancy, increased intracranial pressure, gastric motility disorders, subacute mechanical obstructions (e.g., gastric cancer), and in psychogenic vomiting.

Pain preceding vomiting is a key historical finding that may indicate myocardial or intestinal ischemia, bowel obstruction, or biliary colic. Pain out of proportion to physical signs is suggestive of intestinal ischemia. Pain relieved by vomiting is typical in peptic ulcer disease.

The physical examination of the patient with vomiting should include a careful abdominal examination. In addition, a careful evaluation of cranial nerve function, vestibular function, and eye findings should be documented. Orthostatic vital signs should be tested routinely.

Laboratory adjuncts should be tailored to the patient's age and condition and to the suspected etiology of the vomiting. Serum electrolytes, measures of renal function, urinalysis, and hematologic testing may all prove helpful but will not be required in every patient. In women of childbearing age, pregnancy should be excluded as a potential cause of the vomiting.

Indications for Treatment

The treatment of nausea and vomiting centers on management of the underlying etiology. If the cause has a direct treatment, such as cessation of an emetic drug, then antiemetic therapy may not be indicated. When acute ischemic, obstructive, or other surgical causes of vomiting have been excluded, the physician may elect to use antiemetics for symptomatic relief.

The use of antiemetics requires clinical judgment and is determined on a case by case basis. Antiemetics are indicated when (1) continued symptomatic vomiting is likely, (2) continued vomiting is likely to cause harm to the patient, and (3) no contraindications to their use exist.

The likelihood of continued vomiting may be a difficult prognostication, even for experienced clinicians. The pattern of vomiting in the immediately preceding few hours may prove helpful in predicting continued vomiting.

Vomiting from acute bacterial or viral gastroenteritis, psychogenic causes, hyperemesis gravidarum, or increased intracranial pressure is likely to be intractable, whereas corticobulbar and toxic influences tend to be self-limited. Dehydration, electrolyte imbalance, concomitant illness, and mental status should all be considered when deciding to treat. Patients who are well hydrated and exhibiting clinical improvement with supportive measures need not be medicated.

Treatment is indicated if further episodes of vomiting might reasonably be expected to have deleterious effects on the patient's well-being, such as in intracranial hemorrhage, following ocular surgery, and in Mallory-Weiss tears of the distal esophagus. The routine use of antiemetics postoperatively should be discouraged, as only 3% of postoperative patients vomit.

Known hypersensitivity to the drug and idiosyncratic or severe dystonic reactions represent absolute contraindications to antiemetic use. Altered mental status and head injury are relative contraindications.

The use of antiemetics in pediatric patients and during pregnancy is controversial. Children are more susceptible to the extrapyramidal side effects of the centrally acting antiemetics. Antiemetic use in children can mask the signs and symptoms of Reye's syndrome or serious intracranial infections and may delay appropriate medical intervention. The liver metabolism of most antiemetics is altered in Reye's syndrome, which leads to increased active drug levels. Large doses of antiemetics with anticholinergic properties can induce hallucinations, seizures, and sudden death in children. Therefore, antiemetic use in the pediatric population should be reserved for those patients in whom fasting, rest, and intravenous fluid, electrolyte, and nutritional therapy have failed and in whom continued vomiting is likely to cause harm.

Antiemetics in pregnancy should also be limited to those patients in whom conservative treatment has failed. While the majority of women in the first trimester of pregnancy experience some degree of nausea and vomiting, only 2.5 per 1000 develop hyperemesis gravidarum. Hyperemesis gravidarum is a condition of protracted vomiting during pregnancy. Circulating pregnancy-induced hormones and psychogenic influences have been postulated as its causes. Fluid and electrolyte disturbances are common. Although very small, a risk of congenital malformations exists or is suspected for most antiemetics used in pregnancy. Intensive studies of most antiemetics used in pregnancy have failed to find malformation rates greater than those in the general population. Meclizine and cyclizine were restricted from use in pregnancy by the Food and Drug Administration in 1956. Further studies failed to support initial findings of adverse fetal outcome, and the ban was removed in 1979.

Antiemetic use in pregnancy must be weighed in light of the risks and benefits to the fetus and mother. Discussion with the mother of potential teratogenicity prior to drug administration and documentation of the conversation are recommended. (See boxes, Drug Treatment: Vomiting and Drug Treatment: Special Circumstances.)

Discussion

The antiemetics available in the United States today generally fall into one of two broad categories: antihistamines and dopamine antagonists.

Dopamine antagonists (metoclopramide, phenothiazines, haloperidol) are potent inhibitors of the CTZ and are favored in the management of vomiting due to cancer chemotherapy, radiation sickness, and toxins. Vomiting from diabetic and postvagotomy gastroparesis has also been successfully treated with dopamine antagonists.

Phenothiazines exert their antiemetic action primarily at the level of the CTZ. Promethazine has fewer antidopaminergic properties than other phenothiazines and is therefore usually classified as an antihistamine. As such, it is the only phenothiazine with usefulness in treating vertigo and motion sickness. As a group, the phenothiazines differ little in their general efficacy. They are

DRUG TREATMENT: VOMITING

First-Line Drugs

Promethazine

Initial Dose	12.5–25 mg IV
	25–50 mg IM or by rectum
Repeat Dose	Every 6 hours
End-Point	Cessation of vomiting

OR

Prochlorperazine

Initial Dose	2.5–10 mg IV
	5–10 mg IM
	25 mg by rectum
Repeat Dose	IV or IM q 4 hours
	By rectum q 12 hours
End-Point	Cessation of vomiting

Second-Line Drugs

Thiethylperazine

Initial Dose	10 mg IM or by rectum
Repeat Dose	q 8–12 hours
End-Point	Cessation of vomiting

OR

Trimethobenzamide

Initial Dose	200 mg IM or by rectum
Repeat Dose	q 6 hours
End-Point	Cessation of vomiting

Third-Line Drug

Chlorpromazine

Initial Dose	10–25 mg IV
	25 mg IM or PO (0.5 mg/kg for children)
	100 mg by rectum (1 mg/kg for children)
Repeat Dose	4–6 hours
End-Point	Cessation of vomiting

all highly protein bound and have large volumes of distribution and high lipid solubility. They are metabolized in the liver and have varying degrees of first-pass effect. Anticholinergic and extrapyramidal side effects are common with phenothiazines. Other common side effects include diminished effectiveness of oral anticoagulants, increased prolactin levels, lowered seizure threshold, and altered thermoregulatory patterns. Their use has also been associated with neuroleptic malignant syndrome.

Antihistamines of the H_1 type (hydroxyzine, dimenhydrinate, promethazine, cyclizine, meclizine) are generally useful in the management of nausea and vomiting induced

DRUG TREATMENT: SPECIAL CIRCUMSTANCES

Vomiting as a Result of Cancer Chemotherapy

First-Line Drug

Metoclopramide

Initial Dose	1–2 mg/kg IV infusion
Repeat Dose	In 8 hours if needed
End-Point	Cessation of vomiting

Second-Line Drugs

Prochlorperazine

Initial Dose	2.5–10 mg IV
	5–10 mg IM
	0.1 mg/kg in children >2 years
Repeat Dose	In 3–4 hours if needed
End-Point	Cessation of vomiting

Haloperidol

Initial Dose	2–10 mg IV
Repeat Dose	In 1–2 hours if needed
End-Points	Cessation of vomiting
	Sedation

Vomiting in Pediatric or Pregnant Patients

First-Line Therapy

Fasting
IV hydration

Second-Line Drug

Promethazine

Initial Dose	1 mg/kg IV or per rectum for children
	25 mg IM or IV for pregnant patients
Repeat Dose	In 4–6 hours
End-Point	Cessation of vomiting

by vestibular stimulation. Vertigo, motion sickness, and hyperemesis gravidarum can be successfully managed with antihistamines.

As a group, the antihistamines have side effects that may limit their usefulness. These side effects include drowsiness, blurred vision, urinary retention, and exacerbation of glaucoma.

Treatment of a vomiting patient will vary depending on the suspected cause. When toxins, drugs, chemotherapy, or radiation sickness is suspected, antidopaminergic drugs are the drugs of choice. Metoclopramide, in doses much higher than recommended for gastroparesis, has been shown to be particularly beneficial in the management of cancer chemotherapy emesis. Prochlorperazine is a good alternative choice in the acute care setting. Marijuana and its metabolites have also been used in the management of cancer chemotherapy emesis.

Antidopaminergic drugs, as well as promethazine, are useful in treating the nausea and vomiting from suspected toxic, metabolic, or infectious causes. Promethazine and prochlorperazine should be considered first-line drugs in this scenario. Promethazine has a lower incidence of extrapyramidal side effects, especially in younger patients, although it is less potent than prochlorperazine. Thiethylperazine and trimethobenzamide have no advantages over first-line drugs and have some dosing disadvantages. In addition, thiethylperazine and promethazine contain metabisulfite and may induce severe allergic reactions in susceptible individuals. Chlorpromazine is a potent antidopaminergic antiemetic. As such, it may be useful when other regimens have failed. Its side effects limit its usefulness as either a first- or second-line medication.

As outlined earlier, use of antiemetics in children or in pregnant women should be approached with caution. When conservative measures have failed, promethazine can be used in children. Its low incidence of extrapyramidal side effects makes it the drug of choice in this situation. Both promethazine and meclizine are useful in the treatment of hyperemesis gravidarum. The wider experience with use of promethazine in pregnancy and the option of intravenous or intramuscular administration make this drug first-line treatment for hyperemesis gravidarum.

Repeat dosing of any antiemetic should be approached with caution. Sedation and incidence of side effects increase as dose and duration of therapy increase. Repeat examination is strongly advised before repeat doses are administered in the acute care setting.

Vertigo

Diagnosis

Vertigo occurs when there are incongruous signals to the brain via the labyrinthine afferent pathways. True vertigo is a sensation of rotational movement either of the patient himself or of the surrounding environment and needs to be distinguished from lightheadedness and near-syncopal sensations. Vertigo implies labyrinthine dysfunction, whereas lightheadedness and syncope suggest cardiovascular etiologies. Vertigo is exacerbated by head movements and improved by closing the eyes and keeping the head motionless. The patient may describe a sensation of pulling to one side. Vertigo is often

accompanied by autonomic symptoms such as sweating, pallor, nausea, and tachycardia.

The physical examination in the vertiginous patient should focus on the head and neck region. Cranial nerve function, otologic examination, cerebellar function, and extraocular movement for the detection of nystagmus should all be documented. Caloric testing is a good test of gross vestibular function. Position testing (right ear down, left ear down, etc.) may be useful in the evaluation of nystagmus. Central lesions have short latencies (delay from change in position to onset of nystagmus), whereas peripheral lesions have long (> several seconds) latencies.

Vertigo and nausea associated with a gait disturbance and exacerbation with head movements suggest a disturbance of the vestibular portion of the eighth cranial nerve. Tinnitus connotes peripheral derangement of the auditory portion of the same nerve. Hearing loss is also found in lesions of the cochlear division and is characterized by bone conduction greater than sound conduction. Brain stem lesions rarely result in hearing loss.

Nystagmus is traditionally symmetrical in vestibular disorders, with the fast component in the same direction for all directions of gaze. Vertigo without nystagmus can be seen in cases of central brain stem infarction; however, most cases of vertigo from brain stem lesions will demonstrate asymmetrical nystagmus or nystagmus in which the fast component changes will change in gaze direction.

Few laboratory tests of vertigo will prove useful in the acute evaluation setting. Hematologic testing and serologic tests for syphilis are beneficial in selected cases. Imaging studies such as computed tomography (CT) and magnetic resonance imaging (MRI) are useful when tumor or vascular insult is suspected.

Indications for Treatment

Treatment of vertigo is indicated when it is severe enough to produce intolerable anxiety, when vomiting predominates the clinical picture, and when no contraindications to drug use exist. Treatment is symptomatic and should not preclude a reasonable search for potential etiologies of vertigo (Table 14–2).

Contraindications to treatment of vertigo include known hypersensitivity to the drugs

TABLE 14–2. Causes of Vertigo

Benign positional vertigo
Cerebellar hemorrhage
Cerebellopontine angle tumors
Cervical vertigo (whiplash)
Diabetes mellitus
Drug- or toxin-induced vertigo
    Aminoglycosides
    Furosemide
    Lead
    Arsenic
    Zinc
Epilepsy
Ménière's syndrome
Motion sickness
Multiple sclerosis
Neurosyphilis
Perilymphatic fistula
Post-traumatic
Subclavian steal
Vertebrobasilar insufficiency
Vertebrobasilar migraine
Vestibular neuronitis

used to treat it. Relative contraindications are those for anticholinergic medications and include prostatic hypertrophy, glaucoma, and bowel obstruction. (See box.)

Discussion

The four main vertiginous syndromes presenting in the acute care setting are benign positional vertigo, vestibular neuronitis, Ménière's syndrome, and cerebellopontine tumors.

Vestibular neuronitis (acute labyrinthitis) results in sudden vertigo, nausea, and nystagmus. The etiology of the disorder is unknown although it is thought to be viral. Tinnitus and hearing loss are usually minimal or absent. Photophobia and headache may be present. Severe symptoms persist for several days. Gradual improvement is noted over the next two weeks. Recurrent attacks can occur rarely. Multiple sclerosis should be suspected if the nystagmus persists after the vertigo subsides.

The treatment of vestibular neuronitis is case dependent. Low-grade symptoms and anxiety can often be treated conservatively with rest and limitation of head motion. For those requiring acute intervention, cyclizine, dimenhydrinate, and diazepam offer the advantages of parenteral therapy and should be employed first. When mild sedation is beneficial and anticholinergic side effects limit therapy, hydroxyzine is a useful alternative. Long-term therapy of acute lab-

yrinthitis should employ meclizine, since it is equally efficacious and offers the benefit of once-daily dosing.

Benign positional vertigo is characterized by vertigo that lasts 3 seconds or less, is initiated by head movement, and occurs without an identifiable etiology. Most common in middle age, it has also been seen in younger patients following head trauma. Since duration of symptoms is short, medical therapy is not recommended. Treatment is limitation of rapid head movements.

Ménière's syndrome is a clinical triad of vertigo, tinnitus, and hearing loss. Attacks of vertigo are sudden and last 10 minutes to 2 hours. Tinnitus and hearing loss persist between the attacks of vertigo. Nausea, vomiting, and profuse sweating are prominent features of the acute attacks. During the vertiginous attacks, nystagmus, veering gait, and past-pointing are the hallmarks of the physical examination. The disease typically occurs in the fifth to sixth decade of life and has a male predominance. Treatment may prove difficult as the vertiginous attacks are intermittent and unpredictable. Because of the short duration of symptoms, medical therapy may not be required. In cases of acute vertigo, the short-acting cyclizine, dimenhydrinate, or diazepam may prove beneficial. Long-term therapy with meclizine has not proved to be beneficial.

Cerebellopontine angle tumors are most commonly acoustic neuromas. These tumors generally appear in the fifth decade of life but may be seen earlier in cases of von Recklinghausen's disease. The presenting signs and symptoms of these tumors are often vertigo, tinnitus, and progressive hearing loss. Palsies of the fifth and seventh cranial nerves may be present. True vertigo is sometimes absent. A suspicious clinical evaluation should be followed up with contrast CT or MRI studies of the brain stem. Treatment is surgical, though the medications described above may be useful in short-term therapy.

SPECIFIC AGENTS

Chlorpromazine (Thorazine)

Pharmacology

Phenothiazine derivative with anticholinergic, antidopaminergic, and antiadrenergic activities

DRUG TREATMENT: VERTIGO

First-Line Drugs

Cyclizine

Initial Dose	50 mg IM
Repeat Dose	50 mg PO q 4–6 hours

OR

Dimenhydrinate

Initial Dose	50 mg diluted in 10 ml saline IV over 2 minutes 50 mg IM
Repeat Dose	50–100 mg PO q 4 hours
End-Point	Relief of symptoms

Second-Line Drugs

Meclizine

Initial Dose	50 mg PO
Repeat Dose	50 mg qd

OR

Hydroxyzine

Initial Dose	50–100 mg IM or PO
Repeat Dose	50–100 mg q 6 hours

OR

Diazepam

Initial Dose	2 mg by IV push
Repeat Dose	2–5 mg by IV push q 6 hours

OR

Promethazine

Initial Dose	12.5–25 mg IV 25–50 mg IM, PO, or by rectum
Repeat Dose	In 4–6 hours
End-Points	Relief of symptoms Excessive sedation (especially with hydroxyzine)

Mechanism of Action

Antiemetic activity through inhibition of the CTZ

Kinetics

Onset—30 to 60 minutes following oral administration

Duration—4 to 6 hours following oral administration, 3 to 4 hours following rectal administration

Metabolism

Liver and kidney with large first-pass effect in liver

Indications

Intractable hiccoughs
Intermittent porphyria
Tetanus
Psychotic disorders
Nausea and vomiting

Cautions

Use in pregnancy—Category C; not recommended

Use in lactation—minimally excreted in breast milk

Use in childhood—not under 6 months; generally not used in pediatric population, but if used, dose is 0.5 mg/kg IM or PO, 1.0 mg/kg by rectum

Contraindications

Coma
Central nervous system depression
Age less than 6 months

Dosage Adjustments in Organ Failure

Renal failure—none
Liver failure—reduce dose.
Cardiac failure—none
Elderly—reduce dose.

Dosage

Initial: 10 to 25 mg PO; 25 mg IM, 100 mg by rectum
Repeat: q 6 to 8 hours

Toxicity

Adverse Effects

Common: hypotension, especially after intravenous use; extrapyramidal effects; photosensitivity

Uncommon: neuroleptic malignant syndrome; can mask signs and symptoms of Reye's disease; some forms contain sulfites, which can cause allergic reactions; cholestatic jaundice; agranulocytosis

Life-threatening: sudden death from cardiac arrest reported

Drug Interactions

Decreased digoxin uptake
Use with narcotics can cause marked sedation.
Avoid central nervous system depressants.
Antacids may decrease absorption.
Diminished effect of oral anticoagulants
Seizure with metrizamide (Amipaque)

Treatment of Toxicity

Supportive

Cyclizine (Marezine)

Pharmacology

Piperazine antihistamine, anticholinergic, antispasmodic

Mechanism of Action

Decreased labyrinthine excitability, exact mechanism unknown, some antiemetic effect through CTZ

Kinetics

Onset—30 minutes
Duration—4 hours

Metabolism

Probably liver

Indications

Motion sickness

Cautions

Use in pregnancy—Category B; use with caution, but probably safe
Use in lactation—not recommended; no data available
Use in childhood—not recommended

Contraindications

Glaucoma
Prostatic hypertrophy
Gastrointestinal obstruction

Dosage Adjustments in Organ Failure

Renal failure—none
Liver failure—reduce dose.
Cardiac failure—none

Dosage

Initial: 50 mg IM or 50 mg PO $\frac{1}{2}$ hour prior to departure
Repeat: 4 to 6 hours

Toxicity

Adverse Effects

Common: restlessness, excitation, nervousness, insomnia, euphoria, anorexia, nausea, vomiting, diarrhea, constipation, blurred vision, drowsiness

Uncommon: reversible agranulocytosis, cholestatic jaundice, hypotension

Life-threatening: drug hypersensitivity

Drug Interations

Potentiates alcohol and central nervous system depressants

Treatment of Toxicity

Symptomatic
Supportive

Dimenhydrinate (Dramamine)

Pharmacology

Ethanolamine derivative
Well absorbed after oral or parenteral administration
Central nervous system depressant
Anticholinergic
Antiemetic
Antihistaminic
53 to 55% diphenhydramine
44 to 47% chlorotheophylline

Mechanism of Action

Inhibits vestibular stimulation via acetylcholine inhibition

Kinetics

Onset—15 to 30 minutes following oral administration; 20 to 30 minutes following intramuscular administration; immediate following intravenous administration
Duration—3 to 6 hours

Metabolism

Little information available; well distributed; crosses placenta

Indications

Motion sickness
Treatment of vestibular disturbances (not approved by the Food and Drug Administration for this use)

Cautions

Use in pregnancy—yes; Category B; remote chance of harm°
Use in lactation—small amounts in breast milk; decide on case-by-case basis
Use in childhood—yes; dose 1 mg/kg q 6 hours

Contraindications

Seizure Disorder
Narrow-angle glaucoma
Prostatic hypertrophy
Gastrointestinal obstruction

Dosage Adjustments in Organ Failure

None

°Rat studies using 20 to 25 times the human dose show no harm to fetus.

Dosage

Initial: adults—50 to 100 mg PO; 50 mg IV; dilute in 10 ml saline over 2 minutes.
Repeat: in 3 to 4 hours, same dose

Toxicity

Adverse Effects

Common: palpitations, drowsiness, paradoxical central nervous system stimulation in children, headache, blurred vision, tinnitus, dryness of mouth, hypotension
Uncommon: anorexia, constipation, diarrhea, urinary frequency
Life-threatening: anticholinergic crisis with overdose, seizures

Drug Interactions

Enhances central nervous system depressants
Enhances anticholinergics
May mask symptoms of otoxicity of aminoglycosides

Treatment of Toxicity

Symptomatic
Supportive
Seizure control with diazepam and phenobarbital

Hydroxyzine (Atarax, Vistaril)

Pharmacology

Piperazine derivative
Antihistamine with principal effects of subcortical depression of central nervous system activity

Mechanism of Action

Antiemetic effects are primarily through antihistaminic effects at local gastrointestinal and VC levels.

Kinetics

Onset—15 to 30 minutes following oral administration
Duration—4 to 6 hours

Metabolism

Liver, with elimination in feces

Indications

Antihistamine
Analgesic adjunct
Sedation
Antiemetic

Cautions

Use in pregnancy—Category C; contraindicated in first trimester
Use in lactation—contraindicated
Use in childhood—0.6 mg/kg IM or PO q 6 hours

Contraindications

Early pregnancy
Central nervous system depressants
Previous reactions to medication
Do not administer subcutaneously, intravenously, or intra-arterially.

Dosage Adjustments in Organ Failure

Renal failure—none
Liver failure—reduce dose.
Cardiac failure—none

Dosage

Initial: 25 to 100 mg IM, PO
Repeat q 6 hours.

Toxicity

Adverse Effects

Common: local discomfort at site, dry mouth, sedation
Uncommon: hypotension, nausea, wheezing, flushing, seizures
Life-threatening: thrombosis/gangrene following intra-arterial use, phlebitis/hemolysis after intravenous injection

Drug Interactions

Potentiates central nervous system depressants
Use with epinephrine may cause paradoxical decrease in blood pressure
May inhibit antipsychotic effects of phenothiazines
May cause neurotoxicity with metoclopramide

Treatment of Toxicity

Supportive

Ipecac

Pharmacology

Derivative of dried root of the South American plant *Cephaelis ipecacuanha*
The primary active ingredient is the alkyloid emetine, although other alkyloids are present.

Mechanism of Action

Emetine has direct effect on the CTZ and also strong local gastrointestinal irritative effects.

Kinetics

Onset—10 to 30 minutes
Duration—up to 6 hours

Metabolism

Renal excretion of absorbed alkyloids

Indications

Induction of nausea and vomiting

Cautions

Use in pregnancy—safety not established but recommended for use in pregnancy when clinical needs outweigh risk
Use in lactation—safety not established
Use in childhood—yes; see Dosage, below.

Contraindications

Altered mental status
Some caustic and petroleum distillate ingestions
Use in camphor, cyclic antidepressant, and phenol ingestion is relatively contraindicated due to rapid decrease in mental status associated with these medications.

Dosage Adjustments in Organ Failure.

None

Dosage

Initial: 5+ years, 30 ml PO; 1 to 5 years, 15 ml PO; 6 to 12 months, 10 ml PO
Repeat: in 30 minutes if no vomiting; do not repeat more than once. If failure to produce vomiting after second dose, lavage should be instituted.

Toxicity

Adverse Effects

Common: protracted vomiting, lethargy, diarrhea
Uncommon: Mallory-Weiss tears, intracranial hemorrhage, pneumomediastinum
Life-threatening: overdose leads to cardiac dysrhythmias and death; hypotension; seizures

Drug Interactions

Activated charcoal may bind ipecac and reduce its efficacy.

Treatment of Toxicity

Supportive
Cardiac monitoring

Meclizine (Antivert)

Pharmacology

Piperazine derivative has marked antihistamine and mild anticholinergic activity that predominates the pharmacologic picture.
Has a long duration of action—24 hours—that allows once-daily dosing

Mechanism of Action

Depresses labyrinthine conduction

Kinetics

Onset—1 hour
Duration—24 hours
Half-life—6 hours

Metabolism

Distributed to most tissues
Excreted in urine after liver metabolism

Indications

Effective treatment of motion sickness
Possibly effective in treatment of vertigo associated with disorders of the vestibular system

Cautions

Use in pregnancy—Category B
Use in lactation—use in nursing mother not recommended
Use in childhood—do not use in children under 12 years old.

Contraindications

Previous hypersensitivity to drug
Asthma
Glaucoma
Prostatic hypertrophy

Dosage Adjustments in Organ Failure

Renal failure—none
Liver failure—reduce dose.
Cardiac failure—none

Dosage

Vertigo

Initial: 25 to 200 mg per day, adjusted in divided dosage for maximum benefit
Repeat: 25 to 100 mg daily

Motion Sickness

Initial: 25 to 50 mg 1 hour before embarkation
Repeat: 25 to 50 mg daily

Toxicity

Adverse Effects

Common: drowsiness, fatigue, dry mouth, blurred vision
Uncommon: exacerbation of asthma, bronchospasm
Life-threatening: allergic reactions (uncommon)

Drug Interactions

Potentiation of central nervous system depressants

Treatment of Toxicity

Supportive

Metoclopramide (Reglan)

Pharmacology

Synthetic substituted benzamide that stimulates gastric emptying, increases lower esophageal sphincter tone

Mechanism of Action

Potent dopamine antagonist with main antiemetic effect on CTZ

Kinetics

Onset—wide variation: 1 to 3 minutes following intravenous administration; 10 to 15 minutes following intramuscular administration; 30 to 60 minutes following oral administration
Duration—1 to 2 hours

Metabolism

85% renal

Indications

Diabetic gastric stasis
Chemotherapy-induced nausea and vomiting
Adjunct for x-ray studies
Gastroesophageal reflux

Cautions

Use in pregnancy—yes; Category B
Use in lactation—increased concentrations in milk; usage cautioned
Use in childhood—2.5 to 5 mg/dose if 6 to

14 years old, 0.1 mg/kg dose if less than 6 years old

Use in neonates—no; may cause methemoglobinemia

Contraindications

Bowel obstruction
Seizure disorders
Gastrointestinal hemorrhage
Pheochromocytoma
Predisposition to extrapyramidal reactions

Dosage Adjustments in Organ Failure

Renal failure—reduce dose.
Liver failure—none
Cardiac failure—none

Dosage

Initial: 10 mg PO or IV for gastroparesis; 1 to 2 mg/kg IV for cancer chemotherapy
Repeat: q 6 to 8 hours

Toxicity

Adverse Effects

Common: restlessness, drowsiness, fatigue, lassitude—10%, diarrhea
Uncommon: insomnia, headache, dizziness, extrapyramidal signs and symptoms (increase with increased dosage), bronchospasm, neuroleptic malignant syndrome
Life-threatening: neuroleptic malignant syndrome, severe bradycardia reported in one patient receiving 15 mg IV

Drug Interactions

May decrease absorption of drugs by the stomach
Increased absorption of drugs by the small intestine
Additive effect with other sedatives
May cause hypertensive crisis with monamine oxidase inhibitors
May necessitate adjustments in insulin dosage and/or timing

Treatment of Toxicity

Supportive
Diphenhydramine for extrapyramidal reactions

Prochlorperazine (Compazine)

Pharmacology

Piperazine phenothiazine with antihistaminic properties; the most studied of all antiemetics and the "benchmark" by which others are compared

Mechanism of Action

Antidopaminergic (CTZ) and antihistaminic (VC)

Kinetics

Onset—30 to 40 minutes, oral; 60 minutes, rectal; 10 to 20 minutes, intramuscular
Duration—3 to 4 hours

Metabolism

Liver

Indications

Severe nausea and vomiting
Nonpsychotic anxiety
Migraine headaches (not approved by the Food and Drug Administration)

Cautions

Use in pregnancy—Category C; not recommended except in severe cases
Use in lactation—not recommended
Use in childhood—do not use if under 2 years old or 9 kg weight; dose in older children is 0.1 mg/kg/dose.

Contraindications

Reye's syndrome
Children under 2 years of age
Hypersensitivity to prochlorperazine
Glaucoma
History of neuroleptic malignant syndrome

Dosage Adjustments in Organ Failure

Renal failure—none
Liver failure—reduce dose.
Cardiac failure—none

Dosage

Initial: 5 to 10 mg IM; 2.5 to 10 mg IV; 25 mg by rectum
Repeat: 12 hours by rectum; 3 to 4 hours PO or IM

Toxicity

Adverse Effects

Common: extrapyramidal side effects, drowsiness, blurred vision
Uncommon: dermatitis, cholestatic jaundice, leukopenia, agranulocytosis
Life-threatening: sulfite allergy, neurolep-

tic malignant syndrome, hypotension with intravenous use

Drug Interactions

Potentiates central nervous system depressants

May see paradoxical drop in blood pressure with epinephrine administration

Increases toxicity of tricyclic antidepressants

Increases beta-blocker effects

Increases valproic acid effects

Increases neurotoxicity of lithium

Decreases levodopa effect

Decreases phenytoin effect

Decreases guanadrel effect

Treatment of Toxicity

Supportive

Diphenhydramine for extrapyramidal reactions

Promethazine (Phenergan)

Pharmacology

Phenothiazine derivative with antihistaminic, anticholinergic properties

Mechanism of Action

A potent H_1 blocker

Antiemetic effects are related to VC depressant effects.

Kinetics

Onset—3 to 5 minutes IV; other routes, 20 minutes

Duration—2 to 8 hours

Metabolism

Liver

Indications

Nausea and vomiting

Anaphylaxis

Pain control adjunct with narcotics

Mild allergic reactions such as urticaria

Dermatographism

Motion sickness

Cautions

Use in pregnancy—Category C

Use in lactation—unknown; use with caution.

Use in childhood—1 mg/kg; q 4 to 6 hours by rectum or IM

Contraindications

Glaucoma

Prostatic hypertrophy

Gastrointestinal obstruction

Asthma

Reye's syndrome

Prior hypersensitivity

Do not give subcutaneously or intra-arterially.

Dosage Adjustments in Organ Failure

Renal failure—none

Liver failure—reduce dose.

Cardiac failure—none

Elderly—reduce dose.

Dosage

Initial: 25 mg IM, PO, or by rectum; 12.5 mg IV

Repeat: q 6 hours

Toxicity

Adverse Effects

Common: sedation, sleepiness, blurred vision, dry mouth

Uncommon: confusion, oculogyric crisis, seizures, cholestatic jaundice; may mask Reye's syndrome

Life-threatening: hypotension (rare), allergic reactions in sulfite-sensitive individuals, agranulocytosis

Drug Interactions

Potentiates central nervous system depressants

With epinephrine may paradoxically decrease blood pressure

May have false Gravindex, Prepurex, and Dap immunologic tests for pregnancy

May interfere with ABO blood typing

Treatment of Toxicity

Supportive

Symptomatic

Thiethylperazine (Torecan)

Pharmacology

Piperazine phenothiazine that is centrally active

Mechanism of Action

Suppresses the CTZ and VC

Exact mechanism of action unknown

Kinetics

Onset—30 minutes, oral
Duration—4 to 8 hours

Metabolism

Unknown

Indications

Antiemetic only

Cautions

Use in pregnancy—contraindicated; limited information
Use in lactation—contraindicated
Use in childhood—usage in children less than 12 years old contraindicated

Contraindications

Depressed level of consciousness
Children
History of phenothiazine reactions
Vertigo

Dosage Adjustments in Organ Failure

Renal failure—none
Liver failure—do not use.
Cardiac failure—none

Dosage

Initial: 10 mg IM, PO, or by rectum
Repeat: q 8 hours

Toxicity

Adverse Effects

Common: drowsiness, postural hypotension after injections
Uncommon: postural hypotension (oral, rectal), extrapyramidal signs and symptoms, seizures, cholestatic jaundice, agranulocytosis, urinary retention, hyperpyrexia
Life-threatening: Injection contains sodium metabisulfite—potential for severe allergic reactions; tartazine (FD & C yellow #5 dye) in tablets—allergic sensitivity possible

Drug Interactions

Potentiates central nervous system depressants
May see paradoxical drop in blood pressure with epinephrine

Treatment of Toxicity

Supportive
Avoid epinephrine in treatment of hypotension.

Trimethobenzamide (Tigan)

Pharmacology

Substituted ethanolamine with antidopaminergic and antihistaminic properties

Mechanism of Action

Antiemetic activity through suppression of CTZ

Kinetics

Onset—10 to 40 minutes, oral; 15 to 35 minutes IM
Duration—3 to 4 hours, oral; 2 to 3 hours IM

Metabolism

Not established but probably *liver*, with urine and feces excretion

Indications

Nausea and vomiting

Cautions

Use in pregnancy—Category C; avoid.
Use in lactation—safety not established; avoid.
Use in childhood—patient less than 30 lb, 100 mg by rectum q 6 to 8 hours; more than 30 lb, 100 to 200 mg by rectum q 6 to 8 hours; do not administer intramuscularly in children; do not use in neonates.

Contraindications

Reye's syndrome
Liver failure
Suppositories contain benzocaine; do not use in patients sensitive to this or similar local anesthetics.

Dosage Adjustments in Organ Failure

Renal failure—none
Liver failure—reduce dose.
Cardiac failure—none

Dosage

Initial: 250 mg PO; 200 mg IM or by rectum
Repeat: q 6 to 8 hours

Toxicity

Adverse Effects

Fewer adverse side effects than phenothiazine antiemetics; side effects are rare.
Common: drowsiness

Uncommon: sensitization, parkinsonian signs and symptoms, blurred vision, coma, seizures, blood dyscrasias, diarrhea, jaundice

Life-threatening: hypotension after intramuscular administration

Drug Interactions

Potentiates alcohol and other central nervous system depressants

Treatment of Toxicity

Supportive
Diphenhydramine for extrapyramidal reactions

REFERENCES

Abdullah AH, Tye A: A comparison of the efficacy of emetic drugs and stomach lavage. Am J Dis Child 113(5):571–575, 1967.

Bakowski MT: Advances in anti-emetic therapy. Cancer Treat Rev 11:237–256, 1984.

Baloh RW: The dizzy patient: Symptomatic treatment of vertigo. Postgrad Med 73(5):317–324, 1983.

Bernardi M, Trevisani F, Gasbarrini G: Metoclopramide administration in advanced liver disease (letter). Gastroenterology 91(2):523, 1986.

Book LS: Vomiting and diarrhea. Pediatrics (Suppl)74: 950–954, 1984.

Borison HL, McCarthy LE: Neuropharmacology of chemotherapy-induced emesis. Drugs (Suppl 1)25:8–17, 1983.

Borison HL, Wang SC: Physiology and pharmacology of vomiting. Pharmacol Rev 5:193–230, 1953.

Chafee-Bahamon C, LaCouture PG, Lovejoy FH: Risk assessment of ipecac in the home. Pediatrics 75(6):1105–1109, 1985.

Chan HSL, Correia JA, MacLeod SM: Nebilone vs prochlorperazine for control of cancer chemotherapy—induced emesis in children: A double-blind, crossover trial. Pediatrics 79(6):946–952, 1987.

Chestnut DH, Vandewalker GE, Owen CL, et al: Administration of metoclopramide for prevention of nausea and vomiting during epidural anesthesia for elective cesarean section. Anesthesiology 66:563–566, 1987.

Clarke RSJ: Nausea and vomiting. Br J Anaesth 56:19–27, 1984.

Czajka PA, Russell SL: Nonemetic effects of ipecac syrup. Pediatrics 75(6):1101–1104, 1985.

Desmond, PV, Watson KJR: Metoclopramide: A review. Med J Aust 144(7):366–369, 1986.

Dipalma JR: Drugs for nausea and vomiting of pregnancy. Am Fam Physician 28(4):272–274, 1983.

Feldman M: Nausea and vomiting. In Sleisenger MH, Fordtran JS (eds): Gastrointestinal Disease, 4th ed. Philadelphia, WB Saunders, 1989, pp 222–238.

Freedman GE, Pasternak S, Krenzelok EP: A clinical trial using syrup of ipecac and activated charcoal concurrently. Ann Emerg Med 16(2):164–166, 1987.

Gilman AG, Goodman LS, Rall TW, Murad F (eds): Goodman and Gilman's The Pharmacological Basis of Therapeutics, 7th ed. New York, Macmillan, 1985.

Grbcich PA, Lacouture PG, Leuander WJ, Lovejoy FH: Effect of milk on ipecac-induced emesis. J Pediatr 110(6):973–975, 1987.

Grbcich PA, Lacouture PG, Lovejoy FH: Effect of fluid volume on ipecac-induced emesis. J Pediatr 110(6):970–972, 1987.

Grbcich PA, Lacouture PG, Kresel JJ, et al: Expired ipecac syrup efficacy. Pediatrics 78(6):1085–1989, 1986.

Griffin JP, D'Arcy PF, Speirs CH: A Manual of Adverse Drug Interactions. London, Wright Publishing, 1988.

Gumbart CH, Sorensen SH, Bickers IN: A comparison of metoclopramide vs droperidol/phenobarbitol for emesis induced by chemotherapy. Am J Med Sci 293(2):90–93, 1987.

Hanson JS, McCalum RW: The diagnosis and management of nausea and vomiting: A review. Am J Gastroenterol 80(3):210–218, 1985.

Hansten PD, Horn JR (eds): Drug Interactions: Clinical Significance of Drug-Drug Interactions, 6 ed. Philadelphia, Lea & Febiger, 1989.

Hill OW: Psychogenic vomiting. Gut 9:348–352, 1968.

Ileh KF, Gibb SM, Unsworth, RW: Syrup of ipecacuanha as an emetic in adults. Med J Aust 2:91–93, 1977.

Joss RA, Galeazzi RL, Bischoff AK, et al: The antiemetic activity of high dose alizapride and high dose metoclopramide in patients receiving cancer chemotherapy: A prospective, randomized, double-blind trial. Clin Pharmacol 39(6):619–624, 1986.

Klebanoff MA, Keslowe PA, Rhoads GG: Epidemiology of vomiting in early pregnancy. Obstet Gynecol 66:612, 1985.

Krenzelok EP, Dean BS: Syrup of ipecac in children less than one year of age. J Toxicol 23:171–176, 1985.

Laszlo J: Closing remarks: Selecting an antiemetic for the individual patient. Drugs (Suppl 1) 25:81–83, 1983.

Laszlo J: Nausea and vomiting as major complications of cancer chemotherapy. Drugs (Suppl 1) 25:1–7, 1983.

Laszlo J, Gralla RJ, Wampler G: Antiemetics: A round table discussion. Drugs (Suppl 1)25:74–80, 1983.

Laszlo J, Lucas VS: Emesis as a critical problem in chemotherapy. N Engl J Med 305(16):948–949, 1981.

Leathem AM: Safety and efficacy of antiemetics used to treat nausea and vomiting in pregnancy. Clin Pharmacol 5(8):660–668, 1986.

Lituvitz TL, Klein-Schwartz W, Oderda GM, et al: Ipecac administration in children younger than one year of age. Pediatrics 76:761–764, 1985.

Lumsden K, Holden WS: The act of vomiting in man. Gut 10:173, 1969.

Macleod J: Ipecac intoxication—use of a cardiac pacemaker in management. N Engl J Med 268(3):146–147, 1963.

Malagelada JR, Camilleri M: Unexplained vomiting: A diagnostic challenge. Ann Intern Med 101:211–218, 1984.

Matsuoka I, Ito J, Takahashi H, et al: Experimental vestibular pharmacology: A mini review with special reference to neuroactive substances and antivertigo drugs. Acta Otolaryngol (Suppl)419:62–70, 1985.

McEvoy GK (Ed): AHFS Drug Information 88. Bethesda, MD, American Society of Hospital Pharmacology, 1988.

Melzack R, Rosberger Z, Hollingsworth ML, et al: New approaches to measuring nausea. Can Med Assoc J 133:755, 1985.

Peroutka SJ, Snyder SH: Antiemetics: Neurotransmitter receptor binding predicts therapeutic actions. Lancet 1:658–659, 1982.

Pyykko I, Schalen L, Jantti V: Transdermally administered scopolomine vs dimenhydrinate I: Effect on nausea and vomiting in experimentally induced motion sickness. Acta Otolaryngol 99:588, 1985.

Reuben DB, Mor V: Nausea and vomiting in terminal cancer patients. Arch Intern Med 146(10):2021–2023, 1986.

Rich CL: Self-induced vomiting—psychiatric considerations. JAMA 239:2688–2698, 1978.

Richards PD, Flaum MA, Bateman M, Kardinal CG: The antiemetic efficacy of secobarbitol and chlorpromazine compared to metoclopramide, diphenhydramine, and dexamethazone: A randomized trial. Cancer 58(4):959–962, 1986.

Rosenthal RH, Webb WL, Wruble LD: Diagnosis and management of persistent psychogenic vomiting. Psychosomatics 21:722–730, 1980.

Schmitt LG, Shaw JE: Alleviation of induced vertigo: Therapy with transdermal scopolomine and oral meclizine. Arch Otolaryngol Head Neck Surg 112 (1):88–91, 1986.

Scobie BA: Recurrent vomiting in adults: A syndrome? Med J Aust April(1):329–331, 1983.

Stein RS, Jenkins D, Korns ME: Death after use of cupric sulfate as emetic. JAMA 235:801–880, 1976.

Tandberg D, Diven BG, McLeod JW: Ipecac-induced emesis versus gastric lavage: A controlled study in normal adults. Am J Emerg Med 4:205–209, 1986.

Tandberg D, Liechty ES, Fishbein D: Mallory-Weiss syndrome: An unusual complication of ipecac-induced emesis. Ann Emerg Med 10:521–523, 1981.

Wampler G: The pharmacology and clinical effectiveness of phenothiazines and related drugs for managing chemotherapy-induced emesis. Drugs (Suppl 1) 25:35–51, 1983.

Wason S: Gastrointestinal decontamination of the poisoned patient—a critical review. Drugs of Today 23(8):455–465, 1987.

Wood CD, Graybiel A: Evaluation of antimotion sickness drugs: A new effective remedy revealed. Aerospace Med 41:932–933, 1970.

Zee DS: Perspectives on the pharmacotherapy of vertigo. Arch Otolaryngol 111(9):609–612, 1985.

CHAPTER 15

Acidifying and Alkalizing Agents

BONITA SINGAL, M.D.

INTRODUCTION

Metabolic acidosis and metabolic alkalosis are common physiologic derangements in severely ill and injured patients. There is abundant experimental and clinical evidence that alterations of hydrogen ion concentration in body fluids can cause central nervous system and cardiovascular dysfunction. Changes occur in membrane binding and transport that alter the distribution and action of pharmacologic agents. Changes in pH can also adversely effect ventilation and oxygen transport. Some controversy remains about what deviation in arterial pH is acceptable and what levels require aggressive treatment. In general, vigorous treatment is indicated to keep the pH above 7.0 to 7.1 and below 7.6.

Any discussion of acidifying and alkalizing agents must begin with the understanding that the treatment of the majority of acid–base disorders involves interventions directed at correcting the underlying cause rather than drug therapy aimed at counteracting the acidic or alkaline state. In fact, rapid and nonphysiologic reversal of acidosis or alkalosis can have adverse consequences for the patient. These include worsening cerebral acidosis, cerebral edema, pulmonary edema, hypokalemia and hyperkalemia, and alterations in serum levels of ionized calcium. In general, when treating severe met-

abolic acidosis or alkalosis, one should aim to bring the abnormalities into a safe range relatively quickly and then allow for a gradual return to a normal pH. This is accomplished by careful dosing of the acidifying or alkalizing agents based on the desired change in serum bicarbonate.

Administration of alkalizing agents may be indicated in the patient with a normal arterial blood pH in order to alter the pH of the urine. This maneuver may be used to increase the solubility of weak acids such as cystine or uric acid that are being excreted in excessively large amounts or to increase the excretory rate of lipid-soluble organic acids such as salicylates and barbiturates. Alkalization is also useful in the urgent treatment of cardiac toxicity caused by severe hyperkalemia and of cardiac and central nervous system toxicity caused by overdose of tricyclic antidepressants. Urinary acidification has been advocated in the past to increase the excretion of weak bases such as phencyclidine and amphetamines. This intervention has not been shown to increase renal clearance rates substantially and can no longer be recommended.

It is necessary to become familiar with only a handful of drugs in order to manipulate the pH of the blood or the urine. Sodium bicarbonate is overwhelmingly the drug of choice for the treatment of metabolic acidosis when drug therapy is indicated. Sodium chloride administration is generally sufficient treatment for metabolic alkalosis. When volume repletion fails to reverse severe metabolic alkalosis, the drug of choice is hydrochloric acid.

Primary respiratory acidosis and alkalosis are not discussed in detail in this chapter. These conditions are treated by optimizing ventilation and controlling the underlying disorder.

CONDITIONS

Metabolic Acidosis

Severe metabolic acidosis is the most serious disturbance of acid–base physiology because it is often the result of a multiorgan failure and because it leads to impaired cardiovascular function. There are four mechanisms that can result in metabolic acidosis: overproduction of endogenous acids, as in diabetic ketoacidosis; underexcretion of endogenous acids, as in renal failure; introduction of an exogenous acid, as in ethylene glycol ingestion; and loss of bicarbonate in the urine from renal tubular acidosis or in the stool from profuse diarrhea.

Diagnosis

One can suspect the presence of a metabolic acidosis from the clinical picture. The patient may present acutely ill with nausea, vomiting, and other nonspecific complaints. The presence of deep regular breathing (Kussmaul respirations) with a normal lung examination is the major clinical clue to the presence of acute metabolic acidosis.

A patient with a pure metabolic acidosis will have a clinical picture consisting of an arterial pH below 7.35, a depressed serum bicarbonate level, and a depressed $paCO_2$. A patient with a serum bicarbonate level of 5 mEq/liter will have an arterial pH of approximately 7.1 and a pCO_2 of about 15 torr if he has full respiratory compensation. Approximately 10 torr is the lower limit of respiratory response to metabolic acidosis. A patient who is unable to mount a respiratory response because of intrinsic lung disease or depressed ventilation from other causes, or because he is on controlled mechanical ventilation, will manifest more severe pH abnormalities and may, in fact, show a combined disturbance of both metabolic and respiratory acidosis. If the $paCO_2$ is significantly below that which is expected given the serum level of bicarbonate, one may postulate either a combined metabolic acidosis–respiratory alkalosis as seen in salicylate ingestion or hyperventilation from other causes such as central nervous system disease or controlled mechanical ventilation.

Once a picture of pure or mixed metabolic acidosis has been established, it is very helpful to calculate the anion gap from the serum electrolyte levels as follows:

$$\text{Anion gap} = Na^+ - (Cl^- + HCO_3)$$

The anion gap should normally be <12. Conditions that present with and without an anion gap acidosis are listed in Table 15–1.

Indications for Treatment

In general, alkali therapy is recommended in the treatment of metabolic acidosis when the pH falls below 7.0 to 7.1. This corresponds to a serum bicarbonate level of 5 mEq/liter in the fully compensated patient. The goal of treatment is the achievement of a "safe pH" of approximately 7.1 to 7.2.

Exceptions to this general approach require special mention. The acidosis of acute and chronic renal failure and that of renal tubular acidosis are usually treated when the serum bicarbonate level falls below 15 mEq/liter or when Kussmaul respirations are present.

Victims of cardiac arrest may be treated empirically with sodium bicarbonate when determination of arterial pH is not feasible and when adequate cardiac and pulmonary function has not been restored after 10 minutes of advanced cardiac life support measures. In these cases, sodium bicarbonate may be administered at a dose of 1 mEq/kg of the 8.4% solution in adults and the 4.2%

TABLE 15–1. Causes of Metabolic Acidosis

Anion Gap Acidosis	Non–Anion Gap Acidosis
Diabetic ketoacidosis	Prolonged severe diarrhea
Alcoholic ketosis	Renal tubular acidosis
Starvation ketosis	HCl, NH$_4$Cl, NaCl
Ethylene glycol	infusions
poisoning	Carbonic anhydrase
Methanol poisoning	inhibitor
Salicylate poisoning	
Renal failure	
Lactic acidosis	

solution in children. Effective ventilation and restoration of circulation are emphasized, whereas the routine use of bicarbonate in repeated doses is no longer recommended by the American Heart Association.

Severe hyperkalemia with serum potassium levels greater than 7.0 mEq/liter and evidence of evolving cardiac conduction abnormalities such as widening of the QRS complex require urgent treatment, which may include alkalization with sodium bicarbonate even in the presence of a normal arterial pH.

Tricyclic antidepressant overdose with cardiac toxicity, either severe tachydysrhythmia or evolving conduction abnormalities, should be treated with alkalization to bring the arterial pH to 7.5.

Alkalization is also recommended as adjunctive treatment in symptomatic salicylate intoxication as long as arterial pH is below 7.5. The goal of therapy is an alkaline diuresis with urine pH ranging from 7.5 to 8.0. Severe overdose with long-acting barbiturates such as phenobarbital is another indication for alkaline diuresis. (See boxes, Drug Treatment: Metabolic Acidosis and Drug Treatment: Urinary Alkalization.)

Discussion
Ketoacidosis

It is generally agreed that sodium bicarbonate should be used to treat ketoacidosis of any cause if the pH of the arterial blood is below 7.0. The goal of treatment is to bring the pH into the "safe range" of 7.1 to 7.2. One can estimate the dose of bicarbonate needed using the formula in the flow sheet on drug treatment of metabolic acidosis with a desired bicarbonate of 5 to 8 mEq/liter. A nearly isotonic solution can be prepared by adding 150 mEq of sodium bicarbonate to 850 ml of sterile water; and this can be infused in place of normal saline as the initial

---

DRUG TREATMENT: METABOLIC ACIDOSIS

First-Line Drug
Sodium Bicarbonate

Preparation	50–150 mEq/liter
Initial Dose	mEq NaHCO$_3$ = (desired HCO$_3^-$ − measured HCO$_3^-$)(weight[kg] $\times$ 0.5) by IV infusion over 1–2 hours

or

Adults:

If arterial pH = 7.0–7.1, give 50–100 mEq by IV infusion over 1–2 hours.

If arterial pH <7.0, give 100–150 mEq by IV infusion over 1–2 hours.

Children:

If arterial pH = 7.0–7.1, give 1 mEq/kg by IV infusion over 1–2 hours.

If arterial pH <7.0, give 2 mEq/kg by IV infusion over 1–2 hours.

Repeat Dose	Repeat measurement of pH and HCO$_3^-$ and recalculate as above.
End-Point	Arterial pH >7.1

Second-Line Drug
Tromethamine (THAM, Tris)

Preparation	150 mEq/500 ml (0.3 M)
Initial Dose	Number of milliliters of 0.3 M solution = (desired HCO$_3^-$ − actual HCO$_3^-$)(weight[kg] $\times$ 1.1) by central venous infusion over 1–2 hours
Repeat Dose	Repeat measurement of pH and HCO$_3^-$. Recalculate as above.
End-Point	pH >7.1

DRUG TREATMENT: URINARY ALKALIZATION (Urine pH <7.5 and Blood pH <7.5)

Drug of Choice

Sodium Bicarbonate

Preparation	50–150 mEq/liter
Initial Dose	*Adult:* 50–150 mEq over 1–2 hours

OR

	Adult or Pediatric: 1–2 mEq/kg over 1–2 hours
Repeat Dose	If blood pH <7.50 and urine pH <7.5 may repeat as above
End-Point	Urine pH = 7.5–8.0 or blood pH >7.55

intravenous fluid for patients with diabetic ketoacidosis. In severe ketoacidosis secondary to starvation or alcoholism, 50 to 150 mEq of sodium bicarbonate can be added to 5% dextrose in water (D_5W). Keep in mind that treatment of the underlying condition will result in the metabolism of ketone bodies and the generation of bicarbonate, so the risk of "overshoot alkalosis" increases as treatment proceeds.

The treatment of all forms of metabolic acidosis usually requires treatment of accompanying potassium depletion. Potassium should be supplemented as soon as the serum level falls into the normal range and should be monitored closely as treatment proceeds.

Lactic Acidosis

The administration of sodium bicarbonate in the treatment of lactic acidosis is more problematic and less satisfactory than in treatment of other forms of metabolic acidosis. Although not known to alter the outcome of this condition, it is reasonable to try to keep the arterial pH in the range of 7.1 to 7.2, which is safer from a cardiovascular standpoint, while other more definitive measures are ongoing. Since lactic acid continues to be generated as long as anaerobic metabolism is occurring, prolonged and generous administration of sodium bicarbonate may be needed. The amount of fluid delivered can be tailored to the patient's needs by varying the concentration of bicarbonate from 50 to

150 mEq in 850 to 950 ml of D_5W or sterile water. The adverse consequences of solute and volume overload can be controlled to some extent by monitoring pulmonary capillary wedge pressure and by using diuretics and vasodilators where indicated. In cases in which these maneuvers fail to minimize complications, a novel approach has been to use peritoneal dialysis with a bicarbonate-buffered dialysate, which obviates the problem of fluid overload and corrects the acidosis.

Another drug, tromethamine, more commonly known as tris or THAM, was introduced about 25 years ago as an alternative to sodium bicarbonate in the treatment of metabolic acidosis. Tromethamine is a hydrogen ion acceptor that acts directly on the carbonic acid buffer system. It has the effect of reducing pCO_2 and may cause respiratory depression. The use of the drug has been limited mainly because of its highly alkaline pH and its propensity to cause vascular damage. Its use is contraindicated in pregnancy, uremia, and chronic respiratory acidosis. It should be delivered via a central venous catheter. It is the general feeling that this drug offers no significant benefit over sodium bicarbonate as a first-line drug. It may be indicated, however, in patients in whom sodium overload precludes further administration of sodium bicarbonate in the face of a persistent severe metabolic acidosis.

Swedish investigators have reported on the use of a new buffer mixture containing tris, acetate, sodium bicarbonate, and disodium phosphate. It can be delivered into a peripheral vein and contains one-third of the sodium of pure sodium bicarbonate. Specific recommendations for the use of this tris buffer mixture await further studies.

Dichloroacetate is a drug that is under investigation as an alternative to sodium bicarbonate in the treatment of severe lactic acidosis. This drug reduces circulating lactate concentrations by stimulating the activity of pyruvate dehydrogenase, the catalyst for the oxidation of lactate and pyruvate. Dichloroacetate has been shown to lower lactate levels in experimental animals and in humans with lactic acidosis resulting from a variety of causes.

Acute Renal Failure

If severe metabolic acidosis develops in the setting of acute renal failure, urgent hemodialysis or peritoneal dialysis should be considered. If these interventions are contraindicated or delayed, it is recommended that medical treatment be instituted when the serum bicarbonate level falls below 15 mEq/liter and is accompanied by Kussmaul respirations. The dosage of bicarbonate can be calculated from the formula given in the drug treatment flow sheet, assuming a desired serum bicarbonate of 15 to 18 mEq/liter. Supplemental calcium gluconate, 1 to 3 g, should be given over the same time period to prevent tetany. Calcium salts and sodium bicarbonate are not compatible in solution and must be given in separate intravenous lines.

Hyperkalemia

Severe hyperkalemia in the setting of acute renal failure or from other causes is another indication for alkalization, especially when dialysis is contraindicated or delayed. If the serum potassium level is above 7.0 mEq/liter or there are electrocardiographic changes of hyperkalemia, such as tall peaked T waves, prolonged PR interval, disappearance of the P wave, or widened QRS, it is prudent to institute treatment. For mild cases where peaking of the T wave is the only abnormality, potassium restriction and possibly Kayexalate enemas are indicated. In more extreme cases where cardiac function is threatened, intravenous calcium, hypertonic glucose, and sodium bicarbonate can be given whether or not the patient is acidotic. It should be given as a bolus dose of 50 mEq IV rapidly, followed by an infusion of 1 to 2 mEq/kg $NaHCO_3$ in 500 to 1000 ml D_5W while monitoring the electrocardiogram (see Chap. 5).

Renal Tubular Acidosis

Patients with renal tubular acidosis often require life-long treatment with alkali to prevent disabling osteomalacia. This can be given as oral bicarbonate or sodium citrate in the form of Shohl's solution. The occasional patient with distal renal tubular acidosis may become profoundly acidotic and require intravenous bicarbonate replacement to bring the arterial pH to above 7.1 and the serum bicarbonate to between 5 and 8 mEq/liter. Dosage is calculated according to the formula in the drug treatment flow sheet.

Ethylene Glycol/Methanol Ingestion

Ethylene glycol and methanol poisoning produce a metabolic acidosis that requires treatment as part of a regimen that also includes the administration of ethyl alcohol and hemodialysis. In contrast to other causes of metabolic acidosis, vigorous efforts to improve the profound pH depression often seen in these cases have been shown to improve outcome. The dose of sodium bicarbonate can be approximated assuming a desired serum bicarbonate level of 5 to 8 mEq/liter (refer to the drug treatment flow sheet). The pH and serum bicarbonate levels should be rechecked after the initial infusion is complete and additional doses administered to maintain a pH of 7.1 to 7.2.

In ethylene glycol poisoning, administration of supplemental calcium should be considered because calcium is being utilized by the precipitation of calcium oxalate as one of the major toxic manifestations of this poisoning. Correction of the acidosis will further decrease the serum level of ionized calcium and may precipitate tetany. From 10 to 30 ml of 10% calcium gluconate should be given intravenously slowly while the patient is under cardiac monitoring. Calcium salts and sodium bicarbonate are not compatible in solution and should be given in separate intravenous lines.

Salicylate Overdose

Unlike other causes of metabolic acidosis in which care is taken to acutely correct the pH only partially, the pH in acidosis of severe salicylate ingestion should be corrected into the normal range. In fact, moderate degrees of alkalosis are acceptable in an effort to produce an alkaline diuresis. Any degree of acidosis is detrimental because it promotes the shift of salicylate from the plasma into the brain and other tissues. Alkaline diuresis favors the elimination of salicylate in the urine and substantially decreases its half-life.

If the patient is acidotic on presentation, the dose of sodium bicarbonate can be estimated assuming a desired serum level of 24 mEq/liter (see drug treatment flow sheet). One-half of that dose should be delivered over 1 to 2 hours. The arterial pH and HCO_3^- level should then be rechecked and the dose recalculated.

If the patient has a normal pH or is mildly alkalotic on presentation, the physician should attempt to bring the pH of the urine to 7.5 to 8 as outlined in the drug treatment flow sheet on urinary alkalization. These patients are often dehydrated and usually require large volumes of fluid to maintain renal perfusion and a brisk diuresis. In the event of supervening renal failure or, less commonly, heart failure, in which fluid and sodium may need to be restricted, hemodialysis or peritoneal dialysis would be the preferred methods of treatment. Maintaining a urine pH of 7.5 to 8 without producing a serious metabolic alkalosis may be difficult but should be attempted.

Metabolic Alkalosis

Metabolic alkalosis has recently been shown to be the most common perturbation of acid–base physiology in hospitalized patients. Combined metabolic and respiratory alkalosis and metabolic alkalosis alone were found frequently in severely ill or injured patients on a shock and trauma unit and were found to correlate with a poor outcome.

Interestingly, the causes of metabolic alkalosis are for the most part iatrogenic. Nasogastric suctioning, prolonged diuretic therapy, excessive administration of bicarbonate or other alkali, fluid and salt restriction, and prolonged use of corticosteroids can all initiate or help sustain a metabolic alkalosis. Under normal conditions the kidney resorbs 100% of filtered bicarbonate. It is effectively able to deal with an alkali load and hydrogen ion deficits by decreasing the resorption of bicarbonate, thus enhancing its excretion and returning the pH to normal.

Bicarbonate excretion is depressed in the presence of contraction of effective arterial blood volume, hypochloremia, hypokalemia, and mineralocorticoid excess. Therefore, the presence of any of these conditions may prevent the kidney from correcting an alkalemic insult.

Diagnosis

Metabolic alkalosis is usually discovered serendipitously when arterial blood gas analysis or serum electrolyte determinations are ordered for other reasons. The characteristic pattern is elevation of the pH, pCO_3, and serum bicarbonate level. The serum chloride level is usually low. Combined metabolic alkalosis and respiratory acidosis are not uncommon in patients with chronic obstructive pulmonary disease who are being treated with diuretics.

It is useful to consider the causes of metabolic alkalosis as being either saline responsive or saline resistant (Table 15–2). Saline-responsive conditions are associated with volume depletion and chloride depletion as mechanisms that prevent the kidney from excreting the excess bicarbonate. In these conditions, even if the initiating insult is corrected, the metabolic alkakosis may not resolve until the volume and chloride deficits are restored.

The causes of saline-unresponsive metabolic alkalosis are listed in Table 15–2. Some experts believe that severe potassium deficiency and severe magnesium deficiency can cause metabolic alkalosis of the saline-unresponsive type. The treatment of these disorders is to correct the underlying condition.

Indications for Treatment

What degree of metabolic alkalosis should be treated is difficult to define. It should definitely be treated aggressively when it results in an adverse clinical consequence such as hypoventilation, tetany, or central nervous system abnormalities, or when the ar-

TABLE 15–2. Causes of Metabolic Alkalosis

Saline Responsive	Saline Resistant
Prolonged severe vomiting	Hyperaldosteronism
Nasogastric suctioning	Cushing's syndrome
Diuretics	Bartter's syndrome
Milk–alkali syndrome	Exogenous steroids
Post-hypercapnea	
Overshoot alkalosis	

terial pH exceeds 7.6. The obvious extension of this is that mild abnormalities should be recognized and controlled in order to avoid progression.

Although it has been widely held that respiratory compensation for a metabolic alkalosis is quite limited, there are abundant reports in the medical literature of respiratory failure caused by hypoventilation secondary to metabolic alkalosis. On average, one can expect a rise in $paCO_2$ of 0.7 torr for each mEq/liter increase in the serum bicarbonate level. This may be especially significant in patients with underlying lung disease in whom the $paCO_2$ is already somewhat elevated and in whom oxygen saturation is tenuous. Respiratory failure has been reported as a complication of severe metabolic alkalosis even in patients with normal pulmonary function, and it has been corrected by treatment of the alkalotic state.

The central nervous system is sensitive to elevations in arterial pH. The manifestations range from lethargy and coma to agitation and grand mal seizures. The cause of this central nervous system dysfunction is not completely clear but may be due in part to impaired oxygen delivery to the brain. Alkalosis has a deleterious effect on the oxyhemoglobin dissociation curve, causes cerebral vasoconstriction, and is associated with volume contraction, all of which may contribute to the central nervous system dysfunction.

Alkalosis itself and some of the causes of metabolic alkalosis can result in hypokalemia. Patients who are alkalotic and receiving digitalis preparations are more prone to cardiac dysrhythmias. Muscle twitching and tetany can be seen in metabolic alkalosis and may be caused by changes in ionized calcium or seen in association with magnesium deficiency. (See box.)

Discussion

When mild metabolic alkalosis is recognized, it is important to search for ways to prevent progression to more serious alkalemia. If nasogastric suctioning cannot be discontinued, it may be helpful to institute an H_2 blocker to decrease hydrochloric acid secretion. Make sure that the patient is getting adequate volume and chloride to replace losses. The use of vasodilators in patients

---

DRUG TREATMENT: METABOLIC ALKALOSIS UNRESPONSIVE TO VOLUME AND CHLORIDE REPLACEMENT

First-Line Drug

Hydrochloric Acid

Preparation	100–300 mEq/liter D_5W (0.1–0.3 N)
Initial Dose	$$mEq\ HCl = \frac{(Actual\ HCO_3^- - 24\ (weight[kg] \times 0.5\ liter/kg)}{2}$$ Injected into a central vein over 12 hours
Repeat Dose	Repeat measurement of pH and HCO_3^-. Recalculate as above.
End-Point	pH <7.5 or relief of symptoms

Second-Line Drug

Acetazolamide

Preparation	250-mg tablets 500-mg injection
Initial Dose	250–500 mg IV or PO
Repeat Dose	Recheck pH and pCO_2 in 8 hours.
End-Point	pH <7.50 or relief of symptoms

with congestive heart failure or hypertension may allow the physician to discontinue or reduce the dose of diuretic without causing decompensation. Replacement of potassium and magnesium is indicated if serum levels of these ions are deficient. Sources of exogenous alkali (e.g., excessive antacid ingestion) should be sought and controlled. Rapid correction of respiratory acidosis in the course of mechanical ventilation should be avoided. Corticosteroids should be tapered where possible.

Intravenous hydochloric acid is the treatment of choice for severe complicated metabolic alkalosis unresponsive to volume and chloride replacement with sodium chloride and where magnesium and potassium deficiencies have been corrected. A 0.2% normal solution is prepared by adding 200 ml of 1N HCl to 800 ml of D_5W or 0.9% NaCl through a 0.22-nm filter. Glass containers should be used, and plastic intravenous tubing should be changed every 12 hours. The solution must be delivered into a carefully placed central venous catheter to prevent phlebitis and sloughing or inadvertent infusion into the mediastinum. The maximum rate of infusion suggested by Worthley is 0.2 mEq/kg/hour. The total calculated dose is usually infused over 24 hours; however, the arterial pH and HCO_3^- level should be reevaluated every 6 to 12 hours.

Acetazolamide is a carbonic anhidrase inhibitor that decreases the rate of aqueous humor formation and causes a sodium bicarbonate diuresis. It is most useful for the treatment of glaucoma and has been effective in the prevention of acute high-altitude sickness, in which the induction of acute metabolic acidosis stimulates respiration and minimizes hypoxemia. It has been suggested for severe refractory metabolic alkalosis when chronic obstructive pulmonary disease predisposes to respiratory failure and congestive heart failure precludes vigorous sodium chloride replacement. In these delicate cases, volume repletion should probably be done with invasive monitoring. However, if this approach is unsuccessful, one can consider acetazolamide in a dose of 250 to 500 mg IV or PO every 8 hours as needed, with careful monitoring of the pH and $paCO_2$. Patients who are unable to increase their minute ventilation are prone to develop metabolic acidosis in addition to their preexisting respiratory acidosis. Acetazolamide is also known to cause a potassium diuresis and

should be given with supplemental potassium.

SPECIFIC AGENTS

Acetazolamide Sodium

Acetazolamide is a sulfonamide that inhibits the enzyme carbonic anhydrase.

Pharmacology

Distribution

Acetazolamide is distributed throughout body tissues and crosses the placenta.

Elimination

The drug is excreted unchanged by the kidneys. About 90% of the administered dose is eliminated within 24 hours.

Actions

Acetazolamide causes a bicarbonate, water, sodium, and potassium diuresis. An increase in minute ventilation results from the drop in bicarbonate. It decreases aqueous humor formation and cerebrospinal fluid formation.

Indications

Glaucoma
Prophylaxis of high-altitude sickness
Treatment of metabolic alkalosis complicated by hypoventilation where vigorous sodium chloride replacement is contraindicated due to sodium and fluid retention
Increased intracranial pressure

Cautions

Hepatic disease—contraindicated
Severe renal disease—contraindicated
Diabetes mellitus—drug may exacerbate hyperglycemia.
Use in pregnancy—acetazolomide is teratogenic in laboratory animals. It should not be administered in the first trimester unless the benefits outweigh calculated risk.

Onset and Duration of Action

See Drug Treatment: Metabolic Alkalosis.
Effects at the nephron begin within 30 minutes, peak at approximately 2 hours, and persist for up to 12 hours.

Toxicity

Drug Interactions

Lithium carbonate	Urinary alkalization may decrease half-life.
Salicylate	
Phenobarbital	
Amphetamine	Urinary alkalization may increase half-life.
Quinidine	
Tricyclic antidepressants	
Thiazide diuretics	May augment effect
Digitalis	May predispose to digitalis toxicity because of potassium depletion, especially if patient is also taking a diuretic, amphotericin-B, or corticosteroids

Adverse Effects

The side effects described with the use of acetazolamide include

Nausea, vomiting, diarrhea, and altered taste and smell

Drowsiness, headache, irritability, confusion, depression, dizziness, seizures, paresthesias, weakness, and tremor

Hypersensitivity reactions

Aplastic anemia, thrombocytopenia, and leukopenia

Renal calculi

Hypokalemia, hypoglycemia, and metabolic acidosis

Hepatic coma

Treatment of Toxicity

Mild side effects like nausea may respond to a decrease in the dose. More severe reactions including hypersensitivity require discontinuation of the drug.

Hydrochloric Acid

Pharmacology

Distribution

The estimated chloride space is 200 ml/kg.

Elimination

Hydrochloric acid is eliminated via the body buffer system and the kidneys.

Actions

This acid directly provides hydrogen and chloride and lowers the pH of the blood.

Indications

Hydrochloric acid is indicated for severe complicated metabolic alkalosis unresponsive to volume, chloride, and potassium replacement.

Cautions

Hydrochloric acid must be prepared in a 0.1 to 0.3 normal solution in the pharmacy using a 0.22-nm filter. It must be delivered via a carefully placed central venous line.

Studies of the use of this drug in pregnancy have not been done. Risk–benefit considerations must dictate treatment.

Onset and Duration of Action

See Drug Treatment: Metabolic Alkalosis.

Toxicity

Adverse Effects

Too vigorous admistration may result in metabolic acidosis. The infusion may cause vascular damage or tissue necrosis.

Treatment of Toxicity

If extravasation occurs, stop the infusion immediately and restart the central venous line at another site. Metabolic acidosis should be avoided by careful dosing according to serum bicarbonate or chloride levels and by frequent monitoring during the infusion period.

Sodium Bicarbonate

Pharmacology

Distribution

Sodium bicarbonate dissociates to provide sodium and bicarbonate ions. The volume of distribution is approximately 500 ml/kg.

Elimination

In the healthy patient with normal renal function, nearly all of the filtered bicarbonate is reabsorbed. Excess bicarbonate is excreted by the kidneys.

Actions

Sodium bicarbonate is an alkalizing agent. It causes an increase in pH in blood and urine and potassium to shift intracellularly.

Indications

Sodium bicarbonate is indicated for the treatment of severe metabolic acidosis. It can be used to akalize the urine for the purpose of increasing the excretion of weak acids. It is also useful in the treatment of life-threatening hyperkalemia and in cardiotoxicity from tricyclic antidepressant overdose.

Cautions

Congestive heart failure—cautious administration is indicated to minimize further fluid and solute load. Consider concomitant use of diuretics, vasodilators, and invasive monitoring if sodium bicarbonate must be given to these patients.

Oliguria, anuria—extreme caution is advised to avoid fluid and sodium overload.

Hypokalemia—alkalization exacerbates hypokalemia because of intracellular ion shifts. It is necessary to correct hypokalemia before or during alkalization.

Use in pregnancy—Category C. Studies to define risk of hypertonic sodium bicarbonate therapy in pregnancy have not been done. Risk–benefit must be evaluated.

Use in pediatrics—rapid injection of hypertonic sodium bicarbonate may cause hypernatremia and possibly intracranial hemorrhage in children under 2 years of age. The rate of administration should not exceed 8 mEq/kg/day.

Onset and Duration of Action

See Drug Treatment: Metabolic Acidosis.

Toxicity

Drug Interactions

Corticosteroids	May enhance fluid overload
Calcium salts	May precipitate if administered in same intravenous line
Quinidine	Bicarbonate-induced
Amphetamine	urinary alkalization
Ephedrine	may increase half-life.
Tetracycline	Urinary alkalization may
Salicylate	decrease half-life.

Adverse Effects

Extravasation of hypertonic solutions may cause tissue damage. Overshoot alkalosis may adversely affect ventilation and oxygen delivery to the tissues.

Treatment of Toxicity

If extravasation occurs, stop infusion immediately and restart the intravenous line at another site. Overshoot alkalosis is managed by stopping the infusion and allowing for renal bicarbonate excretion. Chloride deficits must be replaced for this to occur. Rarely, dialysis or acidification may be indicated.

Tromethamine (TRIS, THAM)

Pharmacology

Distribution

Tromethamine distributes both intracellularly and extracellularly. The ionized fraction, approximately 70% of the dose, distributes to the extracellular compartment, and approximately 30% of the administered dose, which represents the un-ionized fraction, is distributed intracellularly.

Elimination

The drug is excreted by the kidneys, 50 to 75% being eliminated in 24 hours.

Actions

Tromethamine is a direct hydrogen ion acceptor that increases the pH of the blood and the urine.

Indications

This agent appears to have no advantage over sodium bicarbonate in the management of severe metabolic acidosis or for urinary alkalization. Its use may be indicated in some cases where acidosis persists and sodium overload precludes further administration of sodium bicarbonate.

Cautions

Use in pregnancy—Category C. Safety has not been established.

Use in children—hepatic necrosis and hypoglycemia have been observed in newborns treated with tromethamine.

Uremia—contraindicated

Chronic respiratory acidosis—contraindicated

Drug must be administered into a large peripheral intravenous line or preferably into a well-placed central line.

Drug should not be given for longer than 1 day.

Onset and Duration of Action

See Drug Treatment: Metabolic Acidosis.

Toxicity

Adverse Effects

Highly alkaline pH may cause severe vascular reaction and necrosis. Extravasation may result in inflammation and sloughing of overlying skin. Hemorrhagic hepatic necrosis has occurred in newborns when a hypertonic solution of tromethamine with electrolytes was administered via the umbilical vein. Hypoglycemia may occur as a result of too large a dose or too rapid administration of the drug. Respiratory depression may occur especially in patients with chronic hypoventilation or in whom respiratory drive is depressed for other reasons. Hyperkalemia may occur in patients with decreased renal function.

Treatment of Toxicity

If perivascular infiltration occurs, discontinue the infusion immediately. Infiltration of the affected area with 1% procaine hydrochloride to which hyaluronidase has been added may be efficacious in minimizing tissue damage. Local infiltration of alpha-blocking agents such as phentolamine mesylate into vasospastic area has been recommended.

REFERENCES

Abouna GM, Veazy PR, Terry DB: Intravenous infusion of hydrochloric acid for treatment of severe metabolic alkalosis. Surgery 75(2): 194–202, 1974.

Albert MS, Dell RB, Winters RW: Quantitative displacement of acid-base equilibrium in metabolic acidosis. Ann Intern Med 66(2):312–321, 1967.

Anderson RJ, Potts DE, Gabow PA, et al: Unrecognized adult salicylate intoxication. Ann Intern Med 85:745–748, 1976.

Arieff AI, Leach W, Park R, Lazarowitz VC: Systemic effects of NaHCO$_3$ in experimental lactic acidosis in dogs. Am J Physiol 242:F586–591, 1982.

Assal J, Aoki TT, Manzano FM, Kozal GP: Metabolic effects of sodium bicarbonate in management of diabetic ketoacidosis. Diabetes 23(5):405–411, 1974.

Barton CH, Vaziri DV, Ness RL, et al: Cimetidine in the management of metabolic alkalosis induced by nasogastric drainage. Arch Surg 114:70–74, 1979.

Batlle DC, Sehy JT, Roseman MK: Clinical and pathophysiologic spectrum of acquired distal renal tubular acidosis. Kidney Int 20:389–396, 1981.

Bear R, Goldstein M, Phillipson E, et al: Effect of metabolic aklalosis on respiratory function in patients with chronic obstructive lung disease. Can Med Assoc J 117:900–903, 1977.

Bellingham AJ, Detter JC, Lenfant C: The role of hemoglobin affinity for oxygen and red-cell 2,3-diphosphoglycerate in the management of diabetic ketoacidosis. Association of American Physicians 83:113–120, 1970.

Bia M, Thier SO: Mixed acid base disturbances: A clinical approach. Med Clin North Am 65(2):347–361, 1981.

Bleich HL, Schwartz WB: Tris buffer (THAM): An appraisal of its physiologic effects and clinical usefulness. N Engl J Med 274(14):782–787, 1966.

Bloom WL: Fasting ketosis in obese men and women. J Lab Clin Med 59:605–612, 1962.

Brater DC, Morrelli HF: Arrhythmias. Acta Med Scand 647(Suppl):79–85, 1981.

Brenes LG, Brenes JN, Hernandez MM: Familial proximal renal tubular acidosis: A distinct clinical entity. Am J Med 63:244–252, 1977.

Brimioulle S, Vincent JL, Dufaye P, et al: Hydrochloric acid infusion for treatment of metabolic alkalosis: Effects on acid-base balance and oxygenation. Crit Care Med 13(9):738–742, 1985.

Bushinsky DA, Gennari FJ: Life-threatening hyperkalemia induced by arginine. Ann Intern Med 89(1):632, 1978.

Chew WB, Berger EH, Brines OA, Capron MJ: Alkali treatment of methyl alcohol poisoning. JAMA 130(2):61–64, 1946.

Cingolani HE, Faulkner SL, Mattiazzi AR, et al: Depression of human myocardial contractility with "respiratory" and "metabolic" acidosis. Surgery 77(3):427–432, 1975.

Cogan MG, Rector FC, Seldin DW: Acid–base disorders. In Brenner E, Rector FC Jr (eds): The Kidney. Philadelphia, WB Saunders, 1981, pp 841–907.

Cooperman MT, Davidoff F, Spark R, Pallotta J: Clinical studies of alcoholic ketoacidosis. Diabetes 23(5):433–439, 1974.

Croog SH, Levine S, Testa MA, et al: Effects of antihypertensive therapy on the quality of life. N Engl J Med 314(26):1657–1664, 1986.

Cumming G, Dukes DC, Widdowson G: Alkaline diuresis in treatment of aspirin poisoning. Br Med J 2:1033–1036, 1964.

Davies DG, Fitzgerald RS, Gurtner GH: Acid–base relationships between CSF and blood during acute metabolic acidosis. J Appl Physiol 34(2):243–248, 1973.

Davis PR, Burch RE: Pulmonary edema and salicylate intoxication (letter). Ann Intern Med 80(4):553–554, 1974.

De Graeff J, Struyvenberg A, Lameijer LDF: Role of chloride in hypokalemic alkalosis: Balance studies in man. Am J Med 37:778–788, 1964.

DiBona FJ, Kelsch RC: Severe uncompensated metabolic acidosis secondary to ammonium chloride loading. J Pediatr 91(2):263–265, 1977.

Done AK, Temple AR: Treatment of salicylate poisoning. Mod Treatment 8:528–551, 1971.

Douglas JB, Healy JK: Nephrotoxic effects of amphotericin B, including renal tubular acidosis. Am J Med 46:154–162, 1969.

Drug Information for the Health Care Provider. Rockville, MD, United States Pharmacopeal Convention, Inc., 1985

Duck SC, Weldon VV, Pagliara AS, Haymond MW: Cerebral edema complicating therapy for diabetic ketoacidosis. Diabetes 25(2):111–115, 1976.

Dukes DC, Blainey JD, Cumming G, Widdowson G: Treatment of severe aspirin poisoning. Lancet 2:329–331, 1963.

Editorial: Diabetic ketoacidosis—The bicarbonate controversy. J Pediatr 87(1):156–159, 1975.

Editorial: Lactate versus bicarbonate. Am J Med 32(6):831–832, 1962.

Editorial: Sodium bicarbonate in cardiac arrest. Lancet 1:946–947, 1976.

Editorial: Lactic acidosis and a possible new treatment. N Engl J Med 298:564–566, 1978.

Editorial Review: The maintenance of metabolic alkalosis: Factors which decrease bicarbonate excretion. Kidney Int 25:357–361, 1984.

Eichenholz A, Mulhausen RO, Redleaf PS: Nature of acid–base disturbance in salicylate intoxication. Metabolism 12(2):164–175, 1963.

Elkinton JR: Renal acidosis: Diagnosis and treatment. Med Clin North Am 47:935–958, 1963.

Epstein FB, Eilers MA. Poisoning. In Rosen P, et al (eds): Emergency Medicine Concepts and Clinical Practice. St Louis, CV Mosby, 1988.

Erlanson P, Fritz H, Kagstam KE, et al: Severe methanol intoxication. Acta Med Scand 177(4):393–408, 1965.

Fencl V, Vale JR, Broch JA: Respiration and cerebral blood flow in metabolic acidosis and alkalosis in humans. J Appl Physiol 27(1):67–76, 1969.

Frommer JP, Ayus JC: Acute ethylene glycol intoxication. Am J Nephrol 2:1–5, 1982.

Fulop M: Serum potassium in lactic acidosis and ketoacidosis. N Engl J Med 300(19):1087–1089, 1979.

Fulop M, Hoberman HD: Alcoholic ketosis. Diabetes 24(9):785–790, 1975.

Gabow PA, Moore S, Schrier RW: Spironolactone-induced hyperchloremic acidosis in cirrhosis. Ann Intern Med 90:338–340, 1979.

Garella S, Chang BS, Kahn SI: Dilution acidosis and contraction alkalosis: Review of a concept (editorial review). Kidney Int 8:279–283, 1975.

Garella S, Chazan JA, Cohen JJ: Saline-resistant metabolic alkalosis or "chloride-wasting nephropathy." Ann Intern Med 73:31–38, 1970.

Garella S, Dana CL, Chazan JA: Severity of metabolic acidosis as a determinant of bicarbonate requirements. N Engl J Med 289(3):121–126, 1973.

Gilman AG, Goodman LS, Gilman A: The Pharmacologic Basis of Therapeutics. New York, Macmillan, 1980.

Golding PL: Renal tubular acidosis in chronic liver disease. Postgrad Med J 51:550–556, 1975.

Gonda A, Gault H, Churchill D, Hollomby D: Hemodialysis for methanol intoxication. Am J Med 64:749–757, 1978.

Grace WJ, Barr DP: Complications of alkalosis. Am J Med 4:331–337, 1948.

Guisado R, Arieff AI: Neurologic manifestations of diabetic comas: Correlation with biochemical alterations in the brain. Metabolism 24(4):665–679, 1975.

Györy AZ, Stewart JH, George CRP, et al: Renal tubular acidosis, acidosis due to hyperkalaemia, hypercalcaemia, disordered citrate metabolism and other tubular dysfunctions following human renal transplantation. Q J Med 38(15):231–254, 1969.

Halperin ML: Lactic acidosis and ketoacidosis: Biochemical and clinical implications. Can Med Assoc J 116:1034–1038, 1977.

Hertz P, Richardson JA: Arginine-induced hyperkalemia. Arch Intern Med 130:778–784, 1972.

Hill JB: Experimental salicylate poisoning: Observations on the effects of altering blood pH on tissue and plasma salicylate concentrations. Pediatrics 47(4):658–664, 1971.

Hilton JG, Goodbody MF, Kruesi OR: Effect of prolonged administration of ammonium chloride on the blood acid–base equilibrium of geriatric subjects. J Am Geriatr Soc 3:697–703, 1955.

Hodgkin JE, Soeprono FF, Chan DM: Incidence of metabolic alkalemia in hospitalized patients. Crit Care Med 8(12):725–728, 1980.

Huff BB (ed): Physicians Desk Reference. Oradell, NJ, Medical Economics, 1988.

Hrnicek G, Skelton J, Miller WC: Pulmonary edema and salicylate intoxication. JAMA 230(6):866–867, 1974.

Huth EJ, Mayock RI, Kerr RM: Hyperthyroidism associated with renal tubular acidosis: Discussion of possible relationship. Am J Med 26:818–826, 1959.

Irvine ROH, Dow J: Sodium bicarbonate, sodium lactate and Tris in the treatment of metabolic acidosis: Effects on intracellular pH and electrolyte content of voluntary muscle. Metabolism 15:1011–1019, 1966.

Jacobsen D, Jansen H, Wiik-Larsen E, et al: Studies on methanol poisoning. Acta Med Scand 212:5–10, 1982.

Jacobsen D, Ostby N, Bredesen JE: Studies on ethylene glycol poisoning. Acta Med Scand 212:11–15, 1982.

James JA, Kimbell L, Reed WT: Experimental salicylate intoxication: I. Comparison of exchange transfusion, intermittent peritoneal lavage, and hemodialysis as means for removing salicylate. Pediatrics 29:442–447, 1962.

Jarboe TM, Penman RW, Luke RG: Ventilatory failure due to metabolic alkalosis. Chest 61(2):61S–63S, 1972.

Kassirer JP: Serious acid–base disorders. N Engl J Med 291:773–776, 1974.

Kassirer JP, Berkman PM, Lawrenz DR, Schwartz WB: Critical role of chloride in the correction of hypokalemic alkalosis in man. Am J Med 38:172–189, 1965.

Kassirer JP, London AM, Goldman DM, Schwartz WB: On the pathogenesis of metabolic alkalosis in hyperaldosteronism. Am J Med 49:306–314, 1970.

Kassirer JP, Schwartz WB: Correction of metabolic alkalosis in man without repair of potassium deficiency: A re-evaluation of the role of potassium. Am J Med 40:19–25, 1966.

Kastrup EK: Drug Facts and Comparisons. Philadelphia, JB Lippincott, 1988.

Katzung BG: Basic and Clinical Pharmacology. Norwalk, CT, Appleton and Lange, 1989.

Kheirbek AO, Ing, TS, Viol GW, et al: Treatment of metabolic alkalosis with hemofiltration in patients with renal insufficiency. Nephron 24:91–92, 1979.

Knutsen OH: New method for administration of hydrochloric acid in metabolic alkalosis. Lancet April:953–956, 1983.

Kreisberg RA: Lactate homeostasis and lactic acidosis. Ann Intern Med 92(Part 1):227–237, 1980.

Lawson AAH, Proudfoot AT, Brown SS, et al: Forced diuresis in the treatment of acute salicylate poisoning in adults. Q J Med 38(149):31–48, 1969.

Levinsky NG: Acidosis and alkalosis. In Braunwald E, et al (eds): Harrison's Principles of Internal Medicine. New York, McGraw-Hill, 1987.

Lifschitz MY, Brasch R, Cuomo AJ, Menn SJ: Marked hypercapnia secondary to severe metabolic alkalosis. Ann Intern Med 77:405–409, 1972.

Madias NE, Ayus JC, Adrogué HJ: Increased anion gap in metabolic alkalosis: The role of plasma-protein equivalency. N Engl J Med 300(25):1421–1423, 1979.

Marton WJ, Matzke GR: Treating Severe Metabolic Alkalosis. Clinic Pharmacol 1:42–47, 1982.

Massry SG, Preuss HG, Maher JF, Schreiner GE: Renal tubular acidosis after cadaver kidney homotransplantation: Studies on mechanism. Am J Med 42:284–292, 1967.

McCoy HG, Cipolle RJ, Ehlers SM, et al: Severe methanol poisoning: Application of a pharmacokinetic model for ethanol therapy and hemodialysis. Am J Med 67:804–807, 1979.

McEvoy GK: Drug Information 88. Bethesda, MD, American Society of Hospital Pharmacists, 1988.

Mennen M, Slovis CM: Severe metabolic alkalosis in the emergency department. Ann Emerg Med 17(4):354–357, 1988.

Miller PD, Berns AS: Acute metabolic alkalosis perpetuating hypercarbia: A role for acetazolamide in chronic obstructive pulmonary disease. JAMA 238(22):2400–2401, 1977.

Morgan AG, Polak A: Acetazolamide and sodium bicarbonate in treatment of salicylate poisoning in adults. Br Med J 1:16–19, 1969.

Moriarty RW, McDonald RH: Spectrum of ethylene glycol poisoning. Clin Tox 7(6):583–596, 1974.

Morris RC: Renal tubular acidosis (editorial). N Engl J Med 304:418–420, 1981.

Narins RG, Emmett M: Simple and mixed acid–base disorders: A practical approach. Medicine 59:161–187, 1980.

Oh MS, Carroll HJ: Anion Gap. N Engl J Med 297(15):814–817, 1977.

Oliva PB: Severe alveolar hypoventilation in a patient with metabolic alkalosis. Am J Med 52:817–821, 1972.

Parry MF, Wallach R: Ethylene glycol poisoning. Am J Med 57:143–150, 1974.

Peterson CD, Collins AJ, Himes JM, et al: Ethylene glycol poisoning. N Engl J Med 304(1):21–23, 1981.

Poppell JW, Vanamee P, Roberts KE, Randall HT; Effect of ventilatory insufficiency on respiratory compensations in metabolic acidosis and alkalosis. J Lab Clin Med 47(6):885–890, 1956.

Posner JB, Plum F: Spinal-fluid pH and neurologic symptoms in systemic acidosis. N Engl J Med 277:605–613, 1967.

Relman AS: Metabolic consequences of acid–base disorders. Kidney Int 1:347–359, 1972.

Rothe KF, Heisler N: Correction of metabolic alkalosis by HCl and acetazolamide: Effects on extracellular and intracellular acid–base status in rats in vivo. Acta Anaesthesiol Scand 30:566–570, 1986.

Rowlands BJ, Tindall SF, Elliott DJ: The use of dilute hydrochloric acid and cimetidine to reverse severe metabolic alkalosis. Postgrad Med J 54:118–123, 1978.

Sanders AB, Otto CW, Kern KB, et al: Acid–base balance in a canine model of cardiac arrest. Ann Emerg Med 17(7):667–671, 1988.

Seldin DW: Metabolic alkalosis. In Brenner E, Rector FC Jr (eds): The Kidney. Philadelphia, WB Saunders, 1981, pp 661–702.

Stacpoole PW, Harman EM, Curry SH, et al: Treatment of lactic acidosis with dichloroacetate. N Engl J Med 309:390–396, 1983.

Taradash MR, Jacobson LB: Vasodilator therapy of idiopathic lactic acidosis. N Engl J Med 293:468–471, 1975.

Unger A, Rhenman B, Fuller JK, et al: Treatment of severe metabolic alkalosis in a neonate with hydrochloric acid infusion. Clin Pediatr 24:444–446, 1985.

van Goidsenhoven GM-T, Gray OV, Price AV, Sanderson PH: The effect of prolonged administration of large doses of sodium bicarbonate in Man. Clin Sci 13:383–401, 1954.

Vaziri ND, Ness R, Wellikson L, et al: Bicarbonate-buffered peritoneal dialysis: An effective adjunct in the treatment of lactic acidosis. Am J Med 67:392–396, 1979.

Wiklund L, Öquist L, Skoog G, et al: Clinical buffering of metabolic acidosis: Problems and a solution. Resuscitation 12:279–293, 1985.

Wilson RF, Gibson D, Percinel AK, et al: Severe alkalosis in critically ill surgical patients. Arch Surg 105:197–203, 1972.

Worthley LIG: Intravenous hydrochloric acid in patients with metabolic alkalosis and hypercapnia. Arch Surg 121:1195–1198, 1986.

Worthley LIG: The rational use of I.V. hydrochloric acid in the treatment of metabolic alkalosis. Br J Anaesth 49:811–817, 1977.

CHAPTER 16

Antidotes

LOUIS J. LING, M.D.

INTRODUCTION

Gastric decontamination and good supportive care are the primary means of managing poisoned and overdosed patients, and these measures suffice in the vast majority of cases. A few poisons, however, have very specific antidotal therapy that can dramatically reduce their toxicity and reverse otherwise fatal exposures. Since poisonings with such agents are rare, it is not necessary to commit the details of each antidote to memory; however, one should be able to recognize such poisonings so that the antidotes can be utilized when necessary. Once the specific agent involved in a poisoning has been recognized, the proper references can be consulted to determine the need for antidotes, the method of using the antidotes, and the anticipated side effects. Regional poison centers may have more experience and may be a helpful resource in these situations.

Because antidotes are used relatively infrequently, much of the literature is based on case reports and small series with recommendations based on somewhat limited experience. As a result, there are often variations in recommended doses. The most widely used regimens are discussed in this chapter.

CONDITIONS

Iron Poisoning

Diagnosis

Iron intoxication is usually diagnosed by the history but should be suspected in patients with abdominal pain, bloody diarrhea, and access to iron supplements (e.g., pregnant women, patients being treated for anemia, and children receiving vitamin supplements). The classic course of iron toxicity includes five stages: (1) gastrointestinal irritation, which can occur within 30 minutes of a serious ingestion; (2) improvement and quiescence occurring 6 to 24 hours after ingestion; (3) shock; (4) hepatic necrosis; and (5) gastric scarring appearing 2 to 6 weeks later.

Indications for Treatment

An estimate of the amount of elemental iron ingested can be calculated if the iron content of the involved medication is known. There is a wide variation in the iron content of different preparations, as shown in Table 16–1.

In general, ingestion of 10 to 20 mg/kg of elemental iron results in minimal irritative toxicity and will not require treatment. As noted in Figure 16–1, ingestion of greater

TABLE 16–1. Iron Content of Some Different Iron Supplements

Product Name	Iron Salt	Elemental Iron
Bugs Bunny Plus Iron		15 mg
C-Ron	Ferrous fumarate, 200 mg	66 mg
C-Ron Freckles	Ferrous fumarate, 100 mg	33 mg
Centrum Multiple Vitamins		27 mg
Centrum Jr.		18 mg
Chocks Bugs Bunny Plus Iron		15 mg
Feosol Elixir	Ferrous sulfate	44 mg/5 ml
Feosol Spansules	Ferrous sulfate, 150 mg	47 mg
Feosol Tablets	Ferrous sulfate, 325 mg	65 mg
Fergon Capsules	Ferrous gluconate, 435 mg	50 mg
Fergon Elixir	Ferrous gluconate, 300 mg/5 ml	33 mg/5 ml
Fergon Tablets	Ferrous gluconate, 320 mg	36 mg
Fer-In-Sol Capsules	Ferrous sulfate, 190 mg	60 mg
Fer-In-Sol Drops		15 mg/0.6 ml
Fer-In-Sol Syrup	Ferrous sulfate, 90 mg	18 mg/5 ml
Ferro-Sequels	Ferrous fumarate, 150 mg	50 mg
Ferrous fumarate, 300 mg		100 mg
Ferrous gluconate, 325 mg		40 mg
Ferrous sulfate, 325 mg		65 mg
Filibon Forte Prenatal		45 mg
Flintstones Chewable Plus Iron		15 mg
Flintstones Plus Iron		4 mg
Geritol Liquid	Ferric ammonium citrate, 100 mg/30 ml	571 mg/30 ml
Geritol Tablets		50 mg
Myadec		20 mg
Natabec	Ferrous sulfate, 150 mg	30 mg
Natalins Rx (Fumerate)		60 mg
Norlac		60 mg
One-A-Day Plus Iron		13 mg
One-A-Day Plus Minerals		18 mg
Os-Cal Forte		5 mg
Os-Cal Plus		16.6 mg
Pac-Man Children's Chewables With Iron		18 mg
Pac-Man Pre-Schooler's Vitamins Plus Iron		10 mg
Poly-Vi-Flor Drops With Iron (sulfate)		10 mg/ml
Poly-Vi-Flor Tablets With Iron (fumarate)		12 mg
Poly-Vi-Sol Drops With Iron (sulfate)		10 mg/ml
Poly-Vi-Sol With Iron, Chewable Tablets		12 mg
Poly-Vi-Sol With Iron Drops		10 mg/ml
Spiderman Vitamins With Iron		18 mg
Stresstabs 600 With Iron		27 mg
Stuart Formula Tablets (fumarate)		18 mg
Stuart Prenatal		60 mg
Stuartinic Tablets (fumarate)		100 mg
Stuartnatal 1 + 1		65 mg
Theragran-M Tablets (carbonate)		12 mg
Theragran-M		12 mg
Tri-Vi-Sol Drops With Iron (Sulfate)		10 mg/ml
Tri-Vi-Sol With Iron Drops		10 mg/ml
Unicap M Plus Iron (Sulfate)		10 mg
Unicap Plus Iron (Sulfate)		18 mg

than 35 mg/kg requires a serum iron level determination to predict the need for chelation. Serum iron levels should be obtained 4 to 6 hours after ingestion. Levels obtained later may not reflect the peak serum level since the iron may have already distributed into the body tissue. In general, if the serum iron level is lower than 300 μg/dl, the risk for toxicity is low, and if the level is greater than 500 μg/dl, the patient should receive chela-

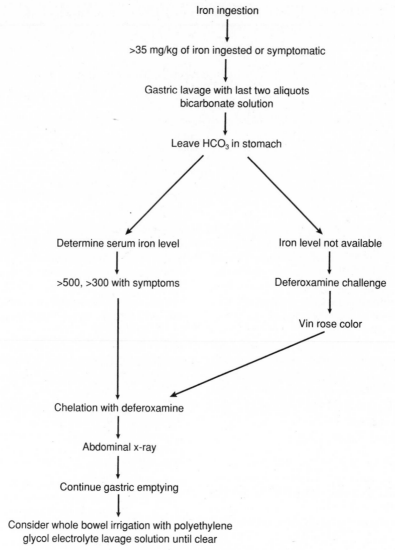

FIGURE 16–1. Treatment algorithm: iron ingestion.

tion therapy. Patients with serum levels between 300 and 500 $\mu g/dl$ may have mild toxicity and should have treatment if symptoms are present.

If a serum iron level is not immediately available, a deferoxamine challenge test should be performed. The patient is given 50 mg/kg of deferoxamine intramuscularly, and if free iron is available in the serum, it binds to the deferoxamine and within 4 hours is excreted in the urine, where it appears as a vin rose color. Since the color may be very faint, the urine should be examined against a white background in good lighting. A positive test indicates the presence of free iron and the need for continued chelation. (See box.)

Discussion

Gastric emptying with gastric lavage should be performed with a large gastric tube and fundal massage to attempt to break up any iron tablet bezoars. The last one or two aliquots of lavage fluid should be with 3% sodium bicarbonate, and then 100 ml of the sodium bicarbonate solution should be left in the stomach. Activated charcoal does not effectively adsorb iron and should not be used. Abdominal radiographs can confirm the presence of intact iron tablets and the need for further gastric decontamination. Whole bowel irrigation with isotonic solutions such as polyethylene glycol may be useful in cleansing the bowel of remaining

---

DRUG TREATMENT: IRON POISONING

First-Line Drug

Deferoxamine

Initial Dose 15 mg/kg/hour IV until clinical improvement
90 mg/kg IM, up to 2 g maximum

Repeat Dose 5–10 mg/kg/hour IV, up to 6 g/24 hours maximim
90 mg/kg IM, up to 2 g every 8 hours

End-Point When vin rose color disappears from the urine

---

intact tablets. Gastrotomy has been done in rare instances when a fatal amount of iron remains and other methods of gastric emptying are unsuccessful. Intramuscular deferoxamine should be avoided when hypotension decreases muscle perfusion and prevents distribution of the drug. If deferoxamine therapy is started, it is continued until the vin rose color is cleared from the urine. Although there is still a small amount of ferrioxamine in the clear urine, most experts believe that therapy is adequate at that point.

Heavy Metal Poisoning

Diagnosis

Heavy metals have no known physiologic activity in humans; however, with the advent of the industrial age, all inhabitants of developed countries have measurable serum levels of heavy metals. The diagnosis of heavy metal poisoning is often considered only after a careful history inquiring into the pa-

tient's occupation, hobbies, and other possible sources of heavy metal exposure. Typical symptoms include nausea, vomiting, diarrhea, gastrointestinal hemorrhage caused by the caustic nature of the metals, and a metallic taste in the mouth. Central and peripheral neurologic symptoms may be present. There are sources of high-risk exposure for each metal (Table 16–2) and a variety of symptoms (Table 16–3). Exposure can be

TABLE 16–2. Sources of Exposure to Common Heavy Metals

Common Heavy Metals	Some Sources of Exposure
Arsenic	Ant killer, pesticide, marine paints
Cadmium	Solder, zinc and lead smelting, alkaline batteries
Lead	Gasoline, paint, ceramic glazes, batteries, herbal medications, bullets, solder
Mercury	Coal and fuel production and burning, seafood, felt-making, disk batteries, scientific instruments
Zinc	Soldering flux, dental cement, oil refining, taxidermy

TABLE 16–3. Symptoms of Heavy Metal Poisoning

Common Heavy Metal	Specific Symptoms
Arsenic	Acute: garlic odor of breath, gastrointestinal symptoms, shock, headache, late peripheral neuropathy, hair loss, high body temperature, seizures Chronic: gastrointestinal symptoms, hyperpigmentation, hyperkeratosis, sensory neuropathy, hepatomegaly, edema, mucous membrane irritation, anemia
Cadmium	Acute: flu-like symptoms, pulmonary edema, proteinuria, gastrointestinal symptoms
Lead	Acute: constipation, colic, encephalopathy, behavioral abnormalities Chronic: gastrointestinal symtoms, motor neuropathy, fatigue, arthralgias
Mercury	Acute: gastrointestinal symptoms, mucous membrane irritation, renal failure Chronic: mucous membrane irritation, tremor, neuropathy, behavioral abnormalities
Zinc	Acute: gastrointestinal symtpoms, ataxia, renal failure, pulmonary edema.

acute or chronic and may occur through inhalational or oral routes. The exposure may be to inorganic metal or organic metal salts. All of these factors will influence the presentation of the patient.

Heavy metals cannot be metabolized in the body. When they bind with reactive protein groups and enzymes containing oxygen, sulfur, and nitrogen, they disrupt enzymatic function. Chelating agents bind metals in the same way to decrease their effects on the body. The choice of agent depends on the affinity for the metal, the ability to distribute into areas of metal concentration, and the disposition of the bound metal. Since chelating agents with sulfur and nitrogen bind more strongly to heavy metals than to calcium, these are preferred.

Indications for Treatment

Heavy metal intoxication should be treated if the patient is symptomatic or the body burden of the metal must be decreased based on blood or urine levels.

Patients present with various combinations of acute and chronic exposure from different sources, and the indications for heavy metal chelation are controversial. Because the individual conditions of each case of poisoning may affect the need for chelation, consultation with a regional poison center or a toxicologist experienced in such poisoning is recommended to ensure that each individual patient receives the proper treatment. (See box.)

Discussion

Dimercaprol should be the standard therapy for patients hospitalized with arsenic poisoning. Penicillamine has the advantage of oral administration and can be used on an outpatient basis after initial dimercaprol therapy or in asymptomatic patients with increased urinary arsenic excretion.

The same regimens can be used in mercury and zinc poisonings, although dimercaprol may actually be harmful when mercury is in the organic form.

Cadmium excretion is not increased after chronic poisoning, but chelation is probably of benefit after an acute cadmium exposure. For lead toxicity, removal of the patient from the source of lead is the key intervention. Chelation with larger doses of dimercaprol should be used for children with encephalopathy, whereas smaller doses of dimercaprol are sufficient for less severe symptoms or in asymptomatic children with blood levels

---

DRUG TREATMENT: HEAVY METAL POISONING

Arsenic, Mercury, and Zinc

First-Line Drug
Dimercaprol

Initial Dose	3 mg/kg IM for mild symptoms 5 mg/kg IM for severe symptoms
Repeat Dose	Same dose repeated every 4 hours for 2 days and then twice daily for a week or once daily for 10 days
End-Points	Urinary arsenic level less than 50 μg/24 hours; switch to penicillamine in mild cases when the patient can tolerate oral medications. Reduced urinary mercury and zinc levels

Second-Line Drug
D-*Penicillamine*

Initial Dose	25 mg/kg orally, up to 250 mg in children and 500 mg in adults
Repeat Dose	Same dose every 6 hours for 5 days
End-Points	Observation for five days after treatment with repeat course if symptoms recur Urinary arsenic level lower than 60 μg/24 hours

---

DRUG TREATMENT: HEAVY METAL POISONING Continued

Cadmium

First-Line Drug

Calcium Disodium Edetate

Initial dose	50–75 mg/kg/24 hours by continuous IV infusion
Repeat Dose	Continuous infusion daily
End-Point	Continue treatment for 5-day course.

Lead

First-Line Drugs

Dimercaprol (BAL)

Initial Dose	3–5 mg/kg IM
Repeat Dose	Same dose every 4 hours for 2 days, then every 4–12 hours
End-Points	Continue treatment for 5-day course. Repeat course if blood level >50 μg/dl in 2–5 days after last dose.

Calcium Disodium Edetate

Initial Dose	50–75 mg/kg/24 hours continuous IV infusion
Repeat Dose	Continuous infusion daily
End-Points	Continue treatment for 5-day course. Repeat course if blood level >50 μg/dl after 2–5 days. Negative calcium edetate provocation test

Second-Line Drugs

Penicillamine

Initial Dose	20–40 mg/kg/24 hours, up to 1 g daily
Repeat Doses	May be given in 2–4 daily doses for 2 months
End-Points	Blood levels and urinary excretion

---

greater than 70 μg/dl. Calcium edetate should be given continuously and should not exceed 0.5% concentration in the solution. It may be given without dimercaprol if levels are only moderately elevated. In asymptomatic children with levels lower than 50 μg/dl, a calcium edetate provocation test can help determine if continued treatment is needed. In this test, 500 mg/m^2 calcium edetate is given and the urine is collected for 8 hours. The test is considered positive if the ratio of excreted lead (measured in micrograms) to calcium edetate given (measured in milligrams) is greater than 0.60. Penicillamine may be used for longer treatment after a course of parenteral chelation with dimercaprol and calcium edetate or as primary treatment in asymptomatic patients with mildly elevated blood lead levels. Close weekly follow-up to monitor for toxicity is necessary.

Organophosphate Poisoning

Diagnosis

A history of exposure to organophosphates or occupational risk is usually obtained in poisoned patients. The classic cholinergic symptoms of organophosphate poisoning are listed in Table 16–4. At low doses, musca-

TABLE 16–4. Effects of Organophosphate Poisoning

Muscarinic Effects
Blurred vision, miosis
Nausea, vomiting, increased bowel sounds
Diarrhea, abdominal cramps, fecal incontinence
Salivation, bronchorrhea
Lacrimation, diaphoresis, moist skin
Bradycardia

Nicotinic Effects
Tachycardia
Hypertension
Fasciculations
Muscle weakness
Mydriasis

Central Nervous System Cholinergic Effects
Agitation
Ataxia
Psychosis
Confusion
Coma

rinic symptoms may be prominent, but nicotinic activity predominates at high doses. Thus the actual presentation may be quite variable, and the entire syndrome must be considered. Mydriasis and tachycardia should not be contraindications to treatment if other signs of the cholinergic syndrome are present. The response of signs and symptoms to atropine is extremely helpful in establishing the diagnosis.

Indications for Treatment

Symptomatic patients should be treated, especially if they exhibit increased secretions of the respiratory tract. Respiratory distress is the most common serious management problem. Patients with organophosphate poisoning should be relatively resistant to atropine. If a typical 1 to 2-mg dose of atropine results in an anticholinergic state, the diagnosis should be reconsidered. (See box.)

Discussion

Overly cautious administration of atropine is a common mistake, and it is important to remember that patients exposed to organophosphates will be resistant to atropinization and require much more than the standard doses. The amount required depends on the degree of exposure, so the dose will need to be titrated. The atropine may be needed for several days depending on the dose and the rate of elimination of the specific organophosphate. A typical patient may require 40 mg/day for 2 days, but the need for 1000 mg/day has been reported. Atropine reverses only muscarinic effects, whereas pralidoxime reverses effects at the muscarinic and central sites, including muscle fasciculations, weakness, and sympathetic signs within 30 to 40 minutes. Pralidoxime reactivates acetylcholinesterase but usually only

DRUG TREATMENT: ORGANOPHOSPHATE POISONING

First-Line Drug

Atropine

Initial Dose	1–2 mg IV
Repeat Dose	2 mg IV every 15 minutes
End-Points	Bronchorrhea is controlled. Heart rate is 130–140 beats per minute. Other signs of atropine excess preclude further treatment.

Second-Line Drug

Pralidoxime

Initial Dose	1 g IV over 30–60 minutes
Repeat Dose	1 g in 1 hour if no improvement May be repeated every 12 hours or as an IV infusion at 0.5 g/hour.
End-Points	After 48 hours many organophosphates have become irreversible, but pralidoxime may be continued as long as symptoms respond.

if it is given within the first 24 to 36 hours. After that, the organophosphate becomes irreversibly bound to the cholinesterase. There have been anecdotal reports that late pralidoxime administration more than 48 hours after exposure has resulted in a clinical response, so it may be given as a therapeutic trial. Early administration of pralidoxime also minimizes the amount of atropine needed. Although it is less effective against some specific organophosphates and not effective at all against carbamate insecticides, the clinical presentation for all of these insecticides is identical so that pralidoxime should be given unless there is absolute identification of the toxin as a carbamate.

Acetaminophen Poisoning

Diagnosis

The clinical syndrome of acetaminophen overdose consists of four stages. Initially, the patient may be asymptomatic or have only nausea and vomiting for 24 hours. During the second 24 hours, the patient may have decreased symptoms, but hepatic necrosis will be manifest by increases in liver transaminases. Coagulopathy, jaundice, and associated encephalopathy ensue 72 to 96 hours after ingestion. If the patient survives, recovery is the fourth stage. Because patients lack obvious specific symptoms during the initial phases, the diagnosis is based solely on history or clinical suspicion confirmed by the laboratory. A serum acetaminophen level done 4 hours after an acute ingestion is a reliable predictor of hepatic toxicity. Levels greater than 300 μg/ml are associated with a 90% risk of hepatic encephalopathy, whereas those below 120 μg/ml have almost no risk. Serum levels above 200 μg/ml result in 60% incidence of elevated transaminases and probable hepatotoxicity. Because the exact time between ingestion and the laboratory determination of serum level may not be exact, the Rumack-Matthew nomogram has incorporated a 25% error so that a 4-hour serum level of 140 μg/ml is considered possibly hepatoxic. The levels are extrapolated so that one may predict hepatotoxicity up to 24 hours after an acute ingestion. Because the patient may be asymptomatic or have nonspecific symptoms, there should be a low threshold to use serum acetaminophen levels to guide treatment. This can avoid the tragic return of patients with advanced toxicity after the antidote is no longer effective.

Indications for Treatment

N-acetylcysteine should be given if the acetaminophen level is above the possible hepatotoxicity line on the nomogram following an acute ingestion. An acetaminophen half-life, which can be calculated from two serum levels, greater than 4 hours is associated with hepatotoxicity and greater than 12 hours is associated with hepatic coma. This is especially useful after chronic ingestion of high doses of acetaminophen when the nomogram is not valid. If a severe overdose is suspected by history or if laboratory confirmation is not immediately available, antidotal treatment should be initiated in the interim. N-acetylcysteine is an effective antidote when given within the first 8 hours after acetaminophen ingestion. Because the risk of significant hepatotoxicity is greatly increased if administration of the antidote is delayed longer than 16 hours, every effort should be made to begin antidotal treatment before then, although there is still some benefit up to 24 hours after ingestion. While it appears that children under the age of 5 years are more resistant than are adults to hepatotoxicity, current recommendations are to treat children in a manner similar to adults. (See box.)

Discussion

Acetaminophen toxicity is believed to be caused by an unidentified toxic metabolite produced by the hepatic P-450 enzyme system in the liver. In therapeutic doses, acetaminophen is metabolized to nontoxic metabolites, and any toxic metabolite produced is bound and neutralized by endogenous gluthione. With a large ingestion of acetaminophen, the nontoxic metabolic pathways are saturated, resulting in shunting of the metabolism to the P-450 pathway. Glutathione stores are depleted, allowing the toxic metabolite to accumulate and damage hepatocytes. The mechanism of hepatic protection provided by N-acetylcysteine is uncertain. It may serve as a replacement for glutathione, regenerate glutathione, or prevent saturation of the sulfation pathway.

Gastric decontamination should be performed with a significant ingestion of acetaminophen if spontaneous emesis has not already occurred. The use of activated charcoal in this situation is controversial since the charcoal has been demonstrated to absorb N-acetylcysteine. In cases of multiple drug ingestion or early presentation, activated char-

DRUG TREATMENT: ACETAMINOPHEN POISONING

First-Line Drug

Oral N-Acetylcysteine Loading Dose

Initial Dose	140 mg/kg of 20% solution diluted 1:3 in chilled cola syrup, grapefruit juice, or other diluent to mask the flavor
	Antiemetic if unable to retain N-acetylcysteine, and repeat dose
	Administration by slow nasogastric drip
Repeat Dose	70 mg/kg every 4 hours with a repeat dose if there is emesis within 1 hour
End-Point	Total of 18 doses including the loading dose

Second-Line Drug

Intravenous N-Acetylcysteine

Initial Dose	150 mg/kg in 200 ml 5% dextrose and water (D_5W) over 15 minutes
Repeat Dose	50 mg/kg in 500 ml D_5W over 4 hours, followed by 100 mg/kg in 1000 ml D_5W over 16 hours

coal may be considered while waiting for a 4-hour serum acetaminophen level. If N-acetylcysteine is given after oral charcoal, any remaining charcoal should be removed through nasogastric suction and the oral dose of N-acetylcysteine should be increased by 40% to compensate for the amount absorbed by the activated charcoal. For patients with nausea and vomiting who are unable to retain oral N-acetylcysteine several options are available. An antiemetic may be given, or the antidote may be given slowly through a small nasogastric tube. If both of those options are unsuccessful, intravenous administration of N-acetylcysteine may be considered. Prescott has developed an intravenous protocol frequently used in Europe and Canada, where a pyrogen-free preparation is available, but this route has not been approved in the United States by the Food and Drug Administration, and there is not an approved parenteral product available for commercial use. The inhalational product may contain contaminants and pyrogens, which can cause severe reactions when given intravenously even after filtration through a 0.22-micron filter.

Methemoglobinemia

Diagnosis

When hemoglobin is in the oxidized, ferric Fe^{3+} state, it is not capable of carrying oxygen molecules. The blood normally contains about 1% methemoglobin. Hypoxia is generally not a problem until the methemoglobin level approaches 60%. Concentrations of 70 to 80% are lethal. Many chemicals and drugs can induce methemoglobinemia and are listed in Table 16–5. Infants are much more susceptible since there is less ability to reduce methemoglobin in the first few months of life. Because methemoglobin has a very dark color, patients may appear cyanotic without being dangerously hypoxic or appearing in distress. The mucous membranes are classically a "chocolate brown" color and do not improve with high concentrations of supplemental oxygen. Since the dissolved oxygen tension is unchanged, a measured pO_2 will be normal while the *directly* measured oxygen saturation is low. These blood gas findings suggest the diagnosis, and a specific methemoglobin level will be diagnostic.

Blood containing more than 10 to 15% methemoglobin will appear brown when placed on filter paper next to a drop of known normal blood. Bubbling oxygen through dark venous blood normally changes it to a bright red color but will not affect the color of blood containing methemoglobin. Both of these tests can be done rapidly at the bedside.

Indications for Treatment

Many patients will not be in distress and will not require any treatment. Patients who

TABLE 16-5. Agents That Induce Methemoglobinemia

Acetanilid	Hydroxylacetanilid	Phenols
Acetophenetidin	Hydroxylamine	Phenylazopyridine
Alloxans	Inks, marking	Phenylenediamine
Alpha naphthylamine	Kiszka	Phenylhydrazine
Aminophenols	Lidocaine	Phenylhydroxylamine
Ammonium nitrate	Menthol	Phenytoin (Dilantin)
Amyl nitrite	Meta-chloraniline	Piperzoine
Aniline dyes	Methylacetanilid	Plasmoquine
Anilinoethanol	Methylene blue	Prilocaine
Antipyrine	Monochloroaniline	Primaquine
Arsine	Moth balls	Propitocaine
Benzocaine	Naphthylamines	Pyridium
Bismuth subnitrate	Nitrates	Pyrogallol
Chlorates	Nitrites	Pyridine
Chloranilines	Nitrobenzene	Quinones
Chlorobenzene	Nitrogen oxide	Resorcinol
Chloronitrobenzene	Nitrofurans	Shoe dye or polish
Cobalt preparations	Nitroglycerin	Spinach
Corning extract	Nitrophenol	Sulfonal
Crayons, wax (red or orange)°	Nitrosobenzene	Sulfonamides
Dapsone	Pamaquine	Sulfones
Diaminodiphenylsulfone	Para-aminopropiophenone	Tetranitromethane tetronal
Diesel fuel additives	Para-bromoaniline	Tetralin
Dimethylamine	Para-chloronaniline	Tetranitrate
Dimethyl aniline	Para-nitroaniline	Toluenediamine
Dinitrobenzenes	Para-toluidine	Toluidine
Dinitrophenol	Pentaerythritol	Toluylhydroxylamine
Dinitrotoluene	Phenacetin	Trichlorocarbanilide (TCC)
Hydroquinone	Pheneticin	Trinitrotoluene
		Trional

°No longer manufactured.
Reprinted with permission from Curry S: Methemoglobinemia. Ann Emerg Med, 11:215, 1982.

are in respiratory distress or have cardiac or nervous system symptoms, such as arrhythmias, confusion, lethargy, or chest pain, usually have methemoglobin levels greater than 30% and should receive antidotal therapy. Patients with methemoglobin levels above 60% should also receive methylene blue.

Most experts believe asymptomatic patients may be observed for toxicity and receive the antidote when symptoms develop. Anemic patients will become affected and need treatment at lower methemoglobin levels since they already have a decreased oxygen-carrying capacity. (See box.)

DRUG TREATMENT: METHEMOGLOBINEMIA

First-Line Drug
Methylene Blue

Initial Dose	1–2 mg/kg (0.2 ml/kg) IV of 1% solution over 5 minutes
Repeat Dose	If cyanosis remains after an hour, a second dose can be repeated.
End-Points	Cyanosis resolves. Total dose should not exceed 7 mg/kg.

Second-Line Treatment
Exchange Transfusion

Discussion

In high concentrations, methylene blue itself can oxidize hemoglobin to methemoglobin, worsening the methemoglobinemia. The body normally uses ascorbic acid to reduce methemoglobin, but the conversion is slow and probably not clinically useful. The diagnosis should be reconsidered after failure to respond to two doses since patients with glucose-6-phosphate dehydrogenase (G-6-PD) deficiency, sulfhemoglobinemia, or nicotinamide-adenine dinucleotide phosphate hydrogenase (NADPH) methemoglobin reductase deficiency do not respond to the antidote. G-6-PD deficiency results in a low level of NADPH, which prevents the effectiveness of NADPH methemoglobin reductase. Methylene blue can also induce hemolysis in patients with glucose 6-phosphate dehydrogenase deficiency. Sulfhemoglobinemia is a rare entity and clinically appears similar to methemoglobinemia. It is not life threatening and has no antidote. Exchange transfusion with twice the blood volume has been reported to rapidly reduce the methemoglobin-generating substance, but other data are limited. In addition, this may be the treatment for patients with G-6-PD deficiency.

Digoxin Poisoning

Diagnosis

Because of its narrow low therapeutic index, accidental digoxin poisoning is relatively common in chronically digitalized patients. Acute poisoning is less common but has a mortality estimated to be between 13 and 25%. Symptoms include nausea, vomiting, weakness, drowsiness, visual disturbances, and headaches. Atrial tachycardia with atrioventricular (AV) nodal block is the classic arrhythmia, demonstrating increased automaticity and excitability with decreased conduction, but almost any other arrhythmia may occur. Ventricular arrhythmias may be difficult to control.

Indications for Treatment

Digoxin-specific antibody (Fab) fragments can dramatically reverse digoxin toxicity and should be considered when the initial treatment outlined in Figure 16–2 is unsuccessful. Since there is a cross-reactivity, Fab fragments may also be used for toxicity resulting from digitoxin as well as from the oleander plant and other cardiac glycosides. It should be used whenever serious arrhythmias such as high-grade AV block or frequent ventricular ectopy is resistant to conventional drug therapy. Its safety and risk compared to other modalities, such as cardiac pacing, have not been fully answered. Fab fragments should also be used when hyperkalemia is present that is not controlled with insulin, glucose infusions, and Kayexalate. Patients with renal failure are also candidates. Its use in more moderate toxicity is currently being explored, and as the safety of this drug becomes established, its use will probably increase. An elevated serum digoxin level

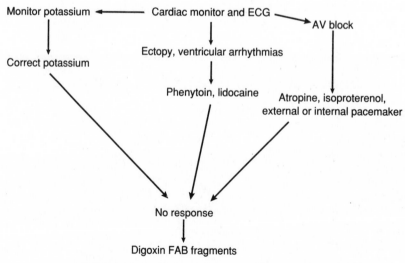

FIGURE 16–2. Treatment algorithm: digoxin toxicity.

without serious clinical manifestations should not be sufficient criteria to use digoxin antibody. Children may tolerate very high serum digoxin levels without toxic side effects. (See box.)

Discussion

An estimated dose of digoxin-specific antibody can be determined from the following data:

Number of 0.25-mg Tablets Digoxin Ingested	Antibody Dose (mg)	Antibody Dose (Vials)
25	340	8.5
50	680	17
75	1000	25
100	1360	34
150	2000	50

A severely symptomatic patient with a life-threatening poisoning requires approximately 10 vials.

Initial therapy should be with standard antiarrhythmic agents, including magnesium sulfate. Control of hyperkalemia may require administration of Kayexalate and insu-

lin. Gastric decontamination should be performed for acute ingestion of digoxin. Bile acid–binding resins, such as cholestyramine or colestipol, may be helpful in disrupting enterohepatic circulation of the digoxin and preventing its reabsorption. Their use has been reported to decrease the serum half-life of digoxin. Fab fragments should be used if there is resistance to these methods. Toxicity will begin to reverse within 30 minutes of the Fab fragment infusion. After all of the accessible digoxin is initially bound, digoxin equilibrates from the tissue, and there may be a delayed rebound elevation in free digoxin. Once digoxin antibody has been given, immunoassay techniques of measuring digoxin will demonstrate an extremely high digoxin level since the method cannot differentiate between free active drug and antibody-inactivated drug. Free digoxin levels can be measured using newer methods such as fluorescence polarization immunoassay of protein-free ultrafiltrates of the serum. Hemodialysis may be necessary to remove the bound complexes in the face of renal failure. Because Fab fragments are sheep protein, the possibility of anaphylactic and allergic reactions should be anticipated.

DRUG TREATMENT: DIGOXIN POISONING

First-Line Drugs

Digoxin-Specific Antibody Fragments

Initial Dose　If a steady-state serum digoxin concentration (SDC) is known, the patient's SDC and the body weight can be entered into the formula below with the following units:

$$\text{Dose in vials} = \frac{(\text{SDC in ng/ml})(5.6 \text{ l/kg})(\text{body weight in kg})}{(1000 \text{ ng/mg})(0.6 \text{ mg/vial})}$$

For digitoxin, the formula is modified to reflect the lower volume of distribution as follows:

$$\text{Dose in vials} = \frac{(\text{SDC in ng/ml})(0.56 \text{ l/kg})(\text{body weight in kg})}{(1000 \text{ ng/mg})(0.6 \text{ mg/vial})}$$

If the estimated ingested amount of digoxin is known, the following formula is used:

$$\text{Dose in vials} = (\text{ingested dose in mg})(0.8)/(0.6 \text{ mg/vial})$$

Repeat Dose　More Fab may be given if needed in rare cases.

End-Point　Therapy should be based on the clinical response, but no clinical improvement should lead to reconsideration of the diagnosis of digoxin poisoning.

Methanol and Ethylene Glycol Poisoning

Diagnosis

Methanol is used in many widely available commercial products such as canned heat (Sterno), windshield washer fluid, solvents, varnishes, antifreeze, and fuel. Poisoning has occurred with accidental contamination of homemade beverages, accidental ingestion of a product containing methanol, or substitution of a methanol-containing product for ethanol. The smallest lethal ingestion reported is 15 ml of a 40% solution. A dose of 1 to 2 ml/kg may be toxic. Symptoms may be similar to ethanol intoxication or may be relatively nonspecific such as headache, dizziness, nausea, and vomiting. There may be hyperpnea as a result of the respiratory compensation for the metabolic acidosis. Decreased visual acuity may also be reported. Severe cases may progress to seizures, coma, severe acidosis, and respiratory arrest. Although patients may have hyperemic optic discs or retinal edema, the physical examination is generally normal except for general acute illness. Patients frequently present late since the toxic active metabolites are not initially present and may be delayed further if there is co-ingestion of ethanol. The diagnosis should be suspected in all patients with a severe metabolic acidosis. Although an anion gap is frequently present, it may not be present until the metabolites are present. An osmolal gap may be helpful if present, but this sign is not sensitive enough to rule out toxic ingestion if it is absent. Therefore, a serum methanol level should be obtained whenever possible.

Ethylene glycol is most commonly found in antifreeze but also as a coolant and in paint, detergent, polishes, and other commercial products. Approximately 100 ml is said to be a lethal dose in an adult. The diagnosis is most readily made by the history or identification of the container. Because of its color, antifreeze excreted in the urine fluoresces under an ultraviolet light. Central nervous system symptoms are similar to those of ethanol intoxication, but the odor of ethanol on the breath is absent. Other manifestations, such as calcium oxalate crystals in the urine, are distinctive. The anion and osmolal gaps are increased, as in methanol poisoning.

Indications for Treatment

The approach to these poisonings is outlined in Figure 16–3. Ethanol therapy should be given for methanol or ethylene glycol levels greater than 25 mg/dl, or when an ethylene glycol or methanol ingestion is

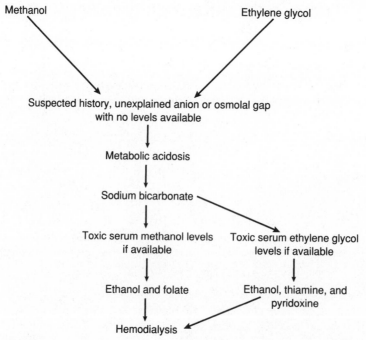

FIGURE 16–3. Treatment algorithm: methanol and ethylene glycol poisoning.

suspected either by history or by the presence of an unexplained anion or osmolal gap and a serum level is not available. Hemodialysis is indicated in methanol poisoning for methanol levels greater than 50 mg/dl, intractable metabolic acidosis, or visual disturbances. Hemodialysis is indicated with an ethylene glycol level greater than 50 mg/dl, uncorrectable acidosis, or renal insufficiency. Jacobsen and associates believe that hemodialysis should be used for all ethylene glycol poisonings. (See box.)

Discussion

Methanol is metabolized by alcohol dehydrogenase and aldehyde dehydrogenase to formaldehyde and formic acid. Formic acid is the metabolite believed to be responsible for methanol toxicity. Ethylene glycol is also metabolized by the same route to glycolic acid, which causes acidosis, and to the final products of oxalate, oxalomate, and several nontoxic metabolites. Ethanol has a higher affinity for alcohol dehydrogenase than does methanol or ethylene glycol, preventing formation of toxic metabolites. It may be given orally, but severe ingestions are frequently associated with nausea and vomiting. If the patient cannot retain oral ethanol, intravenous administration may be required.

Folate protects monkeys from methanol poisoning by increasing formic acid metabo-

---

DRUG TREATMENT: METHANOL AND ETHYLENE GLYCOL POISONING

First-Line Drugs
Oral Ethanol

Initial Dose	2.0 ml/kg of a 50% solution over 1 hour
Repeat Dose	0.33 ml/kg/hour maintenance dose by nasogastric tube 0.78 ml/kg/hour with dialysis
End-Point	Maintain blood ethanol level between 100 and 200 mg/dl until methanol or ethylene glycol is metabolized.

OR

Intravenous Ethanol

Initial Dose	10.0 ml/kg of a 10% solution over 1 hour
Repeat Dose	1.6 ml/kg/hour continuous IV infusion 3.3 ml/kg/hour during dialysis
End-Points	Maintain blood ethanol level between 100 and 200 mg/dl. Methanol or ethylene glycol is metabolized.

Second-Line Drugs
Folate

Initial Dose	50 mg IV to every patient with methanol poisoning
Repeat Dose	50 mg IV every 4 hours
End-Points	Until the poison is metabolized

Thiamine

Initial Dose	100 mg IV to every patient with ethylene glycol poisoning

Pyridoxine

Initial Dose	50 mg IV to every patient with ethylene glycol poisoning
Repeat Dose	50 mg every 6 hours

lism and may also be useful in humans. Because it is safe in the doses recommended, it is recommended as adjunctive therapy.

Pyridoxine and thiamine are cofactors in the metabolism of ethylene glycol to nontoxic metabolites. Supplementation of these vitamins is probably beneficial, especially to alcohol abusers, who may have dietary vitamin deficiencies.

Since ethanol, ethylene glycol, and methanol are easily cleared by hemodialysis, ethanol doses must be increased accordingly to maintain a constant therapeutic serum level during hemodialysis.

Massive ethylene glycol poisoning has also been treated successfully with 4-methylpyrazole, another competitive inhibitor of the alcohol dehydrogenase enzyme. It is protective in animals against both methanol and ethylene glycol poisoning, and single large doses have been safely used in humans. It has a rapid onset of action when administered orally and intravenously and may be given twice daily, avoiding the need for continuous ethanol maintenance. Furthermore, there is no central nervous intoxication as seen with ethanol. Although it is not commercially available in the United States, it is currently undergoing clinical investigation.

Dystonic Reactions

Diagnosis

Extrapyramidal effects may occur acutely after administration of antipsychotic agents such as phenothiazines or haloperidol. This reaction occurs more commonly in younger patients and those who have not been exposed to these drugs in the past. The syndrome occurs 5 to 40 hours after the first dose and classically has the characteristics of (1) abrupt onset, (2) intermittent and bizarre neuromuscular presentations, (3) an otherwise normal physical examination, (4) medication history, and (5) rapid response to treatment. Different types of dystonic reactions include torticollis (spasm of the neck with or without arm involvement), oculogyric crisis (upward gaze with rotation of the globe and spasms of the lids), buccolingual dysarthria (protruding of the tongue, trismus, and facial grimaces), opisthotonos (arching or scoliosis of the back), and tortipelvis (abdominal spasm, bizarre gait, inability to walk). Tetany is almost always accompanied by severe anxiety, agitation, and discomfort. The dystonia may be intermittent and allow for active movement between episodes. The history is not always clear since the syndrome may follow use of an antiemetic or street drugs.

Indications for Treatment

Usually the dystonic reaction is easily recognized and rapidly responds to treatment. Whenever the diagnosis is in question, the antidote should still be used as a therapeutic trial since the antidote is relatively safe, and resolution of the dystonia confirms the diagnosis. (See box.)

DRUG TREATMENT: DYSTONIC REACTIONS

First-Line Drugs

Diphenhydramine

Initial Dose	25–50 mg IM or IV
Repeat Dose	May be given if initial response is inadequate
End-Point	25–50 mg tid should be given orally for 3 days.

Benztropine

Initial Dose	1–2 mg IM or IV
Repeat Dose	May be given if initial response is inadequate
End-Point	1–2 mg tid should be given orally for 3 days.

Discussion

The initial dose should be given parenterally for the fastest onset. In addition, these patients are quite uncomfortable and will not be able to swallow oral medications. A response can be expected within 30 minutes after intramuscular administration and sooner when given intravenously. Oral medications should be continued since the dystonic reaction can recur after the initial dose of antidote has worn off.

Coumarin Poisoning

Diagnosis

Most accidental ingestions of a single dose of coumarin do not cause symptoms and require no treatment. On the other hand, patients chronically taking coumarin may have excessively prolonged prothrombin times and bleeding from various sites, requiring emergency treatment. It should be remembered that coumarin has been used on occasion by malingering patients to simulate illness.

Many rodenticides use anticoagulants as the active ingredient. The warfarin compounds have long been popular, but resistance among rats has lead to the development of a new class of "superwarfarins." Unlike warfarin, these compounds can cause hemorrhage and severe toxicity after a single dose. Brodificoum and difenacoum have an effect that may last up to 6 or 8 weeks. It is extremely important to identify these exposures correctly, and attention to subtle differences in product names is vital since the names can be very similar to warfarin products. For example, D-con contains warfarin, but D-con Mouse Prufe II contains brodifacoum.

Indications for Treatment

Although some bleeding can be controlled with local measures, in cases of cerebral or gastrointestinal hemorrhage, the risk of exsanguination or permanent brain damage outweighs the risk of anticoagulant reversal. Phytonadione, or vitamin K, is a useful treatment in these situations. Poisoning with a "superwarfarin" always requires prolonged monitoring and aggressive treatment. (See box.)

Discussion

The dosage of phytonadione should be increased if active bleeding persists. If anticoagulation will be restarted after phytonadione therapy, the dose of phytonadione should be kept to a minimum since patients receiving phytonadione will be resistant to coumarin effects. Patients with superwarfarin poisoning have been reported to require as much as 125 mg/day of phytonadione in conjunction with fresh-frozen plasma. Because of prolonged effects, they may require oral vitamin K therapy for many weeks after hospital discharge.

Heparin Reversal

Diagnosis

The frequency of bleeding during heparin therapy is approximately 5 to 10%. In most

---

DRUG TREATMENT: COUMARIN POISONING

First-Line Drug

Phytonadione

Initial Dose	2.5–10 mg IM; if given IV, the dose should be given at the rate of 1 mg/min to avoid reactions.
	10 mg should be given for "superwarfarin" poisoning.
	If active bleeding is occurring, 20–50 mg may be needed for an effect.
Repeat Dose	Initial dose may be repeated after 6–8 hours.
	For superwarfarin toxicity, doses should be rapidly increased, and up to 10 times the initial dose may be required for a response.
End-Point	Clinical response or correction of the prothrombin time

DRUG TREATMENT: HEPARIN REVERSAL

First-Line Drug

Protamine Sulfate

Initial Dose	1 mg protamine sulfate for every 100 units of heparin
Repeat Dose	Half the initial dose may be repeated.
End-Point	Cessation of bleeding and correction of the PTT

cases, the bleeding is controlled with local pressure or the cessation of heparin therapy.

Indications for Treatment

For minor bleeding, if the partial thromboplastin time (PTT) is greater than 1.5 to 2 times the normal range, the heparin dose should be reduced. If the bleeding is life threatening or not controlled with local means and the PTT is elevated, heparin should be reversed with protamine sulfate. (See box.)

Discussion

Because protamine sulfate is a basic chemical that itself is an anticoagulant in high doses, it is important to give the proper dose. The full neutralizing dose is 1 mg of protamine sulfate for every 100 units of heparin, but since heparin has a half-life of only 1 hour, the protamine sulfate dose will be lower if heparin has been discontinued. If the last dose of heparin was 1 hour ago, only half the dose, 0.5 mg of protamine sulfate needs to given per 100 units of heparin.

Anticholinergic Toxicity

Diagnosis

A large number of medications have anticholinergic properties either as a therapeutic effect or a side effect. These include antihistamines, antipsychotics, (butyrophenones, phenothiazines, thioxanthines), antispasmodics, belladonna alkaloids, cyclic antidepressants, mydriatics, parkinsonian medications, and over-the-counter medications such as analgesics, cold relief products, and sedatives. Many plants and mushrooms also contain anticholinergic chemicals, which can cause symptoms if ingested or intentionally smoked.

The anticholinergic syndrome consists of easily identified peripheral effects and less specific central nervous system effects. Peripheral signs include tachycardia, hypertension, hyperpyrexia, dry skin, urinary and gastrointestinal retention, and dilated pupils. Central symptoms include confusion, agitation, disorientation, hallucinations, decreased consciousness, and seizures.

Indications for Treatment

The vast majority of patients present with only mild symptoms such as sinus tachycardia and decreased level of consciousness and require observation or standard supportive care. While physostigmine has had widespread use in the past, it is used less frequently now because of the potential complications. Because it can cause seizures, bradycardia, and asystole, physostigmine should be reserved for patients with seizures, arrhythmias, and agitation in whom standard treatment fails, as outlined in Figure 16–4. (See box.)

Discussion

Physostigmine can cause convulsions that may be impossible to distinguish from anticholinergic toxicity. In cyclic antidepressant overdoses, there is a conduction delay that may be additive to the cholinergic effect of the physostigmine and may cause asystole. Since physostigmine has a short-lived effect, the dose may need to be repeated if life-threatening symptoms recur.

Cyanide and Hydrogen Sulfide Poisoning

Diagnosis

Cyanide and hydrogen sulfide are rapidly acting cellular poisons that cause coma and death if prompt treatment is delayed. The diagnosis is almost always based on the history of exposure or circumstances that make exposure likely. Cyanide is used in fumigants,

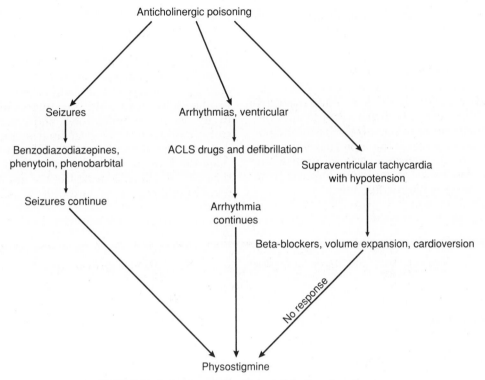

FIGURE 16–4. Treatment algorithm: anticholinergic poisoning.

DRUG TREATMENT: ANTICHOLINERGIC POISONING

First-Line Drug

Physostigmine

Initial Dose	1–2 mg in adults and 0.5 mg in children, diluted in 10 ml and given IV slowly over 3 minutes
Repeat Dose	Initial dose may be repeated every 30–60 minutes.
End-Point	Cessation of life-threatening symptoms or onset of bradycardia or seizures, which may be secondary to physostigmine

ore extraction, photographic processing, electroplating, and manufacture of synthetic rubber products and is liberated by the combustion of plastics, especially acrylonitriles and polyurethane. Hydrogen sulfide is used in preparing animal hides and in the production of rayon, wood pulp, carbon disulfide, coal products, and sulfuric acid. It is found naturally whenever proteins undergo anaerobic decomposition and is also known as "sewer gas."

Typically dyspnea is the initial symptom. Hypoxia may cause a rapid loss of consciousness and seizures. Since there is no cellular uptake of oxygen from the saturated hemoglobin, cyanosis will be absent and there will be a low arterial to venous oxygen saturation gradient. A severe lactic acidosis will be present. A rotten egg smell is typical for hydrogen sulfide, but high concentrations of the gas can cause rapid paralysis of the olfactory nerve. Although a bitter almond odor is classically associated with cyanide, the literature is replete with case reports where this clue was absent. At low concentrations, hydrogen sulfide causes irritation of the mucous membranes of the eyes, pharynx, and respiratory tree. Although cyanide may be measured in the serum, the results are not rapidly available for use in patient care decisions.

Indications for Treatment

Seizures or coma in patients with suspected cyanide or hydrogen sulfide exposure should be treated with the cyanide antidote kit. Since the antidote produces methemoglobin and decreases the blood's oxygen-carrying capacity, it should not be used when carbon monoxide poisoning or hypoxia from other causes is likely. (See box.)

Discussion

Nitrites induce production of methemoglobin, which has a high affinity for both cyanide and hydrogen sulfide, removes them from the cytochrome system, and revives cellular respiration. The sulfmethemoglobin produced has a half-life of 2 hours and naturally decays to hemoglobin and a nontoxic sulfur compound. The cyanomethemoglobin requires the sulfur from thiosulfate to produce the less toxic thiocyanate. The best indicators of clinical response are improved level of consciousness, cessation of seizures,

---

DRUG TREATMENT: CYANIDE AND HYDROGEN SULFIDE POISONING

First-Line Drug

Oxygen

Initial Dose	100% by endotracheal tube or high-flow non-rebreather mask

Second-Line Drugs

Amyl Nitrate

Initial Dose	Inhalation of one perle for 30 seconds
Repeat Dose	Repeat for 30 seconds every minute.
End-Point	Availability of sodium nitrate and IV access

Followed by

Sodium Nitrate

Initial Dose	Adults: 300 mg (10 ml of 3% solution) IV ideally over 20 minutes or at least 2 minutes Children: 10 mg/kg (0.33 ml/kg of 3% solution), up to 300 mg maximum
Repeat Dose	Repeat initial dose if no response.
End-Point	Clinical response or methemoglobin level >40%

Followed by (for cyanide poisoning only)

Sodium Thiosulfate

Initial Dose	Adults: 12.5 g (50 ml of 25% solution) IV over 2 minutes Children: 0.4 g/kg (1.0 ml/kg of 25% solution) In the case of oral exposure, one 50-ml ampule of thiosulfate should be diluted up to 250 ml and left in the stomach after gastric lavage.
Repeat Dose	Repeat initial dose if no response.
End-Point	This should not be given for hydrogen sulfide poisoning.

Third-Line Therapy

Hyperbaric oxygen if readily available

and restoration of normal respirations, pulse, and blood pressure. Specific doses for children should be based on body weight and hemoglobin. The recommendation for children in the drug treatment flow sheet above assumes a hemoglobin of 12.0 g/dl.

Amyl nitrate perles should be broken into a gauze pad and inhaled for 30 seconds of every minute. A good response may be obtained in patients who are intubated by placing a broken perle directly in the ambu bag used to ventilate the patient. It should be used only until intravenous access is secured since the sodium nitrite is a much more potent drug. If patients can tolerate the delay, the 3% sodium nitrite (0.2 ml/kg in children) should be given over 20 minutes in an intravenous drip followed by one 50-ml ampule of the 25% sodium thiosulfate (1 ml/kg in children) over 20 minutes. Although the package insert recommends the drug be given over 3 to 5 minutes, the slower administration will avoid the hypotension commonly seen after nitrite therapy. Children should not receive the adult dose, which may result in an overproduction of methemoglobin. In the case of oral exposure, one 50-ml ampule of thiosulfate should be diluted up to 250 ml with dilute hydrogen peroxide solution and left in the stomach after gastric lavage. The hydrogen peroxide may be mixed by diluting a 3% solution with water 1:5. This lavage fluid theroetically may oxidize the remaining cyanide to cyanate, but its efficacy has never been proved, and its use should not delay the specific intravenous antidotal treatment.

Other Antidotes

Hydrocobalamin is an antidote successfully used in Europe for cyanide poisoning. It binds directly in a one-to-one molecular ratio to form cyanocobalamin, which is excreted in the urine. It may be even more efficacious when combined with thiosulfate. Rhodenase can then extract the cyanide from the cyanocobalamin to form thiocyanate, which is less toxic and excreted. Although hydrocobalamin avoids the vasodilatation and the formation of methemoglobin, which can compromise the blood's oxygen-carrying capacity, it is only available in the United States in dilute solution and the large 4-g dose necessary for its use as an antidote would require a prohibitive amount of fluid. Dicobalt edetate is also used in Europe. It may produce pulmonary and generalized edema.

Isoniazid Poisoning

Diagnosis

The typical presentation of an isoniazid (INH) overdose is nausea and vomiting, followed by decreasing level of consciousness, seizures, lactic acidosis, and hyperglycemia. Seizures are the most dramatic symptom and are frequently resistant to treatment by the usual medications. In addition, phenytoin may interfere with INH metabolism and prolong its half-life. Groups at high risk for poisoning include native Americans and immigrants from areas with a high incidence of tuberculosis, such as Southeast Asia. INH overdose should also be considered in any patient presenting with intractable seizures and lactic acidosis.

Indications for Treatment

After standard gastric decontamination, all patients with a symptomatic INH overdose or a history of ingestion of greater than 2 g should receive pyridoxine. (See box.)

DRUG TREATMENT: ISONIAZID POISONING

First-Line Drug

Pyridoxine

Initial Dose	1 g for every gram of INH ingested
Repeat Dose	Half the initial dose may be repeated if necessary.
End-Point	Cessation of seizures

Discussion

A gram of pyridoxine for every gram of INH ingested should be given intravenously over 15 minutes. If the amount of the INH ingestion is unknown, 5 g of pyridoxine is recommended as a standard dose.

SPECIFIC AGENTS

N-Acetylcysteine (Mucomyst)

Pharmacology

This drug is the amino acid cysteine with an acetyl group added at the nitrogen position. It is water soluble.

Distribution

The drug is well absorbed orally. Oral therapy results in direct delivery to the liver via the portal circulation and probably results in optimal delivery of the drug.

Elimination

The routes of metabolism and elimination are unknown. It may be deacetylated in the liver and metabolized as the amino acid cysteine. A small amount is detectable in the urine.

Actions

Acetaminophen toxicity is thought to be due to an unidentified toxic metabolite produced from the P-450 mixed-function oxidative enzyme system in the liver. Normal doses of acetaminophen are predominantly metabolized through sulfation and glucuronidation to nontoxic metabolites. The small amount of toxic metabolite produced is bound to endogenous glutathione and rendered nontoxic. With a large ingestion of acetaminophen, the nontoxic metabolic pathways are saturated, resulting in more metabolism by the P-450 pathway. Glutathione stores are depleted, allowing the toxic metabolite to accumulate and bind to liver macromolecules, resulting in damage to hepatocytes. The exact mechanism of hepatic protection provided by N-acetylcysteine is uncertain. It may bind to the toxic metabolite with the sulfhydryl group as a replacement for glutathione, or it may regenerate glutathione or act to prevent saturation of the sulfation pathway.

Indications

N-acetylcysteine is indicated for patients following an acetaminophen overdose who are at high risk as predicted by the Rumack-Matthew nomogram or who have a prolonged acetaminophen half-life greater than 4 hours. Oral administration is preferred, but intravenous administration may be considered in severe intoxication when vomiting is present and the risk of hepatotoxicity is greater than the risk incurred by intravenous administration.

Cautions

Cardiac failure—no dosage adjustment is necessary.

Renal failure—no dosage adjustment is necessary.

Hepatic failure—no dosage adjustment necessary.

Use in pregnancy—Category C. Animals exposed to high doses in utero have not sustained ill effects. Acetaminophen toxicity has been reported in the neonate with transplacental exposure, and N-acetylcysteine has been given in individual cases without ill effects.

Use in children—may be used

Onset and Duration of Action

For optimal hepatic protection, the drug should be given within the first 16 hours before a large amount of acetaminophen has been metabolized. It should also be given up to 24 hours or later since the drug is relatively safe and there is little alternative in treatment.

Dosage

Oral N-Acetylcysteine Loading Dose

The loading dose is 140 mg/kg of 20% solution diluted 1:3 in cola syrup, grapefruit juice, or other diluent to mask the sulfur taste.

Oral N-Acetylcysteine Maintenance Dose

Once the loading dose is given, a maintenance dose of 70 mg/kg every 4 hours for 17 additional doses should be given. If there is emesis within 1 hour, the dose should be repeated.

Intravenous N-Acetylcysteine Administration

The loading dose according to Prescott is 150 mg/kg in 200 ml D_5W over 15 minutes, followed by a maintenance dose of 50 mg/kg in 500 ml D$_5$W over 4 hours, followed by 100 mg/kg in 1000 ml D$_5$W over 16 hours. Since a parenteral preparation is not commercially available in the United States, it has been suggested that all solutions should be filtered through a 0.22-micron filter to decrease the amount of contaminants. Although the intravenous route has been used in Europe and Canada, it has not been approved by the Food and Drug Administration for general use in the United States.

Limits

The entire course of therapy should be completed.

Toxicity

Drug Interactions

Hydrogen peroxide, other oxidizing agents—oxidation of acetylcysteine
Metallic iron and copper—hydrogen sulfide is released.

Adverse Effects

Nausea, vomiting, and abdominal discomfort are frequently seen, probably as a result of the odor and taste of the drug. These effects typically last for an hour after drug administration and, for many patients, improve after the first several doses. Urticaria and fever have been reported. Anaphylactic reactions and one death have been reported with intravenous use.

Treatment of Toxicity

Discontinuing the drug and providing standard treatment of urticaria usually suffice. Using a chilled solution may decrease the unpleasant odor and taste and alleviate nausea. If the patient is unable to retain the N-acetylcysteine orally, an antiemetic such as 10 mg of metoclopramide (Reglan) or 200 mg of trimethobenzamide (Tigan) may be given and the dose repeated. Another alternative is to administer the drug by slow nasogastric drip.

Atropine

Pharmacology

Atropine is a racemic mixture of hyoscyamine. L-Hyoscyamine is the major active portion.

Distribution

The drug is widely distributed throughout the body.

Elimination

Hepatic, 60%
Renal, 40% or less

Actions

Atropine competes with and decreases the parasympathetic effect of acetylcholine at the muscarinic receptors. Although it antagonizes muscarinic receptors, it does not reverse anticholinergic activity at nicotinic receptors or neuromuscular junctions.

Indications

Atropine is used to reverse muscarinic signs of organophosphate poisoning.

Cautions

Since the dose is determined by clinical response, it will remain unchanged in renal failure, cardiac failure, and hepatic failure.

Atropine is classified as a Category C drug. The Collaborative Perinatal Project involving 50,282 children had 2323 exposures to parasympatholytics, and a possible association with minor malformations was found. The 1198 exposures that were specifically to atropine were not associated with increased malformations. It has been used during labor without notable effects on the neonate.

Patients can have worsening of their narrow-angle glaucoma because of the anticholinergic-induced mydriasis.

Atropine may be used in children.

Onset and Duration of Action

Onset is within 1 minute and peak effect occurs within 5 minutes. Cardiac effects last 2 hours.

Dosage

Initial dose for symptomatic patients is 0.05 mg/kg or 2 to 4 mg in adults. It should be repeated every 10 minutes until the desired response of drying excess secretions and bronchorrhea occurs or until signs of atropine excess appear.

Limits and Repeat Dose

Atropine should be given until bronchial secretions are controlled. Pupil size and tachycardia alone should not be used as end-points to determine the cessation point for atropine treatment.

Toxicity

Drug Interactions

Sodium bicarbonate, norepinephrine, and isoproterenol are incompatible with atropine.

Adverse Effects

Atropine may cause an elevated temperature as a result of decreased perspiration. There may be a significant anticholinergic rebound effect from residual atropine after pralidoxime therapy regenerates cholinesterase. Thickening of secretions can exacerbate asthma, and increased intraocular pressure may be noted in narrow-angle glaucoma.

Treatment of Toxicity

Patients with glaucoma should also receive myotics to prevent increased intraocular pressure.

Benztropine (Cogentin)

Pharmacology

Distribution

It crosses the blood–brain barrier.

Elimination

Its method of elimination is not well known.

Actions

The drug has anticholinergic and antihistaminic properties and is used on a long-term basis to relieve symptoms of Parkinson's disease as well as to treat extrapyramidal reactions resulting from phenothiazines.

Indications

Extrapyramidal reactions from phenothiazines and butyrophenones are indications for use of benzotropine.

Cautions

Renal failure—no adjustment in dosage is necessary.

Cardiac failure—it should be used cautiously in patients who cannot tolerate an increased heart rate.

Hepatic failure—no adjustment in dosage is necessary.

Use in pregnancy—Category C. Its safe use in pregnancy has not been established.

Other—benztropine should be used carefully in patients who are taking other anticholinergic medications and in patients with prostatic hypertrophy.

Use in children—experience is limited; not recommended

Onset and Duration of Action

It usually offers relief within a few minutes of administration. Its action may persist for 24 to 48 hours after a single 2-mg intramuscular injection.

Dosage

Dosage is 1 to 2 mg IM or IV.

Limits

Clinical response should be evident after one or two doses.

Repeat Dose

A second parenteral dose may be given if there is no initial response. The drug should be continued orally twice a day for 3 days to prevent recurrence of the extrapyramidal reaction.

Toxicity

Drug Interactions

Anticholinergics—increased urinary retention, ileus, hyperpyrexia

Haloperidol—decreased effect of haloperidol

Marijuana—increased heart rate

Adverse Effects

Sedation is the most common side effect. Other side effects are due to the anticholinergic and antihistaminic actions of the drug and include blurred vision, tachycardia, mydriasis, decreased gastrointestinal motility, and urinary retention. Its anticholinergic activity is approximately one-half that of atropine, and its antihistaminic effects are similar to those of pyrilamine in animal studies. The drug may accumulate so that onset of symptoms may be delayed for several days. Toxic psychosis with visual hallucinations, confusion, and speech difficulties have been reported. These effects are reversible after cessation of the drug.

Treatment of Toxicity

Cessation of the drug results in recovery from the adverse affects.

Calcium Disodium Edetate (Calcium Disodium Versenate, Calcium Edetate)

Pharmacology

Distribution

The drug is poorly absorbed from the gastrointestinal tract. It is water soluble and easily administered intravenously. It distributes rapidly through 90% of the extracellular space but crosses the blood–brain barrier slowly and does not cross into red blood cells.

Elimination

The drug is cleared almost completely unmetabolized by the kidneys, with 50% removed within 1 hour and almost complete removal within 1 day.

Actions

Calcium is replaced by heavy metals in the +2 or +3 valence state to form a complex that is excreted in the urine. It works well for lead and zinc. Although theoretically 1 g of calcium binds 620 mg of lead, only 3 to 5 mg of lead is actually measured in the urine for each gram of calcium edetate. Iron, copper, manganese, nickel, chromium, and cadmium are also bound to a lesser degree. The drug is not useful for arsenic, gold, or mercury because it binds calcium preferentially. It may be used after exposure to radioactive or nuclear fission products.

Indications

It should be used in severe lead intoxication with dimercaprol. It may also be used in cadmium poisoning.

Cautions

Disodium edetate is a different drug and should not be used because it may cause severe hypocalcemia when the sodium is displaced by the calcium in the body. Because calcium edetate has a calcium cation, hypocalcemia is avoided. When used intravenously, 1 g should be diluted in 250 to 500 ml D_5W or normal saline.

Renal failure—this drug should not be used in renal failure.
Cardiac failure—no dosage adjustment is necessary.
Hepatic failure—no dosage adjustment is necessary.
Use in pregnancy—it should not be used in pregnancy unless there are significant hazards to the mother or fetus.
Use in children—may be used.

Onset and Duration of Action

Onset of action is within 1 hour, and the effect lasts for 24 to 48 hours. The drug's half-life in the blood is 20 to 60 minutes after intravenous dosing and 90 minutes after an intramuscular dose.

Dosage

The dosage is 17 to 25 mg/kg three times a day IV or IM. Solutions should be diluted to 2 to 4 mg/ml and infused over 1 to 2 hours or given intramuscularly.

Limits

Maximum dose should be 1 g/day. A course should run 5 days and be followed by at least 2 days of rest to allow for excretion of the metal before any repeat treatments. Although the maximum dose is 75 mg/kg/24 hours, there are fewer side effects at 50 mg/kg/24 hours.

Repeat Dose

Repeat doses should be based on clinical improvement and monitoring of blood lead levels.

Toxicity

Drug Interactions

Calcium edetate is incompatible with 10% dextrose, lactated Ringer's solution, sodium lactate, amphotericin B, and hydralazine.

Adverse Effects

Acute tubular necrosis, hematuria, and proteinuria may occur and can be minimized by maintaining a good urine flow. Pain at the intramuscular injection site is common, and the addition of 1 ml of procaine to the injection may be helpful. Other adverse effects include nausea, headache, myalgias, malaise, excessive thirst, chills, hypotension, allergic reactions, and gastrointestinal distress.

Treatment of Toxicity

Adequate hydration is essential; however, this needs to be balanced with overhydration of patients suffering from lead encephalopathy. General support is adequate to treat other reactions.

Cyanide Antidote Kit (Lilly)

The kit contains amyl nitrate, sodium nitrite, and sodium thiosulfate.

Pharmacology

Distribution

Nitrites are rapidly absorbed through the skin, lungs, and gastrointestinal tract.

Elimination

Nitrites are hydrolyzed in the liver, but little is known about metabolism and elimination of nitrites and thiosulfate.

Actions

Nitrites oxidize hemoglobin (Fe^{+2}) to methemoglobin (Fe^{+3}). Amyl nitrate may produce up to 5% methemoglobin, and a single dose of sodium nitrite is estimated to produce a 20% methemoglobinemia; the methemoglobin then competitively binds cyanide to form cyanomethemoglobin. This frees the cytochrome a-a₃ oxidase of the cyanide and allows resumption of cellular respiration. Although this is a possible explanation, there have been cases in which patients with a negligible methemoglobin level have clinically responded to the treatment. In experimental studies animals have also had an antidotal effect despite pretreatment with methylene blue, which prevents methemoglobin formation. Cyanide in the body is normally detoxified by the enzyme rhodenase to form thiocyanate, a nontoxic substance. The rate of this detoxification depends on the availability of sulfur, which can be supplied as thiosulfate.

Indications

Use of the antidote is indicated in patients with a possible history of cyanide or hydrogen sulfide exposure and signs of toxicity.

Cautions

Renal failure—no dosage adjustment is necessary.

Cardiac failure—no dosage adjustment is necessary. Hypotension should be monitored.

Hepatic failure—no dosage adjustment is necessary.

Use in pregnancy—nitrites are Category C. The experience with amyl nitrate is limited. In the Collaborative Perinatal Project, four of fifteen newborns exposed to nitrites and other vasodilators suffered malformations. Because cyanide causes fetal demise, treatment should not be withheld in symptomatic pregnant patients.

Use in children—may be used

Onset and Duration of Action

The clinical response to amyl nitrate and sodium nitrite is rapid and usually seen within 1 hour. Many case reports demonstrate a response even before the infusion is completed.

Dosage

Amyl nitrate perles should be inhaled for 30 seconds every minute until the sodium nitrite is given. A broken perle may be placed in the ambu bag to ventilate the patient. Ideally, one 10-ml ampule of the 3% sodium nitrite (0.2 ml/kg in children) should be given over 20 minutes in an intravenous drip, followed by one 50-ml ampule of the 25% sodium thiosulfate (1 ml/kg in children) over 20 minutes. This will avoid the hypotension commonly seen after nitrite therapy. If the patient is in cardiac arrest or moribund, the package insert recommends the drug be given over 3 to 5 minutes. Patients who are anemic and children require less sodium nitrite. For oral exposures, one 50-ml ampule of thiosulfate should be diluted up to 250 ml of volume and left in the stomach with dilute hydrogen peroxide solution after gastric lavage. Three percent hydrogen peroxide should be diluted with water in a 1:5 ratio. Although this lavage fluid may oxidize some of the remaining cyanide to cyanate, the efficacy of this therapy has never been proved, and the specific intravenous antidotal treatment should not be delayed.

Limits

Methemoglobin levels should be checked shortly after the administration of sodium nitrite and should be <40%.

Repeat Dose

Half of the original dose may be repeated in 30 minutes if there is no response or if the patient's condition deteriorates after initial improvement. The methemoglobin level should be monitored if possible.

Toxicity

Adverse Effects

Nitrites cause vasodilation and hypotension in a patient who already has cardiovascular compromise from decreased oxygen delivery. Headache is a complication, but patients are typically comatose. Methemoglobin formation should be limited to less than 30 to 40% to prevent critical compromise of oxygen-carrying capacity of the erythrocytes. It should not be routinely used in victims of smoke inhalation when there is a suspicion of carbon monoxide poisoning since the limited oxygen-carrying capacity in that condition will be made worse by the formation of methemoglobin.

Treatment of Toxicity

Hypotension should be treated with fluids and vasopressors when necessary. Slower administration of nitrites may avoid hypotension. While methylene blue may be used to treat methemoglobinemia over 40% from overzealous nitrite therapy, it must be used with great care and reluctance because it will liberate the cyanide previously bound to the methemoglobin. The dose for methemoglobinemia is 0.2 ml/kg of a 1% solution.

Deferoxamine Mesylate (Desferal)

Pharmacology

Distribution

The drug is made by the bacteria *Streptomyces pilosus*. Deferoxamine has been widely studied in animals and forms complexes best at an acidic pH.

Elimination

Deferoxamine is metabolized by plasma enzymes. Its half-life is unknown, but 15% is eliminated by renal clearance. Ferrioxamine is mainly eliminated in the urine, resulting in the vin rose tint. As opposed to free iron, the ferrioxamine compound is dialyzable.

Actions

The molecule's three hydroxamic groups bind ferric ions and form ferrioxamine, a compound that is water soluble and renally excreted. Each 100 mg of drug can theoretically bind 8.5 mg of free iron. Deferoxamine has a special affinity for iron over other heavy metals and binds to iron preferentially in the ferric ($^{+2}$) rather than the ferrous ($^{+3}$) state. It does not bind iron present in hemoglobin or in the cytochrome system and has minimal effect on calcium and other trace metals in the body.

Indications

Deferoxamine has the highest affinity for iron of any chelating agent but also chelates aluminum. Ingestion of greater than 300 mg elemental iron/kg is severe. There have been case reports of oral deferoxamine treatment after acute iron poisoning, and one study found an increase in total absorbed iron following oral therapy. The usefulness and safety of oral deferoxamine are currently still unclear.

Cautions

Rapid intravenous infusion can cause flushing, erythema, urticaria, and hypotension. The drug should be given slowly intravenously at a maximum rate of 15 ml/kg/hour. It has fewer side effects when given by the intramuscular route. The drug may also be given subcutaneously.

Renal failure—the drug should be avoided in patients with renal failure. It can be removed by dialysis if necessary. Deferoxamine can cause acute tubular necrosis, which may be prevented by adequate hydration. Renal failure usually resolves with cessation of deferoxamine administration.

Cardiac failure—the drug can cause hypotension and tachycardia if given rapidly intravenously. There is no direct cardiac effect.

Hepatic failure—hepatic disease should not affect the use of deferoxamine.

Use in pregnancy—Category C. Skeletal abnormalities in the fetus have been reported in animal studies. There have been seven clinical cases of deferoxamine treatment during pregnancy with no fetal abnormalities, although low neonatal iron levels in one newborn were thought to have been from fetal iron chelation by transplacental deferoxamine. In near-term gravid sheep, maternal iron poisoning with 20-fold elevations in maternal serum iron increased fetal serum iron by a factor of 2. Miscarriages have followed iron overdose in humans, and women at high risk should be treated. It is unclear if pregnant women at mild risk should receive chelation therapy.

Use in children—may be used

Onset and Duration of Action

The onset of action is variable, but vin rose colored urine should be seen within 4 hours of administration of the drug.

Dosage

The intravenous dosage is 15 mg/kg/hour to 90 mg/kg, then 5 to 10 mg/kg/hour, up to the maximum dose of 6 g/24 hours or 240 mg/kg. The intra-muscular dose is 90 mg/kg, up to a maximum 2 g, every 8 hours for three doses.

Limits

The intramuscular route should not be used when hypotension is present.

Toxicity

Drug Interactions

Deferoxamine should not be mixed with other drugs.

Adverse Effects

Long-term use has been associated with cataract formation. Visual loss, tinnitus, and hearing loss have been reported after high doses in patients with thalassemia and in those with low ferritin levels. Although these effects are mostly reversible, permanent disability may result. Anaphylaxis has been reported with this drug.

Treatment of Toxicity

Anaphylaxis should be treated by the usual means. Cessation of deferoxamine administration results in recovery of most of the visual and hearing loss. There is no other specific treatment.

Digoxin-Specific Antibody

Pharmacology

Distribution

The Fab fragment has a wide distribution and rapidly binds serum digoxin in the extracellular space. The distribution half-life is approximately 30 minutes.

Elimination

Fab fragments are filtered and eliminated from the kidney. They have an elimination half-life of approximately 16 hours in patients with normal renal function.

Actions

Fab fragments have a high affinity for binding digoxin in the interstitial fluid. As digoxin is bound and the free serum digoxin level drops, more digoxin is removed from binding sites in the myocardium and other tissues, with consequent reversal of digoxin toxicity. Most methods of measuring serum digoxin cannot differentiate between free and inactivated, antibody-bound drug and will demonstrate extremely elevated concentrations. Complete resolution can be expected in 80% of severely intoxicated patients. It is important to use the drug before the patient enters a moribund state.

Indications

Initial clinical trials were based on patients with severe symptoms. Antibody fragments should be given to patients with arrhythmias and hyperkalemia (greater than 5 to 6 mEq/liter) not responsive to other treatment. As clinical experience increases, this method of treatment may replace other more conventional therapy. Its use as a diagnostic tool to confirm the diagnosis in patients with possible digoxin-toxic arrhythmias needs further exploration.

Cautions

Renal failure—no adjustment in dosage is necessary. Elimination is approximately two times slower than normal. A rebound in free digoxin levels may occur 40 hours or more after administration of Fab fragments.

Cardiac failure—no adjustment in dosage is necessary. Patients who are dependent on digoxin for its inotropic or rate-limiting effects may need a substitute drug to replace digoxin after it is bound to the Fab fragments.

Hepatic failure—no adjustment in dosage is necessary.

Use in pregnancy—Category C. It crosses the placenta but the effect is unknown. It should not be withheld in severe digoxin poisoning where the effects of hypotension and arrhythmias are dangerous to the fetus.

Other—the antibody is derived from sheep antisera. Fever and hypersensitivity allergic reactions to the antibody fragments are possible.

Use in children—may be used

Onset and Duration of Action

The free digoxin levels drop to unmeasurable levels within 1 minute of administration. Clinical effects are usually observed within 15 to 30 minutes after the infusion, and complete response typically occurs by $1\frac{1}{2}$ hours but may take as long as 4 hours. Digoxin remains bound until it is excreted, but as tissue digoxin slowly equilibrates back into the serum, there may be a delayed rise in free digoxin level if inadequate antibody is present.

Dosage

The antibody comes as a lyophilized powder, which needs to be reconstituted with sterile water. Each vial contains 40 mg of antibody fragments, which will bind 0.6 mg of digoxin or digitoxin. The dosage should be calculated from the estimated total cardiac glycoside present, and the following formulas may be used. If a steady-state serum digoxin concentration (SDC) is known, the patient's SDC and the body weight can be entered into the formula below:

Dose in vials =
(SDC in ng/ml)
(5.6 l/kg)(body weight in kg)/
(1000 ng/mg)(0.6 mg/vial)

For digitoxin, the formula is modified to reflect the lower volume of distribution as follows:

Dose in vials =
(SDC in ng/ml)
(0.56 l/kg)(body weight in kg)/
(1000 ng/mg)(0.6 mg/vial)

If the estimated ingested amount of digoxin is known, the following formula is used:

Dose in vials = (ingested dose in mg)(0.8)/
(0.6 mg/vial)

The other factors in the formula are the volume of distribution (5.6 l/kg), 1000 ng/mg factor to convert units, and 0.6 mg of drug bound by each vial of antibody.

The ingested dose is multiplied by the oral bioavailability of digoxin and divided by the amount of digoxin each vial reverses. This formula results in the following approximations of the dose needed to reverse digoxin poisoning:

Number of 0.25-mg Tablets Digoxin Ingested	Antibody Dose (mg)	Antibody Dose (Vials)
25	340	8.5
50	680	17
75	1000	25
100	1360	34
150	2000	50

Limits

Although an adequate dose is necessary, excessive amounts should be avoided to minimize sensitization. Less than a full neutralizing dose may be used if some inotropic activity of digoxin is desired.

Repeat Dose

Because of possible inaccuracies in the initial dose, the patient's clinical situation should be monitored to ensure that more antibody fragment is given if clinically necessary.

Toxicity

Drug Interactions

No specific drug interactions are known.

Adverse Effects

Animals have developed sensitization after multiple doses of Fab fragments, but to date, several humans who have been treated twice have not become sensitized. Allergic reactions have been reported.

Treatment of Toxicity

Treatment of allergic reactions and substituting other rate-controlling or inotropic drugs may be necessary.

Dimercaprol (BAL)

Pharmacology

This drug was developed as an antidote to Lewisite, a chemical warfare agent containing arsenic. It is soluble in alcohol, vegetable oil, and water. Because it is unstable in the aqueous phase, the commercial product is suspended in peanut oil.

Distribution

Eighty percent of an intramuscular dose appears in the blood within 1 hour. The drug is widely distributed in all tissues including the brain but with highest concentrations in the liver and kidneys.

Elimination

Free dimercaprol is probably metabolized to a glucuronide, which is then excreted, half in the bile and half in urine. Elimination occurs rapidly and is complete within 6 to 24 hours.

Actions

The two sulfhydryl groups compete with sulfhydryl-containing enzymes to bind heavy metals and form a mercaptide that can be excreted. It can remove metals from the sulfhydryl-dependent enzymes essential for cell function. It does not protect against heavy metals, such as selenium, which inhibit oxidative enzymes. Since the degree of dimercaprol affinity for the metal depends on the pH, it is less effective in acidic media. Binding of the drug to the metal requires an excess of free drug and maintenance of a neutral or alkaline environment.

Indications

Dimercaprol is the drug of choice for arsenic, mercury, or gold poisoning. It may be used along with calcium edetate in serious lead poisoning where serum lead levels exceed 100 μg/dl or lead encephalopathy exists.

Cautions

The injections are very painful, and sterile abscesses may form at the injection site. It should not be used for cadmium, iron, selenium, or uranium poisoning because the resulting metal–dimercaprol complex is more toxic than the metal alone.

Renal failure—no dosage adjustment is necessary. The drug can possibly cause nephrotoxicity as the metal–dimercaprol complex dissociates in an acid environment. The urine should be alkalized and the drug discontinued if renal failure ensues.

Cardiac failure—no dosage adjustment is necessary.

Hepatic failure—because it is metabolized by the liver, it is contraindicated in patients with liver dsyfunction.

Use in pregnancy—abnormalities have been reported in mice but normal human infants have been reported after prenatal exposure. The drug should be used only when heavy metal toxicity is a significant risk to the mother and fetus.

Use in children—may be used

Onset and Duration of Action

Onset of action is within minutes, and the peak effect occurs within 30 to 60 minutes. The drug half-life is 4 to 5 hours.

Dosage

In arsenic or gold toxicity, the intramuscular dose is 3 mg/kg every 4 hours for 2 days, then twice a day for a week (or daily for 10 days). It should be given by deep intramuscular injection only. In acute mercury poisoning, the dose should be 5 mg/kg initially and followed by 2.5 mg/kg twice a day for a week. As an adjunctive treatment for severe lead poisoning with encephalopathy or serum levels greater than 100 μg/dl, the dose should be 3 to 5 mg/kg given every 4 hours for 3 to 7 days. Asymptomatic lead poisoning in children with serum levels greater than 70 to 80 μg/dl should also be treated with calcium edetate and dimercaprol followed by penicillamine.

Toxicity

Drug Interactions

Because cadmium, selenium, and iron complexes are toxic, these supplements should not be given. The drug is not soluble in water or aqueous solution.

Adverse Effects

The drug has a foul mercaptan (sulfur-like) odor that is disliked by patients. Increased heart rate and blood pressure can occur within 30 minutes but usually subside in 2 hours without treatment. Nausea and vomiting are common but are usually transient and dose related. Most patients affected are receiving more than 5 mg/kg. Fever is common in children. This drug may interfere with thyroid accumulation of iodine.

Treatment of Toxicity

Reduction of dosage may be necessary in patients experiencing severe adverse effects.

Ethanol

Pharmacology

Distribution

Absorption is rapid after oral administration. The volume of distribution is 0.55 l/kg.

Elimination

The drug is metabolized by alcohol dehydrogenase.

Actions

Methanol and ethylene glycol are metabolized by the enzyme alcohol dehydrogenase (ADH), producing high concentrations of toxic metabolites such as formic and oxalic acids. Ethanol has an affinity for ADH 200 times greater than methanol or ethylene glycol and will decrease the formation of toxic metabolites, allowing urinary excretion.

Indications

Ethanol treatment is indicated for serious methanol and ethylene glycol poisonings. Indications of serious toxicity are metabolic acidosis or serum levels greater than 20 mg/dl for either chemical.

Cautions

Renal failure—no adjustment in dosage is necessary until hemodialysis is started; then the dose needs to be increased.

Cardiac failure—no adjustment in dosage is necessary, although the intravenous route results in delivery of a large fluid volume over a short period of time.

Hepatic failure—chronic alcohol abusers may need increased ethanol dosing to maintain a therapeutic ethanol level.

Use in pregnancy—the ethanol concentrations in the fetus and mother equilibrate within 2 hours. The drug has long been used as a tocolytic to halt premature labor. Long-term use is associated with fetal alcohol syndrome, and the drug is classified as Category D.

Use in children—may be used

Onset and Duration of Action

Onset of activity occurs within minutes.

Dosage and Repeat Dose

The goal is an ethanol level of 100 mg/dl. This can be accomplished through a loading dose of 0.6 to 0.8 g/kg, followed by a maintenance dose of 0.11 g/kg/hour.

The oral loading dose is 2 ml/kg of a 50% solution over 1 hour; the maintenance dose is 0.33 ml/kg/hour.

Orally, 2 ml/kg of a 50% ethanol solution is equivalent to a 0.8 g/kg load. Alternatively, 2 ml/kg of commercial 80-proof (40% ethanol) whiskey is equivalent to 0.6 g/kg. These solutions should be given by nasogastric tube over 1 hour with a maintenance dose of 0.33 ml/kg/hour. The solutions should be diluted to avoid gastritis.

In the patient who is unable to retain oral ethanol because of emesis, 10 ml/kg of a 10% ethanol solution may be given intravenously as a loading dose, followed by a 1.6 mlc/kg/hour intravenous infusion.

Limits

Ethanol levels of >200 mg/dl are not needed and may cause sedation and other signs of intoxication. The intravenous infusion should be maintained until the methanol or ethylene glycol level is below 25 mg/dl.

Toxicity

Adverse Effects

Oral administration frequently results in nausea and vomiting. Fluid overload can occur with the large volumes used in intravenous administration. Complications from intoxication include hypoglycemia, aspiration, arrhythmias, hypertension, and hyperuricemia. Cessation of therapy may induce alcohol withdrawal in chronic alcohol abusers. The respiratory depressant effect may be enhanced if sedatives are present. An "antabuse-like" reaction may occur with metronidazole.

Treatment of Toxicity

Nausea and vomiting may be avoided by using more dilute solutions, which are not as irritating, or by administering by a slow drip through a nasogastric tube. Hypoglycemia can be avoided with continuous intravenous glucose infusion. Benzodiazepine therapy may be required during withdrawal.

Methylene Blue (Methylene Blue Injection, 10 mg/ml)

Pharmacology

Methylene blue, or trimethylthionine chloride, is a dark green crystal.

Distribution

Methylene blue is soluble in water but erratically absorbed following oral administration. Much of it is metabolized in the tissue to leukomethylene blue.

Elimination

The drug is excreted predominantly in the urine but also in the bile. Seventy-five percent of a dose is recovered in the urine over 5 days, with approximately 78% in the leukomethylene blue form and the remainder as unchanged drug. Because leukomethylene blue is colorless, the urine appears normal until it is exposed to ambient oxygen, which oxidizes the drug to a blue-colored methylene blue sulfone. This causes the urine to appear green.

Actions

Methylene blue is reduced to leukomethylene blue by the enzyme NADPH-methemoglobin (MetHb) reductase.

$$\text{Methylene blue} \xrightarrow{\text{NADPH MetHb reductase}}$$
$$+ \text{ NADPH}$$
$$\text{leukomethylene blue}$$
$$+ \text{ NADP}^+$$

The leukomethylene blue is then oxidized back to methylene blue and reduces methemoglobin back to hemoglobin in the process.

Leukomethylene blue $\rightarrow$ methylene blue
+ MetHb   + Hb

This NADPH-methemoglobin reductase is normally active and converts 5% of the methemoglobin back to hemoglobin. The addition of methylene blue greatly speeds up this reaction, resulting in an abundance of leukomethylene blue, which becomes available to reduce the methemoglobin. Because this reaction is reversible, methylene blue in high concentrations can accept electrons from normal hemoglobin to form leukomethylene blue and methemoglobin, thus worsening the clinical condition of methemoglobinemia.

Leukomethylene blue $\leftarrow$ methylene blue
+ MetHb   + Hb

This method has been used in the past to form methemoglobin in the treatment of cyanide poisoning, but it is no longer recommended since treatment with sodium nitrite is much more effective.

Indications

Methylene blue should be used in patients who are symptomatic from methemoglobinemia.

Cautions

The drug should be given slowly to avoid local concentrations high enough to induce methemoglobinemia. If there is subcutaneous extravasation, local necrosis may result.

Renal failure—since the drug is renally excreted, it should not be used in patients with severe renal disease.

Cardiac failure—hypotension and transient hypertension have been reported after rapid intravenous administration.

Hepatic failure—no dosage adjustment is necessary.

Hematologic—this drug should not be used in patients with glucose-6-phosphate dehydrogenase (G-6-PD) deficiency since it is ineffective and may cause hemolysis.

Use in pregnancy—Category C. Its safety in pregnancy is not established since there are no known reports of intravenous use during pregnancy. It has been used to diagnose ruptured membranes by direct injection into amniotic fluid. Case reports of hemolytic anemia, methemoglobinemia, and hyperbilirubinemia have been reported following such use.

Use in children—may be used

Onset and Duration of Action

The symptoms and cyanosis should improve within 1 hour. Once the source generating methemoglobin is removed and the patient has improved, regression will not occur.

Dosage

Dosage is 1 to 2 mg/kg or 0.2 ml/kg of a 1% solution.

Repeat Dose

The dose can be repeated once in 1 hour if there is no improvement or if cyanosis persists.

Limits

The maximum dose should not exceed 7 mg/kg. Above this dose, dyspnea, chest pain, apprehension, and restlessness may occur and methemoglobin concentration may increase.

Toxicity

Adverse Effects

Urine and feces may turn bluish or greenish with excretion of the methylene blue. A delayed hemolytic anemia has been reported to follow methylene blue treatment of methemoglobinemia induced by aniline dye. This may occur several days after initial treatment. Large doses may result in methemoglobin formation, as discussed under Actions, or in hemolysis.

Treatment of Toxicity

Skin exposed to the drug will be stained and may be cleaned with a hypochlorite solution. Exchange transfusion may be necessary for hemolysis resulting from methylene blue.

D-Penicillamine (Cuprimine, Depen Titratabs)

Pharmacology

Penicillamine is a degradation product of penicillin but has no antimicrobial activity. The D-isomer, the active isomer, is synthetically produced for commercial use. The L-isomer inhibits pyridoxine-dependent enzymes.

Distribution

The drug is well absorbed orally with 50 to 70% bioavailability, although decreased absorption occurs after meals and with enteric-coated formulations.

Elimination

One-third of the drug is excreted in the feces and one-half in the urine after metabolism by the liver to inactive disulfides.

Actions

The drug is a monothiol and chelates lead, gold, copper, mercury, and zinc.

Indications

Case reports have demonstrated efficacy in mild arsenic exposures when nausea and vomiting have subsided enough to allow oral therapy. It is also used following initial parenteral treatment of severe lead poisoning, as well as in management of cystinuria, Wilson's disease, and rheumatoid arthritis.

Cautions

Cardiac failure—no dosage adjustment is necessary.
Hepatic failure—no dosage adjustment is necessary.
Renal failure—no dosage adjustment is necessary.
Use in pregnancy—Category D. Penicillamine has been used to treat pregnant patients for a variety of chronic conditions, and several infants of these mothers have had connective tissue abnormalities that might be related to penicillamine.
Use in children—may be used

Onset and Duration of Action

The peak serum levels occur in 1 to 3 hours, and the average half-life varies between 1.5 and 3.1 hours with a biphasic elimination.

Dosage

Penicillamine can be given orally, 20 to 40 mg/kg/day in 2 to 4 doses up to 2 g/day for 5 days. It should be given on an empty stomach, 2 hours before or 3 hours after meals. Pyridoxine, 10 to 25 mg, should be given daily since pyridoxine-dependent enzymes are inhibited by penicillamine.

Limits

The decision to cease treatment is based on blood lead levels or urinary arsenic levels. For lead intoxication, several months of therapy is usually necessary.

Repeat Dose

As above.

Toxicity

Drug Interactions

Milk and food—decreased absorption
Gold, antimalarials, oxyphenbutazone, phenylbutazone, cytotoxic drugs—increased marrow suppression

Adverse Effects

Allergic reactions with a pruritic rash occur in one-third of patients. Because penicillamine is a degradation product of penicillin, it is contraindicated in patients allergic to penicillin. Complications include rash, gastrointestinal discomfort, decreased taste sensation, fever, proteinuria, bone marrow suppression, autoimmune disorders and a lupus-like syndrome, and renal and hepatic impairment.

Treatment of Toxicity

Allergic reactions respond to the usual treatment. Cessation of penicillamine administration will cause reversal of the adverse effects.

Physostigmine Salicylate (Antilirium)

Pharmacology

Physostigmine, a tertiary amine with an ester bond, binds acetylcholinesterase. It interferes with the metabolism of acetylcholine and causes an increase in the amount of acetylcholine at the synapse and the receptor site. This causes an increased acetylcholine or cholinergic effect.

Distribution

The drug is widely distributed. It crosses the placenta and, because it is a tertiary amine, also crosses the blood–brain barrier to allow reversal of central as well as peripheral anticholinergic effects.

Elimination

The drug is metabolized by cholinesterases.

Actions

Physostigmine hydrolyzes the acetylcholinesterase to choline and acetic acid, which results in an increase in acetylcholine at the neuroreceptor site.

Indications

It should be used in life-threatening anticholinergic drug poisoning when the usual treatment is inadequate. It should be avoided in tricyclic antidepressant (TCA) overdose because slowed cardiac conduction from TCAs may be additive to the cholinergic effect of physostigmine. Physostigmine has been used in children intramuscularly to treat delirium caused by anticholinergic preanesthetic agents.

Cautions

Cardiac failure—use with care in patients with heart block or bradyarrhythmias.
Hepatic failure—no dosage adjustment is necessary.
Renal failure—no dosage adjustment is necessary.
Other—patients with asthma, diabetes, bowel obstruction, and hypothyroidism have relative contraindications since the increased cholinergic effect may worsen their medical condition.
Use in pregnancy—Category C. Newborns of mothers treated with physostigmine for myasthenia gravis during pregnancy may have transient muscular weakness.
Use in children—may be used

Onset and Duration of Action

Onset of action and peak activity occur within 5 minutes, and the duration varies from 30 minutes to 5 hours. The half-life is unknown.

Dosage

The dose is 1 to 2 mg for adults and 50 μg/kg for children.

Limits

The drug should be given slowly at a rate less than 1 mg/min. The dose may be slowly increased depending on the patient's clinical response. It should be stopped if signs of cholinergic excess occur.

Repeat Dose

The dose may need to be repeated at 30- to 60-minute intervals.

Toxicity

Drug Interactions

Other cholinergic drugs, Type 1a antiarrhythmics, and beta-blockers cause decreased heart rate and cardiac conduction.

Adverse Effects

This drug can cause cholinergic excess manifested by increased secretions, defecation, urination, bradycardia, seizures, and respiratory paralysis. It has been temporally associated with asystole during the treatment of tricyclic antidepressant overdose.

Treatment of Toxicity

Atropine should be carefully given in doses starting at 0.1 to 0.2 mg, up to one-half the physostigmine dose, to counteract cholinergic excess.

Pralidoxime (Protopam)

Pharmacology

Distribution

The drug is poorly absorbed orally. Pralidoxime is widely distributed in extracellular fluid and is not protein bound. Its volume of distribution is approximately 0.8 l/kg. As a quaternary amine, pralidoxime should not cross the blood–brain barrier, but clinical experience demonstrates a central nervous system effect. Its half-life is reported to be from 1.2 to 2.6 hours.

Elimination

It is probably metabolized in the liver. Unchanged drug and metabolites undergo tubular secretion by the kidney. The amount of unmetabolized drug varies between 20% and 99% of total excretion.

Actions

Pralidoxime will pull the organophosphate from the cholinesterase enzyme and bind it, thereby reactivating the cholinesterase. This can only occur within the first 24 to 36 hours of exposure, since an irreversible change in the organophosphate-cholinesterase bond occurs within that time. It has variable activity with different organophosphate insecticides but should be used in all exposures. Although it has an effect at both muscarinic and nicotinic receptors, the muscarinic effects are more pronounced than the nicotinic effects.

Indications

Although atropine is most available and is given first, pralidoxime should be given as soon as possible after suspected organophosphate poisoning.

Cautions

Studies of animals poisoned with carbamates have shown a higher mortality after treatment with oximes similar to pralidoxime. Because carbamate poisoning also presents with cholinergic signs, it may be difficult to distinguish from organophosphate poisoning. If the exposure is to a known carbamate, pralidoxime may be withheld, but if there are central nervous system symptoms or if the poison may be an organophosphate, most experts believe that the pralidoxime should be given early while it is still effective. If a large amount of atropine has been given before the administration of prolidoxime, there may be a significant anticholinergic response from the residual atropine after the cholinesterase is reversed. Since red blood cell cholinesterase will be reported as falsely normal after pralidoxime administration, a blood sample for red blood cell cholinesterase must be sent before pralidoxime is given.

Renal failure—since the drug is renally excreted, a decrease in dose may be advisable in patients with severe renal insufficiency.

Cardiac failure—no adjustment in dosage is necessary.

Hepatic failure—the effect in the presence of hepatic disease is unknown, but the usual dose is recommended until more information is available.

Use in pregnancy—Category C. The effect in pregnancy is not known. The drug should be used when the toxicity of organophosphate poisoning presents a risk to the fetus and mother.

Use in children—may be used

Onset and Duration of Action

Fasciculations and muscle weakness improve in 10 to 40 minutes after intravenous administration. The half-life is from 0.8 to 2.7 hours with normal renal function.

Dosage

The initial intravenous dose is 25 to 50 mg/kg up to 2 g over 5 minutes or a 200 mg/min infusion.

Limits

Muscle fasciculations and weakness should be monitored for improvement. The drug should be given as soon as possible because organophosphate becomes irreversibly bound to the cholinesterase and not susceptible to reversal within 48 hours. However, a therapeutic trial may be worthwhile even in late cases since each organophosphate has its own characteristics.

Repeat Dose

The dose may be repeated in 1 to 2 hours and every 6 hours thereafter, or it may be given as a continuous infusion of 500 mg/hour.

Toxicity

Drug Interactions

Sympathomimetic drugs and theophylline cause additive side effects.

Adverse Effects

In healthy patients, pralidoxime is generally safe and has minimal side effects when given intravenously. In mice, the LD_{50} is 159 mg/kg. Adverse effects include tachycardia, laryngospasm, hypertension, muscle rigidity, confusion, dizziness, nausea, and headache.

Treatment of Toxicity

Adverse reactions usually resolve with supportive care and may be avoided with slower administration of pralidoxime.

Pyridoxine

Pharmacology

Distribution

Pyridoxine is water soluble and crosses the blood–brain barrier.

Elimination

It is metabolized in the liver and excreted as pyridoxic acid.

Actions

Pyridoxine is active as pyridoxal-5-phosphate, a coenzyme for glutamic acid decarboxylase and gamma-aminobutyric acid (GABA) transaminase. These enzymes are involved in the synthesis and degradation of GABA, a major inhibitory neurotransmitter in the brain. Isoniazid binds with pyridoxine in the body to form inactive isoniazid-pyridoxal hydrazones, which are excreted in the urine. The central nervous system depletion of pyridoxine results in the attenuation of pyridoxine-dependent enzymes and a net decrease in GABA levels, resulting in seizures. In ethylene glycol poisoning, pyridoxine is a cofactor in the metabolism of glyoxylic acid to glycine, a nontoxic end product of ethylene glycol, and may increase the rate of metabolism by this pathway.

Indications

Pyridoxine should be used in symptomatic patients and in all patients who have ingested more than 2 g of isoniazid. Patients symptomatic after ingestion of mushrooms that contain gyromitrin, a toxin metabolized to monomethylhydrazine, should also receive pyridoxine. It should be given as an adjunctive treatment in all patients with ethylene glycol poisoning.

Cautions

Renal failure—no adjustment in dosage is necessary.

Cardiac failure—no adjustment in dosage is necessary.

Hepatic failure—no adjustment in dosage is necessary.

Use in pregnancy—Category C in doses greater than the recommended daily allowance (RDA) minimum. Large doses of pyridoxine given during pregnancy have been suspected of causing seizures in neonates due to a relative pyridoxine deficiency. These infants may require lifetime pyridoxine supplementation. The effects of a single large dose are unknown. Pyridoxine supplementation has been used for both hypertension and glucose intolerance in pregnancy without known harm to the fetus.

Use in children—may be used

Onset and Duration of Action

Most cases report cessation of seizures within 60 minutes of pyridoxine administration, and, once seizures subside, there should be no need for further dosing. Coma usually resolves in 5 to 9 hours but has been reported to last as long as 72 hours.

Dosage

Pyridoxine is usually given in a gram-per-gram dose equivalent to the amount of isoniazid ingested. A suggested protocol is to mix the drug as a 5 to 10% solution and give it over 30 minutes in D_5W as soon as possible after ingestion.

In ethylene glycol poisoning, the recommended dose is 50 mg every 6 hours IV or IM.

After mushroom ingestion with monomethylhydrazine poisoning, a dose of 25 mg/kg is appropriate. For comparison, the RDA is 2 mg/day.

Limits

The drug should not be given in these large doses for long-term therapy.

Repeat Dose

The dose should be repeated if there is no response.

Toxicity

Drug Interactions

Phenobarbital, phenytoin—levels may be decreased with chronic pyridoxine use.
Levodopa—metabolism is increased, resulting in decrease levadopa effects.
Isoniazid, penicillamine, cycloserine, hydralazine—pyridoxine requirements are increased.

Adverse Effects

The drug is nontoxic even at a dosage of 1 g daily. Problems may arise with dosages greater than 2 g daily when used long term. Typical manifestations are peripheral sensory neuropathy with widespread axonal degeneration, which resolves after discontinuation of the drug. Although neuropathy occurs most commonly with chronic therapy, one patient developed a reversible sensory neuropathy after a single 10-g dose of pyridoxine given for an isoniazid overdose. Other possible toxic effects include tachypnea, postural blood pressure changes, paralysis, and convulsions. The LD_{50} in dogs is reported to be 1 g/kg.

Treatment of Toxicity

Discontinuation of the drug results in improvement of neuropathy. Seizures and other adverse effects should be treated with standard methods.

Vitamin K₁ (Aquamephyton, Konakion, Mephyton)

Preparations of phytonadione include Aquamephyton for parenteral use, Konakion for intramuscular use, and Mephyton for oral use.

Pharmacology

Phytonadione is vitamin K_1, a fat-soluble vitamin necessary in the blood clotting cascade.

Distribution

Phytonadione is a cofactor for a carboxylation reaction necessary to activate clotting factors from inactive precursors. Eventually, it is metabolized to more polar, water-soluble metabolites.

Elimination

Elimination of the polar metabolites occurs through the bile and kidneys.

Actions

Vitamin K is a precursor for clotting Factors II, VII, IX, and X synthesized in the liver and is naturally present in adequate amounts in the diet. Warfarin inhibits regeneration of vitamin K_1 from the vitamin K_1 epoxide and slows down the coupled reaction to activate clotting factors. An excessive amount of vitamin K can overcome the warfarin effect. It is thought that water-soluble forms of vitamin K such as menadione are not as efficacious as the fat-soluble phytonadione.

Indications

Phytonadione is indicated for reversal of warfarin anticoagulant toxicity.

Cautions

Renal failure—there is no dosage adjustment necessary.
Cardiac failure—hypotension and shock have been reported after intravenous injection.
Hepatic failure—exogenous phytonadione therapy may not reverse hypoprothrombinemia if the hepatocytes are so damaged that they are unable to synthesize vitamin K–dependent clotting factors when adequate substrate is available. There may be a paradoxical decrease in the amount of prothrombin with vitamin K administration in patients with severe hepatitis or cirrhosis.

Use in pregnancy—Category C. It crosses the placenta and may result in hyperbilirubinemia if given to near-term pregnant women. In a series of pregnant women given oral phytonadione, there was a transient increase in prothrombin time.

Use in children—may be used

Onset and Duration of Action

Onset is within 1 to 2 hours, and the prothrombin time may be normal within 12 hours. The effect can last 1 to 4 days, depending on the dose.

Dosage

The dose should be 2.5 to 10 mg, depending on the urgency of treatment. If given intravenously, the dose should be administered at the rate of 1 mg/min to avoid reactions. If active bleeding is occurring, 20 to 40 mg may be needed. The initial dose may be repeated after 6 to 8 hours. For superwarfarin toxicity, doses 10 times larger may be required for a therapeutic response.

Toxicity

Drug Interactions

The drug is incompatible with many other drugs in solution.

Adverse Effects

Intramuscular and subcutaneous injections may result in hemorrhage or hematoma formation. Severe reactions with hypotension and cardiac arrest resembling hypersensitivity may occur if phytonadione is given rapidly intravenously. Skin lesions, which are localized erythematous and tender plaques, may occur in a delayed fashion after injection. Large doses of phytonadione result in refractoriness to oral anticoagulant therapy.

Treatment of Toxicity

Fluid and vasopressors have been successfully used to reverse hypotension.

REFERENCES

Arena JM, Rourk MH, Sibrack CD: Acetaminophen: Report of an unusual poisoning. Pediatrics 61:68–72, 1978.

Banner WJR, Lund ME, Clawson L: Failure of naloxone to reverse clonidine toxic effect. Am J Dis Child 137:1170–1171, 1983.

Barash P, Kitahata LM, Mandel S: Acute cardiovascular collapse after intravenous phytonadione. Anesth Analg Curr Res 55:304–306, 1976.

Baud FJ, Galliot MG, Astair A, et al: Treatment of ethylene glycol poisoning with intravenous 4 methylpyrazole. N Engl J Med 319:97–100, 1988.

Becker CE: Methanol poisoning. J Emerg Med 1:51–58, 1983.

Bentur Y, Koren G, Klein J, et al: Pharmacokinetics and nephrotoxicity of deferoxamine (abstract). Vet Hum Toxicol 30(4):371, 1988.

Bergstrom RF, Kay DR, Harkcom TM, Wagner JG: Penicillamine kinetics in normal subjects. Clin Pharmacol Ther 30:404–413, 1981.

Berlin CM: Treatment of cyanide poisoning in children (letter). Pediatrics 46:793–796, 1970.

Blanchard PD, Yao JDC, McAlpine DE, Hurt RD: Isoniazid overdose in the Cambodian population of Olmsted County, Minnesota. JAMA 256(12):3131, 1986.

Briggs GG, Freeman RK, Yaffe SJ: Drugs in Pregnancy and Lactation, 2nd ed. Baltimore, Williams & Wilkins, 1986.

Buckler HM, Smith WDF, Rees WDW: Self-poisoning with oral cadmium chloride. Br Med J 292:1559–1560, 1986.

Chisolm JJ: The use of chelating agents in the treatment of acute and chronic lead intoxication. J Pediatr 73:1–38, 1968.

Cohen MR, Cohen RM, Pickar D, et al: Behavioral effects after high dose naloxone administration to normal volunteers. Lancet November 14:1110, 1981.

Curry S: Methemoglobinemia. Ann Emerg Med 11:214–221, 1982.

Curry S, Bond R, Raschke R, et al: Fetal iron kinetics in an animal model of maternal iron poisoning with and without maternal deferoxamine therapy (abstract). Vet Hum Toxicol 30:372, 1988.

Eisen TF, Lacouture PG, Woolf A: Visual detection of ferrioxamine color changes in urine (abstract). Vet Hum Toxicol 30:369, 1988.

Ekins BR, Rollins DE, Duffy DP, Gregory MC: Standardized treatment of severe methanol poisoning with ethanol and hemodialysis. West J Med 3:337–340, 1985.

Ellenhorn MJ, Barceloux DG: Medical Toxicology. New York, Elsevier, 1988.

Fauman BJ: Treatment of acute phenothiazine reaction. Ann Emerg Med 10:228, 1981.

Gentile DA: Severe methemoglobinemia induced by a topical teething preparation. Pediatr Emerg Care 3:171–175, 1987.

Goldfrank L, Weisman RS, Errick JK, Lo MW: A dosing nomogram for continuous infusion intravenous naloxone. Ann Emerg Med 15:566–570, 1986.

Hall AH, Linden CH, Kulig KW, Rimack BH: Cyanide poisoning from laetrile ingestion: Role of nitrite therapy. Pediatrics 78:269–272, 1986.

Hall AH, Rumack BH: Hydrocobalamine/sodium thiosulfate as a cyanide antidote. J Emerg Med 5:115–121, 1987.

Handal KA, Schauben JL, Salamone FR: Naloxone. Ann Emerg Med 12:438–445, 1983.

Hansteen V, Jacobsen D, Knudsen K, et al: Acute massive poisoning with digitoxin: Report of seven cases and discussion of treatment. Clin Toxicol 18:679–692, 1981.

Harris JC, Rumack BH, Peterson RG, McGuire BM: Methemoglobinemia resulting from absorption of nitrates. JAMA 242:2869–2871, 1979.

Heath A: Beta adrenoreceptor blocker toxicity. Am J Emerg Med 2:518–525, 1984.

Henderson RP, Soloman CP: Use of cholestyramine in the treatment of digoxin poisoning. Arch Intern Med 148:745–746, 1988.

Hoidal CR, Hall AH, Robinson MD, et al: Hydrogen sulfide poisoning from toxic inhalations of roofing asphalt fumes. Ann Emerg Med 15:826–830, 1986.

Jacobsen D, Ostby N, Bredsen JE: Studies on ethylene glycol poisoning. Acta Med Scand 212:11–15, 1982.

James JA: Acute iron poisoning: Assessment of severity and prognosis. J Pediatr 77:117–119, 1970.

Jones EC, Growe GH, Naiman SC: Prolonged anticoagulation in rat poisoning. JAMA 252:3005–3007, 1984.

Kukovetz WR, Beubler E, Kreuzig F, et al: Bioavailability and pharmacokinetics of d-penicillamine. J Rheumatol 10:90–94, 1983.

Lee AS: Drug induced dystonic reactions. JACEP 6:351–354, 1977.

Lipton RA, Klass EM: Human ingestion of a superwarfarin rodenticide resulting in a prolonged anticoagulant effect. JAMA 252:304–3005, 1984.

Lotti M, Becker CB: Treatment of acute organophosphate poisoning: Evidence of direct effect on central nervous system by 2-PAM. Clin Tox 19:121–127, 1982.

Mant TG, Tempowski JH, Volans GN, Talbot JC: Adverse reactions to acetylcysteine and effects of overdose. Br Med J 289(6439):217–219, 1984.

McElvoy GK (ed): Drug Information 88. Bethesda, MD, American Hospital Formulary Service, American Society of Hospital Pharmacists, 1988.

McMartin KE, Ambre JT, Tephly TR: Methanol poisoning in human subjects. Am J Med 68:414–418, 1980.

Mofenson HC, Caracio TR: Glucagon for propranolol overdose (letter). JAMA 255:2025–2026, 1986.

Mortenson ML: Management of acute childhood poisoning caused by selected insecticides and herbicides. Pediatr Clin North Am 33:421–445, 1986.

Noker PE, Eells JT, Tephly TR: Methanol toxicity: Treatment with folic acid and 5-formyl tetrafolic acid. Alcoholism: Clin Exp Res 4:378–383, 1980.

North DS, Wieland MJ, Peterson CD, Krenzelok EP: Naloxone administration in clonidine overdosage (correspondence). Ann Emerg Med 10:397, 1981.

Orlowski JP, Paganini EP, Pippenger CE: Treatment of a potentially lethal dose isoniazid ingestion. Ann Emerg Med 17(1):73–76, 1988.

Ott DA, Goeden SR: Treatment of acute phenothiazine reaction. JACEP 8:471–472, 1979.

Panos RJ, et al: Esophageal spasm following propranolol overdose relieved by glucagon. Am J Emerg Med 4:227–228, 1986.

Perrett D: An outline of d-penicillamine metabolism. Proc R Soc Med 70(Suppl 3):61–64, 1977.

Pentel PR, Peterson CD: Asystole complicating physostigmine treatment of tricyclic antidepressant overdose. Ann Emerg Med 9:588, 1980.

Peterson CD, Leeder SJ, Sterner S: Glucagon therapy for beta blocker overdose. Drug Intell Clin Pharm 18:394–398, 1984.

Peterson RG, Rumack BH: D-penicillamine therapy of acute arsenic poisoning. J Pediatr 91:661–666, 1977.

Prescott LF, Illingworth RN, Critchley JAJH, et al: Intravenous N-acetylcysteine: The treatment of choice for paracetamol poisoning. Br Med J 2:1097–1100, 1979.

Robotham JL, Lietman PS: Acute iron poisoning. Am J Dis Child 134:875–879, 1980.

Rumack BH: Anticholinergic poisoning: Treatment with physostigmine. Pediatrics 52:449, 1973.

Seiden BS, Curry SC: Prolonged succinylcholine induced paralysis in organophosphate insecticide poisoning. Ann Emerg Med 16:215–217, 1987.

Smilkstein MJ, Knapp GL, Kulig KW, Rumack BH: Efficacy of oral N-acetylcysteine in the treatment of acetaminophen overdose. N Engl J Med 319:1557–1562, 1988.

Smith RP, Gosselin RE: Hydrogen sulfide poisoning. J Occup Med 21:93–97, 1979.

Smith RP, Gosselin RE: On the mechanism of sulfide inactivation by methemoglobin. Toxicol Appl Pharmacol 8:159–172, 1966.

Stine RJ, Slosberg B, Beacham BE: Hydrogen sulfide intoxication. Ann Intern Med 85:756–758, 1976.

Tafuri J, Roberts J: Organophosphate poisoning. Ann Emerg Med 16:193–201, 1987.

Tenenbein M: Whole bowel irrigation in iron poisoning. J Pediatr 111:142–145, 1987.

Thompson D, Thompson GD, Greenwood RB, et al: Therapeutic dosing of pralidoxime chloride. Drug Intell Clin Pharm 21:590–593, 1987.

Vitale LF, Rosalinas-Bailon A, Folland D, et al: Oral penicillamine therapy for chronic lead poisoning in children. J Pediatr 83:1041–1045, 1984.

Wason S, Lacouture PG, Lovejoy FH: Single high dose pyridoxine treatment for isoniazid overdose. JAMA 246:1102–1104, 1981.

Wiesner RH, Dickson ER, Go VLW, Carlson GL: Pharmacokinetics of d-penicillamine in normals and primary biliary cirrhosis. Gastroenterology 76(5, Part 2):1270, 1979.

Yarbrough BE, Wood JP: Isoniazid overdose treated with high dose pyridoxine. Ann Emerg Med 12(5):303–305, 1983.

Zaritsky AL, Horowitz M, Chernow B: Glucagon antagonism of calcium channel blocker induced myocardial dysfunction. Crit Care Med 16:246–251, 1988.

CHAPTER 17

Antivenins and Antitoxins

EDWARD J. OTTEN, M.D.

Antivenins

INTRODUCTION

Venomous animals are those that have evolved specific venom glands and a venom delivery system that is used either for food gathering, defense, or, in some cases, for both. Humans are generally accidental recipients of the venom but may nonetheless be at great risk from certain envenomations. In the United States three types of antivenin are currently available for venomous animal injuries. Many more antivenins are available worldwide, and several experimental antivenins also exist.

Antivenin is a suspension of antibodies prepared from the serum of animals hyperimmunized against a specific venom or venoms. The French microbiologist Calmette developed the first antivenin in 1892 while working at the Pasteur Institute in Saigon by inoculating rabbits with Indian cobra venom and using the serum from the recovered rabbits to treat humans bitten by the cobra. Antivenin may be derived from venom of one species of animal, monovalent antivenin, or from venom of several species of animals, polyvalent antivenin. For example, coral snake antivenin is a monovalent antivenin and will only neutralize venom from *Micrurus* species found in the southeastern United States. Crotalidae antivenin is a polyvalent antivenin made from the venom of four different pit vipers, but because of the large

number of similar substances in the venom of pit vipers, this antivenin will neutralize over a hundred different varieties of snake venom found throughout the world.

Most antivenins are derived from horse serum because horses are readily available and their large size allows a large amount of antivenin to be produced from a single animal. The problem of allergic reactions to horse serum can be serious and has been the driving force behind the development of recombinant deoxyribonucleic acid (DNA)-produced antisera for other diseases such as rabies and tetanus. However, there has not been the economic incentive for the development of an antiserum such as snake antivenin because it is rarely used in most hospitals. No human serum antivenins are commercially available, but research is being done in this area. There is also current research to develop active immunization against snakebite for use in underdeveloped countries where venomous snakebite is a significant medical problem.

It is likely that the only antivenin the clinician will be using in the next few years will be of horse serum derivation. The incidence of immediate allergic reaction is 3 to 5% and may not be related to previous exposure but rather to the amount of serum given. The incidence of late serum sickness type reactions approaches 100% in patients given more than 10 vials of antivenin. It is not known whether the immediate reaction is a Type I or anaphylactic reaction or whether it is complement mediated.

Because of the possibility of anaphylaxis, an intradermal skin test is recommended prior to the administration of the antivenin. The patient should be questioned prior to skin testing concerning allergy to horses or horse serum, history of hay fever or urticaria, or history of prior injections of horse serum. The patient should not be skin tested unless the decision has been made to administer the antivenin. The skin test may precipitate an allergic reaction and may also sensitize the patient to horse serum and cause future problems with allergic reactions. If the patient is known to be allergic to horse serum or has a positive skin test and the antivenin must be given, special precautions must be taken to avoid a serious allergic reaction. Administering the antivenin in small aliquots and administering antihistamines and epinephrine concurrently may reduce the risk of allergic reaction and allow sufficient antivenin to be absorbed. It is important to remember that a negative skin test does not guarantee that an allergic reaction will not occur. All antivenin should be diluted in normal saline and administered intravenously. Antivenin may be administered intramuscularly in a large muscle mass, but this should only be done if intravenous access cannot be obtained. Any patient receiving antivenin should have two intravenous lines in place so that one can be used for the administration of medications in the event of an allergic reaction. Antivenin should be given in an intensive care unit setting where the patient's response to the antivenin and possible adverse reactions can be constantly monitored. Any decision to administer antivenin should take into account the size, species, and condition of the animal as well as the number and location of the bites, the general health and size of the patient, and, most importantly, the clinical response of the patient to the bite.

CONDITIONS

Pit Viper Bite

Diagnosis

The diagnosis of venomous snakebite can be made on clinical examination or by enzyme-linked immunosorbant assay (ELISA).

However, there are no ELISA tests currently marketed for species of pit vipers found in the United States. The diagnosis is therefore made by history and physical examination. The patient will usually give a history of either handling a snake or being involved in some outdoor activity such as hiking or gardening. Pit vipers include rattlesnakes, copperheads, and water moccasins. They are found throughout the United States except in Maine, Hawaii, and Alaska. They may also be found in zoos, laboratories, and private collections. The pit viper can be easily identified by the presence of a small pit midway between the nostril and the eye of the snake. Nonvenomous snakes will not have this pit. If there is any question concerning the identification of the snake, expert advice should be obtained. Under no circumstances should a live snake be handled. In addition, careless handling of recently expired snakes has been reported to result in envenomation.

If positive identification of the snake is not possible, the decision to use antivenin must be made on clinical grounds. A sharp, intense pain usually occurs in the area of the bite and moves proximally. The pain may be accompanied by nausea, vomiting, light-headedness, numbness, weakness, and a metallic taste in the mouth in the case of pit viper envenomation. The bite occurs on the extremities 98% of the time. On physical examination the patient will usually have fang mark puncture wounds but in some cases may have only a scratch. The pit viper bite may show a large amount of edema, ecchymosis, bleb formation, and tissue destruction. Hypotension, renal failure, disseminated intravascular coagulation, pulmonary edema, and coma may be seen in severe envenomation.

Indications for Treatment

The severity of the bite should be graded to determine if antivenin should be given and how much is needed. Most crotalid species have a number of toxins capable of producing local pain, edema, and ecchymosis as well as systemic signs and symptoms. Therefore, a grading system has been developed to help decide if antivenin is necessary. This system can only be used for crotalids or pit vipers; it should not be used for other types of snakes (see Table 17–1 for a list of crotalid snakes). In a few species of pit viper, such as the Mojave rattlesnake *(Crotalus scutulatus)* whose bite may cause significant neurologic

TABLE 17–1. Venomous Snakes Neutralized by Crotalid Polyvalent Antivenin

Scientific Name	Common Name
Agkistrodon bilineatus	Cantil
A. contortrix	American copperhead
A. halys	Mamushi
A. piscivorus	Cottonmouth water moccasin
A. rhodostoma	Malayan pit viper
A. acutus	One hundred pace snake
Bothrops atrox	Fer-de-lance or Barba Amarilla
B. alternatus	Yarara or urutu
B. neuwiedi	Weid's lance head
B. venezuelae	Tigra-mariposa
B. jararaca	Jararaca
B. cotiara	Cotiara
Crotalus adamanteus	Eastern diamondback
C. atrox	Western diamondback
C. cerastes	Sidewinder
C. durissus	Cascabel, tropical
C. horridus	Timber rattlesnake
C. molossus	Black tailed
C. scutulatus	Mojave rattlesnake
C. tigris	Tiger rattlesnake
C. ruber	Red diamond rattlesnake
C. viridis abyssus	Grand Canyon
C. viridis helleri	Southern Pacific
C. lepidus	Rock rattlesnake
Lachesis muta	Bushmaster
Sistrurus catenatus	Massasauga
S. miliarius	Pigmy rattlesnake
Trimeresurus flavoviridis	Habu
T. gramineus	Green tree viper

symptoms without any local signs or symptoms, the grading system is not useful. With most pit viper bites, minimal envenomation is considered to be pain and edema localized to the bite area with little or no proximal spread, no systemic signs or symptoms, and no laboratory abnormalities. Patients with minimal envenomation can be observed for 24 hours and, if no further signs or symptoms develop, can be discharged without antivenin treatment. Effects of moderate envenomation would include extensive pain and edema and/or systemic signs and symptoms. Patients with moderate envenomation should be given 5 vials of antivenin intravenously over 1 hour and reevaluated. If their condition does not improve or worsens, 3 to 5 more vials should be given. The end-point in treatment is indicated by the clinical condition of the patient. In some cases, 30 or more vials of antivenin have been administered before the patient's condition improved. Severe envenomation manifests with extensive tissue destruction along with signs of hypotension, pulmonary edema, renal fail-

ure, severe coagulopathy, hemolysis, hemorrhage, or coma. Patients with severe envenomation should be given 10 vials of antivenin in the first hour and, depending on the patient's response, 3 to 5 additional vials each additional hour. The earlier the antivenin is given, the more efficacious it is.

For a variety of reasons, 30 to 40% of all bites by venomous snakes may not cause significant envenomation and are referred to as "dry bites." All patients bitten by pit vipers should be observed for at least 4 hours and, if no sign of envenomation has occurred, can be discharged with instructions to return if any signs or symptoms develop. Once the bite has been graded, the antivenin should be reconstituted and administered. Additional antivenin should be administered depending on the clinical response of the patient. Persistent hypotension, disseminated intravascular coagulation, renal failure, and coma may require large amounts of antivenin. Children may need larger amounts of antivenin than adults owing to their smaller volume and available protein binding sites. Antivenin should usually not be administered for more than 24 hours or more than 24 hours after a bite has occurred. However, in severe envenomations when the patient's clinical status has not responded, antivenin may be given for a longer period. Most patients receiving more than 7 vials of antivenin will develop serum sickness days to weeks later, which usually responds to systemic steroids. Figure 17–1 outlines the

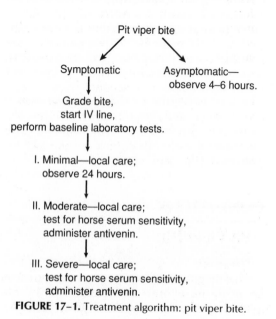

FIGURE 17–1. Treatment algorithm: pit viper bite.

DRUG TREATMENT: MODERATE PIT VIPER ENVENOMATION

First-Line Drug

Crotalid Polyvalent Antivenin

Initial Dose	5 vials IV diluted in 500 ml normal saline over 60 minutes
Repeat Dose	If condition not improved or worse, 3–5 vials IV diluted in 500 ml normal saline each hour
End-Point	Resolution of symptoms

DRUG TREATMENT: SEVERE PIT VIPER ENVENOMATION

First-Line Drug

Crotalid Polyvalent Antivenin

Initial Dose	10 vials IV diluted in 500 ml normal saline over 60 minutes
Repeat Dose	3–5 vials IV diluted in 500 ml normal saline every 60 minutes until symptoms and signs resolve
End-Point	Resolution of symptoms and signs

treatment approach for pit viper bites. (See boxes, Drug Treatment: Moderate Pit Viper Envenomation and Drug Treatment: Severe Pit Viper Envenomation.)

Discussion

There are many other types of treatment of pit viper envenomation referred to in the literature (e.g., excision of the bite area, incision and suction, and compression and immobilization), but these should be considered first-aid measures and not definitive treatment. Antivenin is the only specific treatment currently available for venomous snakebite.

Patients who are allergic to horse serum have been successfully treated by administration of aliquots of the antivenin in very low concentrations (e.g., 1:10,000) and pretreatment with antihistamines and concomitant infusion of intravenous epinephrine. This therapy would be analogous to treating someone who is allergic to penicillin with intravenous penicillin for meningitis. Expert advice should be obtained prior to attempting this procedure.

Crotalid polyvalent antivenin is a lyophilized, concentrated antivenin derived from the serum of healthy horses that have been injected with the venom of the eastern dia-

mondback rattlesnake *(Crotalus adamanteus)*, the western diamondback rattlesnake *(Crotalus atrox)*, the Cascabel rattlesnake *(Crotalus durissus)*, and the Fer-de-lance *(Bothrops atrox)*. This antivenin is capable of neutralizing venom from most of the crotalids or pit vipers found throughout the world (see Table 17–1).

Coral Snake *(Micrurus)* Bite

Diagnosis

The coral snake is found throughout the southeastern United States from Texas to Georgia and Florida. Although it is similar in appearance to the Sonoran coral snake found in Arizona and New Mexico, it is not related, and *Micrurus* antivenin may not be used for bites from the Sonoran coral snake. The coral snake may be identified by the colored bands on its body and the black tip of its head. The bands are arranged red next to yellow, whereas the similar appearing scarlet king snake has red next to black bands. This system should not be used to identify coral snakes from other parts of the world. Coral snake envenomation may produce weakness, diplopia, lethargy, headache, and paralysis. One or two fang marks are usually present; however, even a scratch may cause serious

DRUG TREATMENT: CORAL SNAKE BITE

First-Line Drug

***Micrurus fulvius* Antivenin**

Initial Dose	3–5 vials by IV piggyback
Repeat Dose	3–5 additional vials by IV piggyback
End-Point	Based on clinical response, neurologic improvement may take weeks.

envenomation. Coral snake envenomations usually have few local signs but may present with systemic signs such as ptosis, gaze paralysis, respiratory paralysis, and coma.

Indications for Treatment

Coral snakes are members of the Elapidae family, and their venom contains mainly neurotoxic substances. Therefore, there may be little or no local reaction to the bite, and the first manifestation of envenomation may be respiratory arrest. For this reason, all patients bitten by an eastern coral snake should receive antivenin. The dose is 3 to 5 vials given as soon as possible after the bite. If bulbar paralysis is present, 5 to 10 vials should be given intravenously over an hour. Because of the small size of this snake, this amount of antivenin should neutralize the total amount of venom injected. (See box.)

Discussion

Micrurus fulvius antivenin is a lyophilized, concentrated antivenin derived from horses hyperimmunized by injecting them with venom derived from the eastern coral snake *(Micrurus fulvius)*. It will neutralize venom from only two varieties of *Micrurus: Micrurus fulvius fulvius* (eastern coral snake) and *Micrurus fulvius tenere* (Texas coral snake). It should not be used for the Arizona or Sonoran coral snake *(Micruroides euryxanthus)* or the various species of Mexican, Central American, or South American coral snakes. The same precautions for administering crotalid antivenin apply to *Micrurus* antivenin. The patient should be skin tested for horse serum sensitivity as noted at the beginning of this chapter. The antivenin should be reconstituted, and 3 to 5 vials should be given intravenously. The dose should be adjusted to the response of the patient, and if paralysis is present after the initial dose, 3 to 5 additional vials should be given.

Black Widow Spider Bite *(Latrodectus)*

Diagnosis

There are over 20,000 species of spiders in the world, and nearly all are venomous. Most do not pose a danger to humans because their fangs are not long enough to penetrate human skin. An exception is the black widow spider, which is found throughout the United States. Its bite can be fatal. The victim usually complains of a rather mild pain initially at the bite site. This pain increases in intensity over about an hour and is accompanied by severe muscle spasms that begin in the area of the bite and move proximally. The patient may also complain of headache, paresthesias, weakness, chest pain, and abdominal pain. Physical examination reveals tachycardia, hypertension, muscle spasm, abdominal pain without tenderness, and increased salivation.

Indications for Treatment

Most black widow spider bites will not require antivenin but can be treated with calcium gluconate and muscle relaxants. If the patient does not respond to this conservative therapy, 1 vial of antivenin should be administered intravenously over 15 minutes. If the patient continues to be symptomatic, another cause of the symptoms should be sought. Patients over 65 years of age or under 6 years of age are the usual candidates for antivenin. Other patients with severe hypertension, uncontrolled muscle spasm pain, hypotension, neurologic signs, or organ failure should be given antivenin. (See box.)

Discussion

Black widow spider antivenin is a lyophilized, concentrated antivenin obtained from the serum of horses injected with black widow spider *(Latrodectus mactans)* venom.

DRUG TREATMENT: BLACK WIDOW SPIDER BITE

First-Line Drug

Calcium Gluconate 10%

Initial Dose	10 ml by IV push
Repeat Dose	10 ml by IV push, up to 100 ml
End-Point	Relief of muscle spasms

Second-Line Drug

Diazepam

Initial Dose	1–5 mg by IV push
Repeat Dose	1–5 mg by IV push
End-Point	Relief of muscle spasm

Third-Line Drug

Black Widow Spider Antivenin

Initial Dose	1 vial (2.5 ml) diluted in some saline over 30 minutes
Repeat Dose	Usually not indicated May repeat initial dose if patient symptomatic after 1 hour
End-Point	Relief of symptoms, normalization of vital signs

It can be used to neutralize the effects of envenomation by black widow spiders if the patient does not respond to more conservative measures. Most patients envenomated by black widow spiders will complain of severe muscle spasms beginning in the area of the bite and moving proximally; diaphoresis, nausea, weakness, and headache are also common. A few patients may present with seizures, severe hypertension, or hypotension. This more severe reaction is usually seen in children or in adults with underlying health problems such as hypertension or cardiovascular disease. The majority of patients with muscle spasms can be treated with intravenous calcium gluconate and diazepam. Patients who do not respond and those who have hypertension, hypotension, or other major complications should be given 1 vial of reconstituted antivenin after being tested for horse serum sensitivity. There is usually a rapid response to the antivenin. A second vial may be necessary in children. The antivenin may be given intramuscularly in a large muscle group, but the preferred route is intravenous administration of antivenin in 50 ml of normal saline over 30 minutes. Because of the possibility of allergic reactions to the horse serum, the antivenin should be reserved for the pediatric patient, the geriatric patient, and the patient in extremis.

Exotic Animal Envenomation

Discussion

Exotic Snakes

Thousands of non-native snakes are imported, raised, and sold in the United States annually. A number of collectors, zoos, and laboratories have these snakes in captivity. Unfortunately, a large percentage of these non-native or exotic snakes are venomous and the people who come in contact with them are at risk for envenomation. Most zoos and research facilities keep antivenin for these exotic species on hand in case of envenomation, but most private collectors cannot afford to do this and those who are bitten may present to an emergency department with a venomous bite and no antivenin. If this occurs, the physician should contact the local Drug and Poison Information Center for help in locating the nearest appropriate antivenin. The Arizona Poison and Drug Information Center (telephone 1-602-626-6016) maintains a 24-hour service called the Antivenin Index that will aid in locating the nearest antivenin. However, it is up to the physician to obtain the antivenin once it has been located. Most antivenin manufacturers will include a package insert to aid in administering the antivenin, but if they do not, expert advice should be obtained from consultants familiar with venomous animal injuries.

Other Animals

A number of other antivenins are manufactured outside the United States for use in treating various envenomations from spiders, ticks, marine animals, and scorpions. One antivenin is manufactured and available in Arizona for use against the Arizona bark scorpion *(Centruroides scupturatus)*. If it would become necessary to use any of these antivenins, expert help should be obtained from the local Drug and Poison Information Center, zoo, or toxicology consultant.

Antitoxins

INTRODUCTION

Antitoxins are solutions of immunoglobulins obtained from the serum of humans or animals hyperimmunized against various viral and bacterial toxins either from the administration of toxoids or from the presence of the disease itself. Antitoxins are usually IgG because IgA does not usually protect against specific toxins. These IgG antibodies must combine with the viral or bacterial toxins in the host before the toxin combines with cell membrane receptors on the target cells. Once the toxins have entered the target cells, specific antitoxins are not effective.

The antitoxins derived from horses have the same caveats associated with them as do the antivenins (see Antivenins, earlier in this chapter). The possibility of developing an acute allergic reaction or serum sickness is always present when these substances are used. Prior to administration of antitoxins, a careful history should be taken especially with regard to previous allergic reactions to antitoxins, prior administration of horse serum, atopy, hay fever, asthma, or other allergies. An intradermal skin test should be done to test for sensitivity before administering any horse serum–derived product. This should only be done if the need for the product has already been determined; otherwise, needless sensitization to horse serum or an anaphylactic reaction may occur. If a patient has a positive skin test, desensitization should be performed prior to administration of the product.

Patients who have a positive skin test should not be given intravenous antitoxin even after desensitization but may be given intramuscular antitoxin. The incidence of serum sickness is related to the amount of serum given and often occurs long after the administration of the serum. For this reason, most horse serum antitoxins have been replaced with human antitoxins. Whenever there is a choice between human and animal-derived antitoxin, the human antitoxin should be used. Pain, tenderness, erythema, and muscle stiffness commonly occur at the site of antitoxin administration and should not be considered a contraindication to its administration.

CONDITIONS

Diphtheria

Diagnosis

Diphtheria is an acute infectious disease caused by *Corynebacterium diphtheriae*, a gram-positive, nonmotile, nonsporulating bacillus. It may be transmitted via air droplets or skin contact and is characterized by a local inflammatory lesion in the upper respiratory tract. Systemic effects are produced by a toxin and affect the heart, kidneys, and nervous system. The local lesions, classically described as gray membranes, may be in the nares, pharynx, larynx, trachea, or bronchi. The more extensive the local lesions, the more severe the systemic intoxication. Myocarditis, peripheral neuritis, renal failure, and ascending paralysis may be complications of the toxin.

Indications for Treatment

The diagnosis of diphtheria should be made on clinical examination. Treatment should not be delayed while waiting for bacterial confirmation by culture. The symptoms and signs of diphtheria, along with the identification of typical gram-positive rods on Gram's stain, will make a presumptive diagnosis. The treatment of diphtheria is with antitoxin; antibiotics will eradicate the organism but not the toxin. The dose of antitoxin is empiric; the more extensive the membrane, the higher the white blood cell count, the longer the duration of the illness, and the more systemic signs, the more antitoxin is needed. The patient should be tested for horse serum sensitivity and questioned concerning allergies, atopy, and prior horse serum therapy before administration of diphtheria antitoxin. Both immediate and delayed allergic reactions are common and appropriate precautions should be taken. Treatment with antitoxin or clinical disease does not confer immunity; immunization is still necessary according to the standard schedule. (See box.)

Discussion

Patients allergic to horse serum may be treated by using aliquots of antitoxin diluted in normal saline. Concomitant treatment with antihistamines and epinephrine is usually necessary. Expert advice should be obtained before attempting this procedure. In patients allergic to penicillin, erythromycin, 40 mg/kg/day for 14 days, may be used.

Hepatitis B Exposure

Persons not immunized against hepatitis B and having parenteral exposure may be at risk for contracting hepatitis B. This exposure may be through body fluids such as blood, semen, vaginal secretions, or saliva; from mother to fetus; or through sexual contact. The incubation period varies from 50 to 150 days and may be related to the size of the inoculum.

Indications for Treatment

Any person not immunized against hepatitis B who has significant exposure to hepa-

---

DRUG TREATMENT: DIPHTHERIA

First-Line Drugs

Diphtheria Antitoxin, Equine

Initial Dose	Given slowly by IV piggyback, entire dose at one time
	40,000 units for mild nasal or pharyngeal diphtheria
	80,000 units for moderate pharyngeal diphtheria
	120,000 units for severe pharyngeal diphtheria, brawny edema of the neck, duration >48 hours, or systemic manifestations
Repeat Dose	Not indicated
End-Point	
	No clinical guidelines

PLUS

Penicillin G

Initial Dose	600,000 units IM
Repeat Dose	600,000 units IM daily for 14 days
End-Point	Three successive negative cultures, 24 hours apart, after treatment has ended

DRUG TREATMENT: HEPATITIS B EXPOSURE

First-Line Drugs

Hepatitis B Immune Globulin (HBIG)

Initial Dose	0.06 ml/kg or 5.0 ml IM for adults
Repeat Dose	0.06 ml/kg or 5.0 ml for adults with continued exposure to heterosexual contacts who remain HB$_s$Ag positive at 3 months
	0.06 ml/kg or 5.0 ml IM for adults 1 month after initial dose if patient elects not to receive hepatitis B vaccine (below).
End-Point	No clinical guidelines

PLUS

Hepatitis B Vaccine

(For those in high-risk groups who have significant contact, as noted above)

Initial Dose	1.0 ml (0.5 ml for neonates) IM in the deltoid region (may be given at the same time as HBIG in a different site)
Repeat Doses	1.0 ml (0.5 ml for neonates) IM 1 month after initial dose and another 1.0 ml IM 6 months after initial dose
End-Point	Adequate anti-HB$_s$ titers

titis B, or anyone who has inadequate titers of anti-HB$_s$ and significant exposure to hepatitis B should receive hepatitis B immune globulin (HBIG). Significant exposure includes sexual contact with hepatitis B carriers or those with acute hepatitis B, infants born to mothers at high risk of hepatitis B or who are positive for hepatitis B surface antigen (HB$_s$Ag), or body fluid exposure to anyone who is positive for HB$_s$Ag. Body fluid exposure includes needlestick from a contaminated needle and contact with mucous membranes or open skin lesions. (See box.)

Discussion

Immune globulins may interfere with the normal immune response of live virus vaccines. Therefore immunization with live vaccines should not be done within 3 months of administering hepatitis-B immune globulin. Hepatitis B vaccine should be given intramuscularly only in the deltoid muscle. Inadequate anti-HB$_s$ titers have been seen when the vaccine is given intramuscularly in the gluteal region.

Rabies

Diagnosis

Rabies is an acute viral disease caused by a ribonucleic acid (RNA) virus of the rhabdo-virus group that affects the central nervous system and is transmitted by mammals. The usual mode of transmission is by contact with an infected animal's saliva, but it may be acquired by inhalation, ingestion, or even organ transplant. Wild animals such as skunks, foxes, bats, and raccoons and non-immunized dogs and cats have been the primary carriers in the United States. Human rabies is fortunately rare in the United States (from 1980 to 1988 there were a total of 9 cases) but remains a major problem in underdeveloped countries. The incubation time after exposure is quite variable (10 days to 12 months), and a history of animal exposure may not be obtained. The early symptoms are nonspecific and may resemble a viral upper respiratory infection. Encephalitis and finally brain stem dysfunction and death follow. The diagnosis can be made by rabies fluorescent antibody test either from the infecting mammal or the symptomatic patient. There is no specific treatment, but postexposure prophylaxis will usually prevent the disease.

Indications for Treatment

Any person coming in contact with the saliva of a rabid animal, anyone accidentally exposed to aerosolized fluids containing rabies virus in the laboratory or in caves, or

DRUG TREATMENT: RABIES

First-Line Drugs

Human Rabies Immune Globulin (HRIG)

Initial Dose	20 IU/kg body weight One-half of this infiltrated around the wound area if feasible One-half given IM in thigh or gluteal region
Repeat Dose	Not indicated
End-Point	No clinical guidelines

PLUS

Human Rabies Diploid Cell Vaccine (HDCV)

Initial Dose	1.0 ml IM in deltoid region (do not give in same extremity as HRIG)
Repeat Dose	1.0 ml IM in deltoid region on days 3, 7, 14, and 28 following initial dose
End-Point	No guideline for this usage of HDCV

Second-Line Drugs

(Use only if HRIG is not available.)

Antirabies Serum, Equine (ARS)

Initial Dose	40 IU/kg body weight One-half of the dose should be infiltrated around the wound if feasible. One-half should be given IM in the thigh or gluteal region.
Repeat Dose	Not indicated
End-Point	No clinical guidelines

PLUS

Human Rabies Diploid Cell Vaccine

Guidelines are the same as above.

---

anyone receiving donor organs from a person with rabies (e.g., cornea transplants) should receive both passive and active immunization against rabies. Regulations vary from state to state, but any domestic animal that bites someone, even if immunized against rabies, should be closely observed for 10 days for signs of illness. Any wild animal should be sacrificed and its brain examined for rabies antibodies since wild animals may not exhibit symptoms of rabies or may have prolonged incubation periods. If the biting animal cannot be located, rabies prophylaxis should be given. Public health officials should be consulted for recommendations concerning domestic animals and the incidence of rabies in the community. (See box.)

Discussion

The diagnosis and treatment of rabies can be extremely difficult. The last two cases of human rabies in the United States were both diagnosed at autopsy. The signs and symptoms of rabies are protean, and without a clear history of exposure to an animal, the diagnosis is usually missed. Even when the diagnosis is made, once the symptoms of rabies appear the patient usually deteriorates rapidly. However, HRIG should be given and supportive therapy instituted.

Tetanus

Diagnosis

Tetanus is an acute disease caused by an anaerobic, gram-positive, spore-forming rod, *Clostridium tetani*, that gains access to tissue and locally produces an exotoxin, tetanospasmin, which causes systemic effects. The incubation period is from 2 to 60 days. The symptoms of tetanus are due to the effect of the toxin on central motor neuron synapses, peripheral neuromuscular blockade, and autonomic dysfunction. Pain and stiffness, difficulty swallowing, and severe muscle spasms of several muscle groups are noted. The disease does not confer immunity, and persons who have had tetanus still require active immunization. Tetanus is rare in the United States because of widespread immunization, but it remains a major cause of morbidity and mortality, especially in neonates, in underdeveloped countries. Many patients with tetanus have no history of trauma, and only 30% of patients with tetanus have *Clostridium tetani* cultured from a wound.

Indications for Treatment

Any person with symptoms of trismus, intermittent severe spasms of multiple muscle groups, restlessness, irritability, and profuse sweating in whom meningoencephalitis and strychnine poisoning have been ruled out should be treated for tetanus. This is especially true if the tetanus immunization status of the patient is either inadequate or unknown. The presence of a tetanus-prone wound or a culture growing *Clostridium tetani* is helpful but not necessary. There is increased mortality with delayed treatment, short incubation time, or rapidly progressing symptoms. The specific treatment is administration of tetanus immune globulin. Antibiotics should be used if wound infection is present, but they do not eliminate the need for meticulous debridement. Muscle relaxants, neuromuscular blockers, and sympathetic blockers may be needed to control symptoms and assist ventilation. (See box.)

Discussion

The treatment of tetanus may include the use of muscle relaxants such as diazepam to

---

DRUG TREATMENT: TETANUS

First-Line Drug

Tetanus Immune Globulin (Human) (TIG[H])

Initial Dose	3000–6000 units IM (optimum dose not established)
Repeat Dose	Not indicated
End-Point	No clinical guidelines

OR

Tetanus Antitoxin, Equine

(Should only be used if TIG[H] not available)

Initial Dose	50,000–100,000 units IV or IM
Repeat Dose	Not indicated
End-Point	No clinical guidelines

PLUS

Tetanus Toxoid

0.5 ml IM at time zero, 1 month, and 6 months (total 3)

Second-Line Drug

Penicillin G

(Will not affect formed toxin)

Initial Dose	2 million units by IV piggyback
Repeat Dose	2 million units by IV piggyback every 6 hours
End-Point	Pending culture and sensitivity

control muscle spasms that become problematic. Labetolol can be used to control sympathetic hyperactivity, which may become life-threatening especially in the elderly. Pancuronium or other paralyzing agents may be needed to facilitate ventilatory support in the intubated patient. Some neurologic symptoms may persist after adequate treatment of the acute episode of tetanus.

Botulism

Diagnosis

Botulism is caused by the ingestion of food containing either the gram-positive, anaerobic, spore-forming rod *Clostridium botulinum* or the preformed toxin. The spores of *C. botulinum* are heat resistant but the toxin itself is heat-labile, and most cases of adult or food-borne botulism are caused by eating foods not heated properly before ingestion. Infant botulism is usually caused by ingestion of spores, often found in honey. Rarely, botulism can be acquired through wound infection. There are seven types of antigenically distinct toxins, but types A, B, and E account for 99% of human intoxications. The toxin acts at the myoneural junction, binding irreversibly to prevent the presynaptic release of acetylcholine. The symptoms and signs of food-borne botulism include onset 18 to 36 hours following ingestion, dry mouth, diplopia, nausea, vomiting, abdominal cramps, dysphagia, cranial nerve paralysis, and symmetrical descending weakness, which may proceed to respiratory paralysis. Level of consciousness is usually not impaired until late in the course of the illness. Wound botulism is similar in its presentation but without the gastrointestinal symptoms. Infant botulism usually presents with constipation, cranial nerve paralysis, descending symmetrical weakness, autonomic dysfunction, and respiratory paralysis. The diagnosis can be confirmed by identification of the organism or toxin in the stool, gastric contents, or serum.

Indications for Treatment

Adults, often presenting in clusters, with symptoms of botulism should be admitted to the hospital because of the possibility of respiratory paralysis and given antitoxin. Antibiotics are not necessary for food-borne botulism but should be used along with debridement for wound botulism. Aminoglycosides should not be used because they may increase neuromuscular blockade. The mainstay of infant botulism therapy is hospitalization and respiratory support. Antitoxin is not currently recommended for infant botulism nor are antibiotics. The possibility of allergic reaction from the antitoxin and the potential for release of more toxin by killed bacteria negate the use of antibiotics. (See box.)

Discussion

Trivalent antitoxin is available from the Centers for Disease Control or one of its distribution centers. A polyvalent antitoxin is also available for specific outbreaks due to C, D, or F botulism. The antitoxin may still be of benefit when administered several weeks after the toxin was ingested. Circulating toxin has been detected 30 days after ingestion. Guanidine has been anecdotally shown to increase acetylcholine release from terminal nerve endings. However, its effectiveness in botulism toxicity is unproved and it cannot be recommended at this time.

DRUG TREATMENT: BOTULISM, FOOD-BORNE

First-Line Drug

Botulism Antitoxin Trivalent (A,B,E), Equine

Initial Dose	1 vial IV 1 vial IM
Repeat Dose	1 vial IV if symptoms worsen
End-Point	Antitoxin will only neutralize unbound toxin; therefore, neurologic signs will not improve immediately.

DRUG TREATMENT: VARICELLA ZOSTER

First-Line Drug

(For immunocompromised patient with exposure)

Varicella Zoster Immune Globulin (VZIG)

Initial Dose	1 vial (125 units)/10 kg body weight IM
Repeat Dose	Not indicated
End-Point	No clinical guidelines

Varicella/Zoster

Varicella or chickenpox is usually a benign, febrile illness seen in preschool children. It is caused by the herpes zoster virus and is highly contagious. Clinical disease is thought to confer lifetime immunity, although reinfection is possible and latent viral infection is common (shingles). The usual childhood course is a short febrile illness followed by the appearance of erythematous papules that progress to vesicles, then pustules. The rash starts on the scalp, face, and trunk and proceeds distally. All three stages of the rash may be present at one time, and the patient complains of intense pruritus. Complications are rare in children and may include encephalitis, pneumonia, purpura, and Reye's syndrome. Because of the increasing association of the latter with aspirin ingestion, aspirin should not be given to patients with varicella. Adults have a more severe course with a higher incidence of complications, especially pneumonia. Immunocompromised patients are at greatest risk for fatal complications.

Indications for Treatment

Immunocompetent patients with varicella pneumonia or purpura fulminans should be treated with acyclovir. Immunosuppressed patients who are susceptible to varicella and have had exposure to varicella should receive varicella zoster immune globulin (VZIG). Neonates whose mothers develop varicella 5 days before or 2 days after delivery should be given VZIG and should be isolated in the nursery. Premature infants less than 28 days old who have been exposed to varicella and premature infants more than 28 days old exposed to varicella in whom the mother has not had varicella should be given VZIG. (See box.)

Discussion

Patients who are immunocompetent but have complications associated with varicella such as encephalitis or pneumonia should be treated with acyclovir. Immunocompromised patients with varicella should also be treated with acyclovir. The usual dose is 1500 mg/m^2 of body surface area every 8 hours for 7 days.

Other Antiserums

Discussion

Immune globulin is used as prophylaxis against hepatitis A virus, measles (rubeola), rubella, varicella-zoster, antibody-deficiency diseases, idiopathic thrombocytopenic purpura, and Kawasaki syndrome. The efficacy of its use in these diseases is unproved. Vaccinia immune globulin and western equine encephalitis immune globulin are used for the treatment of specific diseases that are rarely encountered.

Specific Agents

Antirabies Serum

Pharmacology

Antirabies serum is a protein solution obtained from the serum of horses hyperimmunized with rabies vaccine.

Antirabies serum contains rabies antibodies, which neutralize rabies virus and inhibit its spread from the initial incubation site and along neural pathways toward the central nervous system. The antibodies will not neutralize virus that has entered nervous tissue or when clinical symptoms of rabies are present.

Indications

Antirabies serum is used in prophylaxis of rabies when rabies immune globulin cannot be obtained.

Cautions

Because of the danger of allergic reaction to this horse serum derivative, prior to administration a history of allergy to horses or horse serum, hay fever, asthma, atopy, or prior administration of horse serum should be obtained. Sensitivity testing should be done prior to administering this drug.

Use in pregnancy—not contraindicated
Use in childhood—not contraindicated

Dosage Adjustment in Organ Failure

Renal failure—none
Cardiac failure—none
Hepatic failure—none

Dosage

40 IU/kg body weight, one-half infiltrated around wound area if feasible and one-half given IM in the thigh or gluteal region

Toxicity

Anaphylaxis is always a possibility when administering a horse serum derivative, even if the results of a skin test are negative. Therefore, oxygen, epinephrine, and intubation equipment should be available when administering this drug.

Corticosteroids and other immunosuppressive drugs may interfere with the activity of rabies antibody. If possible, these drugs should be avoided during rabies prophylaxis. If this is not possible, serologic testing for rabies antibody should be done. These antibody titers should be 1:5 or greater.

Approximately 40% of patients receiving this drug will develop serum sickness and should be treated appropriately; however, corticosteroids should be avoided. Local pain and erythema may develop in the area of the injection.

Antivenin, Crotalidae, Polyvalent

Pharmacology

Crotalid antivenin is a protein solution made by freeze drying the serum of horses hyperimmunized against the venom of four pit viper snakes.

This antivenin contains antibodies capable of neutralizing the venom of most pit vipers found throughout the world (see Table 17–1). The distribution and elimination of this drug are unknown.

Indications

Antivenin should be used to treat moderate to severe bites from snakes listed in Table 17–1. The use of this antivenin to treat other than pit viper bites is not recommended.

Cautions

This product is a horse serum derivative and precautions should be taken as for all horse serum antivenins or antitoxins.

Use in pregnancy—not contraindicated
Use in childhood—not contraindicated

Dosage Adjustments in Organ Failure

Renal failure—none
Cardiac failure—none
Hepatic failure—none

Dosage

5 to 15 vials IV initial dose diluted in 500 ml saline over 60 minutes
5 to 15 additional vials based on clinical response

The dosage is not dependent on weight or body surface area. In many cases the pediatric dose may be larger than the adult dose.

Patients who are allergic to horse serum may still be treated with antivenin if the antivenin is administered in small aliquots along with the simultaneous administration of diphenhydramine and epinephrine. Treatment with antivenin in allergic patients should only be done in life-threatening circumstances where the risk of the snakebite outweighs the risk of anaphylaxis, and expert consultation should be obtained before attempting it.

Toxicity

Corticosteroids theoretically may interfere with the action of the antivenin, but there are currently no controlled studies to verify this. There is always a possibility of anaphylaxis and serum sickness when administering horse serum. Resuscitation equipment, including epinephrine, oxygen, and intubation equipment, should be available before this drug is administered. Serum sickness occurs 5 to 7 days later in up to 90% of patients receiving more than 10 vials of antivenin. These patients usually respond to corticosteroid therapy, which is not contraindicated this remote from antivenin therapy.

Antivenin, *Latrodectus mactans* (Black Widow Spider)

Pharmacology

This antivenin is a freeze-dried protein solution of venom-neutralizing antibodies obtained from the serum of horses hyperimmunized with the venom from black widow and other related spiders.

The antivenin is used to treat the symptoms associated with the bite of black widow spiders presumably by neutralizing unbound venom.

Indications

The antivenin is indicated for patients with severe symptoms due to a black widow spider bite not controlled by conservative therapy (calcium, diazepam).

Cautions

This product is a horse serum derivative, and precautions should be taken before administration.

Use in pregnancy—not contraindicated
Use in childhood—not contraindicated

Dosage Adjustments in Organ Failure

Renal failure—none
Cardiac failure—none
Hepatic failure—none

Dosage

1 vial by IV piggyback in 50 ml 0.9% saline
May repeat 1 vial by IV piggyback if symptoms worsen

Toxicity

Precautions should be taken when administering this horse serum derivative. Anaphylaxis and serum sickness can occur and should be treated by the usual methods. Epinephrine, oxygen, and intubation equipment should be available when administering the antivenin. Serum sickness may occur 7 to 10 days after administration and usually responds to corticosteroid therapy.

Antivenin *Micrurus fulvius* (Coral Snake)

Pharmacology

Coral snake antivenin is a freeze-dried protein solution of antibodies derived from the serum of horses hyperimmunized with the venom of *Micrurus fulvius fulvius* (eastern coral snake).

This antivenin contains antibodies that will neutralize venom of the eastern coral snake *(Micrurus fulvius fulvius)* and the Texas coral snake *(Micrurus fulvius tenere)*. It will not neutralize the venom from the Arizona or Sonoran coral snake *(Micruroides euryxanthus)*.

Indications

Bite by the eastern or Texas coral snake

Cautions

This antivenin is a horse serum derivative, and precautions should be taken with this and all drugs derived from horse serum.

Use in pregnancy—not contraindicated
Use in childhood—not contraindicated

Dosage Adjustments in Organ Failure

Renal failure—none
Cardiac failure—none
Hepatic failure—none

Dosage

3 to 5 vials by IV piggyback in 100 ml 0.9% saline over 1 hour

3 to 5 additional vials may be given if signs of paralysis are present or if the patient's condition does not improve.

Toxicity

Same as other horse serum–derived antivenins

Botulism Equine Antitoxin (ABE)

Pharmacology

This antitoxin is a protein solution of immunoglobulins derived from the serum of horses hyperimmunized against Types A, B, and E of *Clostridium botulinum* toxin. It is believed to contain adequate amounts of antibody to neutralize A and B toxins and more than adequate amounts to neutralize E toxins.

Indications

Adult food-borne botulism or wound botulism

Cautions

This is a horse serum derivative and appropriate precautions should be followed. This antivenin is not currently recommended for infant botulism.

Use in pregnancy—not contraindicated
Use in childhood—not contraindicated except for infant botulism

Dosage Adjustments in Organ Failure

Renal failure—none
Cardiac failure—none
Hepatic failure—none

Dosage

1 vial IV and 1 vial IM
1 additional vial IV if symptoms worsen in 4 hours

Toxicity

The possibility of anaphylaxis and serum sickness exists when administering horse serum derivatives. Epinephrine, oxygen, and intubation equipment should be available when using this drug. Serum sickness can appear 5 to 10 days following administration and can be treated with corticosteroids.

Note: **Botulism equine antitoxin must be obtained from the Centers for Disease Control or one of its distribution centers, telephone 404-329-2888**

Diphtheria Antitoxin

Pharmacology

This antitoxin is a protein solution of immunoglobulins derived from the serum of horses hyperimmunized against diphtheria toxin.

The antibodies in this product combine with and neutralize unbound toxins produced by toxic strains of *Corynebacterium diphtheriae.*

Indications

This antitoxin should be administered as soon as possible after the clinical diagnosis of diphtheria is made. Bacteriologic confirmation is not necessary and will delay the treatment and thus worsen the outcome.

Cautions

This product is a horse serum derivative and precautions should be taken.

Use in pregnancy—not contraindicated
Use in childhood—not contraindicated

Dosage Adjustments in Organ Failure

Renal failure—none
Cardiac failure—none
Hepatic failure—none

Dosage

40,000 units by IV piggyback for mild nasal or pharyngeal diphtheria

80,000 units for moderate pharyngeal diphtheria

120,000 units for severe pharyngeal diphtheria, brawny edema of the neck, duration greater than 48 hours, or systemic manifestations

Toxicity

Anaphylaxic reactions occur in 7% of patients receiving this drug, and 5 to 10% will develop serum sickness. Precautions should be taken while administering this drug to treat anaphylaxis. Epinephrine, oxygen, and intubation equipment should be available during treatment. There are no known drug interactions.

Note: **Diphtheria antitoxin must be obtained from the Centers for Disease Control or one of its distribution centers, telephone 404-329-2888.**

Hepatitis B Immune Globulin (HBIG)

Pharmacology

This protein solution of immunoglobulin G is obtained from the plasma of humans with high titers of antibody to hepatitis B surface antigen and who are hepatitis B surface antigen negative. All donors of plasma must also be human immunodeficiency virus (HIV) negative. The preparation process inactivates all known viruses, including HIV.

The hepatitis B surface antigen antibodies in this product combine with hepatitis B surface antigen and neutralize the hepatitis B virus. If clinical hepatitis B is present or the patient is hepatitis B surface antigen positive, then HBIG may not provide protection.

Distribution

Crosses placenta
Excreted in breast milk
Elimination half-life—approximately 21 days

Indications

Patients at risk for acquiring hepatitis B who have had significant exposure to the virus or hepatitis B surface antigen–positive body fluids

Cautions

Patients with allergies to immune globulins or with specific IgA antibodies may develop anaphylaxis to HBIG. Epinephrine, oxygen, and intubation equipment should be available when administering this drug.

Use in pregnancy—not contraindicated, but there are no studies on the effects of HBIG on the fetus
Use in childhood—not contraindicated
Use in bleeding disorders—intramuscular administration may cause bleeding

Dosage Adjustments in Organ Failure

Renal failure—none
Cardiac failure—none
Hepatic failure—none

Dosage

0.06 ml/kg body weight IM in deltoid or anterior lateral thigh

Drug Interactions

Should not be given in same syringe or same extremity as hepatitis B vaccine
HBIG may interfere with the immune response of live vaccines, and these vaccines should not be given until 3 months after HBIG has been given.

Rabies Immune Globulin (RIG)

Pharmacology

This protein solution of immunoglobulin G is obtained from the plasma or serum of healthy humans who have been hyperimmunized with rabies vaccine.

This drug contains rabies antibody, which can neutralize rabies virus and inhibit its spread and pathologic effect.

Its elimination half-life is approximately 24 days. It crosses the placenta and is excreted in breast milk.

Indications

RIG is indicated for prophylaxis in anyone exposed to rabies virus who has not been immunized to rabies as demonstrated by adequate rabies antibody (1:16 or greater). RIG may inhibit the normal anamnestic response.

Cautions

Use in pregnancy—not contraindicated; however, there are no studies indicating whether fetal effects occur.
Use in childhood—not contraindicated
Use in bleeding disorders—bleeding may follow intramuscular injection.

Patients with allergies to immunoglobulins or with specific IgA antibodies may have an allergic reaction to RIG. Epinephrine, oxygen, and intubation equipment should be available when RIG is administered.

Dosage Adjustments in Organ Failure

Renal failure—none
Cardiac failure—none
Hepatic failure—none

Dosage

20 IU/kg body weight
One-half infiltrated around the wound if
feasible
One-half IM

Drug Interactions

Doses of RIG greater than 20 IU/kg may
suppress the active antibody response to rabies vaccine. RIG may also interfere with the
response of live vaccines, and these products
should not be administered within 3 months
of RIG. Corticosteroids and other immunosuppressive drugs may interfere with the response of rabies vaccine and if possible
should be discontinued during rabies prophylaxis.

Tetanus Antitoxin

Pharmacology

This protein solution of immunoglobulins
is derived from the serum of horses hyperimmunized with tetanus toxin or toxoid.
The antibodies in this product neutralize
the unbound toxin produced by *Clostridium
tetani.*

Indications

Following exposure to tetanus
Treatment of tetanus

Note: **Tetanus antitoxin product should
be used to provide passive immunization against tetanus only when tetanus
immune globulin, human (TIG[H]) is
not available. When TIG(H) is available, it should be used preferentially.**

Cautions

This antitoxin is derived from horse serum
and precautions should be followed.

Use in pregnancy—not contraindicated
Use in childhood—not contraindicated

Dosage Adjustments in Organ Failure

Renal failure—none
Cardiac failure—none
Hepatic failure—none

Dosage

For postexposure prophylaxis: 3000 to
5000 units IM for weight >30 kg; 1500
units IM for weight <30 kg
For treatment of tetanus: 50,000 to
100,000 units, one-half IV and one-half
IM

Tetanus antitoxin should not be given in
the same syringe or in the same extremity as
tetanus toxoid.

Toxicity

Anaphylaxis and serum sickness may occur
after the administration of this horse serum
derivative. Standard precautions of epinephrine, oxygen, and intubation equipment
should be available when administering this
drug. Serum sickness will occur in 10% of
patients receiving this drug and may occur
several weeks after its administration. Corticosteroids may be used to treat this condition.

Note: **Tetanus antitoxin must be obtained from the Centers for Disease
Control or one of its distribution centers, telephone 404-329-2888.**

Tetanus Immune Globulin
(TIG)

Pharmacology

This protein solution of immunoglobulins
is derived from the plasma of humans hyperimmunized with tetanus toxoid.
Its elimination half-life is approximately
28 days.
TIG contains tetanus toxin antibodies,
which neutralize unbound toxin produced
by *Clostridium tetani.*

Indications

Postexposure prophylaxis of tetanus
Treatment of tetanus

Cautions

Use in pregnancy—not contraindicated
Use in childhood—not contraindicated

Dosage Adjustments in Organ Failure

Renal failure—none
Cardiac failure—none
Hepatic failure—none

Dosage

For postexposure prophylaxis: 250 units IM

For the treatment of tetanus: 3000 to 6000 units IM

TIG should not be given intravenously or in the same syringe or in the same extremity as tetanus toxoid.

Toxicity

Allergic reactions are possible after administration of any immunoglobulin, and standard precautions should be taken.

Varicella-Zoster Immune Globulin (VZIG)

Pharmacology

This protein solution of immunoglobulin G is derived from the plasma of humans with titers of antibody to varicella of 1:32 or greater. It has replaced zoster immune globulin (ZIG).

VZIG is used to provide passive immunity to susceptible individuals exposed to the herpes zoster virus by combining with and neutralizing the virus.

Indications

VZIG is used for postexposure prophylaxis of susceptible individuals exposed to the disease or virus. Susceptible individuals include:

Neonates born to mothers who develop varicella 5 days before or 48 hours after delivery

Premature infants <28 days old or premature infants >28 days old whose mothers are not immune to varicella

Immunocompromised individuals

Note: VZIG is not useful in treating clinical Herpes zoster infections.

Cautions

Use in pregnancy—it is not known if VZIG can cause fetal abnormalities. It is currently not recommended for use in pregnancy to prevent congenital varicella

syndrome, but it may be used to prevent varicella complications in the mother.

Use in childhood—not contraindicated

Use in bleeding disorders—intramuscular administration may cause bleeding.

Patients with allergies to immunoglobulins or with specific IgA antibodies may have severe allergic reactions to VZIG.

Dosage Adjustments in Organ Failure

Renal failure—none
Cardiac failure—none
Hepatic failure—none

Dosage

125 units/10 kg body weight IM (usual maximum dose 625 units)

This dose can be repeated at 3-week intervals if the patient has continued exposure to varicella.

Not more than 125 units at any one site

Note: VZIG must be obtained from the Centers for Disease Control or one of its distribution centers, telephone 404-329-2888 or 614-449-0773 (Massachusetts Red Cross).

Drug Interactions

VZIG may interfere with the immune response of live vaccines, and these products should not be administered within 3 months of VZIG. There is always a possibility of allergic reaction to any immunoglobulin, and epinephrine, oxygen, and intubation equipment should be available when administering this product.

REFERENCES

Arnon SS: Infant botulism. Annu Rev Med 31:541, 1980.

Centers for Disease Control: Human rabies diagnosed two months postmorten—Texas. MMWR 34:700, 705, 1985.

Centers for Disease Control: Immunobiologic Agents and Drugs Available from the Centers for Disease Control—Descriptions, Recommendations, and Adverse Reactions, 2nd ed. Atlanta, Centers for Disease Control, 1979.

Hattwick MAW: Human rabies. Public Health Rev 3:229, 1974.

Immunization Practices Advisory Committee: Recommendations for protection against viral hepatitis. MMWR 34:313, 329, 1985.

Immunization Practices Advisory Committee: Rabies prevention—United States 1984. MMWR 33:393, 407, 1984.

Immunization Practices Advisory Committee: Varicella-zoster immune globulin for the prevention of chickenpox. MMWR 33:84, 95, 100, 1984.

Immunization Practices Advisory Committee: Supplement. MMWR 33:1S, 1984.

Immunization Practices Advisory Committee: Diphtheria, tetanus, and pertussis: Guidelines for vaccine prophylaxis and other preventive measures. MMWR 30:392, 401, 1981.

Kitchens CS, Van Mierop LH: Envenomation by the eastern coral snake *(Micrurus fulvius fulvius):* A study of 39 victims. JAMA 258:1615, 1987.

Otten EJ: Antivenin therapy in the emergency department. Am J Emerg Med 1:83, 1983.

Rauber A: Black widow spider bites. J Toxicol Clin Toxicol 21:473, 1984.

Seef LB, Koff RS: Passive and active immunoprophylaxis of hepatitis B. Gastroenterology 86:958, 1984.

Shill M, Baynes RD, Miller SD: Fatal rabies encephalitis despite appropriate post-exposure prophylaxis. N Engl J Med 316:1257, 1987.

Stevens CE, Toy PT, Tong MJ, et al: Perinatal hepatitis B transmission in the United States: Prevention by passive immunization. JAMA 253:1740, 1985.

Sullivan JA, Russell FE: Isolation and purification of antibodies to rattlesnake venom by affinity chromatography. Proc West Pharmacol Soc 25:185, 1982.

Wingert WA, Chan L: Rattlesnakes in southern California and rationale for recommended treatment. West J Med 148:37, 1988.

CHAPTER 18

Respiratory Drugs

WILLIAM G. BARSAN, M.D.

INTRODUCTION

The pulmonary tree extends from the pharynx to the alveoli of the lungs. Respiratory difficulty may be caused by any condition that leads to air flow obstruction in the pulmonary tree. Although obstruction to air flow is a common cause of respiratory difficulty, other nonrespiratory disorders may be involved. Abnormal oxygen-carrying capacity of the blood resulting from anemia or methemoglobinemia can cause dyspnea with no air flow obstruction. Abnormal gas diffusion across the alveoli or ventilation–perfusion mismatching with shunting can also cause dyspnea and hypoxemia without air flow obstruction. Although these nonobstructive causes of dyspnea are common and often severe, drug therapy is not the definitive treatment in most cases. Most causes of reversible airway obstruction are amenable to drug therapy and will be the emphasis of this chapter.

Upper Airway Obstruction

The laryngeal airway is of sufficient size in adults that only severe degrees of obstruction are life threatening. However, infants and small children are susceptible to upper airway obstruction that may develop and progress rapidly. Since the extrathoracic airways narrow during inspiration, upper airway obstruction is more pronounced during inspiration, producing stridor. Although there are numerous causes of upper airway obstruction in children, croup is a common cause for which emergency drug treatment is effective in reversing the obstruction (Table 18–1). Upper airway obstruction with angioedema from allergic reactions is also amenable to drug therapy and may occur in both children and adults.

The croup syndrome has been subdivided into three disorders: (1) viral croup, (2) spasmodic croup, and (3) bacterial tracheitis. In each, edema and inflammation in the subglottic area produce the clinical syndrome of inspiratory stridor and barking cough. In viral croup and bacterial tracheitis, there is usually a prodrome of nonspecific upper respiratory infection symptoms. Croup has a highly variable course in which symptoms wax and wane over several days, followed by complete recovery. Symptoms are usually worse at night. Obstruction occurs only in severe cases. The peak onset is in the second year of life, and boys are affected more com-

TABLE 18–1. Causes of Upper Airway
Obstruction in Children

Croup
Allergic angioedema
Epiglottitis
Retropharyngeal abscess
Foreign bodies
Postinstrumentation
Diphtheria
Trauma

monly than girls. The etiologic agent in viral croup is usually parainfluenza virus. Bacterial tracheitis resembles viral croup except that high fever, toxicity, and a higher incidence of airway obstruction are observed. Spasmodic croup is a less common entity in which the child develops sudden onset of stridor without prodromal symptoms or fever. Symptoms usually subside during the day but may recur for several nights. The etiology is unclear.

It is important to distinguish croup from other causes of upper airway obstruction. Causes such as epiglottitis or foreign body aspiration require very different treatment and invasive procedures, whereas most cases of croup are managed more conservatively. When in doubt, radiographs or laryngoscopy may be indicated to establish the diagnosis.

Upper airway obstruction from allergic angioedema may be caused by either a local allergic reaction (e.g., swallowing a bee) or as part of a systemic reaction (anaphylaxis) to an antigenic stimulus. Anaphylaxis is an immediate Type I hypersensitivity reaction caused by antigen–antibody reaction at the surface of mast cells and basophils. The mast cells and basophils release numerous vasoactive mediators, including histamine, eosinophil chemotactic mediator of anaphylaxis, platelet-activating factor, and slow-reacting substance of anaphylaxis. Histamine is thought to account for the angioedema and urticaria seen in anaphylaxis.

The clinical manifestations of anaphylaxis are variable and may include shock, urticaria, wheezing, and upper airway obstruction. Symptoms usually occur immediately after antigenic exposure but may be delayed for some hours. The clinical manifestations may occur singly or in combination. Despite the variable presentation, a good history will usually reveal the source of antigenic exposure. Any case of rapidly developing upper airway obstruction in a child or adult without signs of respiratory infection should suggest the possibility of an allergic reaction with laryngeal edema.

Asthma and Chronic Obstructive Pulmonary Disease

Asthma is the most common respiratory disease for which drug therapy is used. It is estimated that asthma affects 5% of adults and up to 7 to 10% of children. It is characterized by an increased responsiveness of the airways to many different stimuli and produces the clinical symptoms of cough, dyspnea, and wheezing. Symptoms are paroxysmal and there are disease-free intervals between symptomatic relapses. For unknown reasons, attacks are more common at night.

Inciting stimuli may vary among patients, and several stimuli may contribute to an exacerbation of asthma. Infection is the most common stimulus for an acute attack. Respiratory viruses, especially respiratory syncytial virus and parainfluenza virus, are the major etiologic factors in children. In adults, rhinovirus and influenza virus are most common. Drugs may also precipitate an exacerbation of asthma. Aspirin and other non-steroidal anti-inflammatory agents, sulfites, beta-adrenergic blockers, and tartrazine dyes are common inciting agents. Other inciting causes include allergens, exercise, air pollution, cold, occupation factors, and emotional stress.

Regardless of the inciting agent, the main pathophysiologic event is obstruction of airways produced by mucosal edema, bronchial smooth muscle contraction, and thick secretions. Because intrathoracic airway diameter is normally decreased on expiration, obstruction will be more pronounced on expiration, leading to air-trapping, hyperinflation of the lungs, and decreased forced expiratory volumes and flow rates. Hypoxia will commonly occur during acute attacks. Patients usually respond by increasing their respiratory rate, leading to hypocapnia and respiratory alkalosis. Normocapnia or hypercapnia during an asthmatic exacerbation usually indicates impending ventilatory failure.

Bronchospasm may occur in chronic obstructive pulmonary disease and lead to clinical deterioration and respiratory failure in these patients. Athough the pathophysiology of the underlying disease state is different, bronchospasm usually requires treatment in these patients. Treatment of any reversible airway obstruction can help avert respiratory failure and alleviate symptoms.

Other conditions that should be considered in patients with wheezing are endobronchial lesions, foreign bodies, carcinoid tumors, congestive heart failure, and recurrent pulmonary emboli.

CONDITIONS

Upper Airway Obstruction

Diagnosis

Croup is probably the most common cause of upper airway obstruction for which drug treatment is indicated. Diagnosis is usually not difficult. Typically, patients will present at night with the sudden onset of inspiratory stridor and barking cough. Prodromal symptoms of upper respiratory infection are usually present. Patients are usually 3 months to 3 years of age, and males predominate. High fever may be seen with bacterial tracheitis, although fever is usually low grade. It is most important to differentiate croup from epiglottitis, foreign body aspiration, retropharyngeal abscess, and peritonsillar abscess. When in doubt, lateral neck radiographs and/or laryngoscopy in a conrolled environment are indicated.

Angioedema of the larynx from an allergic reaction may also cause reversible upper airway obstruction. Prodromal symptoms of infection are absent. A history of bee sting, swallowing a bee, or other drug or food exposure can usually be elicited. Patients present with stridor and varying degrees of respiratory distress. If a generalized anaphylactic reaction is present, wheezing and cutaneous flushing may also occur.

Indications for Treatment

Drug treatment for croup should be reserved for those patients with moderate to severe symptoms. Categorizing the severity of symptoms can be easily accomplished using a croup scoring system (Fig. 18–1). Using this system, drug treatment should be reserved for patients with scores >7. When-ever racemic epinephrine is used to treat croup, most authors recommend that the patient should be admitted to the hospital for observation because there may be a rebound effect after the patient initially improves. Cool mist should be used in all patients regardless of their croup score (see Fig. 18–1). Many patients with mild to moderate croup will improve with cool mist alone.

Patients with allergic angioedema should be treated if symptoms are present. Symptoms that deserve treatment are hoarseness, a feeling of "lump in the throat," stridor, or any degree of respiratory distress. Even if the patient has only mild respiratory distress or subjective air hunger, it is difficult to predict the subsequent course. These patients may deteriorate abruptly after presenting with only mild symptoms. If symptoms resolve totally after treatment, several hours of observation or hospital admission is indicated to observe for recurrence of symptoms. (See boxes, Drug Treatment: Croup and Drug Treatment: Laryngeal Edema.)

Discussion: Croup

Racemic epinephrine is a mixture of the D and L isomers of epinephrine, but only the L isomer causes α- and β-adrenergic effects. Therefore, either racemic epinephrine (2.25%) or L-epinephrine (1%) should be equivalent in action. Although epinephrine often has dramatic effects in the treatment of croup, cool mist should be the mainstay of therapy unless the patient is in moderate to severe distress.

The use of steroids in the treatment of croup is controversial. Some studies have shown beneficial effects when steroids are given early in spasmodic or viral croup. Steroids may be detrimental in the treatment of

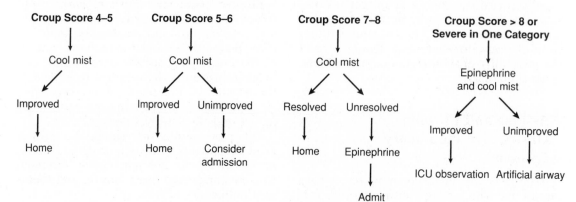

FIGURE 18–1. Treatment algorithm: croup.

DRUG TREATMENT: CROUP

First-Line Drug
Racemic Epinephrine (2.25%) or L-Epinephrine (1%)

Initial Dose	0.5 ml in 4 ml saline by aerosol
Repeat Dose	0.5 ml in 4 ml saline by aerosol
	May repeat in 30 minutes
End-Point	Improvements in croup score to <7

Second-Line Drug
Dexamethasone

Initial Dose	1.0–1.5 mg/kg IM
Repeat Dosing	Not indicated
End-Point	No clinical guidelines

DRUG TREATMENT: LARYNGEAL EDEMA

First-Line Drug
Epinephrine 1:1000

Initial Dose	0.01 ml/kg, up to 0.5 ml subcutaneously
Repeat Dose	Same
	May be repeated in 20–30 minutes
	Not to exceed three doses in 60 minutes
End-Point	Improvement in symptoms

Second-Line Drugs
Diphenhydramine

Initial Dose	1 mg/kg, up to 50 mg IV or IM
Repeat Dose	Same
	May repeat every 6 hours
End-Points	No clinical end-points
	Continue for 24–72 hours

Third-Line Drugs
Methylprednisolone

Initial Dose	1–2 mg/kg IV
Repeat Dose	No known guidelines
	Suggest 1 mg/kg every 8 hours × 3
End-Points	No clinical end-points

bacterial tracheitis. Prednisolone and dexamethasone have been used most often. No data exist to suggest that repetitive doses are beneficial.

Discussion: Laryngeal Edema

Epinephrine should always be the first drug given to a patient with symptomatic allergic laryngeal edema. Although the subcutaneous route is preferred, nebulized epinephrine (either L-epinephrine or racemic epinephrine) may be given in older patients with coronary artery disease in whom cardiac arrhythmias are a concern with parenteral administration. Epinephrine doses may be repeated in 20 to 30 minutes, although this is usually not required. Epinephrine suspension (Sus-Phrine) may also be given in a single dose for a longer-lasting effect. This usually is given after an initial epinephrine dose has produced clinical improvement.

Although the value of H_1 blocking agents in the treatment of symptomatic allergic reactions is questionable, most authors recommend at least an initial dose of antihistamines in patients with an acute allergic reaction. Corticosteroids have no proven value in anaphylactic reactions but have been used frequently. There is no known advantage of one corticosteroid compound over another for this purpose.

Bronchospasm

Diagnosis

The combination of dyspnea and wheezing indicates the presence of airway obstruction but not necessarily bronchospasm. The causes of dyspnea and wheezing are listed in Table 18–2. Symptomatic bronchospasm is most commonly seen in asthma, chronic obstructive pulmonary disease (COPD), infection with hyperactive airways, and exposure to industrial and environmental toxins.

The patient with asthma usually has a prior

TABLE 18–2. Causes of Dyspnea and Wheezing

Asthma
Chronic obstructive pulmonary disease (COPD)
Foreign bodies
Endobronchial neoplasms
Acute left ventricular failure
Carcinoid tumors
Recurrent pulmonary emboli
Eosinophilic pneumonias
Systemic vasculitis

history of symptomatic bronchospasm, and the episodes occur paroxysmally with interceding symptom-free intervals. Infection is a common precipitating factor for an acute attack, as is allergen exposure, physical exercise, or emotional excitement. Tachypnea, tachycardia, systolic hypertension, and cough are common findings. Measurements of air flow obstruction, such as forced expiratory volume in 1 second (FEV_1) and peak expiratory flow rate (PEFR), will be decreased from normal. It is not usually difficult to differentiate asthma from other causes of wheezing.

The diagnosis of COPD is also not difficult in most cases. The patient usually gives a history of emphysema, chronic bronchitis, or "breathing problems" and will not have symptom-free intervals like the patient with asthma. Patients will have the body habitus of the "pink puffer" or "blue bloater." There is often a history of recent respiratory infection causing a deterioration from baseline symptoms. Decreased air movement is evident by auscultation, and wheezing, rhonchi, or rales may be detected. Unlike the patient with asthma, auscultation of these patients is usually not "normal" even when they are at their "baseline." If right heart failure is present, peripheral edema, liver enlargement, and neck vein distention may be present. Heart examination may reveal a retrosternal heave, an S_4 or S_3 gallop, and tricuspid insufficiency.

Indications for Treatment

The presence of wheezing alone on physical examination does not necessarily dictate immediate treatment. Patients should be treated when they have *symptomatic* dyspnea regardless of the degree of wheezing. The patient with COPD who is always symptomatic should be treated when the clinical condition deteriorates from baseline.

A rationale for single drug or multiple drug therapy in bronchospasm is shown in Figure 18–2. Patients who are mildly symptomatic and have a PEFR above 200 liters/min may initially receive single drug therapy and then be reevaluated for improvement. If improvement is minimal, other agents need to be added.

The patient with COPD may not have a significant degree of reversible airway obstruction, but a trial of bronchodilating agents is still indicated during acute exacerbations. (See box.)

DRUG TREATMENT: BRONCHOSPASM

First-Line Drugs

Albuterol Solution 0.083%

Initial Dose	3 ml
Repeat Dose	Every 20–30 minutes $\times$ 2, then every 2–3 hours
End-Points	Resolution of symptoms
	Drug toxicity

OR

Metaproterenol Solution 5%

Initial Dose	0.3 ml in 2.5 ml saline by aerosol
Repeat Dose	Every 20–30 minutes $\times$ 2, then every 2 hours
End-Points	Resolution of symptoms
	Drug toxicity

OR

Isoetharine Solution 1%

Initial Dose	0.5 ml in 2.5 ml saline by aerosol
Repeat Dose	Same dose every 20–30 minutes $\times$ 2, then every 2 hours
End-Points	Resolution of symptoms
	Drug toxicity

OR

Epinephrine 1:1000

Initial Dose	0.01 ml/kg subcutaneously (not to exceed 0.5 ml)
Repeat Dose	Same dose every 20–30 minutes
End-Points	Resolution of symptoms
	3 doses
	Drug toxicity

OR

Terbutaline sulfate

Initial Dose	0.25 mg subcutaneously
Repeat Dose	Same dose in 30–60 minutes
End-Points	Resolution of symptoms
	2 doses
	Drug toxicity

OR

Isoproterenol Solution 1:200 (By Inhalation) (Children Only)

Initial Dose	0.5 ml in 2.5 ml saline
Repeat Dose	Every 2 hours
End-Points	Resolution of symptoms
	Five doses
	Drug toxicity

Chart continued on following page

DRUG TREATMENT: BRONCHOSPASM Continued

Second-Line Drug

Aminophylline

Initial (Loading) Dose	5.5 mg/kg infusion over 30 minutes
Repeat (Maintenance) Dose	Child or adult smoker: 0.9 mg/kg/hour
	Adult nonsmoker: 0.7 mg/kg/hour
	Age >50, COPD, liver disease, congestive heart failure: <0.5 mg/kg/hour
End-Points	Resolution of symptoms
	Drug level >20 mg/liter
	Drug toxicity

Third-Line Drugs

Methylprednisolone

Initial Dose	2 mg/kg infusion over 10 minutes
Repeat Dose	Every 6 hours
End-Points	Resolution of symptoms
	Drug taper over 1–2 weeks with oral prednisone

OR

Hydrocortisone Sodium Succinate

Initial Dose	5–7 mg/kg IV infusion
Repeat Dose	Every 4–6 hours
End-Points	Resolution of symptoms
	Drug taper over 1–2 weeks with oral prednisone

OR

Dexamethasone

Initial Dose	0.25 mg/kg IV infusion
Repeat Dose	Every 8–12 hours
End-Points	Resolution of symptoms
	Drug taper over 1–2 weeks with oral prednisone

Fourth-Line Drugs

Atropine Sulfate

Initial Dose	0.025 mg/kg in 3 ml saline by aerosol
Repeat Dose	Every 2 hours
End-Points	Resolution of symptoms
	Drug toxicity

OR

Ipratropium Inhaler

Initial Dose	Two metered dose inhalations
Repeat Dose	Every 4 hours
End-Points	Resolution of symptoms
	Drug toxicity

DRUG TREATMENT: BRONCHOSPASM Continued

Fifth-Line Drug

Isoproterenol

(Children Only)

Initial Dose	0.05 μg/kg/min IV infusion
Repeat Dose	Double dose every 15–20 minutes to 0.8 μg/kg/min. Increase 0.2 μg/kg/min thereafter.
End-Points	Decreasing pCO_2
	Tachycardia >200 beats/min
	Cardiac arrhythmias
	6 μg/kg/min maximum

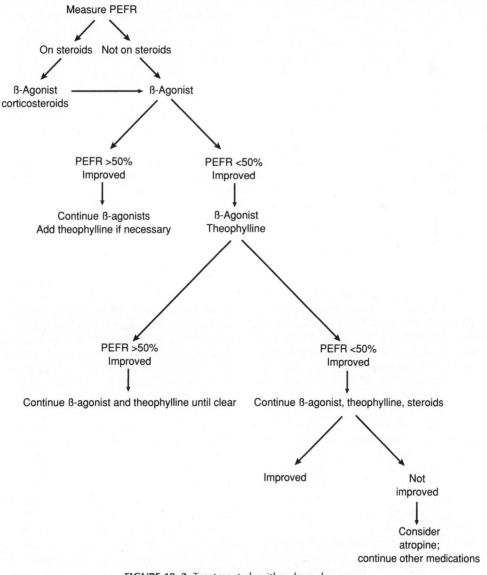

FIGURE 18–2. Treatment algorithm: bronchospasm.

Discussion

The choice of a first-line agent depends on the patient's age and general medical condition. Subcutaneous epinephrine and terbutaline should be avoided in any patient with significant risk factors for coronary artery disease. This would include, in general, adults >35 years of age and patients with diabetes, hypertension, cigarette smoking, known hyperlipidemia or hypercholesterolemia, or a strong family history of coronary artery disease. Isoproterenol aerosol is likewise avoided in adults because of its prominent beta$_1$ activity. Albuterol may be preferred for its longer duration of action, but the other agents are probably equally effective. One may give repeat doses of beta-adrenergic aerosols every 20 to 30 minutes for three doses as initial treatment.

In starting aminophylline therapy, a serum theophylline level should be obtained in all patients chronically taking theophylline prior to a loading dose. The presence or absence of side effects does not accurately predict the serum theophylline level. If the serum theophylline level is subtherapeutic, a modified loading dose may be given. A dose of 1 mg/kg should raise the serum theophylline level approximately 2 mg/liter. One should aim to produce a serum theophylline level of 10 to 12 mg/liter to avoid overdosing. During the first 6 hours of treatment, the maintenance dose chosen is probably not crucial because the drug should not accumulate rapidly in this short period of time. When maintenance doses are continued for a longer time, the exact dose will be more important and repeat theophylline levels should be obtained to avoid drug toxicity.

Steroid treatment should be started when the patient is refractory to standard therapy. If a patient is on chronic steroids and has an exacerbation of bronchospasm, high-dose intravenous steroids are indicated early in treatment. Patients with severe respiratory distress with high degrees of air flow obstruction should also receive steroids early. Patients with moderate obstruction that does not improve significantly with beta-agonists are also candidates for steroid therapy. In the outpatient setting, it should be possible within the first hour of treatment to identify the majority of patients who will require steroid therapy.

Atropine should be considered when patients are not improving significantly with beta agonists and theophylline. Although atropine may cause drying of secretions and tachycardia, these effects are lessened with aerosol treatment. Ipratropium, which has minimal systemic effects, should be available in the future in a solution form for aerosol treatment. It can be used as a metered dose inhaler in acute asthmatic attacks.

Intravenous isoproterenol has been used in children with severe asthma and respiratory failure. Its use should only be considered when one wishes to avoid mechanical ventilation and the child is refractory to beta agonists, theophylline, and steroids. It is usually used when the pCO$_2$ is elevated and respiratory acidosis is present. Mechanical ventilation may be more advisable in these patients.

In the patient with COPD or pickwickian syndrome in whom one wishes to avoid tracheal intubation, doxapram, which is a centrally acting respiratory stimulant, may be helpful if the acute exacerbation is felt to be reversible. Arterial blood gases should be monitored carefully in all cases. Doxapram infusion should not be given for longer than 2 hours and should not be used during mechanical ventilation. There are multiple side effects from doxapram, and it should be used judiciously if at all. Patients who respond to doxapram may benefit from chronic therapy with progesterone.

Neonatal Apnea

Apnea of prematurity is frequently encountered in premature infants. Apnea may be defined as cessation of breathing for more than 20 seconds with or without accompanying bradycardia or cyanosis. Apnea is also considered pathologic if it lasts less than 20 seconds but is accompanied by bradycardia. Such apnea may be a significant contributor to morbidity and mortality in the premature neonate and should be treated aggressively. The incidence is highest in newborns of gestational age less than 36 weeks. Only a minority of such newborns will actually demonstrate "normal" breathing patterns, and apnea of prematurity is a severe reflection of the inherent immaturity of breathing in these infants. Apnea in the newborn may be primarily central in origin, obstructive, or mixed.

Initial evaluation of apnea includes specific therapy for predisposing factors such as infection, seizures, hypoglycemia, anemia, atelectasis, and hypoxemia. Other manage-

DRUG TREATMENT: NEONATAL APNEA

First-Line Drug

Aminophylline

Initial Dose	6.0 mg/kg IV over 20–30 minutes
Repeat Dose	1.5 mg/kg every 8 hours
End-Points	Serum theophylline level >15 mg/liter
	Reduction in apnea of >50%
	Theophylline toxicity

ment techniques include tactile stimulation, mechanical ventilation, maintenance of normal body temperature, and respiratory stimulant drugs.

Indications for Treatment

Pharmacologic treatment for apnea should only be given after other contributory conditions have been treated or excluded (Table 18–3). Significant apnea (as defined above) that occurs more than three times in an 8-hour period is an indication for pharmacologic therapy. Parenteral treatment of apnea with aminophylline should only be undertaken in a neonatal intensive care setting with appropriate monitoring and skilled nursing care. (See box.)

Discussion

Aminophylline must be used with great caution in the premature neonate. The mean serum half-life of theophylline in neonates is 30 hours and may be prolonged to up to 100 hours in some infants. This is more than a five-fold increase in the half-life compared to that in healthy adults. Serum theophylline levels should be monitored at least once daily during intravenous treatment.

The therapeutic serum theophylline level in adults ranges from 10 to 20 mg/liter, but

TABLE 18–3. Treatable Causes of Infant Apnea

Hypoxemia	Infection
Seizures	Intracranial hemorrhage
Hypothermia	Polycythemia
Hypoglycemia	Anemia
Hypocalcemia	Patent ductus arteriosus
Congenital airway obstruction	

it may be lower in preterm neonates with apnea. Most data would suggest that serum theophylline levels of 5 to 15 mg/liter are therapeutic in these children.

Other agents for treatment of apnea of prematurity that have been used outside the United States include caffeine and doxapram. Doxapram in the United States contains benzyl alcohol as a preservative and should not be used in premature infants. Doxapram with chlorobutanol 0.5% as a preservative is probably safe for use in preterm infants.

SPECIFIC AGENTS

Albuterol (Proventil, Ventolin)

Pharmacology

Distribution

After inhalation treatment, systemic concentrations are very low. Albuterol does not cross the blood–brain barrier.

Elimination

Albuterol is metabolized in the liver to an inactive metabolite. Twenty-eight percent of an inhaled dose is excreted unchanged in the urine and 44% is excreted in the urine as metabolite.

Actions

A direct-acting sympathomimetic amine, albuterol acts relatively selectively on beta$_2$-adrenergic receptors in recommended dosages. It produces bronchodilation and also causes uterine smooth muscle relaxation.

Indications

Bronchial asthma

Reversible bronchospasm from acute or chronic airway disease

Cautions

Renal failure—no dosage adjustment necessary

Cardiac failure—no dosage adjustment necessary. However, excess adrenergic stimulation may be detrimental in congestive heart failure. Caution should be utilized when concomitant sympathomimetic agents are used.

Hepatic failure—no dosage adjustment necessary

Use in pregnancy—Category C. Albuterol has been shown to be teratogenic in mice. Risk–benefit must be considered. Albuterol may inhibit uterine contractions when given orally. It is not known whether inhalation therapy will do the same. It is unknown whether albuterol is excreted in breast milk. However, animal studies have shown albuterol to be potentially tumorigenic, and it probably should not be used in nursing mothers.

Onset and Duration of Action

Dosage

The dosage is 0.5 ml of 5% solution diluted with 2.5 ml saline. Improvement of pulmonary function is evident within 5 to 15 minutes. Peak improvement will be seen in 60 to 90 minutes.

Limits

The limits are determined by development of toxicity or clinical improvement.

Repeat Dosing

The duration of action after an inhaled dose is 4 to 6 hours. In emergency situations, the initial dose may be repeated in 30 to 60 minutes if toxicity is not evident. Thereafter, doses are given every 3 to 4 hours.

Toxicity

Drug Interactions

Anesthetics—may increase arrhythmias

Central nervous system (CNS) stimulants—may increase CNS stimulation

Beta-adrenergic blockers—may increase bronchospasm

Monoamine oxidase (MAO) inhibitors and tricylic antidepressants—may increase or potentiate vascular effects

Levodopa—may increase arrhythmias

Sympathomimetics—may increase toxicity

Xanthines—may increase toxicity

Specific Adverse Effects

Tremor, 20%

Headache, 7%

Tachycardia, palpitations, 5%

Muscle cramps, 3%

Nausea, weakness, 2%

Treatment of Toxicity

Reduction of dosage: Cardioselective beta-blockers may be used but may increase bronchospasm.

Aminophylline

Pharmacology

Chemical Structure

Aminophylline is a 2:1 complex of theophylline and ethylenediamine. Approximately 80% of a given aminophylline dose is theophylline. The bronchodilating effect of aminophylline is from theophylline alone.

Distribution

Theophylline is distributed into all body compartments. The apparent volume of distribution is 400 to 600 ml/kg. Theophylline is about 60% bound to plasma proteins, although this is less in newborns and adult cirrhotics.

Elimination

Primarily by metabolism in the liver. About 10% of theophylline is excreted unchanged in the urine. Mean half-life of the drug is decreased in smokers.

Half-Life

Premature infants, 20 to 36 hours

Children, 3.5 hours

Adults, 8 to 9 hours

Cirrhosis, congestive heart failure, up to 60 hours

Actions

Theophylline inhibits phosphodiesterase and increases cAMP, thereby directly relaxing the smooth muscle of bronchial airways and pulmonary vessels. It also increases the capacity for muscular work by the diaphragm and other skeletal muscles. It produces coronary vasodilation, cardiac stimulation, cerebral stimulation, and diuresis.

Indications

Acute bronchial asthma
Reversible bronchospasm in acute or chronic airway disease
Apnea of prematurity

Cautions

Renal failure—no dosage adjustment necessary
Cardiac failure—maintenance infusion should be decreased; adjust to serum theophylline level.
Hepatic failure—maintenance infusion should be decreased; adjust to serum theophylline level.
Use in pregnancy—Category C. Theophylline will cross the placenta and is present in breast milk. No teratogenic effects are documented but risk versus benefit must be weighed prior to use.

Onset and Duration of Action

Dosage

Loading dose: 5 to 6 ml/kg total body weight
Maintenance dose: child or adult smoker, 0.9 mg/kg/hour; adult nonsmoker, 0.7 mg/kg/hour; age >50 years, COPD, liver disease, congestive heart failure, < 0.5 mg/kg/hour

Limits

The dose of aminophylline must be adjusted using the serum theophylline level. Therapeutic levels are 10 to 20 mg/liter. Each 1 mg/kg IV dose of aminophylline will raise the serum theophylline level about 2 mg/liter. This will increase with increasing serum theophylline levels.

Repeat Dosing

For patients already taking theophylline preparations, a loading dose should not be given until the serum theophylline level is known. Infusion rates should be adjusted based on the serum theophylline level.

Toxicity

Drug Interactions

Lithium carbonate—increased lithium excretion
Propranolol—antagonism of propranolol effects
Cimetidine—increased theophylline level
Troleandomycin, erythromycin—increased theophylline level
IV isoproterenol—decreased theophylline level

Adverse Effects

Adverse effects may occur with normal serum theophylline levels. Seizures will occur with levels >40 mg/liter. The most common adverse effects are nausea, vomiting, tremor, restlessness, palpitations, and tachycardia. Life-threatening reactions include ventricular arrhythmias and seizures.

Treatment of Toxicity

For symptoms with a "normal" serum theophylline level, a decrease in dose is necessary until symptoms are gone or are tolerable to the patient. If the serum theophylline level is elevated, drug administration should be stopped. Repeated oral activated charcoal can aid in lowering serum levels. Theophylline is dialyzable. In severe reactions with high serum levels, charcoal hemoperfusion may be used. Treatment for theophylline-induced seizures is with parenteral benzodiazepines, phenytoin, and barbiturates if necessary.

Atropine

Pharmacology

Chemical Structure

dl-Hyoscyamine

Distribution

Atropine is widely distributed and crosses the blood–brain barrier.

Elimination

Atropine is hydrolyzed in the liver; 13 to 50% of an administered dose is excreted in the urine unchanged. The excretion of atropine after inhalation therapy is not known.

Actions

Atropine inhibits the muscarinic effects of acetylcholine on smooth muscles and structures innervated by postganglionic cholinergic nerves. In bronchial smooth muscles, antimuscarinic effects will promote bronchodilation.

Indications

Bronchial asthma
Reversible bronchospasm with COPD

Bradycardia

Toxicity from cholinesterase inhibitors, organophosphate poisoning

Prophylaxis of arrhythmias with succinylcholine use

Cautions

Renal failure—may need to decrease frequency of administration secondary to impaired excretion. This may not be an issue with intrapulmonary use.

Cardiac failure—after intrapulmonary use, increase in heart rate should be minimal. Repetitive dosing and additive effects on heart rate from sympathomimetics may be harmful.

Hepatic failure—may need to decrease frequency of administration. This may not be an issue with intrapulmonary use.

Use in pregnancy—Category B. In animals, atropine is not harmful to the fetus in large doses. Small amounts of atropine are excreted in breast milk, but problems in humans have not been documented. Atropine may inhibit lactation.

Other—atropine may impair bronchial mucociliary function and produce drying of secretions. This has not been documented to be a significant problem with intrapulmonary use.

Onset and Duration of Action

Dosage

The dose is 0.025 mg/kg atropine sulfate in 3 ml saline via nebulizer.

Limits

The limits are determined by development of toxicity or clinical improvement.

Repeat Dosing

If there is a documented improvement in respiratory function, the initial dose may be repeated every 2 to 5 hours.

Toxicity

Drug Interactions

When intrapulmonary atropine is used, drug interactions should be minimal because of limited systemic absorption. With greater systemic absorption, the following interactions are noteworthy:

Haloperidol—decreased antipsychotic effect

Alkalizing agents, amantadine, antihistamines—may decrease excretion of atropine

Antimuscarinics, buclizine, cyclizine, cyclobenzaprine, disopyramide, loxapine, maprotiline, meclizine, methylphenidate, nomifensine, orphenadrine, phenothiazine, pimozide, procainamide, thioxanthenes, tricyclic antidepressants—may increase antimuscarinic effects

Metoclopramide—may antagonize effects of metoclopramide on gastric motility

MAO inhibitors—may increase antimuscarinic effects

Opioids—may increase constipation, urinary retention

Specific Adverse Effects

With intrapulmonary use, adverse effects should be minimal because of reduced systemic absorption. If absorption is considerable, the effects that may occur include blurred vision, tachycardia, dryness of mouth and eyes, fever, flushing of skin, and drowsiness. More severe toxicity will produce confusion, delirium, convulsions, respiratory depression, and hallucinations. Atropine may exacerbate narrow-angle glaucoma and cause eye pain.

Treatment of Toxicity

Reduce frequency of administration or reduce dose.

Diphenhydramine (Benadryl)

Pharmacology

Distribution

It is widely distributed through the body and crosses the blood–brain barrier.

Elimination

Very little of the administered dose is excreted unchanged in the urine. Most of the drug is metabolized in the liver.

Actions

Diphenhydramine is an H_1-receptor blocking agent that competes with histamine for sites on effector cells. It prevents, but will not reverse, the responses mediated by histamine alone. Diphenhydramine also possesses antimuscarinic effects and will cause central inhibition of the actions of acetylcholine mediated through muscarinic receptors.

Indications

Anaphylactic reactions

Drug-induced extrapyramidal reactions

Cautions

Renal failure—no dosage adjustment necessary

Cardiac failure—no dosage adjustment necessary

Hepatic failure—half-life will be prolonged with hepatic failure. Decrease in dosage or dosage intervals may be required.

Use in pregnancy—Category B. No evidence of teratogenicity in animal studies. Human studies are lacking. Diphenhydramine is excreted in breast milk and its use may be dangerous in newborn and premature children. Its use is contraindicated in nursing mothers.

Onset and Duration of Action

Dosage

The dosage is 25 to 50 mg IM or IV. Onset of action is evident within minutes. The usual duration of action is 3 to 6 hours.

Limits

The upper limit for a single dose is 100 mg. The dosage should not exceed 400 mg/day.

Repeat Dosing

The initial dose is repeated every 6 hours.

Toxicity

Drug Interactions

Alcohol, CNS depressants—increased CNS depression

MAO inhibitors—prolonged and increased anticholinergic effects

Antimuscarinics, haloperidol, phenothiazines, procainamide—increased anticholinergic effects

Specific Adverse Effects

Most frequent: dizziness, sedation, disturbed coordination, epigastric distress, thickening of secretions

Less frequent: tachycardia, palpitations, hypotension, difficult urination, confusion, restlessness, blurred vision

Treatment of Toxicity

Reduction in dosage. Volume expansion or vasopressors may be used to treat hypotension.

Doxapram (Dopram)

Pharmacology

Distribution

Doxapram readily crosses the blood–brain barrier and is probably widely distributed.

Elimination

Renal

Actions

Doxapram stimulates all levels of the cerebrospinal axis. In therapeutic doses, it stimulates respiration by an action on carotid chemoreceptors and by direct action on the medullary respiratory centers. It produces an increase in tidal volume and a slight increase in respiratory rate.

Indications

Doxapram is rarely indicated. However, selected patients with COPD or pickwickian syndrome and *acute* respiratory insufficiency may benefit from short-term doxapram therapy. In these patients, doxapram may prevent an elevation of pCO_2 when oxygen is administered. It should not be used when ventilatory failure is caused by airway obstruction, bronchial asthma, pulmonary embolus, or neuromuscular disorders.

Cautions

Renal failure—should not be used

Cardiac failure—should not be used in uncompensated heart failure

Hepatic failure—no dosage adjustment necessary

Use in pregnancy—Category B. This drug should only be used in pregnancy if *clearly* indicated. It is not known whether doxapram is excreted in breast milk.

Other—doxapram is contraindicated in patients with epilepsy, head injury, cerebrovascular accidents, coronary artery disease, or severe hypertension.

Onset and Duration of Action

Dosage

Administration is by intravenous infusion with 400 mg doxapram in 180 ml saline (2.0 mg/ml concentration). Infusion should be started at 1 mg/min and may be increased to a maximum of 3 mg/min.

Limits

Doxapram infusion should not be continued beyond 2 hours.

Repeat Dosing

Repeat dosing is not recommended. Increases in the infusion rate during the 2-hour infusion should be determined by measurement of arterial pCO_2 at least every 30 minutes.

Toxicity

Drug Interactions

Anesthetics—may increase arrhythmias
CNS stimulants—may increase seizures
MAO inhibitors—may increase blood pressure
Vasopressors—may increase blood pressure

Specific Adverse Effects

The most important adverse effects are uncontrolled trembling or movements and unusual increase in reflexes, which may precede generalized seizures. Doxapram may also cause bronchospasm, laryngospasm, hiccoughs, elevation in blood pressure, chest pain, nausea, vomiting, urinary retention or incontinence, phlebitis, sweating, flushing, and hyperpyrexia.

Treatment of Toxicity

Stop infusion. Seizures may be treated with short-acting barbiturates, benzodiazepines, and respiratory support.

Epinephrine (Adrenalin, Sus-Phrine, Asthmanefrin, Micronefrin, Vaponefrin)

Pharmacology

Chemical Structure

Racemic epinephrine contains both the active (−) and inactive (+) isomers of epinephrine. Epinephrine suspension contains epinephrine and ascorbic acid, thioglycolic acid, phenol, and glycerin.

Distribution

Epinephrine is slowly absorbed following subcutaneous injection and more rapidly absorbed following intramuscular injection. Inhaled epinephrine has limited systemic absorption in conventional doses.

Elimination

Epinephrine is metabolized in sympathetic nerve endings, liver, and other tissues. Very little is excreted unchanged in the urine.

Actions

Bronchial—will relax bronchial smooth muscle and constrict bronchial arterioles
Cardiovascular—in low doses may elevate systolic and decrease diastolic pressure. In higher doses it will increase both. It will increase inotropy and chronotropy in the heart.

Indications

Bronchial asthma
Reversible bronchospasm with acute or chronic airway disease
Croup
Anaphylaxis
Cardiac arrest
Low cardiac output (selected cases)

Cautions

Renal failure—no dosage adjustment necessary
Cardiac failure—will increase myocardial oxygen consumption and demand. This may precipitate arrhythmias. Epinephrine treatment for bronchospasm is contraindicated in heart failure or patients with suspected coronary artery disease.
Hepatic failure—no dosage adjustment necessary
Use in pregnancy—Category C. Has been shown to be teratogenic in animals in large doses. May slow labor. Epinephrine is excreted in breast milk and should not be used for treatment of asthma in nursing mothers.
Other—epinephrine treatment for asthma is contraindicated in patients known or suspected to have coronary artery disease or pheochromocytoma.

Onset and Duration of Action

Dosage

Subcutaneous epinephrine 1:1000, 0.2 to 0.5 ml (children, 0.01 ml/kg, up to 0.5 ml)
Epinephrine suspension, 0.2 ml (0.005 ml/ kg in children, up to 0.2 ml)
Inhalation epinephrine 1% or racemic epinephrine 2.25%, 0.5 ml in 4 ml saline

Onset of action is within minutes with subcutaneous or inhaled epinephrine. The duration of action of subcutaneous epinephrine 1:1000 and inhaled epinephrine is 2 to 3 hours. Epinephrine suspension will be active for 4 to 6 hours.

Limits

Limits are determined by development of toxicity or clinical improvement.

Repeat Dosing

Subcutaneous aqueous epinephrine: may repeat initial dose in 30 to 60 minutes if toxicity not present. Thereafter, repeat doses are given every 3 to 4 hours

Subcutaneous epinephrine suspension: every 6 hours

Inhalation epinephrine: repeat in 30 minutes if toxicity absent. Thereafter, repeat every 2 to 4 hours.

Toxicity

Drug Interactions

Alpha-adrenergic blockers, haloperidol, labetalol, loxapine, phenothiazines, prazosin, thioxanthenes, vasodilators—may cause decreased blood pressure and tachycardia

Anesthetics—may increase arrhythmias

Antidiabetics—may increase serum glucose

Beta-adrenergic blockers—may increase blood pressure and decrease heart rate

Digitalis glycosides—may increase arrhythmias

Ergot alkaloids—may increase vasoconstriction

Guanethidine—may increase blood pressure

Maprotiline, nomifensine—may increase arrhythmias, blood pressure, and heart rate

Sympathomimetics, xanthines—may increase toxic side effects

Specific Adverse Effects

Anxiety, headaches, fear, and palpitations are most common. More serious side effects are chest pain, hypertension, arrhythmias, nausea, vomiting, seizures, pounding heart beat, and severe anxiety.

Treatment of Toxicity

Reduction in dosage or discontinuation of drug. Pressor effects may be treated with vasodilators, but prolonged hypotension may result.

Arrhythmias may be treated with beta-adrenergic blockers, but caution should be used because hypertension may occur.

Ipratropium Bromide (Atrovent)

Pharmacology

Chemical Structure

Ipratropium is a synthetic quaternary ammonium compound.

Distribution

Ipratropium has its major effect locally and is not well absorbed systemically from the lungs or gastrointestinal tract.

Elimination

The half-life is 2 hours following intravenous administration

Actions

Inhaled ipratropium has a local, site-specific effect. It antagonizes acetylcholine and prevents increase in intracellular cyclic guanosine monophosphate, producing bronchodilation. It has minimal if any systemic effects.

Indications

Bronchial asthma
Bronchospasm with chronic airway disease

Cautions

Dosage adjustments in organ failure—none

Use in pregnancy—Category B

Use during lactation—probably not excreted in breast milk. Use with caution.

Use in children—use in children under 12 years of age has not been studied.

Onset and Duration of Action

Dosage

The dosage is 2 metered dose inhalations every 4 to 6 hours.

Duration of Action

Improvement in pulmonary function occurs within 15 minutes and persists for 3 to 4 hours in most patients.

Toxicity

Drug Interactions

None known

Specific Adverse Effects

Cough, 6%
Nervousness, 3%
Nausea, 3%
Dizziness, headache, dry mouth, <2.5%

Treatment of Toxicity

Discontinue administration.

Isoetharine (Bronkosol)

Pharmacology

Chemical Structure

1-(3,4   Dihydroxyphenyl)-2-isopropyl-amino-1-butanol

Distribution

The distribution of isoetharine is not known.

Elimination

Isoetharine is metabolized in the liver, lungs, gastrointestinal tract, and other tissues. About 10% of an administered dose is excreted unchanged in the urine.

Actions

A direct-acting sympathomimetic agent. It will relax bronchial smooth muscle and is preferentially a $beta_2$-adrenergic agonist. There may be some $beta_1$ effects although less than with isoproterenol.

Indications

Bronchial asthma
Reversible bronchospasm in acute or chronic airway diseases

Cautions

Renal failure—no dosage adjustment necessary
Cardiac failure—no dosage adjustment necessary. However, excess adrenergic stimulation may be detrimental in congestive heart failure. Caution should be used when concomitant sympathomimetic agents are administered.
Hepatic failure—no dosage adjustment necessary.
Use in pregnancy—Category C. There is no evidence of teratogenic effects in animals or humans. It is not known whether isoetharine is excreted in breast milk. Risk–benefit must be considered in nursing mothers and pregnant patients.

Onset and Duration of Action

Dosage

The dose is 0.5 ml of 1% solution diluted with 2.5 ml saline. Onset of action is evident within 1 minute and the peak effect occurs in 15 to 60 minutes.

Limits

Limits are determined by development of toxicity or clinical improvement.

Repeat Dosing

Initial dose may be repeated in 30 to 60 minutes in emergency situations if toxicity is not present. Thereafter, doses may be given every 2 to 4 hours.

Toxicity

Drug Interactions

Anesthetics—may increase arrhythmias
CNS stimulants—may increase CNS stimulation
Beta-adrenergic blockers—may increase bronchospasm
MAO inhibitors and tricyclic antidepressants—may potentiate vascular effects
Levodopa—may increase arrhythmias
Sympathomimetics—may increase toxicity
Xanthines—may increase toxicity

Specific Adverse Effects

Isoetharine may cause tachycardia, palpitations, tremor, restlessness, nausea, vomiting, and headache.

Treatment of Toxicity

Reduction of dosage. Cardioselective beta-blockers may be used but may increase bronchospasm.

Isoproterenol (Aerolone, Isuprel, Vapo-Iso)

Pharmacology

Chemical Structure

3,4-Dihydroxy-α-[(isopropylamino) methyl]benzyl alcohol hydrochloride

Distribution

It is readily absorbed when given by aerosol and is distributed widely.

Elimination

It is metabolized primarily in the liver and other tissues by catechol-O-methyl transferase (COMT). After intravenous administration, 40 to 50% of the dose is excreted unchanged in the urine. After inhalation, 5 to 15% of the dose is excreted unchanged in the urine.

Actions

Direct-acting sympathomimetic drug on beta-adrenergic receptors. Isoproterenol has potent beta$_1$- and beta$_2$-adrenergic actions. It will produce bronchodilation, peripheral vascular dilation, increased inotropy, and chronotropy.

Indications

Reversible bronchospasm
Bradycardia unresponsive to atropine
Torsades de pointes

Cautions

Renal failure—no dosage adjustment necessary
Cardiac failure—no dosage adjustment necessary but monitoring for arrhythmias indicated
Hepatic failure—no dosage adjustment necessary
Use in pregnancy—Category C. It should be used in pregnancy only if the potential benefits outweigh the risks. It is not known whether isoproterenol is excreted in breast milk.

Onset and Duration of Action

Dosage

Inhalation solution: 0.5 ml of 0.5% solution in 2.5 ml of saline or water over 10 to 20 minutes.
Intravenous: 0.05 mg/kg/min infusion initially; may double the dose every 15 to 20 minutes to 0.8 mg/kg/min. Increase by 0.2 mg/kg/min thereafter.

Limits

No more than 5 treatments/24 hours. Dosing is also limited by development of toxicity or increased bronchospasm due to accumulation of metabolite with beta-blocking actions.

Repeat Dosing

The initial dose may be repeated every 4 hours, not to exceed 5 doses/24 hours.

Toxicity

Drug Interactions

Anesthetics—may increase arrhythmias
Beta-adrenergic blockers—may decrease bronchodilation
Levodopa—may increase arrhythmias
Tricyclic antidepressants—may increase arrhythmias
Sympathomimetics, xanthines—may increase toxic side effects

Specific Adverse Effects

Because isoproterenol has beta$_1$-adrenergic effects, it may precipitate angina and arrhythmias. These will be more likely to occur in patients with preexisting coronary artery disease or myocardial ischemia. Other effects include nausea, vomiting, tremor, tachycardia, "pounding" heart beat, and restlessness.

Treatment of Toxicity

Reduction in dosage. For severe toxicity, beta-adrenergic blockers may be indicated although they may worsen bronchospasm. Use of cardioselective beta-blockers may be useful in treatment of toxicity without causing bronchospasm.

Metaproterenol (Metaprel, Alupent)

Pharmacology

Chemical Structure

Metaproterenol is quite similar to isoproterenol except for the position of two hydroxyl groups. It is resistant to methylation by COMT.

Distribution

Absorption, biotransformation, and excretion studies are not available for inhalational use.

Elimination

After oral administration, the drug is excreted primarily as glucuronic acid conjugates. Half-life for intrapulmonary use is unknown.

Actions

Primarily a beta$_2$-adrenergic agonist. When administered by inhalation, there are minimal cardiac beta$_1$ effects. Metaproterenol will produce bronchial airway relaxation.

Indications

Bronchial asthma

Reversible bronchospasm with acute or chronic airway disease

Cautions

Renal failure—no dosage adjustment necessary

Cardiac failure—elimination of the drug is not affected. However, excess adrenergic stimulation may be detrimental in congestive heart failure. Caution should be exercised when repeated dosing is used, especially when combined with other sympathomimetic agents.

Hepatic failure—no dosage adjustment necessary

Use in pregnancy—Category C. There are teratogenic and embryocidal effects in animals at high doses, but controlled human studies are lacking. It should be used in pregnancy only if the potential benefit outweighs the risk.

Onset and Duration of Action

Dosage

The dose is 0.3 ml of 5% solution diluted with 2.5 ml of saline. Improvement should be apparent within 1 minute. Peak effect occurs at 1 hour.

Limits

Limits will be determined by development of side effects or clinical improvement.

Repeat Dosing

For emergency use, initial dose may be repeated within 30 to 60 minutes if there is no evidence of toxicity. Thereafter, repeat initial dose every 2 to 3 hours.

Toxicity

Drug Interactions

Anesthetics—may increase arrhythmias

Beta-adrenergic blockers—may prevent bronchodilation

Sympathomimetics—additive toxicity

Levodopa—may increase arrhythmias

Xanthines—additive toxicity

Specific Adverse Effects

Nervousness, tachycardia, 14%

Tremor, 5%

Nausea, 2%

Hypertension, tachycardia, <2%

Treatment of Toxicity

Reduction of dosage. Use of beta-adrenergic blockers may worsen bronchospasm.

Terbutaline (Brethine, Bricanyl)

Pharmacology

Distribution

Terbutaline is probably widely distributed and absorbed well following oral or subcutaneous administration.

Elimination

Terbutaline is partially metabolized in the liver to an inactive sulfate conjugate. Excretion is primarily renal.

Actions

Terbutaline is a direct-acting sympathomimetic agent. When given by inhalation, it is relatively $beta_2$ selective but appears to have more $beta_1$ effects when given parenterally. It will relax bronchial smooth muscle and uterine muscle.

Indications

Bronchial asthma

Reversible bronchospasm in acute or chronic airway disease

Cautions

Renal failure—no dosage adjustment necessary

Cardiac failure—no dosage adjustment necessary. However, excess adrenergic stimulation may be detrimental in patients with heart failure. Caution is advised in these patients.

Hepatic failure—no dosage adjustment necessary

Use in pregnancy—Category B. Terbutaline has not been shown to have adverse effects on the fetus in experimental animals. Human studies are lacking. It is excreted in breast milk and must be used with caution in nursing mothers. Terbutaline may inhibit labor and may cause hypokalemia, pulmonary edema, and hypoglycemia in the mother and hypoglycemia in the neonate when given during labor.

Onset and Duration of Action

Dosage

The subcutaneous dose is 0.25 mg. The onset of action is apparent within 5 to 15 minutes with the peak effect occurring in 30 to 60 minutes.

Limits

Limits are determined by development of toxicity or clinical improvement. Dose should not exceed 0.5 mg in 4 hours.

Repeat Dosing

A dose of 0.25 mg may be repeated 15 to 30 minutes after the initial dose. No more than 0.5 mg should be given every 4 hours. The duration of action is 1.5 to 4 hours after subcutaneous administration.

Toxicity

Drug Interactions

Anesthetics—may increase arrhythmias

CNS stimulants—may increase CNS stimulation

Beta-adrenergic blockers—may increase bronchospasm

MAO inhibitors and tricyclic antidepressants—may potentiate vascular effects

Levodopa—may increase arrhythmias

Sympathomimetics—may increase toxicity

Xanthines—may increase toxicity

Specific Adverse Effects

Most commonly observed are tremor and nervousness. Other adverse effects include tachycardia, palpitations, dizziness, headache, nausea, and vomiting.

Treatment of Toxicity

Reduction in dosage. Cardioselective beta-adrenergic blockers may be used but may worsen bronchospasm.

REFERENCES

Avanda JV, Grondin D, Sasyniuk BI: Pharmacologic consideration of the therapy of neonatal apnea. Pediatr Clin North Am 28:113–133, 1981.

Chermack RM: Comprehensive approach to asthma. Chest 87(1):94S–97S, 1985.

Cohen RM: A pharmacokinetic approach to the use of theophylline in status asthmaticus. Ann Allergy 54:11, 1985.

Denny FW, Murphy TF, Clyde WA Jr, et al: Croup: An 11-year study in a pediatric practice. Pediatrics 71:871–876, 1983.

Drugs for asthma. The Medical Letter 29(732):11–16, 1987.

Eyal F, Alpan G, Sagi E, et al: Aminophylline vs. doxapram in idiopathic apnea of prematurity: A double-blind controlled study. Pediatrics 75:709–713, 1985.

Fanta CH, Rossing TH, McFadden ER Jr: Treatment of acute asthma. Am J Med 80:5–10, 1986.

Greenberger PA, Patterson R: Management of asthma during pregnancy. N Engl J Med 312:897–902, 1985.

Ingram RH Jr: "Chronic bronchitis, emphysema, and airways obstruction. In Braunwald, E, Isselbacher, KJ, Petersdorf, RG, et al (eds): Principles of Internal Medicine. New York, McGraw-Hill, 1987.

Karpel FP, Appel D, Breidbart D, Fusio MJ: The use of atropine sulfate and metaproterenol sulfate in the emergency treatment of asthma. Am Rev Respir Dis 133:727–729, 1986.

Koren G, Frand M, Barzilay Z, MacLeod SM: Corticosteroid treatment of laryngotracheitis vs. spasmodic croup in children. Am J Dis Child 137:941–944, 1983.

Maze A, Block E: Stridor in pediatric patients. Anesthesiology 50:132–145, 1979.

McFadden ER Jr: Asthma. In Braunwald E, Isselbacher KJ, Petersdorf RG, et al (eds): Principles of Internal Medicine. New York, McGraw-Hill, 1987.

Morris HG: Review of ipratropium bromide in induced bronchospasm in patients with asthma. Am J Med 81 (Suppl 5A):36–44, 1986.

Myers DL: Pharmacologic therapy of respiratory failure. In Kirby RR, Taylor RW (eds): Respiratory Failure. Chicago, Year Book, 1986.

Reed CE: New therapeutic approaches in asthma. J Allergy Clin Immunol 77:537–543, 1986.

Remington S, Meakin G: Nebulized adrenaline 1:1000 in the treatment of croup. Anesthesia 41:923–926, 1986.

Robertson C, Levison H: Broncodilators in asthma. Chest 87(1):64S–68S, 1985.

Schlueter DP: Ipratropium bromide in asthma. Am J Med 81(Suppl 5A):55–60, 1986.

Spitzer AR, Fox WW: Infant apnea. Pediatr Clin North Am 33:561–581, 1986.

Summer W: Status asthmaticus. Chest 87(1):87S–94S, 1985.

CHAPTER 19

Osmotic Agents

LEO C. ROTELLO, M.D.

INTRODUCTION

Osmotic diuresis is a phenomenon observed most commonly in the diabetic patient with an uncontrolled blood glucose level. When the load of glucose delivered to the renal system exceeds the reabsorptive ability of the kidneys, the glucose is excreted into the urine. Because of the relatively high osmolarity of the glucose, water reabsorption is hindered and the volume of the urine is increased. In this scenario the effect is detrimental, but in certain clinical situations this type of osmotic diuresis can produce a favorable therapeutic effect. Glucose is the least effective of the available agents because of its high level of reabsorption by the kidney. The osmotic agents that are used therapeutically are intravenous mannitol, oral glycerol, and oral sorbitol. Glycerol and sorbitol are also available as intravenous preparations but are rarely used in this form because of the popularity of mannitol. Urea is very rarely, if ever, used clinically because of its excessive rebound effect and will not be discussed here.

An osmotic agent/diuretic is basically any substance that prevents or hinders water (as well as sodium and chloride) reabsorption solely on the basis of its osmotic contribution to the tubular fluid. The major site of action of these agents is at the proximal tubule. There is also some action at the loop of Henle, but this is less potent and occurs by a different mechanism. To illustrate the mechanisms by which osmotics act in the kidney, we will consider mannitol, the most commonly used of these agents (Fig. 19–1). Mannitol is a six-carbon sugar that is freely filtered at the glomerulus but, unlike glucose, is not reabsorbed. Therefore, whatever amount of mannitol is filtered for a given volume of fluid contributes directly to the osmotic load in the proximal tubule at that time. Normally, sodium is actively reabsorbed in the proximal tubule and water follows passively. When mannitol is present in the proximal tubular fluid, the active reabsorption of sodium continues, but as the water leaves, the concentration of the mannitol in the proximal tubule fluid rises because the mannitol is not reabsorbed. The osmolarity of this fluid subsequently rises and retards the further passive reabsorption of water. The active transport of sodium still proceeds, causing a low intraluminal concentration of sodium due to increased intraluminal water. The result is a large volume of nearly isotonic urine.

It should be understood that although the urine is isotonic, large amounts of sodium and chloride are also excreted. Although the main transport of sodium and chloride in the proximal tubule is actively out of the lumen, some passive diffusion along the concentration gradient of sodium does occur, and the direction is opposite to the direction of the active transport. When mannitol is present, the concentration gradient of sodium is enhanced by the dilute urine, and the passive

Normal

With Mannitol

Proximal tubule with mannitol filtered at the glomerulus

Proximal tubule

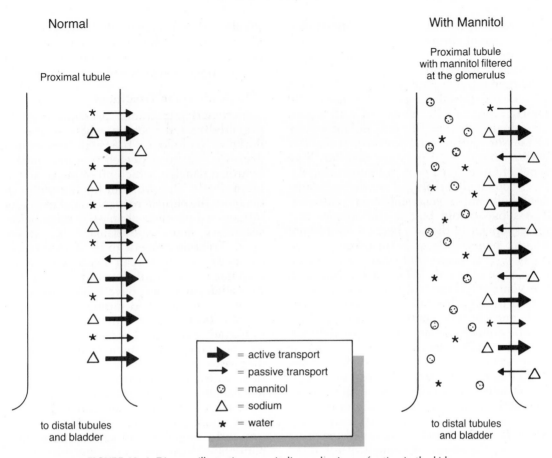

= active transport
→ = passive transport
⊙ = mannitol
△ = sodium
★ = water

to distal tubules and bladder

to distal tubules and bladder

FIGURE 19–1. Diagram illustrating mannitol's mechanisms of action in the kidney.

diffusion of sodium back into the lumen is increased. This accounts for a higher *net* amount of sodium (and chloride) loss in the urine than occurs normally, even though the osmolarity of the urine is actually lower.

CONDITIONS

Increased Intracranial Pressure

Diagnosis

The syndrome of increased intracranial pressure is considered to be a medical emergency. It is imperative that therapy be quick and effective. The first component of therapy is recognition of the condition at a stage when brain salvage is still possible. To begin an intensive treatment protocol in a patient with an already fatal cerebral insult is an exercise in futility that benefits neither the patient nor his or her family.

There are several clinical situations and syndromes in which increased intracranial pressure should be suspected. The most obvious of these is the patient who arrives in the emergency department with head trauma. Increased intracranial pressure can also occur in conjunction with any type of neurologic event, such as a cerebrovascular accident (hemorrhagic, thrombotic, or embolic), subdural or epidural hematoma, prolonged seizures, meningitis (bacterial or viral), and Reye's syndrome. Not all causes of increased intracranial pressure present as an acute or catastrophic emergency. Malignant or nonmalignant tumors may be a cause of chronic or progressive increased intracranial pressure. Cerebral perfusion pressure and intracranial pressure are both determined in part by vascular factors. Any pathology causing vascular obstruction or increases in cerebral blood flow and volume can play a significant role in the etiology of increased intracranial pressure, for example, superior vena cava syndrome or hypercapnia. Another cause of chronic increased intracranial pressure is seen in patients who develop pseudotumor cerebri.

Normal intracerebral pressure is less than 15 mmHg. Sustained pressures above 30 mmHg are generally associated with a poor neurologic outcome. The only definitive way to measure intracranial pressure is directly with an intracranial pressure monitor. Two types of intracranial pressure monitoring devices commonly employed are the subarachnoid bolt and a ventriculostomy catheter. The subarachnoid bolt is the simpler and more popular of the two because it does not require penetration of brain tissue, is relatively easy to place, and carries a lower incidence of infection. When monitoring with the ventriculostomy catheter, a catheter is passed through the brain tissue into the lateral ventricle. The ventriculostomy catheter may be difficult to place in patients who have altered cerebral anatomy (e.g., trauma or mass lesion) or in situations in which cerebral edema has caused compression or shift of the lateral ventricles. The major advantage of the ventriculostomy catheter is that it allows drainage of cerebrospinal fluid (CSF), which is a very effective means of lowering intracranial pressure. Although direct measurement of the intracranial pressure is the most accurate method of detecting increased intracranial pressure, it is not always the most feasible in an acute situation. The diagnostic procedure of choice in most emergent situations is computed tomography (CT) scanning of the head, which can detect noninvasively the presence of increased intracranial pressure in many cases. The most common symptom of increased intracranial pressure is progressively worsening headache. The brain has no pain receptors, and the sensation of pain resulting from increased intracranial pressure comes from compression of surrounding pain-sensitive structures such as the vasculature and meninges. Progressive symptoms are vomiting (more common in children) and worsening mental status, progressing from irritability to coma. Late changes are manifestations of brain stem compression (coning) and usually present as hypertension with bradycardia (the Cushing response), coma with rostal to caudal loss of brain stem reflexes, and, finally, death. By the time there is clinical evidence of increased intracranial pressure, the situation may already be far advanced. Papilledema is a specific sign of increased intracranial pressure but is often not present when intracranial pressure increases acutely.

Indications for Treatment

Increased intracranial pressure must be urgently treated because, whatever the underlying pathology, the high intracranial pressure can be expected to cause further neuronal damage, which often progresses to brain death. The problem for the physician becomes the clinical recognition of increased intracranial pressure at an early stage before secondary neurologic damage has developed. Treatment needs to be started before a definitive diagnosis can be obtained by CT scanning or intracranial pressure monitoring. The clinician should have a high degree of suspicion of increased intracranial pressure in patients presenting with conditions known to elevate intracranial pressure. The threshold for initiating treatment before obtaining diagnostic studies should be low in any patient with an appropriate insult and an abnormal neurologic examination.

As a general set of guidelines, I recommend empiric treatment with hyperventilation and a single dose of an osmotic agent in patients with an acute neurologic insult and any mental status changes or acute neurologic deficits or who have the physical finding of papilledema. After these temporizing measures, a CT scan should be obtained immediately to provide a definitive diagnosis and indicate the need for acute surgical intervention. Those patients who present with headache, with or without vomiting, but no alteration in level of consciousness and no neurologic deficits can be managed with immediate CT scanning to obtain a definitive diagnosis before beginning treatment. (See box.)

Discussion

Three volumes combine within an inelastic cranial vault to account for intracranial pressure. These are the brain, the blood, and the CSF. An increase in the volume of any of these compartments or the addition of an abnormal compartment (tumor, clot) will cause a subsequent increase in intracranial pressure, and, furthermore, the increased volume of one compartment must be at the expense of the other two (Monroe-Kellie hypothesis). The corollary of this is the basis

DRUG TREATMENT: INCREASED INTRACRANIAL PRESSURE*

First-Line Drug
Mannitol

Initial Dose	1–2 g/kg IV over 5–10 minutes
Repeat Dose	0.5–1 g/kg every 4–6 hours
End-Points	Improvement in clinical status Measured decrease in intracranial pressure Titrated to serum osmolality of not greater than 310 mOsm

Second-Line Drug
Glycerol

Initial Dose	IV: continuous infusion or repeated hourly doses of 0.2–1 g/kg/hour Oral: 1 g/kg
Repeat Dose	IV: 0.2–1 g/kg/hour Oral: 0.5–1 g/kg every 3–4 hours
End-Points	Improvement in clinical status Measured decrease in intracranial pressure Titrated to serum osmolality of not greater than 310 mOsm or serum level of 10–30 mOsm/liter

Third-Line Drug
Loop Diuretics: Furosemide

Initial Dose	20 mg IV
Repeat Dose	As tolerated by the patient (see end points, below) up to a total dose of 60–100 mg/24 hours
End-Points	Improvement in clinical status Measured decrease in intracranial pressure Hemodynamic compromise Titrated to serum osmolality of not greater than 310 mOsm

Fourth-Line Drug
Acetazolamide

Initial Dose	500 mg IV
Repeat Dose	125–250 mg every 4 hours
End-Point	Improvement in clinical status

*A urinary catheter should be in place before any osmotic agents are used.

for the treatment of increased intracranial pressure—a decrease in the volume of any compartment will decrease intracranial pressure. In patients with mass lesions, the definitive treatment of increased intracranial pressure is surgery. With subdural and epidural hematomas, it is clear that the degree of neurologic recovery is directly related to

the rapidity of surgical intervention. It is important to realize that the medical management of intracranial hypertension represents a temporizing action until definite diagnostic and, if indicated, surgical therapy can be accomplished. Clinical improvement with medical therapy does not lessen the urgent need for CT scanning. Only a limited number of medical methods are available that can be used in the treatment of increased intracranial pressure.

The first medical treatment modality to use is hyperventilation, which has a rapid but often transitory effect. This may be accomplished by either an increase in respiratory rate or tidal volume. Hyperventilation causes a decrease in pCO_2 and a rise in serum pH, which secondarily cause cerebral vascular constriction and thereby decreases the size of the vascular compartment and intracranial pressure. Hyperventilation to arterial pCO_2 levels less than 25 torr should be avoided because excess vasoconstriction with the potential for regional cerebral ischemia may occur.

The second form of effective medical treatment for increased intracranial pressure is osmotic diuresis. Mannitol is most often utilized for this purpose, but glycerol is sometimes used for children with Reye's syndrome. Mannitol and glycerol should be viewed as methods of temporizing the lethal progression of increased intracranial pressure until definitive treatment can be accomplished. These agents lower intracranial pressure by creating an osmotic gradient between the brain tissue and the intravascular space, thereby decreasing cerebral edema. It is generally accepted that an osmotic gradient of at least 20 mOsm between the vascular space and the intracerebral compartment must be present to relieve cerebral edema. Osmotic agents will not cross an intact blood–brain barrier, but in situations where the blood–brain barrier has been disrupted either chemically (e.g., toxins) or physically (i.e., trauma), care should be taken in administering osmotic agents because there may be some leakage or penetration of these substances into the brain tissue, which may actually increase brain edema. This can become a fatal complication in the treatment of critically ill patients. Mannitol is given initially in a dose of 1 to 2 g/kg. It is given as an intravenous bolus over 5 to 10 minutes by either a peripheral or central vein. A urinary catheter should be in place because the brisk diuresis can cause urinary retention and painful bladder distention. The peak action occurs at 5 to 15 minutes following administration. Repeated doses of 0.5 to 1 g/kg can be administered every 4–6 hours. The dosing of the osmotic agents should be titrated to serum osmolality. Levels of greater than 310 mOsm should be avoided because this

may cause osmotically active particles to be driven into the brain tissue. Levels of greater than 340 mOsm are damaging to the kidneys and other organs.

Glycerol is an oral osmotic agent similar to mannitol but has a slower onset of action (10 to 12 hours). It is given as an oral dose of 1 g/kg or as an intravenous infusion of 0.2 to 1 g/kg/hour. The oral dose can be repeated as needed every 3 to 4 hours. Prior to the widespread institution of mannitol, glycerol had been the major intravenous drug used in the treatment of increased intacranial pressure. Because of its longer onset of action, it is rarely used in the acute treatment of increased intracranial pressure, but it is employed in the treatment of more chronic syndromes of increased intracranial pressure (e.g., following neurosurgical procedures, cerebrovascular accident with prolonged cerebral edema, pseudotumor cerebri, chronic mass effect secondary to tumor, and Reye's syndrome). Glycerol may have some advantage over mannitol in situations in which repetitive doses of osmotic agents are needed. It is metabolized and is less likely to accumulate and produce dangerously high serum osmolarities. For glycerol to reduce intracranial pressure effectively, serum levels need to be maintained between 10 and 30 mOsm/ liter, which relates to a dose of approximately 0.2 to 1 g/kg/hour.

Care must be used in administering osmotic agents because "rebound" may occur. After the administration of the osmotic agents, the intravascular volume rises acutely, secondary to redistribution of fluid from the extracellular and cellular compartments into the intravascular space. This rise may actually cause a transient "rebound" rise in the intracranial pressure. Ultimately, this reverts when the diuresis begins and circulating vascular volume decreases. This rebound phenomenon may also be potentially dangerous in those patients with renal or cardiac failure and a predisposition to pulmonary edema. Of all the osmotic agents, mannitol has the least rebound effect. Urea is no longer utilized as an osmotic agent because of its potent rebound effect.

If there is no response to mannitol, or if there is danger of systemic fluid overload, furosemide should be administered in conjunction with the osmotic agent. Furosemide should be administered carefully and in small doses (i.e., 20 mg of furosemide). It should never be given if the patient is in shock because the vasodilatation and diuresis may further compromise systemic perfusion of vital organs.

A drug that has some role in the management of intracranial hypertension is acetazolamide. Acetazolamide lowers the intracranial pressure by decreasing production of CSF. Acetazolamide is useful in the management of patients with chronic increased intracranial pressure. It is available in intravenous and oral formulations and is administered by either route, using a regimen of 250 mg every 4 to 6 hours.

Renal Failure with Pulmonary Edema

Diagnosis

Renal failure patients are likely to develop pulmonary edema because of an inability to excrete salt and water, coupled with the propensity of these patients to develop cardiac dysfunction due to coronary artery disease or hypertension. These patients present with all the usual symptoms and signs of pulmonary edema. They will be dyspneic and orthopneic with tachypnea, tachycardia, hypertension, cyanosis, jugular venous distention, rales, gallops, and peripheral edema. The unique problem posed by these patients is the absence of a mainstay in the usual treatment of pulmonary edema: functional kidneys that can be stimulated by diuretics to eliminate volume.

Indications for Treatment

Any patient with renal failure and pulmonary edema will need urgent therapy. The definitive treatment for the renal failure patient presenting in pulmonary edema is dialysis. This modality is not always immediately available or is precluded for technical reasons in some patients with end-stage renal

---

DRUG TREATMENT: RENAL FAILURE WITH PULMONARY EDEMA

First-Line Drugs

Oxygen

Initial Dose	60% or greater
Repeat Dose	Continuous

AND

Nitroglycerin

Initial Dose	1/150 tablet sublingual
Repeat Dose	1/150 tablet sublingual every 5 minutes until hypotension or relief of symptoms
Maintenance Dose	Nitroglycerin by continuous titrated IV infusion
End-Points	Relief of symptoms SaO$_2$ greater than 95% Hypotension

Second-Line Drug

Sorbitol

Initial Dose	50 g of a 70% solution orally or as a retention enema
Repeat Doses	50 g of a 70% solution orally or as a retention enema every 30 minutes for four doses, then every 2–4 hours
End-Points	Diarrhea averaging 100–200 ml/hour Relief of symptoms Institution of dialysis Hypotension

disease. Therefore, alternative treatment modalities are necesary until dialysis can be implemented or for definitive management if dialysis is not possible. Standard immediate therapy with oxygen, ventilatory support if needed, placing the patient in the sitting position, and vasodilation with morphine and nitrates are immediately indicated.

Phlebotomy is indicated in patients with acute renal failure who have a normal hematocrit. This modality should not be used in patients with chronic renal failure because of their significant anemia. Lowering the hematocrit further in these patients may be detrimental to tissue oxygen delivery and worsen the situation.

The gastrointestinal tract should be utilized in these renal failure patients who do not promptly improve with the immediate measures outlined above and who cannot be on dialysis within 1 to 2 hours. (See box.)

Discussion

The bowel, and especially the colon, can be utilized as an effective organ of fluid elimination in patients who are unable to excrete fluid via the kidneys. Water will be passively transferred from the vascular space to the lumen of the bowel if an osmotic gradient is established. Sorbitol is an osmotically active six-carbon sugar alcohol with no gastrointestinal absorption. Sorbitol produces a voluminous osmotic diarrhea that may fully resolve the problem or at least acutely remove enough fluid to stabilize the situation until dialysis can be initiated. Clinical (subjective relief, slower respiratory rate) and hemodynamic (lowering of the pulmonary artery wedge pressure) improvement occurs in 15 to 30 minutes and precedes the onset of diarrhea. The sorbitol dosing regimen outlined above can be expected to produce 400 to 500 ml of diarrhea in the first hour and 4000 to 5000 ml within the first 24 hours.

It is important to remember that *intravenous* osmotic agents are specifically contraindicated in pulmonary edema, especially with coexisting renal failure. Intravenous osmotic agents acutely increase intravascular volume and thus worsen pulmonary edema.

Large doses of a loop diuretic may be tried in patients not known to have fixed anuria and may provide some immediate relief due to vasodilation and induce a diuresis if the renal failure is not fixed. A dose of 100 mg of furosemide is given initially, and the dose is doubled to 200 mg if there is no increase in urine output after 1 hour.

SPECIFIC AGENTS

Diuretics

Acetazolamide

Pharmacology

Sulfonamide

Mechanism

Inhibits carbonic anhydrase present in kidneys, choroid plexus, and ciliary body.

Kinetics (IV)

Onset	Minutes
Peak	15 minutes
Duration	4–5 hours
Half-life	4–10 hours

Metabolism

Renal excretion of unaltered drug

Indications

Acute angle-closure glaucoma
Increased intracranial pressure
Metabolic alkalosis
Prevention of acute mountain sickness

Cautions

Use in:
   Pregnancy—Category C
   Lactation—avoid if possible
   Childhood—yes

Contraindications

Severe hypokalemia or hyponatremia
Adrenal insufficiency
Hyperchloremic acidosis
Liver failure

Dosage

Initial 500 mg IV over 20 to 30 minutes
Subsequent 250 to 500 mg every 4 to 6 hours

Dosage Adjustments in Organ Failure

Renal failure: glomerular filtration rate (GFR) 10 to 50—increase dosing interval to 12 hours; GFR < 10—do not use.
Hepatic failure: do not use.

Toxicity

Side Effects

Common: fatigue, anorexia, headache, nervousness, nausea and vomiting, diarrhea, paresthesias, hypokalemia (usually minor), kidney stones, metabolic acidosis

Uncommon: convulsions, hepatic failure, paralysis, thrombocytopenia

Dangerous: thrombocytopenia, convulsions, acute allergic syndromes in patients allergic to other sulfa drugs

Treatment of Acute Toxicity

Stop drug.
For convulsions, IV diazepam
For allergy, epinephrine, diphenhydramine, methylprednisolone

Interactions

Increases toxicity of lithium, quinidine, salicylates, sympathomimetic amines

Furosemide

Pharmacology

Mechanism

Inhibits reabsorption of sodium and chloride in loop of Henle and proximal and distal tubules

Kinetics (IV)

Onset   5 minutes
Peak   10–30 minutes
Duration   2 hours
Half-life   1 hour

Metabolism

35% hepatic metabolism to glucuronide
65% renal excretion
95% protein bound

Indications

Diuresis
Intracranial hypertension
Increased intraocular pressure
Hypertension
Hypercalcemia

Cautions

Use in:
  Pregnancy—Category C
  Lactation—no; appears in breast milk
  Childhood—yes; dose 1 mg/kg initial to maximum of 6 mg/kg

Contraindication

Anuria

Dosage

Initial: 20 to 40 mg by IV bolus over 1 to 2 minutes
Repeat: Every 2 hours. Increase dose if no or minimal response to initial dose.

Dosage Adjustment in Organ Failure

Renal failure: increase dose to 100 to 200 mg.

Toxicity

Side Effects

Common: hypokalemia, hypomagnesemia, hyperuricemia, hyponatremia, hypochloremic alkalosis, hypocalcemia, hyperglycemia, gastrointestinal upset, rash/pruritus, headache, dizziness (may be postural), paresthesias

Uncommon: pancreatitis, deafness, marrow suppression, exacerbation of lupus, cholestatic jaundice

Dangerous: hypovolemia, hypokalemia, pancreatitis, aplastic anemia

Treatment of Acute Toxicity

Stop drug.
Replace potassium.
Trendelenburg position
Volume infusion

Note: Patients who are allergic to sulfonamides may also have serious allergic reactions to furosemide.

Interactions

Increases digoxin toxicity
Increases lithium toxicity
Increases salicylate toxicity
Enhances neuromuscular blockade of succinylcholine
Increases nephrotoxicity and ototoxicity of aminoglycosides
Increases nephrotoxicity of cephalosporins
Increases captopril-induced renal failure
Vasomotor instability with chloral hydrate
Nonsteroidals decrease furosemide effects.
Phenytoin decreases furosemide effects.
Furosemide decreases theophylline effects.

Osmotic Agents

Glycerol

Pharmacology

Simplest of the trihydric sugar alcohols
Chemical formula $C_3 H_8 O_3$
Molecular weight 92.09

Kinetics

Onset of action: oral—10 to 12 hours;
IV—related to attainment of serum levels of 10 to 30 mOsm/liter

Metabolism

Converted to glucose; provides 4.32 kcal/g

Indications and Uses

Reduction of increased intracranial pressure
Reduction of increased intraocular pressure
Topical agent
Evacuant (as a 50 to 75% solution)
As a vehicle for other medications

Dosage and Administration

Intravenous: 0.2 to 1.0 g/kg/hour (or the dose that attains plasma concentrations of 10 to 30 mOsm/liter); mixed in isotonic saline so final concentration is 40% or less
Oral: initial dose of 1 g/kg followed by 0.5 to 1.0 g/kg every 3 to 4 hours as an oral evacuant; used as a 50 to 75% solution

Cautions

Dosage adjustment in organ failure—do not use intravenously in renal or cardiac failure.
Use in:
   Pregnancy—yes; Category C
   Lactation—yes
   Childhood—yes

Toxicity

Glycerol is a simple sugar and has little toxicity of its own. The main toxicity is secondary to its osmotic effect:

Fluid and electrolyte imbalances
Dehydration
Mild hemolysis (with intravenous concentrations greater than 40% administered at a rate of infusion exceeding 4 to 5 ml/min)

Gastric irritation (with oral preparation of 50 to 75%)

Mannitol

Pharmacology

Six-carbon sugar alcohol
Molecular weight 182.17
Chemical formula $C_6 H_{14} O_2$
Occurs naturally in fruits and vegetables

Kinetics

Supersaturated at room temperature
Only for intravenous use
Must be warmed before given intravenously
Only minimal metabolism

Onset	Approximately 1 minute
Peak	5–15 minutes
Duration	2–4 hours

Metabolism

Freely filtered at the glomerulus
Less than 10% reabsorption by tubules
Not secreted by tubules
80% of intravenous dose appears in the urine within 3 hours

Indications

Promotion of diuresis
Prevention or treatment of oliguric phase of acute renal failure
Reduction of increased intracranial pressure
Reduction of intraocular pressure
Promotion of urinary excretion of toxic substances
Irrigating solution during transurethral surgical procedures (as a 2.5% solution)

Dosage and Administration

Prepared only as an intravenous medication

Prevention of Acute Renal Failure

Test dose: 0.2 mg/kg
Initial dose: 50 to 100 g (20 g if secondary to acute hemolysis)

Reduction of Intracranial Pressure or Intraocular Pressure

Initial dose: 1 to 2 g/kg over 5 to 10 minutes
Repeat dose: 0.5 to 1 g every 4 to 6 hours

Cautions

Dosage adjustments in organ failure—do not use in cardiac or renal failure.
Use in:
Pregnancy—no data on fetal effects; Category C
Lactation—yes, if necessary for the mother
Childhood—yes

Contraindications

Fluid overload (due to rebound phenomenon)
Evidence of disruption of the blood–brain barrier (may leak into tissue and cause fluid influx into the intracranial cavity)
Severe dehydration states (as it may still cause diuresis and further dehydration)
Not contraindicated in diabetics as its metabolism is minimal

Toxicity

Mannitol is a simple sugar with minimal metabolism and in itself is basically not toxic. Side effects due to mannitol are infrequent and may include the following:

Metabolic: fluid and electrolyte imbalance, dehydration, acidosis (packaging solution has a pH of 4.5 to 7.0)
Cardiovascular: pulmonary edema, systemic edema, hypotension (based on dehydration), angina-like chest pain
Central nervous system: headaches, dizziness, convulsions
Genitourinary: osmotic nephrosis, urinary retention (should always have a urinary catheter in place)
Gastrointestinal: dry mouth, nausea/vomiting, diarrhea
Dermatologic: skin necrosis, thrombophlebitis
Miscellaneous: urticaria, blurred vision, rhinitis, arm pain, fever and chills

Treatment of Acute Toxicity

Stop mannitol.
For pulmonary edema, oxygen, nitroglycerin, diuretic
For hypotension, Trendelenburg position, dopamine, volume infusion

Sorbitol

Pharmacology

Six-carbon sugar
Molecular weight 182.17
Chemical formula $C_6 H_{14} O_6$

Kinetics

Available as an oral or intravenous preparation (rarely used in intravenous form)
Minimal metabolism by gastrointestinal tract
Almost totally excreted via the colon
Onset, peak, and duration of action depend on the gastrointestinal function of the particular patient.

Indications and Uses

Main use is presently as a vehicle for other medications, i.e., Kayexalate.
Pulmonary edema in anuric patient

Dosage and Administration

Oral (as a laxative): 30 to 50 g, with frequency titrated to desired effect
IV (as an intravenous osmotic agent): 50 to 100 ml of a 50% solution, titrated to response and serum osmolarity

Cautions

Dosage adjustments in organ failure—none
Use in:
Pregnancy—yes; Category C (no data)
Lactation—yes
Childhood—yes

Toxicity

Sorbitol is basically a nontoxic substance, but, as with the other osmotic agents, abnormalities can occur secondary to the effects of its osmotic actions (in this case, the osmotic diarrhea). During administration, fluid and electrolyte status should be monitored closely.

REFERENCES

Anderson C, Shahvari M, Zimmerman J: The treatment of pulmonary edema in the absence of renal function. A role for sorbitol and furosemide. JAMA 241:1008–1010, 1979.
Buckell M, Walsh L: Effect of glycerol by mouth on intracranial pressure in man. Lancet 2:1151–1152, 1964.
Cantore GP, Guidetti B, Virno M: Oral glycerol for the reduction of intracranial pressure. J Neurosurg 21:278–283, 1965.
Cottrell JE, Robustelli A, Post K, Turndorf H: Furosemide and mannitol induced changes in intracranial pressure and serum osmolality and electrolytes. Anesthesiology 47:28–30, 1977.
Ellis FW, Krantz JC: Sugar alcohols: Metabolism and toxicity studies with mannitol and sorbitol in man and animals. J Biol Chem 141:147–154, 1941.
James HE, Langfitt TW, Kumar VS: Analysis of the response to therapeutic measures to reduce intracranial

pressure in head injured patients. J Trauma 16:437–441, 1976.

Javid M, Gilboe D, Cesario T: The rebound phenomenon and hypertonic solutions. J Neurosurg 21:1059–1066, 1964.

Levin AB, Duff TA, Javid MJ: Treatment of increased intracranial pressure: A comparison of different osmotic agents and the use of thiopental. Neurosurgery 5:570–575, 1979.

Marshal LF, Smith RW, Rausher LA, Shapire HM: Mannitol dose requirements in brain-injured patients. J Neurosurg 48:169–172, 1978.

Meyer JS, Charney IZ, Rivera VM: Treatment with glycerol of cerebral edema due to cerebral infarction. Lancet 2:993–997, 1971.

Mickell JJ, Cook DR, Reigel DH, et al: Intracranial pressure monitoring in Reye-Johnson syndrome. Crit Care Med 4:1–7, 1976.

Miller JD, Leech P: Effects of mannitol and steroid therapy on intracranial volume-pressure relationships in patients. J Neurosurg 42:274–281, 1975.

Peters R: Laxative effect of sorbitol. Br Med J 677–678, 1958.

Pitlich W, Pirikitakulr P, Painter MJ, Wessel HB: Effects of glycerol and hyperosmolality on intracranial pressure. Clin Pharmacol Ther 131:466–471, 1982.

Reinglass J: Dose response curve of intravenous glycerol in the treatment of cerebral edema due to trauma. Neurology 24:743–747, 1984.

CHAPTER 20

Ophthalmic Agents

DOUGLAS EVANS, M.D.
JOHN HOEPNER, M.D.

CONDITIONS

Angle-Closure Glaucoma

Diagnosis

Although this vision-threatening disorder is responsible for only a small percentage of the cases of glaucoma diagnosed in the United States, the acuteness of its presentation causes patients to seek help at the hospital emergency department more frequently than is the case with the much more common primary open-angle glaucoma. Patients with the most severe form of acute angle-closure glaucoma (ACG) experience pain, nausea, and visual disturbance. Each of these symptoms is directly related to the elevated intraocular pressure (IOP). Pain secondary to ACG can be localized to the involved eye and orbit, or it can present simply as a diffuse headache. The elevation in IOP causes stimulation of visceral afferent fibers, which can produce marked nausea and vomiting. Occasionally, the prominence of the gastrointestinal symptoms in relation to the ocular signs and symptoms may distract the physician away from the correct diagnosis. The visual symptoms are most commonly related to corneal edema caused by the elevated IOP. Corneal edema will alter the refraction of light as it passes through the cornea and results in blurred vision and the appearance of "halos" around lights.

The ocular signs include an elevation in IOP, which may be as high as 60 to 80 mmHg, the normal reading being lower than 22 mmHg. Whereas pressure elevations in open-angle glaucoma are characteristically small in scale, the IOP elevation in ACG is dramatic. A simple technique to screen for the disease in the emergency setting is to press gently on both eyes simultaneously through closed lids. The eye with ACG will feel rock hard compared to the firm but more rubbery consistency of the normal eye. This is a crude test, and IOP should be confirmed with a Schiøtz or applanation tonometer. Characteristically, there is a conjunctival vascular injection. The pupil is typically mid-dilated and nonreactive or poorly reactive. The view of the iris and pupil is often obscured by corneal edema, which results in a grayish-white haziness to the normally clear cornea. These signs can often be noted with a penlight examination. If a slit lamp is available, it may be used to examine the depth of the anterior chamber. The anterior chamber is usually shallow peripherally, and aqueous cells and flare are usually present.

The increased IOP in ACG is caused by apposition of the peripheral iris to the trabecular meshwork, which is the normal site of aqueous drainage from the eye. Aqueous humor is produced by the ciliary body epithelium just behind the iris in the posterior chamber of the eye. In order for this fluid to drain from the eye, the aqueous must circulate forward through the pupil into the anterior chamber (AC). When the pupil is mid-dilated, as occurs in a dark environment or as a result of pharmacologic treatment, the iris is in close apposition to the anterior lens capsule. This "pupillary block" creates a resistance to flow from the posterior chamber of the anterior segment, allowing pressure to build up in the posterior chamber. As the posterior chamber (PC) pressure rises, the differential in PC/AC pressure allows the iris to bow forward (a sign referred to as *iris*

bombé). As the peripheral iris bows forward, it is placed in apposition to the trabecular meshwork, causing it to occlude the angle structures. This closure of the angle causes the IOP to rise over a period of 30 minutes to 2 hours.

Indications for Treatment

Treatment of ACG should begin promptly as soon as the condition is diagnosed. Although surgical or laser iridotomy is the definitive curative procedure in ACG, the initial treatment should be medical. (See box.)

DRUG TREATMENT: ACUTE ANGLE-CLOSURE GLAUCOMA

First-Line Drugs
Pilocarpine 1%

1 drop every 10 minutes for 1 hour

AND

Timolol 0.5%

1 drop every 15 minutes for 1 hour

AND

Acetazolamide

500 mg by IV push

AND

Glycerin Solution

1 g/kg PO

OR

Mannitol

1 g/kg IV over 30–60 minutes

Second-Line Drugs
Isosorbide

Used instead of glycerin, especially in diabetics
1.5 g/kg (Do not confuse with isosorbide dinitrate[Isordil].)

Betaxolol 0.5%

Used instead of timolol or levobunolol in asthmatics

End-Points

Relief of symptoms
Reduction in IOP to < 22 mmHg.

Discussion

The objectives in the initial treatment of ACG are to stop the attack and reopen the angle structures. Topical 1 or 2% pilocarpine is given in a dose of 1 drop every 10 minutes until the pupil constricts.

Pilocarpine is a direct-acting cholinergic agonist that, when used in the eye topically, produces miosis, contraction of the ciliary muscle and pupillary sphincter, and a fall in IOP associated with an increase in the facility of outflow of aqueous humor from the eye. It is believed that miotics produce a lower IOP by placing tension on the trabecular meshwork and opening the trabecular spaces to fluid outlow. In ACG treated with pilocarpine, the contraction of the pupillary sphincter muscle places tension on the peripheral iris, flattening the "bombé" configuration, reducing the area of lens and iris contact, and pulling the iris away from the angle structures where it is blocking the aqueous outflow. The stronger miotics can potentially aggravate pupillary block. Contraction of the ciliary muscle allows the lens to ride forward and can bring it in closer apposition to the iris. It is for this reason that the stronger miotic agents such as echothiophate, carbachol, and the 4 and 6% solutions of pilocarpine should be avoided in treating ACG.

Echothiophate and isoflurophate are long-acting miotic agents. They are organophosphorus compounds that have irreversible effects and are used in the treatment of severe primary open-angle glaucoma. There is no use for these agents in the setting of ACG. Likewise, carbachol, a miotic agent that combines the direct-acting properties of pilocarpine with the anticholinesterase effects of the organophosphorus compounds, is not used in the treatment of ACG. It penetrates the eye poorly and can also potentially aggravate pupillary block.

Topical beta-blockers are also used in the initial management of ACG. Timolol 0.5% (Timoptic) or levobunolol 0.5% (Betagan) or, in asthmatic patients, the beta$_1$-selective betaxolol 0.5% (Betoptic) can be given to decrease ciliary body production of aqueous humor and can thereby lower IOP. The primary indication for the use of each of the drugs is primary open-angle glaucoma; however, in the acute ACG setting, these drugs can be helpful as a fast, easily administered adjunct to the carbonic anhydrase inhibitors and miotics. Their use, however, must be followed promptly by the administration of acetazolamide or a hyperosmotic agent if the attack of ACG is not easily broken (10 to 15 minutes) by the use of beta-blockers and pilocarpine.

Timolol 0.5% or levobunolol 0.5% is given in doses of 1 to 2 drops every 15 minutes over the first 30 to 60 minutes of an acute attack of ACG. Betaxolol, a beta$_1$-selective agent, is preferred in patients with a known history of asthma or bronchitis, but as with all beta$_1$-selective agents, this property is dose dependent, and a beta$_2$ effect is produced with higher levels of the drug. Side effects have been reported related to systemic beta blockade, and this possibility must be kept in mind when the drug is given more frequently than the usual open-angle glaucoma dose of twice a day, as it may be in treatment of ACG.

Useful systemic medications include the carbonic anhydrase inhibitors and the osmotic agents. Acetazolamide (Diamox), the most commonly prescribed carbonic anhydrase inhibitor, can be given both orally and parenterally.

The carbonic anhydrase inhibitors, as a group, inhibit the enzyme carbonic anhydrase, which catalyzes the reaction

$$CO_2 + H_2O \rightarrow H_2CO_3 \rightarrow H^+ + HCO_3^-$$

It is known that the enzyme carbonic anhydrase is present in the ciliary processes and that there is a high concentration of bicarbonate in aqueous humor. The exact relationship between the inhibition of the enzyme and the lowering of IOP has yet to be worked out. It is known, however, that the IOP-lowering effect is independent of the diuresis produced.

The initial dosage of acetazolamide for acute ACG, when given orally in tablet form, is 250 to 500 mg. This dose may be repeated after several hours, if necessary. The usual maximum daily dosage is 1 g. Acetazolamide is also supplied in a timed-release 500-mg capsule; this form of the drug should be reserved for the chronic treatment of primary open-angle glaucoma. Acetazolamide given orally reaches peak blood levels approximately 2 hours after ingestion, and it has a duration of action of 24 hours. The half-life of the drug is 5 hours, and since it is not metabolized, over half of the drug can be recovered in the urine within 24 hours. If intravenous acetazolamide is given, the usual adult dose is 500 mg. The drug should be reconstituted in 5 ml of sterile water prior to injection and given over 20 to 30 minutes. The usual adult dosage of methazolamide is 50 mg given orally.

In severe cases of ACG associated with nausea and vomiting, acetazolamide is best given intravenously in adults at a dose of 500 mg. It can also be given orally in doses of 250 to 500 mg. Acetazolamide, like methazolamide (Neptazane), which can be given only orally, produces a more significant fall in IOP than the topical beta-blocking drugs.

The hyperosmotic agents used either orally or parenterally are potentially the most effective in lowering IOP in the setting of acute ACG. They are, in general, believed to be more effective than the carbonic anhydrase inhibitors because they decrease vitreous volume and thereby diminish the forward pressure on the iris, which is closing the angle. These solutions work by increasing plasma osmolarity and inducing free water to move from the globe to the intravascular fluid compartment. Various agents are available. The most common agent used orally is glycerin (glycerol and Osmoglyn). Glycerin is supplied in 50% and 75% solutions and is given full strength over cracked ice or with a small amount of juice. The advantages of glycerin are that it is a nontoxic, well-tolerated agent that is rapidly metabolized and therefore produces little diuresis. The chief disadvantage is that it is a significant calorie load and can produce hyperglycemia in diabetic patients. The other agent available for oral administration is isosorbide (Ismotic), which should not be confused with isosorbide dinitrate (Isordil). Isosorbide is a nonmetabolized agent similar to mannitol. It does not provide a calorie load or cause hyperglycemia, but it does produce significant diuresis. In general, the advantages of the oral agents are that they can be given in the office setting with a greater margin of safety than can the intravenous osmotic agents. The chief disadvantage is that patients with acute ACG may already be nauseated and vomiting and may not be able to drink these syrup-like agents, let alone keep them down long enough to be absorbed.

The usual oral dose of glycerin is 1.0 to 1.5 g/kg. A reduction in IOP occurs within 30 minutes of ingestion and lasts approximately 4 to 5 hours, at which time the dose of glycerin may be repeated if necessary. Isosorbide can be given in doses of 1.5 g/kg. It is supplied in a 45% solution. The maximum decrease in IOP is achieved within 1 hour of administration and lasts approximately 4 to 6 hours.

Side effects associated with the oral hyperosmotic agents include headache, which is related to decreased intracranial pressure and is minimized in the supine position. Nausea and vomiting may also be produced by the agents themselves because they provide a large osmotic load.

Mannitol is the agent of choice when an intravenous osmotic agent is required. It is a large molecule and is confined to the extracellular fluid compartment. It is not absorbed through the gastrointestinal tract and cannot be given orally. It is not metabolized and can be given safely in diabetics. Mannitol produces a maximal decrease in IOP within 30 to 60 minutes, and the effect lasts for 6 hours. The usual dosage is 1 g/kg IV given in a 20% solution over 30 minutes. Diuresis is a prominent feature. The chief side effects associated with the use of mannitol are similar to those seen with the oral agents. In addition, with the use of an intravenous agent, there is a greater risk of dehydration. The risk to those patients whose cardiopulmonary status is compromised is high, since mannitol produces a large shift of fluid into the intravascular compartment, creating a volume load on the heart. Pulmonary edema can occur.

Ideally, an ophthalmologist should be consulted at the time a diagnosis of ACG is first considered, and he or she should be on hand to oversee the above treatment regimen. In the case where a non-ophthalmologist is faced with treating this condition alone, after the acute episode is broken, the patient should be maintained on topical pilocarpine 1%, 1 drop four times a day, and a referral should be made to an ophthalmologist so that definitive laser iridotomy or surgical iridectomy can be performed.

Central Retinal Artery Occlusion

Diagnosis

Central retinal artery occlusion (CRAO), like acute ACG, is a true ophthalmologic emergency. Occlusion of the central retinal artery, however, unlike acute ACG, causes painless loss of vision. It commonly occurs secondary to thrombosis of the central retinal artery at the level of lamina cribrosa in association with arteriosclerosis or embolization. There is a high incidence of occlusive vascular disease such as hypertension, carotid artery disease, giant cell arteritis, and diabetes mellitus in patients who develop CRAO.

The typical patient presents with a history of sudden painless loss of vision in a previously healthy eye. The vision is usually dramatically decreased often to the "counting fingers" level. The pupil on the affected side is fixed or sluggish when stimulated directly but will respond briskly to consensual stimulation. This is a manifestation of a severe afferent pupillary defect or Marcus Gunn pupil, and paradoxical dilation is easily demonstrated with the swinging flashlight test. The anterior segment is otherwise typically unremarkable. The funduscopic examination shows a boggy, pale, edematous retina. The classic "cherry-red spot" is seen at the fovea. Since the retina is very thin at the fovea and the outer retina gets its blood supply from the choroid, the perfused choroid is seen through the outer retina at the fovea. The edematous milky-colored retina obscures the perfused choroid elsewhere. Inspection of the blood vessels will often demonstrate sludging and "box caring" of the blood in the veins secondary to the slow transport in these vessels. The veins also appear dark in color because of the deoxygenated blood they carry. Retinal hemorrhages are not a prominent feature of CRAO.

Indications for Treatment

Diagnosis is based on the patient's history and the above-mentioned features on the fundus examination. Once the diagnosis is established, treatment should begin promptly. (See box.)

Discussion

Treatment is aimed at restoring blood flow through the central retinal artery. A simple, fast, initial maneuver that occasionally helps restore blood flow is digital massage of the globe. Massage is believed to help dislodge an embolus at the level of the lamina cribrosa. Other measures such as the administration of agents such as acetazolamide to lower the IOP will reduce the resistance to perfusion of the retinal arterial tree.

The use of a mixture of 95% oxygen and 5% carbon dioxide is also of value in the acute phase of CRAO. The rationale for the use of this gas mixture is to elevate alveolar pCO_2 to a level sufficient to increase cerebral arteriolar pCO_2 enough to dilate the intracranial arteriole tree. The high oxygen level will also ensure adequate arteriole pO_2. Most hospital respiratory therapists are familiar with this form of treatment and can assist in its administration. The gas mixture is given via face mask for a 10-minute period every waking hour and every 4 hours at night. Blood pressure monitoring during administration is essential. An ophthalmologist should be consulted immediately to aid in the management of this condition. Surgical decompression to lower IOP by anterior chamber paracentesis may be sight saving.

Corneal Abrasion

Diagnosis

One of the most common ophthalmologic diagnoses is the corneal abrasion. This problem occurs when minor trauma to the eye

---

DRUG TREATMENT: CENTRAL RETINAL ARTERY OCCLUSION

First-Line Treatment

1. Digital massage of the globe
   and
2. Acetazolamide, 500 mg by IV push
   and
3. 95% O_2 with 5% CO_2 via mask given for 10 minutes every hour
   and
4. Call ophthalmologist

disrupts the corneal epithelium. Ocular foreign bodies that gain entry to the conjunctival surface of the eye can abrade the cornea as they are pushed across the epithelial surface of the cornea by the lids. Smaller particles that may spray into the eyes can become embedded in the corneal surface, creating an abrasion with a retained corneal foreign body. Contact lenses are also a common cause of corneal abrasions. Contact lenses can cause corneal abrasions by preventing adequate oxygen delivery to the corneal surface. This occurs if the patient wears the older hard contact lenses, which are not gas permeable, for an extended period. Abrasions can also occur if particles or debris are trapped beneath a contact lens while it is worn. Finally, chemicals are another important cause of a loss of corneal epithelium. An alkaline injury is potentially the most threatening to vision.

The most important diagnostic clue to be obtained in the history is that of trauma. The possibility of a penetrating injury must be considered when the history suggests injury by a high velocity particle (e.g., while the patient was hammering steel). If the history does not reveal any prior trauma, other causes such as conjunctivitis and keratitis should be considered. When a patient presents with a corneal abrasion, typical symptoms include pain, photophobia (light sensitivity), and tearing. The pain is often severe, and the patient's reaction may be dramatic, with significant blepharospasm (forceful lid closure) hindering examination of the eye. An attempt should be made to document the visual acuity. If this cannot be done because of blepharospasm, it is helpful to administer a drop of topical anesthetic. Of the three topical anesthetics commonly used in ophthalmology, proparacaine is used most often because it is the one that produces the least discomfort when instilled. After the visual acuity has been recorded, a funduscopic and slit-lamp examination should be performed, paying particular attention to signs of serious trauma (anterior or posterior chamber hemorrhage or secondary iritis). Finally, the ocular surface should be stained with fluorescein. If the patient wears contact lenses, they should be removed prior to instilling fluorescein. The cornea should then be viewed under blue illumination as provided by a Wood's lamp or the cobalt blue filter on a penlight or a slit lamp.

On examination, a corneal abrasion will show up as a punctate, linear, or geographic area of yellow fluorescein stain. Often the appearance and location of the stain will provide clues to the etiology of the abrasion. Typically, a foreign body under the lids will cause vertical linear abrasions. The finding of such an abrasion should reinforce the importance of careful inspection of the conjunctival surface of the upper and lower lids. Both upper lids should be everted and inspected for foreign bodies in every patient with a history of injury to the eye. Contact lenses will often produce an abrasion that stains at the 3 and 9 o'clock positions as well as centrally. An "exposure pattern" is seen when the staining is confined to the central area of the cornea that is not covered by the lids; this pattern suggests an airborne agent. Diffuse punctate staining is commonly see with viral keratoconjunctivitis. Geographic abrasions that involve a majority of the corneal surface are often caused by chemicals.

If a history of chemical injury to the eye is obtained, further history and examination should be delayed, and immediate ocular irrigation should be started. The goal of irrigation is dilution of the injurious chemical and removal of any particulate matter. Topical anesthetics, such as proparacaine, should be instilled in the eyes and a lid speculum or a paper clip retractor should be used to hold the eyes open. The eyes are then irrigated with Ringer's lactate solution for a minimum of 15 to 20 minutes using at least 2 liters of fluid in each eye. An 18-gauge plastic catheter connected to intravenous tubing is ideal for irrigation. Once irrigation is complete, pH paper applied gently to the conjunctival surface should be used to check for the adequacy of dilution of an alkaline agent. If the paper reveals an alkaline pH, more irrigation is required until adequate dilution is achieved. After the irrigation is complete, the visual acuity should be documented. The cornea should then be examined for residual foreign material and stained with fluorescein to document the extent of the loss of epithelium.

Indications for Treatment

Corneal abrasions that cause the patient enough discomfort to seek medical advice should be treated. Simple corneal abrasions can be managed by the primary care physician according to the guidelines listed in the flow sheet that follows. In cases of chemical contamination, the eye should be immediately irrigated and then examined and treated. Severe chemical injuries, particularly alkaline burns, require immediate ophthalmologic consultation, as do penetrating corneal injuries with perforation of the globe. (See box.)

Discussion

Fluorescein ophthalmic strips should be moistened with any sterile ophthalmic irrigating solution. If the eye can be examined without the use of the topical anesthetic, this is preferred, especially if the suspected abrasion is caused by a foreign body underneath the upper lid. Once this is removed with a cotton-tipped swab, the patient will immediately be able to appreciate the difference and can tell you whether or not all foreign bodies have been removed. If, however, there is difficulty in performing the examination because of discomfort and blepharo-

spasm, instill 1 drop of proparacaine. The area of fluorescein staining is usually apparent when illuminated with a white light; however, it is definitely enhanced by the use of a white light and a cobalt filter. Cobalt filters can attach to the end of pocket penlights, hand-held Wood's light, or to a slit lamp.

If the ocular examination does not reveal a foreign body and there is no other serious damage other than a corneal abrasion, the particular therapy chosen will depend on the size of the abrasion and the degree of discomfort. If the abrasion is less than 3 to 4 mm in diameter, the application of a broad-spectrum antibiotic ointment such as an aminoglycoside or Neosporin (or Polysporin) is sufficient. This should be applied every 4 to 6 hours in either drop or ointment form. Follow-up should be obtained within 24 hours. If the abrasion is larger than 3 to 4 mm, or if other signs of inflammation (i.e., a small pupil on that side or flare and cells in the an-

---

DRUG TREATMENT: CORNEAL ABRASION

First-Line Drugs

Proparacaine

1 or 2 drops. *Never* dispense to patient!

End-Point	Provides pain relief to allow adequate examination

THEN

Gentamicin Ophthalmic Ointment

Repeat application twice daily until cornea is healed.
   and
Administer systemic analgesic (i.e., acetaminophen with codeine).

End-Points	Pain relief
	Infection prophylaxis
	Corneal healing

Second-Line Drug

Cyclopentolate

(Use if ciliary spasm is present.)

Initial Dose	2 drops of a 1% solution
Repeat Dose	2 drops every 6 hours
End-Points	Pupillary dilatation
	Pain relief
	Corneal healing

terior chamber), a dilating agent should be administered in addition to the antibiotics. Twenty-four to thirty-six hours of dilatation and cycloplegia (to reduce ciliary spasm) can be obtained with cyclopentolate, 1 or 2 drops every 6 to 8 hours; or homatropine 5%, 1 drop in each eye twice a day. Scopolamine may also be used.

Patching of small corneal abrasions (i.e., those less than 3 to 4 mm in diameter) probably is not necessary. Patching should never be performed unless a broad-spectrum antibiotic ointment has been instilled. If the abrasion is large and the discomfort severe, relief can often be obtained by instilling an antibiotic ointment and putting a moderate pressure dressing over that eye. The dressing should be tight enough to keep the lid firmly closed over the globe but not so tight as to compromise ocular circulation and raise intraocular pressure. No pressure dressing should ever be left on longer than 24 hours. The patient should be instructed that if the discomfort increases or if the eyelid can be felt to move underneath the dressing, the dressing should be removed.

It is difficult to apply a pressure dressing properly. The normal procedure is to apply the dressing and have the patient leave it in place, except for the above-noted exceptions, until seen by the ophthalmologist the following day. An occasional alert patient may be able to remove the dressing and reapply the ointment every 8 hours. This, however, would be the exception rather than the rule. One of the authors (JAH) applies pressure dressings to far fewer than 10% of corneal abrasions. Others make wider use of this particular modality.

The end-point of therapy is lack of corneal staining with fluorescein, improved visual acuity, and resolution of ocular discomfort. No fluorescein staining of the cornea should be remaining. Healing of abrasions in young people occurs quite rapidly. Lesions as large as 3 to 4 mm in diameter will often cover over within 12 to 24 hours. Delayed healing or increased ocular discomfort should be an indication for an immediate visit to an ophthalmologist. Any lesion treated in the emergency department should be seen in a follow-up visit to an ophthalmologist within 24 hours. Increasing discomfort is an indication for earlier or immediate referral.

Iritis

Diagnosis

An area of difficulty in emergent ophthalmologic evaluation is the distinction between iritis and conjunctivitis (Table 20–1). It is not uncommon for a patient to be given a diagnosis of conjunctivitis, and only later in a follow-up examination by the ophthalmologist is the correct diagnosis discovered to be iritis. This delay in treatment can be avoided by the physician understanding the pathophysiology of iritis, knowing the signs to look for on examination, and being familiar with the basic principles of treatment.

The uveal tract gets its name from the Greek work *uva*, or grape, because the inner coat of the eye is a blue-pigmented structure. The uveal tract consists of three structures: the iris, the ciliary body, and the choroid. Inflammation in these structures is termed *iritis, cyclitis,* and *choroiditis,* respectively. In practice, it is often difficult to separate an iritis from a cyclitis, hence the term *iridocyclitis. Uveitis* is a general term used to indicate inflammation of the uveal tract at any location. Inflammation of the uveal tract can occur as a result of various pathophysiologic processes. Systemic disease, often autoimmune in nature, is a common cause of uveitis, as is infection caused by viruses, bacteria, and parasites; more rarely, neoplastic disease can produce intraocular inflammation. Although each of the various etiologies of uveal inflammation has a char-

TABLE 20–1. Differential Diagnosis of The Red Eye

Sign	Conjunctivitis	Uveitis	Angle-Closure Glaucoma
Vision	Normal	Mildly blurred	Marked blurring
Pain	Mild	Moderate	Severe
Discharge	Moderate	None	None
Injection	Diffuse	Ciliary flush	Mixed
Pupils	Normal	Slight constriction, variable	Mid-dilated, poorly reactive
Intraocular pressure	Normal	Variable/normal	Very high
Cornea	Clear	Hazy/variable	Very hazy

acteristic presentation, it is not within the scope of this chapter to deal with each of them individually. Rather, it is important to make the correct general diagnosis, initiate treatment, and make the appropriate referral.

A patient with intraocular inflammation of the uveal tract will typically present with complaints of photophobia, pain, decreased vision, and a red eye. Increased tearing is also noted frequently by patients. One of the most characteristic signs in iritis, and one that is helpful in differentiating this condition from conjunctivitis, is the ciliary flush. This is a perilimbal injection of the deep vessels of the sclera and episclera at the border of the cornea. This injection gives the perilimbal region a violaceous color, which is not present more peripherally on the surface of the globe. In conjunctivitis, the injection is more uniform and extends from the pericorneal region to the fornices. The injection is also in the more superficial conjunctival layer of the eye and hence has a brighter reddish color. It is usually possible to make the distinction between a ciliary flush and a superficial conjunctival injection with only a hand-held penlight. However, a slit lamp is required to evaluate a patient for intraocular inflammation.

The characteristic findings on slit-lamp examination for anterior segment inflammation include anterior chamber flare and cells. The terms *flare* and *cells* refer to inflammatory products, specifically protein and inflammatory cells that are released from the uveal tract vasculature into the aqueous humor. These signs can be noted best with a slit lamp narrowed to a thin beam, aimed at a 45-degree angle to the examiner's visual axis. A darkened room and a dilated pupil facilitate the examination. When protein is present in the anterior chamber, it reflects light much like water vapor reflects a spotlight on a foggy night. If cells have been released into the aqueous, with sufficient magnification they can also be seen floating in the aqueous. If either of these signs is present, you can be sure that the disorder is more than a simple conjunctivitis.

Additional findings, which can be seen in uveal tract inflammation, are keratitic precipitates. These are deposits of inflammatory debris on the endothelial surface of the cornea. They can vary in size and pigmentation but always signify the presence of intraocular inflammation. With prolonged inflamma-

tion, adhesions between the various anterior segment structures begin to occur. These adhesions or synechiae can occur between the iris and lens (posterior synechiae) and between the iris and cornea (anterior synechiae).

Vitreous cells typically are seen in a severe cyclitis or posterior uveitis. Extensive cellular debris in the vitreous can cause considerable visual loss and can obscure funduscopic changes. Chorioretinal inflammation often takes the form of retinal infiltration, vasculitis, edema, and scarring. Cystoid macular edema can cause significant visual loss and is a major cause of visual loss in retinal and vitreal inflammatory processes.

Indications for Treatment

Usually, a consulting ophthalmologist should be called if there is concern that the ocular condition is more than a simple conjunctivitis. Well-trained physicians who are comfortable with the diagnosis of uveitis should begin therapy and initiate an ophthalmologic referral when the diagnosis is made. (See box.)

Discussion

Nonspecific agents are used in the initial management of a uveitis until a more specific diagnosis can be made. It is appropriate in the emergency setting to begin treatment with topical steroids and cycloplegic mydriatic agents. In the emergency setting, it would be wise to use shorter-acting agents, such as cyclopentolate 1%, thereby allowing the ophthalmologist the choice of continuing the short-acting agent or switching to longer-acting agents. It should also be pointed out that angle-closure glaucoma is a rare but serious complication of the use of mydriatic ocular preparations. The physician should be comfortable with the slit-lamp examination for anterior chamber depth prior to use of topical mydriatic-cycloplegic agents.

The purpose of mydriasis in the setting of uveal tract inflammation is to prevent adhesions between the iris and the lens. These adhesions are termed *posterior synechiae*. Additionally, ocular injury or inflammation is often associated with spasm of the ciliary muscle, which can produce severe ocular discomfort. Cycloplegic agents relax the ciliary muscle and contribute to patient comfort.

Topical steroids are used to minimize the ocular inflammatory response and prevent

DRUG TREATMENT: UVEITIS

First-Line Drugs

Cyclopentolate 1% Solution

Initial Dose	2 drops
Repeat Dose	2 drops every 12–24 hours
End-Point	Mydriasis

AND

Dexamethasone Phosphate 0.1%

Initial Dose	1 drop
Repeat Dose	1 drop every 6 hours
End-Point	Healing

Alternative Drugs

Prednisolone Acetate 1%

Initial Dose	1 drop
Repeat Dose	1 drop every 6 hours
End-Point	Healing

Fluorometholone 0.1% or 0.25%*

Initial Dose	1 drop
Repeat Dose	1 drop every 6 hours
End-Point	Healing

*Note: First choice if patient has had steroid-induced glaucoma.

scarring and resultant visual loss. The most commonly used agents in the treatment of uveal tract inflammation are dexamethasone phosphate 0.1%, prednisolone acetate 1%, prednisolone phosphate 1%, and fluorometholone 0.1% or 0.25%. Less potent agents that have been used in the treatment of mild anterior segment inflammation include prednisolone 0.125% preparations. This strength is less effective and therefore used more commonly when treating superficial inflammatory conditions.

The frequency with which topical steroids are prescribed varies and is dependent on the severity of the anterior chamber reaction. Generally, for a mild anterior chamber reaction, the patient can be started on a regimen of 1 drop of prednisolone acetate 1% or dexamethasone 0.1% four times a day in the affected eye. More severe inflammation requires an increased frequency of administra-tion, and ophthalmologists have used potent topical steroids as frequently as every hour in the appropriate setting. Fluorometholone 0.1% and 0.25% can be used in patients with a history of steroid-induced glaucoma. An increased intraocular pressure in response to topical steroid administration is seen most commonly in patients with open-angle glaucoma and in diabetics. Fluorometholone is a topical steroid that does not penetrate the eye as well as the other agents do. It has also been associated with less significant increases in intraocular pressure and therefore is used in patients who are known steroid responders or who fall into a category of patients likely to have an increase in pressure related to topical steroids.

Of all the side effects associated with the use of topical steroids, the one that is of most importance is the danger of exacerbating a preexistent herpes simplex virus infection.

Careful slit-lamp examination of the cornea for dendritic figures with fluorescein stain and a cobalt blue light is an essential prerequisite for the use of topical steroid medications. In addition, the use of steroids can blunt the eye's resistance to fungal or bacterial infection and also mask the signs and symptoms of such infections. Prompt ophthalmic follow-up (within 24 hours), in addition to prior slit-lamp examination, should accompany the use of topical steroids in the emergency setting. Other side effects of ocular topical steroids include the development of posterior subcapsular cataracts and delayed wound healing after ocular surgery.

Herpes Simplex Virus Keratitis

Diagnosis

Every acute care physician should be familiar with the diagnosis of herpes simplex virus (HSV) ocular infection. HSV can cause conjunctivitis, keratitis, iritis, or any combination of these processes. Primary ocular infection typically occurs in children or young adults. Often patients complain of fever and malaise in association with a red, watery, irritated eye. On examination, vesicles can usually be found in the periocular skin or at the mucocutaneous borders of the mouth or nose. A preauricular lymph node can often be palpated. The conjunctiva is typically laden with follicles. The corneal findings classically show dendritic branching figures in the epithelium that stain with fluorescein. However, the corneal staining pattern is variable, and the clinician can be easily fooled by HSV.

The diagnosis is most often made clinically on the basis of the above-mentioned findings. If in doubt, the patient should have a viral culture taken. Once a patient has had an initial ocular infection with HSV, the virus remains latent in the trigeminal ganglion, and the patient is susceptible to subsequent recurrences. The signs and symptoms of recurrent infections are similar to those of the initial infection except that the constitutional symptoms are usually absent. Corneal hypesthesia may be noted owing to the recurrent inflammation. Treatment is similar to that for the primary infection.

Indications for Treatment

The physician should begin treatment for herpes simplex keratitis at the time of diag-

nosis. The patient should receive ophthalmologic follow-up in 1 or 2 days. (See box.)

Discussion

A variety of agents are useful in the treatment of ocular HSV infections. These agents shorten the course of the infection by interfering with viral deoxyribonucleic acid (DNA) synthesis. The three medications available for ocular instillation are idoxuridine, vidarabine, and trifluridine. Trifluridine is the most recent addition to the pharmacologic armamentarium and has less side effects and better ocular penetrance than do the other agents. Acyclovir, another excellent agent used against HSV, is available for topical application to skin lesions but not for ocular instillation.

Idoxuridine is a pyrimidine analogue that resembles thymidine. It is incorporated into DNA and causes it to be unstable. The drug is available in a 1 mg/ml solution, which is given every 1 to 2 hours until healing is complete. The ointment is applied five times per day. Side effects include discomfort upon instillation and irritation and edema of the conjunctiva and lids.

Vidarabine was originally developed as an antineoplastic agent. It is an analogue of adenosine and inhibits the viral DNA polymerase. It is available only as an ointment in 30 mg/g concentration. It is applied five times per day until healing is complete. As with the other agents, local irritation, punctate keratopathy, and, rarely, punctal occlusion may occur.

Trifluridine, or triflurothymidine, another analogue of thymidine, is the third agent useful in the treatment of ocular HSV infections. It inhibits both mammalian and viral DNA synthesis. It has better penetration than do the other agents and is less toxic to the corneal epithelium. It is currently the topical drug of choice for the treatment of HSV keratitis. Trifluridine is available as a 10 mg/ml solution. It is given initially nine times per day until healing is complete. The side effects of trifluridine are similar to, but less severe than, those associated with idoxuridine or vidarabine.

Acyclovir, another highly effective agent, is not yet available for ocular instillation. Its action is specific for viral DNA. It is available in ointment form for use topically in the treatment of skin vesicles associated with primary herpetic infections. The drug should be prescribed in association with one of the

DRUG TREATMENT: HERPES SIMPLEX KERATITIS

First-Line Drug

Trifluridine Ophthalmic Solution 1%

Initial Dose	1 drop
Repeat Dose	1 drop every 2 hours while awake (maximum 9 drops daily) until corneal ulcer healed; then 1 drop every 4 hours while awake (minimum dose 5 drops daily) for 7 days
End-Point	Healing

Second-Line Drug

Idoxuridine Ophthalmic Solution 0.1% and Ophthalmic Ointment 0.5%

Initial Dose	Solution: 1 drop Ointment: 0.5 inch in conjunctival sac
Repeat Dose	Solution: 1 drop every hour during day and every 2 hours at night until corneal ulcer heals; then increase interval to 2 hours during day and 4 hours at night for 5 days Ointment: 0.5 inch 5 times daily, continued for 5 days after corneal ulcer healed
End-Point	Healing

Vidarabine Ophthalmic Ointment 3%

Initial Dose	0.5 inch into conjunctival sac
Repeat Dose	0.5 inch 5 times daily at 3-hour intervals until cornea healed; then 0.5 inch twice daily for 7 days
End-Point	Healing

other ocular medications in cases where skin involvement is present.

Conjunctivitis

Diagnosis

The most common eye disease in the United States is conjunctivitis. The conjunctiva is a smooth transparent tissue that lines the posterior surface of the lids and is reflected in the fornices back over the sclera of the eye. The tissue terminates at the lid margin and at the limbus. The conjunctiva that lines the posterior surface of the lids is termed the *palpebral conjunctiva,* and the tissue that covers the sclera is called the *bulbar conjunctiva.* The tissue is highly vascularized and has many lymphoid elements that serve to protect the eye from pathogens. In addition, the tears that bathe the ocular and conjunctival surfaces contain lysozyme and immunoglobulins, which inhibit the growth

of pathogens. The presence of these protective barriers keeps the incidence of serious ocular infection as a result of conjunctivitis low. However, when a patient presents with a complaint of a red eye, it is important that the more serious causes of conjunctival injection be ruled out (see Table 20–1). Keratitis, iritis, and acute glaucoma can all be misdiagnosed as a simple conjunctivitis if the physician is unfamiliar with the diagnosis of these conditions.

The symptoms and signs of conjunctivitis vary depending on the agent or mechanism causing the conjunctival inflammation. Bacteria, chlamydial organisms, viruses, and fungi are all common pathogens in conjunctivitis. In addition to these agents, conjunctivitis can be caused by allergens or toxic irritants or may result from systemic inflammatory disease.

The ocular symptoms associated with conjunctivitis include itching, which is most common with allergy; a burning or scratchy foreign body sensation; and increased tearing or mucus production. The signs of conjunctivitis include injection, which is most prominent away from the limbus as opposed to the perilimbal ciliary flush seen in iritis. Chemosis or edema of the conjunctiva can cause the tissue to balloon up off the sclera in multiple folds. Drainage from the eye occurs and can take the form of a watery transudate, as in viral conjunctivitis, or a more purulent exudate, as in bacterial conjunctivitis.

Papillary or follicular hypertrophy can provide helpful diagnostic clues to the cause of the conjunctival inflammation. Conjunctival papilla are vascular tufts in the conjunctiva that can produce exudate and cellular infiltration in a characteristic pattern. The presence of papillae is a nonspecific sign, but they occur most commonly in bacterial and allergic conjunctivitis. Follicles are accumulations of lymphoid cells, and their presence can give the conjunctiva a cobblestone-like appearance. Follicles are most commonly seen in viral and toxic conjunctivitis. In addition, all patients should be examined for the presence of preauricular adenopathy, which is a helpful sign in the diagnosis of viral conjunctivitis.

Once the more serious ocular conditions, such as glaucoma and iritis, have been ruled out, an attempt should be made to determine the etiology of the conjunctival inflammation. General classification of conjunctivitis into the categories of viral, bacterial, allergic, or chlamydial can often be made on clinical grounds. The laboratory investigation of ophthalmic infections is usually the responsibility of the ophthalmologist. However, there are several situations that call for an investigation that can be handled by the acute care physician. These are conjunctivitis caused by chlamydial organisms or *Neisseria*. The gonococcus and meningococcus organisms can cause a severe bilateral hyperpurulent conjunctivitis both in neonates and adults.

Chlamydia is also a common cause of ophthalmia neonatorum but can infect all ages. Chlamydial conjunctivitis can be caused by the trachoma organism, which is rare in the United States, or by the chlamydial agent that causes neonatal and adult inclusion conjunctivitis. The value of recognizing and properly diagnosing these conditions is important because *Neisseria* conjunctivitis requires systemic therapy as well as topical treatment in both adults and infants, and chlamydial ocular infection requires systemic therapy in infants because it can be associated with a pneumonitis. A history of venereal disease or urogenital symptoms can be very helpful in the diagnosis of either of these conditions. In patients in whom there is suspicion of infection by either of these organisms, cultures of the conjunctiva can be obtained for chlamydial, bacterial, and viral isolation. In addition, a conjunctival scraping can be done and sent for Gram and Geimsa stains. *Chlamydia* can be diagnosed on Geimsa stain by finding intracytoplasmic inclusions in epithelial cells.

Other organisms known to cause bacterial conjunctivitis include *Staphylococcus aureus*, *Staphylococcus epidermidis*, *Streptococcus*, *Pneumococcus*, *Moraxella*, and *Hemophilus influenzae*. Gram-negative organisms, which are rare causes of conjunctivitis, include *Proteus*, *Klebsiella*, *Serratia*, and *Pseudomonas*. Viral conjunctivitis is most often caused by the adenovirus and occasionally by herpes simplex virus.

Indications for Treatment

It should be recognized that most cases of bacterial, viral, and allergic conjunctivitis are self-limited. Although many cases of conjunctivitis do not have a bacterial etiology, it is prudent for the primary physician to begin antibiotic therapy in all cases because an untreated bacterial conjunctivitis represents some threat to sight. Therefore, those patients who do not give a history suspicious for gonococcal or chlamydial infection, who are not in the neonatal period, who do not have a hyperpurulent presentation, and who have intact corneal epithelium can be treated empirically with a broad-spectrum topical antibiotic and followed up by an ophthalmologist. When treating a patient empirically for conjunctivitis with topical agents, or when these agents are used prophylactically after a corneal abrasion, a broad-spectrum agent that is not irritating to the ocular tissues should be used. Antibiotic and steroid combinations are to be avoided.

Systemic antibiotic therapy should be added to topical therapy if there is a high index of suspicion for chlamydial or gonococcal infection.

The coadministration of an antihistamine-decongestant with the topical antibiotic provides symptomatic relief in allergic or viral conjunctivitis and is recommended when a viral infection or an allergy is a strong etiologic consideration.

Patients who present with unilateral conjunctivitis should be warned that the infection may spread to the uninvolved eye and advised to begin treating the other eye with the prescribed medications when symptoms begin in that eye. (See box.)

Discussion

Gentamicin and tobramycin are excellent broad-spectrum bactericidal antibiotics that

---

DRUG TREATMENT: CONJUNCTIVITIS

First-Line Agents

Gentamicin Ophthalmic Solution or Ointment

Initial Dose	2 drops of solution 0.5 inch of ointment
Repeat Dose	4 times daily

OR

Sulfacetamide Solution or Ointment 10% (in Infants and Adolescents)

Initial Dose	2 drops of solution 0.5 inch of ointment
Repeat Dose	4 times daily
End-Point	Healing Continue antibiotics for 2 days after resolution of symptoms.

PLUS, if allergic or viral conjunctivitis is likely

Naphcon A

Initial Dose	2 drops in affected eye
Repeat Dose	1–2 drops every 3–6 hours
End-Point	Relief of symptoms

Second-Line Agents

Bacitracin Ointment

Provides poor gram-negative coverage

Initial Dose	0.5 inch of ointment
Repeat Dose	0.5 inch every 8–12 hours

OR

Erythromycin Ophthalmic Ointment

Good for *Chlamydia;* no gram-negative coverage

Initial Dose	0.5 inch of ointment
Repeat Dose	5 times daily for 3 weeks

OR

Tetracycline 0.5% or 1.0% Ointment or Suspension

Initial Dose	2 drops of suspension 0.5 inch of ointment
Repeat Dose	5 times daily for 3 weeks
End-Point	Healing

are available topically as both ointments and solutions. They are active against most gram-negative and gram-positive organisms and cause minimal ocular irritation at qid or less frequent dosing intervals. The aminoglycosides are not very effective against chlamydial organisms. Side effects known to be associated with systemic use of these antibiotics, such as ototoxicity and nephrotoxicity, are usually not a consideration in the absence of concurrent systemic treatment.

Sulfacetamide 10% in drops or ointment is a good broad-spectrum agent against gram-positive and some gram-negative organisms. It is also effective against many chlamydial organisms. It should not be used in patients with a known sensitivity to sulfa preparations.

Bacitracin is an antibiotic that is bactericidal against most gram-positive organisms, and it works well against the gonococcus but poorly against other gram-negative organisms. Bacitracin solutions are unstable, and it is available commonly as an ointment. Erythromycin is a very well tolerated ointment that is effective against many gram-positive organisms and *Chlamydia*, although staphylococcal resistance develops easily. It is a bacteriostatic antibiotic that is available only in ointment form. Erythromycin ointment is a good agent to use in the treatment of chlamydial conjunctivitis when used five times daily for a period of 3 weeks.

Tetracycline is available as a 0.5 to 1.0% ointment or suspension and is effective against many gram-negative and gram-positive pathogens as well as *Chlamydia*. When used in the treatment of chlamydial infections, it should be given five times per day for 3 weeks. Although systemic tetracycline should not be given to children, the same restrictions do not apply to topical preparations.

Neomycin is a widely used broad-spectrum bactericidal antibiotic that has a very high incidence of allergic reactions. Chloramphenicol is another antibiotic whose usage has fallen off because of an association with bone marrow depression. However, the incidence of severe aplastic anemia occurring as a result of topical chloramphenicol use is controversial. It remains an excellent broad-spectrum bacteriostatic antibiotic that is effective against gram-positive, gram-negative, and chlamydial organisms. It is particularly useful against *Moraxella* and *Hemophilus influenzae*. The availability of so many other equieffective antibiotics that do not cause these adverse reactions has decreased the use of these drugs in the treatment of conjunctivitis.

Any of these antibiotics can be used empirically in the initial treatment of conjunctivitis. For gonococccal and chlamydial conjunctivitis, particularly in the neonate, specific topical therapy should be combined with systemic antibiotics. Systemic treatment for chlamydial conjunctivitis in children is erythromycin, 30 to 50 mg/kg/day given orally given every 6 to 8 hours. Adults can be given 1 g every 6 hours.

For gonococcal conjunctivitis, the choices for systemic treatment are (1) ceftriaxone, 250 mg IM once; (2) aqueous procaine penicillin G, 4.8 million units IM in two divided doses, given together with probenecid, 1 g orally; (3) ampicillin, 3.5 g orally with 1 g of probenecid; (4) spectinomycin, 4 g IM in two divided doses; or (5) 1.5 g of tetracycline orally, followed by 500 mg four times a day for 4 days. Recently ceftriaxone, given as a single 125-mg IM dose, has been shown to be effective in ophthalmia neonatorum against both *Chlamydia* and the gonococcus.

Naphcon A is a combination of an antihistamine and a decongestant that may provide symptomatic relief from the tearing, itching, and discomfort of conjunctivitis, especially if it is allergic in nature. It may be used in conjunction with antibiotics in those patients who do not have clear-cut bacterial conjunctivitis. A dose of 1 or 2 drops is applied in the affected eye every 3 to 6 hours as required to relieve symptoms. This medication should not be used in infants, children, hypertensive patients, patients receiving monoamine oxidase inhibitors, or patients predisposed to glaucoma or cardiac arrhythmias. Systemic analgesia with aspirin, acetaminophen, or diphenhydramine may increase patient comfort and is recommended.

SPECIFIC AGENTS

Acetazolamide (Diamox)

Pharmacology

Sulfonamide

Mechanism

Inhibits carbonic anhydrase present in kidneys, choroid plexus, and ciliary body

Kinetics (IV)

Onset   Minutes
Peak   15 Minutes
Duration   4–5 hours
Half-life   4–10 hours

Metabolism

Renal excretion of unaltered drug

Indications

Acute angle-closure glaucoma
Increased intracranial pressure
Metabolic alkalosis
Prevention of acute mountain sickness

Contraindications

Severe hypokalemia or hyponatremia
Adrenal insufficiency
Hyperchloremic acidosis
Liver failure

Dosage

Initial: 500 mg IV over 20 to 30 minutes
Subsequent: 250 to 500 mg every 4 to 6
   hours

Cautions

Dosage adjustments in renal failure:
GFR 10 to 50—increase dosing interval to
   12 hours.
GFR < 10—do not use.
Dosage adjustment in hepatic failure—do
   not use.
Use in:
   Pregnancy—no; Category C
   Lactation—avoid if possible.
   Childhood—yes

Toxicity

Side Effects

Common: fatigue, anorexia, headache,
   nervousness, nausea and vomiting, diarrhea, paresthesias, hypokalemia (usually minor), kidney stones, metabolic acidosis
Uncommon: convulsions, hepatic failure,
   paralysis, thrombocytopenia
Dangerous: thrombocytopenia, convulsions, acute allergic syndromes in patients allergic to other sulfa drugs

Treatment of Acute Toxicity

Stop drug.
For convulsions, intravenous diazepam

For allergy, epinephrine, diphenhydramine, methylprednisolone

Interactions

Increases toxicity of lithium, quinidine, salicylates, sympathomimetic amines

Anesthetics

Proparacaine Ophthalmic Solution

Pharmacology

Rapidly acting topical anesthetic

Kinetics

Onset: immediate
Duration: 15 to 30 minutes

Indication

Ocular anesthesia for short diagnostic or
   therapeutic procedures

Contraindications

Hypersensitivity
Prolonged use; do not give the patient for
   self-administration.

Dosage

1 or 2 drops in each eye
For deep anesthesia, 1 drop every 5 minutes for 5 to 7 doses

Cautions

Dosage adjustments in organ failure—
   none
Use in:
   Pregnancy—Category C
   Lactation—no data
   Childhood—yes

Do not use if solution is amber colored.

Toxicity

Adverse Reactions

Discomfort with instillation
Hypersensitivity reaction of cornea
Contact dermatitis

Interactions

None reported

Antibiotics: Antibacterial

Erythromycin Ophthalmic Ointment

Pharmacology

Macrolide
Ribosomal binding interferes with protein synthesis.
Bacteriostatic

Spectrum of Activity

Streptococcal species
Neisseria gonorrhoeae
Chlamydia

Not Effective Against

Many staphylococcal species
Many Hemophilus influenzae strains
Any gram-negative organisms

Indications

Chlamydial conjunctivitis (in conjunction with systemic erythromycin)
Neonatal prophylaxis against gonococcal and chlamydial conjunctivitis

Contraindications

History of hypersensitivity to erythromycin
Infection caused by nonsusceptible organisms

Dosage (5 mg Erythromycin/g Ointment)

0.5 inch in lower conjunctival sac of affected eye five times daily for 3 weeks

Cautions

Dosage adjustments in organ failure—none
Use in:
    Pregnancy—yes
    Lactation—yes
    Childhood—yes

Adverse Reactions

Minimal systemic absorption
Local hypersensitivity reactions

Gentamicin Ophthalmic Ointment and Solution

Pharmacology

Aminoglycoside
Ribosomal binding blocks protein synthesis.
Bactericidal

Spectrum of Activity

Most gram-negative organisms
Coagulase-negative and coagulase-positive staphylococci
Many streptococci
Neisseria gonorrhoeae

Not Effective Against

Chlamydia
Anaerobes
Some gram-negative organisms

Indications

Bacterial conjunctivitis, keratitis, and blepharitis
Prophylaxis of corneal abrasions

Contraindications

History of hypersensitivity to aminoglycosides
Infection with nonsusceptible organism, especially Chlamydia
Warning: Solution should not be injected into the eye or parenterally.

Dosage

Solution (3.0 mg gentamicin/ml): 1 or 2 drops every 4 hours
Ointment (3.0 mg gentamicin/g): 0.5 inch in conjunctival sac every 8 to 12 hours

Cautions

Dosage adjustment in organ failure—none
Use in:
    Pregnancy—yes
    Lactation—yes
    Childhood—yes

Adverse Reactions

Negligible systemic absorption
Local hypersensitivity reactions
Pain and irritation with instillation

Sulfacetamide Ophthalmic Ointment and Solution

Pharmacology

Sulfa class of antibiotics
Blocks folic acid synthesis by competition with para-aminobenzoic acid
Bacteriostatic

Spectrum of Activity

Many gram-positive and gram-negative bacteria
Chlamydia

Not Effective Against

Neisseria gonorrhoeae

Indications

Conjunctivitis and other superficial ocular infections
Prophylaxis of corneal abrasions

Contraindications

Hypersensitivity to sulfa compounds
Infection with nonsusceptible organism

Dosage

(30% solution contains 300 mg sulfacetamide/ml; 10% solution contains 100 mg sulfacetamide/ml; ointment contains 100 mg sulfacetamide/g)
Solution: 2 drops four times daily until 48 hours after clinical resolution
Ointment: 0.5 inch in lower conjunctival sac four times daily until 48 hours after clinical resolution

Cautions

Dosage adjustments in organ failure—none
Use in:
    Pregnancy—yes
    Lactation—yes
    Childhood—yes

Adverse Reactions

Little systemic absorption
Local hypersensitivity reactions
Pain and irritation when instilled
There is one case report of Stevens-Johnson syndrome following topical ophthalmic use of a sulfonamide.

Tetracycline Ophthalmic Suspension and Ointment

Pharmacology

Inhibits microbial protein synthesis
Bacteriostatic

Spectrum of Activity

Staphylococcal species
Streptococcal species
Neisseria gonorrhoeae
Chlamydia
Escherichia coli

Not Effective Against

Most gram-negative organisms, including Hemophilus influenzae and Pseudomonas

Indications

Superficial ocular infection caused by a susceptible organism
Prophylaxis of neonatal gonococcal and chlamydial conjunctivitis

Contraindication

Hypersensitivity

Dosage

Suspension (10 mg tetracycline/ml): 2 drops four times daily until 48 hours after resolution of symptoms
Ointment (10 mg tetracycline/g): 0.5 inch to affected area every 2 hours while awake until symptoms absent for 48 hours

Cautions

Dosage adjustments in organ failure—none
Use in:
    Pregnancy—no
    Lactation—no
    Childhood—no (except for single dose newborn prophylaxis)

Adverse Reactions

Hypersensitivity
Local dermatitis

Tobramycin Ophthalmic Ointment and Solution

No clinically important differences from gentamicin
Some gram-negative organisms may be sensitive to tobramycin and resistant to gentamicin and vice versa.

Antibiotics: Antiviral

Idoxuridine Ophthalmic Solution and Ointment

Pharmacology

Replaces thymidine in viral DNA, causing faulty replication

Spectrum of Activity

Herpes simplex

Indication

Herpes simplex keratitis

Contraindication

Hypersensitivity

Dosage

Solution (1 mg idoxuridine/ml): 1 drop in affected eye every hour during day and every 2 hours at night, or 1 drop a minute for 5 minutes every 4 hours around the clock

Ointment (5 mg idoxuridine/g): 0.5 inch in lower conjunctival sac of affected eye five times daily

Continue treatment with either formulation for 3 to 5 days after healing appears to be complete. Consider resistance if no improvement after 1 week of therapy.

Cautions

Dosage adjustments in organ failure—none

Use in:

Pregnancy—avoid if possible; Category C

Lactation—avoid

Childhood—safety not established. Use if clinically indicated.

Toxicity

Adverse Reactions

Local hypersensitivity
Pain, irritation, pruritus
Corneal clouding
Edema of lids or eye
Photophobia

Interactions

Do not coadminister boric acid as this is a very irritating combination.

Trifluridine Ophthalmic Solution

Pharmacology

Trifluorothymidine
Interferes with DNA synthesis

Spectrum of Activity

Herpes simplex 1 and 2
Some adenoviruses

Indication

Herpes simplex keratitis

Contraindication

Hypersensitivity

Dosage

Solution contains 10 mg trifluridine/ml.
1 drop in affected eye every 2 hours while awake (maximum daily dose is 9 drops) until cornea healed

Then continue 1 drop every 4 hours while awake for 7 more days.

Cautions

Do not use for more than 21 days.

Consider other therapy if there is no healing in 7 days or if complete reepithelialization is not present by day 14.

Dosage adjustments in organ failure—none

Use in:

Pregnancy—yes, if clinically necessary
Lactation—yes
Childhood—yes

Toxicity

Adverse Reactions

Burning with instillation
Edema of lids
Hypersensitivity
Increased intraocular pressure

Interactions

None reported with a variety of topical optic antibiotics, steroids, mydriatics, and miotics

Vidarabine Ophthalmic Ointment

Pharmacology

9-β-D-Arabinofuranosyladenine
Interferes with DNA synthesis

Spectrum of Activity

Herpes simplex 1 and 2
Vaccinia
Varicella-zoster

Indication

Herpes simplex keratitis

Contraindication

Hypersensitivity

Dosage

Ointment contains 30 mg vidarabine/g.

0.5 inch in lower conjunctival sac of affected eye five times daily at 3-hour intervals

After reepithelialization is complete, continue 0.5 inch twice daily for another week.

Cautions

Dosage adjustments in organ failure—
none
Use in:
Pregnancy—yes
Lactation—yes
Childhood—yes

Toxicity

Adverse Reactions

Burning, irritation, and pain with instillation
Lacrimation
Foreign body sensation
Photophobia
Hypersensitivity

Interactions

None reported

Antihistamines

Naphcon A Ophthalmic Solution

Pharmacology

Combination of naphazoline (a decongestant) and pheniramine (an antihistamine)

Kinetics

Onset: 30 to 60 minutes
Duration: 3 to 6 hours

Indication

Symptomatic relief in acute conjunctivitis

Contraindications

Hypertension
Cardiac arrhythmias
Concomitant MAO inhibitor use
Narrow-angle glaucoma
Infants and children

Dosage

1 or 2 drops every 3 to 6 hours

Cautions

Dosage adjustments in organ failure—
none
Use in:
Pregnancy—Category C
Lactation—no
Childhood—no

Toxicity

Adverse Reactions

(Systemic absorption occurs.)
Local: pupillary dilation, increased intraocular pressure
Systemic: hypertension, cardiac arrhythmias, coma, and hypothermia in infants

Interactions

Hypertensive crisis with MAO inhibitors

Beta-Blockers

Betaxolol Ophthalmic Solution

Pharmacology

Cardioselective beta-blocker
No membrane-stabilizing or intrinsic sympathomimetic action
Reduces intraocular pressure by reducing aqueous humor production

Kinetics

Onset: 30 minutes
Peak: 2 hours
Duration: 12 hours

Indications

Acute angle-closure glaucoma
Chronic open-angle glaucoma

Betaxolol is the ocular beta-blocker of
choice in asthmatic patients because of
its cardioselectivity.

Contraindications

Heart block greater than first degree
Cardiac failure
Hypersensitivity

Dosage (5.6 mg Betaxolol/ml)

Acute glaucoma: 1 drop every 15 minutes
for 1 hour
Chronic administration: 1 drop twice daily

Cautions

Dosage adjustments in organ failure—
none
Use in:
Pregnancy—Category C
Lactation—no data
Childhood—no data

Toxicity

Adverse Reaction

(Minimal systemic absorption)
Common: local irritation
Rare: insomnia, depression
Theoretical: cardiac failure, heart block, masked signs of hypoglycemia or hyperthyroidism, bronchospasm

Interactions

Potential additive effect with systemic beta-blockers
Mydriasis with epinephrine

Timolol Ophthalmic Solution

Pharmacology

Nonselective beta-blocker affecting both beta$_1$ (cardiac) and beta$_2$ (pulmonary) receptors
No membrane-stabilizing or intrinsic sympathomimetic activity
Reduces intraocular pressure by reducing aqueous humor production

Kinetics

Onset: 30 minutes
Peak: 2 hours
Duration: up to 24 hours

Indications

Acute angle-closure glaucoma
Chronic glaucoma

Contraindictions

Bronchospastic history
Chronic obstructive pulmonary disease (COPD)
Cardiac failure
Heart block greater than first degree
Hypersensitivity

Dosage

The 0.25% solution contains 2.5 mg timolol/ml, and the 0.5% solution contains 5 mg timolol/ml.

Acute glaucoma: 1 drop of 0.5% solution every 15 minutes for 1 hour
Chronic glaucoma: 1 drop twice daily

Cautions

Dosage adjustments in organ failure—none. Do not use in asthma or chronic obstructive pulmonary disease.

Use in:
  Pregnancy—Category C
  Lactation—no data
  Childhood—no data

Toxicity

Adverse Reactions

(Systemic absorption occurs.)
Bradyarrhythmias
Cardiac failure
Cardiac arrest
Bronchospasm
Headache
Nausea
Diarrhea
Nasal congestion
Local irritation
Hives
Depression
Paresthesias

Interactions

Additive adverse cardiovascular effects with systemic beta-blockers, calcium blockers, digoxin, and reserpine
Mydriasis with epinephrine

Fluorescein Ophthalmic Strips

Fluorescein is a fluorescent dye that is used for detecting corneal injury. It stains disrupted areas of the cornea bright yellow when viewed in ultraviolet light. The only precaution to take when using fluorescein is to remove soft contact lenses first because the fluorescein will discolor them.

Miotics

Pilocarpine Ophthalmic Solution

Pharmacology

Cholinergic parasympathetic stimulator
Causes pupillary constriction by direct stimulation of smooth muscle
Lowers intraocular pressure by opening trabecular spaces with direct traction

Kinetics

Onset: 10 to 20 minutes
Maximum effect: 30 to 60 minutes
Duration: 6 to 8 hours

Indication

Acute angle-closure glaucoma

Contraindications

Iritis
Hypersensitivity
Do not use 4% or 6% solution in acute
 glaucoma.

Cautions

Use in:
 Pregnancy—Category C
 Lactation—no data
 Childhood—no data

Dosage

Acute glaucoma: 1 drop of 1% solution in
 both eyes every 10 minutes for 1 hour
Chronic glaucoma: 1 drop three times a
 day

Toxicity

Adverse Reactions

Local irritation: loss of dark adaptation,
 lacrimation, myopia, retinal detachment
 (especially in myopes)
Systemic reactions very rare: hypertension, tachycardia, bronchospasm, nausea
 and vomiting, salivation, diarrhea

Interactions

None reported

Mydriatics

Topical anticholinergic agents produce
mydriasis and cycloplegia. They are clinically useful for the examination of the fundus
and the therapy of iritis and corneal abrasion. The available agents differ widely in
their kinetics, as is summarized in Table 20–
2. Patients with heavily pigmented irides
usually require larger doses of these agents.

Atropine Ophthalmic Ointment and Solution

Pharmacology

Alkaloid derived from poisonous night-
 shade plant
Blocks action of acetylcholine on ciliary
 muscle and iris sphincter

Kinetics

Onset: 15 to 90 minutes
Duration: 7 to 14 days

Indication

Iritis/uveitis; however, agents with a
 shorter duration of action are recommended for emergency use.

Contraindications

Glaucoma
Children who have experienced severe
 systemic reaction from ocular atropine

Dosage

Solution (0.125%, 0.5%, 1.0%): 1 drop
 three times daily
Ointment (0.5% and 1%): 0.5 inch in
 lower conjunctival sac twice daily

Cautions

Dosage adjustments in organ failure—
 none
Use in:
 Pregnancy—Category C
 Lactation—no data; avoid.
 Childhood—yes, but use lower con-
  centration.

Toxicity

Adverse Reactions

(Systemic absorption may occur, particularly in children.)

TABLE 20–2. Mydriatic and Cycloplegic Properties of Topical
Anticholinergic Agents

Drug	Concentration	Onset	Duration
Tropicamide	1%	20–30 min	2–6 hours
Cyclopentolate	1%	30–60 min	6–24 hours
Homatropine	2%	45–60 min	24–72 hours
Scopolamine	¼%	30 min	48–72 hours
Atropine	1%	60–90 min	7–14 days

Local: acute glaucoma, allergic conjunctivitis, contact dermatitis of periocular tissues, loss of accommodation

Systemic (more likely in children and the elderly; use lower concentration in these age groups): tachycardia, dry mouth, fever, delirium, somnolence, urinary retention, constipation

Interactions

None reported

Cyclopentolate Ophthalmic Solution

Pharmacology

Direct-acting anticholinergic that blocks the responsiveness of the iris sphincter and ciliary body to acetylcholine, resulting in pupillary dilation and paralysis of accommodation

Kinetics

Onset: 30 minutes
Duration: 6 to 24 hours

Indications

Iritis/uveitis
Corneal abrasion with ciliary spasm

Contraindications

Glaucoma
Prior systemic toxicity with this agent
Hypersensitivity

Dosage (0.5%, 1.0%, and 2% solutions available)

Adults: 1% solution, 2 drops two or three times daily as needed
Children: 0.5% solution, 2 drops two or three times daily
Infants: 0.5% solution, 1 drop two or three times daily with pressure applied over nasolacrimal sac for several minutes after each instillation to minimize absorption

Cautions

Dosage adjustments in organ failure—none
Use in:
Pregnancy—Category C
Lactation—no data; avoid if possible.
Childhood: yes; use lower concentration.

Toxicity

Adverse Reactions

Of all the mydriatics, cyclopentolate has the greatest potential for systemic absorption.

Local: acute glaucoma, loss of accommodation, burning and irritation, conjunctivitis

Systemic (especially in children): central nervous system dysfunction—ataxia, disturbed behavior, convulsions, coma, tachycardia, fever, constipation, urinary retention, dry mouth

Interactions

None reported

Homatropine Ophthalmic Solution

Pharmacology

Direct-acting anticholinergic that blocks the responsiveness of the iris sphincter and ciliary body to acetylcholine, resulting in pupillary dilation and paralysis of accommodation

Kinetics

Onset: 45 to 60 minutes
Duration: 24 to 72 hours

Indications

Iritis/uveitis
Corneal abrasion with ciliary spasm

Contraindications

Glaucoma
Hypersensitivity

Dosage

Solution of 2.0% for children or 5.0% for adults

1 or 2 drops every 3 to 4 hours
Compress lacrimal sac for several minutes after instillation in an infant or child to decrease systemic absorption.

Cautions

Dosage adjustments—larger doses may be required if irides are heavily pigmented.
Use in:
Pregnancy—no; Category C
Childhood—yes
Lactation—no data

Adverse Reactions

Local: acute glaucoma, burning and irritation, conjunctivitis, periorbital dermatitis, loss of accommodation

Systemic (rare): tachycardia, dry mouth, delirium, urinary retention, constipation, fever

Scopolamine Ophthalmic Solution

Pharmacology

Alkaloid derived from the shrub *Hyoscyamus niger*

Direct-acting anticholinergic that blocks the responsiveness of the iris sphincter and ciliary body to acetylcholine, resulting in pupillary dilation and paralysis of accommodation.

Kinetics

Onset: 30 minutes
Duration: 48 to 72 hours

Indications

Iritis/uveitis
Corneal abrasion with ciliary spasm

Contraindications

Glaucoma
Hypersensitivity

Dosage (0.25% Solution)

1 or 2 drops four times daily
Compress lacrimal sac for several minutes after administration to an infant or child to prevent systemic absorption.

Cautions

Dosage adjustments in organ failure—none
Use in:
    Pregnancy—no; Category C
    Lactation—no data
    Childhood—yes

Adverse Reactions

Local: glaucoma, loss of accommodation, burning and irritation, conjunctivitis, periorbital dermatitis

Systemic (rare, more likely in children): tachycardia, dry mouth, delirium, urinary retention, constipation, fever

Tropicamide Ophthalmic Solution

Pharmacology

Direct-acting anticholinergic that blocks the responsiveness of the iris sphincter and ciliary body to acetylcholine, resulting in pupillary dilation and paralysis of accommodation

Mydriatic with quickest onset and shortest duration of action

Kinetics

Onset: 20 to 30 minutes
Duration: 2 to 6 hours

Indication

Funduscopic examination

Contraindications

Glaucoma
Hypersensitivity

Dosage (0.5% and 1.0% Solutions)

For funduscopy, 1 or 2 drops of 0.5% solution 15 minutes before the examination

This produces pupillary dilatation with only minimal cycloplegia, thus preserving accommodation.

Cautions

Dosage adjustments in organ failure—none
Use in:
    Pregnancy—yes, if necessary
    Lactation—yes, if necessary
    Childhood—yes

Toxicity

Adverse Reactions

Local: glaucoma, local irritation
Local hypersensitivity: loss of accommodation with 1% solution
Systemic: unlikely, but anticholinergic syndrome theoretical possibility

Interactions

None reported

Osmotic Agents

Glycerol

Pharmacology

Simplest of the trihydric sugar alcohols
Chemical formula $C_3H_8O_3$

Kinetics

Onset of action: oral, 10 to 12 hours; intravenous, related to attainment of serum levels of 10 to 30 mOsm/liter

Metabolism

Converted to glucose; provides 4.32 kcal/g

Indications and Uses

Reduction of increased intracranial pressure

Reduction of increased intraocular pressure

Topical agent

Evacuant (as a 50 to 75% solution)

As a vehicle for other medications

Dosage and Administration

Intravenous: 0.2 to 1.0 g/kg/hour (or the dose that attains plasma concentrations of 10 to 30 mOsm/liter); mixed in isotonic saline so final concentration is 40% or less

Oral: initial dose of 1 g/kg, followed by 0.5 to 1.0 g/kg every 3 to 4 hours as an oral evacuant, used as a 50 to 75% solution

Cautions

Dosage adjustment in organ failure—do not use intravenously in renal or cardiac failure.

Use in:

    Pregnancy—yes; Category C

    Lactation—yes

    Childhood—yes

Adverse Reactions

Glycerol is a simple sugar and has little toxicity of its own. The main toxicity is secondary to its osmotic effect:

Fluid and electrolyte imbalances

Dehydration

Mild hemolysis (with intravenous solution concentrations greater than 40% administered at a rate of infusion exceeding 4 to 5 ml/min)

Gastric irritation (with oral preparation of 50 to 75%)

Isosorbide Solution (Ismotic)

Pharmacology

Dihydric alcohol

Chemical formula $C_6H_{10}O_4$

Rapidly absorbed osmotic agent that reduces intraocular pressure by causing movement of water from ocular to vascular compartment and then out via the kidneys

Kinetics (Oral Administration Only)

Onset: 30 minutes

Maximum: 60 to 90 minutes

Duration: 5 to 6 hours

Metabolism

None; eliminated by renal excretion

Indication

Acute angle-closure glaucoma

Contraindications

Dehydration

Renal failure

Cardiac failure

Dosage (450 mg/ml of Solution)

Initial: 1.5 g/kg body weight

Repeat: 1.5 g/kg every 6 to 12 hours based on intraocular pressure

Cautions

Dosage adjustments in organ failure—do not use in cardiac or renal failure.

Use in:

    Pregnancy—yes; Category B

    Lactation—no data; probably safe

    Childhood—yes

Adverse Reactions

Nausea and vomiting

Dehydration

Pulmonary edema

Headache

Confusion

Hypernatremia

Bladder distention

Mannitol

Pharmacology

Six-carbon sugar alcohol

Chemical formula $C_6H_{14}O_6$

Occurs naturally in fruits and vegetables

Kinetics

Supersaturated at room temperature

Only for intravenous use

Must be warmed before given intravenously

Only minimal metabolism
Onset: approximately 1 minute
Peak: 5 to 15 minutes
Duration: 2 to 4 hours

Metabolism

Freely filtered at the glomerulus
Less than 10% reabsorption by tubules
Not secreted by tubules
80% of intravenous dose appears in the urine within 3 hours

Indications

Promotion of diuresis
Prevention or treatment of oliguric phase of acute renal failure
Reduction of increased intracranial pressure
Reduction of intraocular pressure
Promotion of urinary excretion of toxic substances
Irrigating solution during transurethral surgical procedures (as a 2.5% solution)

Contraindications

Fluid overload (due to rebound phenomenon)
Evidence of disruption of the blood–brain barrier (may leak into tissue and cause fluid influx into the intracranial cavity)
Severe dehydration states (because it may cause diuresis and further dehydration)
Not contraindicated in diabetics because its metabolism is minimal

Dosage and Administration

Prepared only as an intravenous medication

Prevention of Acute Renal Failure

Test dose: 0.2 g/kg
Initial dose: 50 to 100 g (20 g if secondary to acute hemolysis)

Reduction of Intracranial Pressure or Intraocular Pressure

Initial dose: 1 to 2 g/kg over 5 to 10 minutes
Repeat dose: 0.5 to 1 g every 4 to 6 hours

Cautions

Dosage adjustments in organ failure—do not use in cardiac or renal failure.
Use in:
  Pregnancy—yes; no data on fetal effects; Category C
  Lactation—yes, if necessary for the health of the mother
  Childhood—yes

Toxicity

Adverse Reactions and Toxicity

Mannitol is a simple sugar with minimal metabolism that in and of itself is basically not toxic. Side effects due to mannitol are infrequent and may include the following:

Metabolic: fluid and electrolyte imbalance, dehydration, acidosis (packaging solution has a pH of 4.5 to 7.0)
Cardiovascular: pulmonary edema, systemic edema, hypotension (based on dehydration), angina-like chest pain
Central nervous system: headaches, dizziness, convulsions
Genitourinary: osmotic nephrosis, urinary retention (should always have a urinary catheter in place)
Gastrointestinal: dry mouth, nausea/vomiting, diarrhea
Dermatologic: skin necrosis, thrombophlebitis
Miscellaneous: urticaria, blurred vision, rhinitis, arm pain, fever and chills

Treatment of Acute Toxicity

Stop mannitol.
For pulmonary edema, oxygen, nitroglycerin, diuretic
For hypotension, Trendelenburg position, dopamine, volume infusion

Steroids

Dexamethasone Ophthalmic Solution

Pharmacology

Synthetic glucocorticoid
Suppresses the inflammatory response by unknown mechanisms

Indication

Acute iritis/uveitis

Contraindications

Herpetic and other viral infections of the eye
Fungal or mycobacterial ocular infection
Prior hypersensitivity to this drug (if occurs probably due to sulfites in its formulation)

Dosage (0.1% Solution)

1 drop every 6 hours

Cautions

Dosage adjustments in organ failure—
none
Use in:
Pregnancy—no; Category C
Lactation—avoid if possible.
Childhood—yes

Warning: **Do not prescribe steroids if
there is any question of herpes simplex
keratitis.**

Toxicity

Interactions

None reported

Adverse Reactions

Systemic absorption occurs.
Local: glaucoma, secondary infection (especially fungal), cataract, corneal or
scleral perforation
Systemic: anaphylaxis due to sulfite sensitivity, bronchospasm

**Fluorometholone Ophthalmic
Suspension**

Pharmacology

Synthetic glucocorticoid
Suppresses the inflammatory response by
an unknown mechanism
Least ocular penetration of available steroids and thus least likely to increase intraocular pressure

Indication

Acute iritis/uveitis

Contraindications

Herpetic and other viral infections of the
eye
Fungal or mycobacterial ocular infection
Prior hypersensitivity to this agent

Dosage (0.1% Suspension)

1 drop every 6 hours

Cautions

Dosage adjustments in organ failure—
none

Use in:
Pregnancy—no; Category C
Lactation—no data
Children—yes

Toxicity

Interactions

None reported

Adverse Reactions

Local: acute glaucoma, secondary infection (especially fungal), perforation of
globe, cataract
Systemic: highly unlikely; minimal absorption

**Prednisolone Ophthalmic
Suspension**

Pharmacology

Synthetic glucocorticoid
Suppresses the inflammatory response by
unknown mechanisms

Indications

Acute iritis/uveitis

Contraindications

Herpetic and other viral infections of the
eye
Fungal or mycobacterial ocular infection
Prior hypersensitivity to this drug (if occurs probably due to sulfites in its formulation)

Dosage (1.0% Suspension)

1 drop every 6 hours

Cautions

Dosage adjustments in organ failure—
none
Use in:
Pregnancy—yes; Category B
Lactation—yes
Childhood—yes

Toxicity

Interactions

None reported

Adverse Reactions

Systemic absorption occurs.
Local: glaucoma, secondary infection (especially fungal), cataract, corneal or
scleral perforation

Systemic: anaphylaxis due to sulfite sensitivity, bronchospasm

REFERENCES

AMA Drug Evaluations, ed. 6. Chicago, American Medical Association, 1986.

Ellis P: Ocular Therapeutics and Pharmacology, ed. 7. St Louis, CV Mosby, 1985.

Fraunfelder FT, Roy FH: Current Ocular Therapy 3. Philadelphia, WB Saunders, 1990.

Havener W: Ocular Pharmacology. St Louis, CV Mosby, 1990.

Lamberts DW, Potter DE: Clinical Ophthalmic Pharmacology. Boston, Little, Brown & Co, 1987.

CHAPTER 21

Endocrine and Miscellaneous Agents

PETER VAN LIGTEN, M.D.
STEVEN C. CARLETON, M.D., Ph.D.
FREDERICK B. EPSTEIN, M.D.

INTRODUCTION

The endocrine system affects virtually every organ in the body and enables "fine-tuned" homeostasis at all times. Although some endocrine disorders are quite common (e.g., diabetes mellitus), others are fortunately rare. Although acute disorders like thyroid storm or myxedema coma may be encountered infrequently, rapid and accurate treatment is necessary to avoid morbidity and mortality. A high index of suspicion is necessary to accurately diagnose some of these conditions because many of the symptoms may be nonspecific and referable to multiple organ systems.

CONDITIONS

Adrenal Crisis

Adrenal steroids are essential in adaptive responses to acute physiologic stress and have important regulatory effects on intermediary metabolism, electrolyte balance, and extracellular volume status. Destruction or metabolic failure of the adrenal cortex results in primary insufficiency, or Addison's disease. Both glucocorticoid secretion and mineralocorticoid secretion are affected. Secondary adrenal insufficiency is caused by loss of the trophic influence of pituitary adrenocorticotrophic hormone (ACTH); mineralocorticoid secretion is generally preserved. Conditions associated with adrenocortical insufficiency most commonly cause gradual loss of glandular function (Table 21–1), but both primary and secondary adrenal failure can result from acute, catastrophic events. Further, chronic or subclinical hypoadrenalism can present as a medical emergency during the stress of an intercurrent illness. These emergent presentations, termed *adrenal crises*, require rapid recognition and treatment if mortality is to be minimized.

Cortisol stimulates hepatic gluconeogenesis and glycogen synthesis and the mobilization of amino acids and free fatty acids from extrahepatic sources. Glucose utilization is inhibited peripherally, while utilization in liver, cardiac muscle, brain, and red blood cells is preserved. Metabolism in skeletal muscle is shifted to fat as a source of fuel. These catabolic actions ensure a supply of substrate for essential organs in response to trauma, infection, fasting, psychic stress, and other illnesses, comprising a so-called stress reaction. Glucocorticoids also exert permis-

TABLE 21–1. Etiologic Factors of Adrenocortical Insufficiency

I. Primary adrenal failure
  A. Idiopathic
    1. Autoimmune
    2. True idiopathic
  B. Infectious
    1. Granulomatous
      a. Tuberculosis
    2. Protozoal and fungal
      a. Histoplasmosis
      b. Blastomycosis
      c. Coccidiodomycosis
      d. Candidiasis
      e. Cryptococcosis
    3. Viral
      a. Cytomegalovirus
      b. Herpes simplex
  C. Infiltration
    1. Sarcoidosis
    2. Neoplastic (metastatic)
    3. Lymphoma/leukemia
    4. Hemochromatosis
    5. Adrenoleukodystrophy
    6. Amyloidosis
    7. Iron deposition
  D. Postadrenalectomy
  E. Hemorrhage
  F. Congenital adrenal hyperplasia
  G. Congenital unresponsiveness to ACTH
II. Secondary adrenal failure
  A. Pituitary insufficiency
    1. Infarction (Sheehan's syndrome)
    2. Hemorrhage
    3. Pituitary or suprasellar tumor
    4. Isolated ACTH deficiency
    5. Infiltration disease
      a. Sarcoidosis
      b. Histiocytosis X
      c. Hemochromatosis
  B. Hypothalamic insufficiency
  C. Head trauma
III. Functional
  A. Glucocorticoid administration

(Reproduced by permission from Wogan, John M.: Endocrine disorders. In Rosen, Peter, et al., editors: Emergency medicine: concepts and clinical practice, ed. 2. St. Louis, 1988, The C.V. Mosby Co.)

sive effects on the response of cardiac tissue and vascular smooth muscle to catecholamines. In the absence of adequate glucocorticoid, reductions occur in serum glucose, glycogen reserves, peripheral vascular resistance, and myocardial contractility that are inappropriate to the metabolic and hemodynamic needs of the patient.

Secretion of glucocorticoids is under control of the hypothalamopituitary axis. Plasma ACTH levels increase within minutes of the application of physiologic stress, with subsequent enhancement of synthesis and release of cortisol. Under normal circumstances, cortisol secretion averages 20 mg/day, with levels ranging from 5 to 25 μg/dl. In acute stress, production may increase by a factor of 10 to 20. Elevation of plasma cortisol exerts negative feedback on the pituitary secretion of ACTH. This feedback is the basis for the functional secondary adrenal insufficiency in patients receiving chronic exogenous steroids. Functional adrenal insufficiency is currently the most common form of adrenal failure.

Aldosterone promotes sodium reabsorption in the distal convoluted tubule, with resultant expansion of extracellular fluid volume, and stimulates tubular excretion of potassium and hydrogen ions. Secretion is stimulated by hyperkalemia and by decreased renal perfusion pressure via the renin–angiotensin system. Deficient secretion of aldosterone is responsible for the characteristic electrolyte pattern of primary adrenal insufficiency, i.e., hyponatremia, hyperkalemia, and acidemia. Intravascular volume depletion secondary to mineralocorticoid deficiency is the principal contributor to circulatory collapse in addisonian crisis.

Primary adrenal insufficiency is rare, with an incidence of 40 to 50 per million population. Nonetheless, adrenal crisis is more common in primary than in secondary hypoadrenalism. The incidence of secondary adrenal insufficiency is unclear, but the potential for its development is high given the broad use of exogenous steroids. The majority of patients presenting with adrenal crisis have a history of chronic insufficiency. When there is a clear history of chronic insufficiency or exogenous steroid use, the diagnosis of adrenal crisis can be made on historical and clinical grounds. In the absence of such a history, diagnosis is difficult. Because of the urgency of the illness, specific diagnostic tests generally must be postponed in favor of timely empiric therapy.

Diagnosis
The diagnosis of adrenal crisis should be suspected in any patient presenting with unexplained hypotension. Signs and symptoms preceding collapse may include malaise, anorexia, weight loss, generalized weakness, fever, nausea, vomiting, lightheadedness, abdominal pain, salt craving, apathy, and depression. Physical examination demonstrates low-grade temperature and dehydration. Hyperdynamic shock may be present. In patients with chronic primary in-

sufficiency, abnormal mucocutaneous hyperpigmentation can occur in flexion creases, scars, areas of chronic wear, and the mucosa of the gingiva, lips, or buccal surfaces. Mental status examination may demonstrate lethargy, coma, or psychosis. Signs of hypoglycemia may be prominent and include diaphoresis, tachycardia, and seizures.

Laboratory findings include hyponatremia, hyperkalemia, acidemia, and azotemia. The combination of hyponatremia and hyperkalemia strongly supports the diagnosis of Addison's disease. Dehydration and electrolyte disturbances are less dramatic in crises resulting from secondary or functional insufficiency owing to preservation of aldosterone secretion. In addisonian crisis, volume depletion is in the range of 6 to 15% of total body water. Hypercalcemia may be present, and the anion gap will be elevated when peripheral perfusion is compromised by volume depletion. Complete blood count may reveal hemoconcentration and leukocytosis with a predominance of mononuclear cells and an elevated eosinophil count. Electrocardiographic findings can include low voltage, prolonged QT interval, and changes consistent with the degree of hyperkalemia present. Radiographic studies may demonstrate a small cardiac silhouette and occasionally reveal calcification of the pinnae and adrenals. Pituitary adenoma is suggested by enlargement of the sella turcica on skull films.

Serum should be sent for determination of cortisol and ACTH levels prior to treatment. A result for serum cortisol of >25 μg/dl excludes adrenal insufficiency as a cause of hypotension or shock. A value less than 15 μg/dl is inappropriately low in a severely ill patient and strongly suggests adrenal insufficiency, whereas intermediate levels do not contribute to the diagnosis. Markedly elevated pretreatment levels of ACTH suggest the diagnosis of Addison's disease.

When the clinical status of the patient permits a delay in treatment, a short ACTH stimulation test can be performed. Cosyntropin, 250 μg, is administered intravenously after a blood sample has been taken to determine baseline cortisol level. Cortisol level determinations are repeated 30 and 60 minutes after injection. Elevation of serum cortisol by 5 to 8 μg/dl at 30 minutes with a 1-hour peak of 15 to 18 μg/dl is considered a normal test and rules out primary adrenal insufficiency.

Indications for Treatment

Suspicion of adrenal insufficiency in any patient with unexplained hypotension or shock constitutes sufficient indication for initiation of therapy with intravenous steroids. If subsequent studies rule out adrenal insufficiency, steroids can be rapidly tapered with little risk to the patient. (See box.)

DRUG TREATMENT: ADRENAL CRISIS

First-Line Therapy

Hydrocortisone Sodium Phosphate (50 mg/ml)

Initial Dose	100–200 mg by IV push over 30 seconds
Repeat Dose	100 mg by continuous IV infusion every 6–8 hours for 24–48 hours
End-Points	Euglycemia, normalization of serum sodium and potassium, and restoration of hemodynamic stability

OR

Hydrocortisone Sodium Hemisuccinate (100-mg, 250-mg, 500-mg, 1-g vials as sterile powder)

Initial Dose	100–200 mg by IV push over 30 seconds
Repeat Dose	100 mg by continuous IV infusion every 6–8 hours for 24–48 hours. Dilution as above.
End-Points	Euglycemia, normalization of serum sodium and potassium, and restoration of hemodynamic stability

Chart continued on following page

DRUG TREATMENT: ADRENAL CRISIS *Continued*

Second-Line Therapy

Dexamethasone Sodium Phosphate (4 mg/ml)

Dose	4 mg by IV push
Repeat Dose	Hydrocortisone should be started after results of ACTH stimulation test are obtained.
End-Point	Provision of glucocorticoid activity in the patient with suspected acute adrenal insufficiency pending the results of a confirmatory ACTH stimulation test. Dexamethasone does not interfere with determinations of serum cortisol. Because of minimal mineralocorticoid activity, dexamethasone should not be used for replacement therapy in confirmed adrenal crisis.

Discussion

The patient with adrenal crisis should have body weight, urine output, and hemodynamic parameters monitored closely in an intensive care unit (ICU) setting. Determination of renal function, serum electrolytes, and serum glucose should be made every 4 to 6 hours during initial therapy. Potassium replacement should be instituted as needed. The duration of parenteral hydrocortisone treatment will depend on the presence or absence of a precipitating illness, but stress doses can be tapered after 24 to 48 hours in the stable patient. Dosages can be reduced by 20 to 30% daily until maintenance levels (20 to 40 mg/day) are reached. In primary adrenocortical insufficiency, reduction of hydrocortisone dosage below 100 mg/day requires addition of a second agent to maintain mineralocorticoid activity. The agent of choice is fluorocortisone, 0.1 mg/day. Chronic glucocorticoid replacement is generally accomplished with oral hydrocortisone, 20 mg every morning and 10 mg every evening. Fluid resuscitation should be with 5% dextrose in normal saline. From 500 to 1000 ml/hour should be given for the first 2 to 4 hours, with subsequent therapy to be guided by clinical status.

With prolonged therapy, exogenous glucocorticoids can lead to sodium retention and volume overload, peptic ulcer disease, steroid myopathy, osteopenia, cushingoid features, immunosuppression, and a variety of endocrinopathies. These effects can be limited by careful dosing. Therapy with stress doses has few untoward effects when the duration of high-dose treatment is brief.

Acute Gouty Arthritis

Diagnosis

Gout is a disease that primarily afflicts males in the fourth to seventh decades of life. Postmenopausal women are also affected, albeit much less frequently. The proved diagnosis of gout in a younger man or premenopausal woman is sufficiently uncommon to warrant search for one of the rare heredofamilial deficiencies in the enzymatic metabolism of xanthine, the syndromic expression of which includes gout.

The diagnosis of gout more commonly follows a simple clinical evaluation. The natural history of gout is sufficiently characteristic that a new diagnosis may occasionally be made in retrospective review of the history provided by the patient. The first expression of gout is most commonly a sudden attack of acute arthritis in a middle-aged patient otherwise in good health. For reasons elaborated below, the attack often begins at night, and the lower extremity is most commonly involved. This initial attack involves a single joint over 90% of the time; whereas classic podagra involving the metatarsophalangeal joint of the hallux is most specific for the diagnosis, the knee joint may be the site of the initial attack almost as frequently. Within 1 to 2 hours of the onset of symptoms, the involved joint demonstrates the classic rubor and calor of acute inflammation, and occasionally systemic signs such as mild fever and leukocytosis with elevated sedimentation rate may accompany the attack. Left untreated, the attack subsides within two to several days, rarely longer, following which the patient typically enters a quiescent or asymptomatic phase lasting from several months to years. Almost inevitably, the patient begins to experience attacks with escalating frequency and severity if untreated, and the resolution of symptoms following successive attacks becomes incomplete, evolving to chronic, polyarticular disease. Even in the later stage of untreated disease, however, gout has a tendency to remain asymmetric with predilection for lower extremity involvement, which aids in its distinction from rheumatoid arthritis and inflammatory osteoarthritis. Joint radiography in late untreated disease will also typically demonstrate the classic "punched-out" lytic cyst in subchondral bone accompanied by overhanging margins, with a relative tendency to preserve articular cartilage and thus the radiographic joint space. By contrast, the radiographic evaluation of the acute monarthritis characteristic of early presentation most often reveals a normal joint or nonspecific signs of soft tissue swelling or effusion. Although the therapeutic response to a trial of colchicine is often hailed as further diagnostic evidence of gout, other arthropathies, and pseudogout in particular (with which gout is most likely to be confused clinically), may respond to colchicine, and the diagnostic specificity once attributed to this response is now believed unwarranted. Perhaps the greatest clinical benefit of demonstrated response to colchicine is the confidence and propriety with which the physician may use this drug to treat future attacks in the same patient. Conversely, the use of colchicine as a diagnostic trial or in other circumstances in which the diagnosis of crystal-induced arthritis remains speculative is inappropriate. The accurate diagnosis of crystal-induced arthritis, most commonly gout, thus becomes critical.

The gold standard for the diagnosis of gout remains the demonstration by compensated, polarized light microscopy of negatively birefringent, needle-shaped crystals in the synovial fluid aspirate, preferably intracellular within the leukocyte. Unfortunately, arthrocentesis may not be clinically feasible, and crystals may not be detected in up to 15% of cases of aspirates from patients with proven gouty arthritis. In such cases, a presumptive diagnosis may be warranted, based on either prior established diagnosis or the clinical guidelines of the American Rheumatism As-

sociation (Table 21–2). Alternatively, some authorities believe the diagnosis is warranted in the patient with a prior documented history of acute monarthritis subsiding either spontaneously within a few days or in response to therapy and recurring in the presence of demonstrated hyperuricemia. Septic arthritis must be excluded in all cases, however, and especially in a previously undiagnosed patient presenting with acute inflammatory monarthritis accompanied by systemic signs of toxicity. This reinforces the diagnostic importance of arthrocentesis, which may also be therapeutic, as described later. The further differential diagnosis of acute monarthritis is illustrated in Table 21–3.

Indications for Treatment

The pain from gouty arthritis can be severe, and treatment is indicated for the relief of pain. Whether treatment is initiated with parenteral colchicine or oral agents is at the discretion of the treating physician. (See box.)

Discussion

The pathogenesis of gout is relatively well understood and provides rationale for the treatment outlined. Acute gouty arthritis describes the inflammatory synovitis that re-

---

TABLE 21–2. American Rheumatism Association Criteria for the Classification of Gouty Arthritis

○ Presence of urate crystals in the joint fluid
OR
○ Tophus proved by chemical or polarized light microscropy to contain urate crystals
OR
○ Presence of six or more of the following twelve clinical, laboratory, and radiologic findings:
  1. Inflammation a maximum of one day
  2. More than one attack
  3. Monarticular arthritis
  4. Redness
  5. First metatarsophalangeal joint pain or swelling
  6. Unilateral attack involving the first metatarsophalangeal joint
  7. Unilateral attack involving the tarsal joint
  8. Suspected tophus
  9. Hyperuricemia
  10. Asymmetric swelling visualized on roentgenograms
  11. Subcortical cysts, no erosions visualized on roentgenograms
  12. No organisms found on culture

TABLE 21–3. Differential Diagnosis of Acute Monarthritis

Acute hemarthrosis	Acute calcification periarthritis (hydroxyapatite crystals)	Amyloid arthritis
Ankylosing spondylitis	Foreign body	Avascular necrosis of bone
Gout	Hemophilic arthritis	Congenital dysplasia of hip
Localized periarticular syndromes (tendinitis, bursitis, cellulitis)	Juxta-articular bone tumors	Familial Mediterranean fever
	Loose body joint	Gaucher's disease
	Mechanical derangement of joint	Hyperlipoproteinemia
Osteoarthritis	Neuropathic arthropathy	Intermittent hydrarthrosis
Pseudogout	Psoriasis	Juvenile osteochondroses
Reiter's syndrome	Relapsing polychondritis	Osteochondritis dissecans
Rheumatoid arthritis	Sarcoidosis	Pigmented villonodular synovitis
Septic arthritis		Synovioma
Traumatic arthritis		

sults from crystal deposition within a synovial fluid supersaturated with monosodium urate (MSU). The proinflammatory molecules $C1_q$ and IgG adhere to the crystal, triggering the complement cascade by both the direct and alternate pathways. The crystals are thus engulfed by neutrophils, resulting in phagolysosomes. However, the crystal itself is membranolytic to these phagolysosomes, resulting in leakage of the proteolytic enzymes from within the lysosome, causing neutrophil autolysis with liberation of the MSU crystal. Further, a variety of proinflammatory kinins are also released during lysosomal discharge, including leukotrienes and lipoperoxidases, which augment inflammation through the arachidonic acid cascade by generation of prostacyclin. Most notably, however, as regards treatment with colchicine, these leukocytes also release a unique chemotaxin with a mass of 12,000 daltons, known as crystal-induced chemotactic factor

DRUG TREATMENT: ACUTE GOUTY ARTHRITIS

Indomethacin

Initial Dose	100 mg PO or 100 mg by rectal suppository
Repeat Dose	50 mg PO every 6–8 hours, or 100 mg by rectal suppository, not to exceed 300 mg daily
Maintenance Dose	Wean to 25 mg 3–4 times daily as soon as pain relieved, and switch to less potent, less toxic anti-inflammatory agent as soon as feasible.
End-Points	Relief of pain
	Total dose $\leq$ 300 mg daily

AND/OR

Colchicine

Initial Dose	2–3 mg diluted to 20 ml with normal saline, given by slow IV push through secure, medium- to large-bore catheter
Repeat Dose	1 mg IV every 4–6 hours, not to exceed a total of 4–5 mg for duration of any single attack
Alternative Method (not recommended)	0.6 mg PO every 30–60 minutes
End-Points	Relief of pain
	Total dose = 4–5 mg
	Nausea, vomiting

(CCF); an identical glycopeptide has also been recovered following initiation of crystal-induced inflammation by calcium pyrophosphate (pseudogout) crystals. It is this CCF liberation that is specifically blocked by administration of the drug colchicine. Whereas colchicine has been demonstrated to have more general anti-inflammatory effects at supraclinical doses, it is only this specific, CCF-blocking effect that results at clinical doses, thus explaining the relatively specific response of crystal-induced inflammation to this drug. However, the pathogenesis as just explained provides rationale for the treatment of a gouty attack by concomitant administration of both colchicine and any conventional, nonsteroidal anti-inflammatory drug (NSAID). The former inhibits leukocyte chemotaxis by a specific mechanism (as described above), whereas the latter class of drugs modulates the inflammatory cascade associated with generation of prostacyclin. An additive, if not synergistic, result may therefore be expected.

The medicinal use of colchicine long preceded the phase III Food and Drug Administration trials legislated for new drugs introduced since 1969. As such, its use has been well established by precedent, yet there are few scientific studies on which to base treatment decisions. To date, there have been no blinded, controlled studies of the comparative efficacy of colchicine and a representative NSAID, either used alone or in combination. Customary physician practice is thus more the result of individual training or habitual preference than the product of scientific study. Historically, repeated doses of 0.6 mg colchicine tablets have been administered until pain relief results or the patient experiences gastrointestinal toxicity. However, a number of open trials of intravenous colchicine conducted two to three decades ago have demonstrated the benefit and apparent safety of the drug administered by this route without the resulting direct gastrointestinal irritation. A number of authors have nevertheless reported toxicity following cumulative dosing of colchicine by either route, and 16 fatalities as a result of colchicine toxicity have been reported in the English language literature since 1947. The drug elimination depends primarily on hepatic metabolism, but a disproportionate incidence of toxic complications has been reported in patients with mild to moderate renal disease, and the drug should be used with caution in patients with either hepatic or renal insufficiency. A combined hepatorenal insufficiency of any significant degree should probably constitute an absolute contraindication to use of the drug. Interestingly, the drug has never been demonstrated to be teratogenic, but it cannot be recommended for use in pregnancy, in which case the diagnosis of gout should be seriously questioned anyway.

The more recent proliferation of drugs in the NSAID class has been attended by a number of open trials demonstrating successful use of these drugs for treatment of the acute gouty attack. Historically, phenylbutazone or oxyphenbutazone was commonly used because of the anti-inflammatory potency characteristics of these drugs; however, the development of safer drugs with demonstrated benefit has led to relative obsolescence of the former. Whereas a number of these drugs may be equipotent in appropriately adjusted doses, indomethacin is probably the best studied among the higher potency drugs and is generally well tolerated clinically; most patients experience significant relief following administration of 200 to 300 mg over the first 24 hours, as described. Indomethacin also has a relatively rapid onset and adequate therapeutic half-life so that a loading dose is not required. Finally, a rectal suppository of indomethacin is routinely available, which provides a convenient means for NSAID therapy of the patient who has contraindication or intolerance to oral NSAID therapy or enteral feeding. Alternative therapies for the latter patient include intravenous colchicine as described and/or injection of intra-articular steroids, when either of these therapies is feasible and not contraindicated. A number of equivalent NSAID dosing regimens for short-term maintenance exist.

The injection of intra-articular steroids requires arthrocentesis of the affected joint, which is further desirable both for diagnosis by crystal isolation as well as for exclusion of septic arthritis. It is also noteworthy that the process of draining the affected joint results in debulking of the offending crystals, which is therapeutic in itself. Inasmuch as there are no controlled studies by which to refute the benefit of concomitant therapies, it is reasonable to consider administration of intra-articular steroid following evacuation of the inflammatory synovial fluid whenever the physician is certain of both the diagnosis of crystal-induced arthropathy and the absence of joint sepsis. Relatively dramatic benefit may be afforded the appropriately selected patient. It should be recognized that, as regards potential complications, administration of intra-articular steroid to such patients is tantamount to systemic administration of steroids in a patient for whom such systemic therapy is absolutely contraindicated. However, such patients are rare, particularly in view of the short-term nature of this drug use.

As a final comment on the therapy of the acute arthritic attack of gout, the value of narcotic analgesics as an adjunct deserves mention. The celebrated English physician Thomas Sydenham, perhaps better known for his description of the choreiform disorder found in association with the arthritis accompanying rheumatic fever, was himself a victim of gout and described the experience as follows: "The night is passed in torture, sleeplessness, turning of the part affected, perpetual change of posture; the tossing about of the body being as incessant as the pain of the tortured joint, and being worse as the fit comes on." Because it is rare for the victim of gout to report any significant pain relief for a period of at least several hours, regardless of the expediency and propriety of therapies prescribed, some more immediate means of analgesia should be considered. The torment of the acute gouty attack is predictably both severe as well as self-limited by its natural history, and therefore narcotic analgesic therapy may be wholly appropriate for patients whose suffering is evident.

Diabetic Ketoacidosis and Nonketotic Hyperglycemic Hyperosmolar State

Insulin is the hormone of the fed state, in that its principal actions facilitate the incorporation of absorbed nutrients. Insulin stimulates peripheral utilization of glucose and hepatic synthesis of glycogen while inhibiting gluconeogenesis and glycogenolysis. Fat metabolism is shifted toward storage, with inhibition of lipolysis and stimulation of free fatty acid uptake and triglyceride synthesis. Uptake of amino acids is enhanced, and protein synthesis is increased. Proteolysis is inhibited. When fasting, intermediary metabolism is shifted toward catabolism through the effects of relative insulin lack and the actions of glucagon, growth hormone, catecholamines, and cortisol. These counter-regulatory hormones ensure a supply of substrate during periods of physiologic stress and insufficient dietary intake.

Diabetes mellitus represents a state of partial or absolute insulin lack. When deficiency is partial, metabolic derangements are largely limited to carbohydrate handling and are reflected as fasting hyperglycemia and postprandial glucose intolerance. Absolute insulin deficiency compounds these abnormalities with the mobilization of hepatic and peripheral fuel stores liberating glucose, free fatty acids, and amino acids into the serum. In the presence of counter-regulatory hormones, the effects of insulin deficiency are enhanced. Glycogen stores are exhausted, peripheral tissues shift to fat as a source of fuel, and glycerol and amino acids are utilized for gluconeogenesis to provide a carbohydrate source for the central nervous system, cardiac muscle, and red blood cells. Hepatic gluconeogenesis and reduced peripheral glucose utilization result in hyperglycemia. Burning fat results in ketogenesis, and ketonemia and acidosis follow. Diabetic ketoacidosis (DKA) is the clinical expression of this metabolic decompensation. DKA commonly occurs in known diabetics who are on exogenous insulin therapy. In this setting, the effects of the counter-regulatory hormones (particularly glucagon) are thought to overwhelm the actions of available insulin.

As DKA develops, hyperglycemia leads to osmotic diuresis and cellular dehydration. Fluid losses result in intravascular volume depletion and electrolyte abnormalities. Ketonemia and acidemia cause ileus and vomiting with reduction of fluid intake and additional water losses. In the absence of intervention, death occurs secondary to cardiovascular collapse.

When insulin deficiency is incomplete, sufficient hormone may exist to inhibit lipolysis, proteolysis, and ketogenesis. If the patient is able to take fluids, hyperglycemia is generally limited to a range of 400 to 450mg/dl. In the presence of debilitating illness or vomiting, fluid intake will be insufficient to hold hyperglycemia in check. As glycemic control worsens, osmotic diuresis leads to dehydration, hyperosmolality, and prerenal azotemia. This situation is termed *nonketotic hy-*

perglycemic hyperosmolar state (NHHS). Frequently, hyperosmolality may result in coma. The elevation of counter-regulatory hormones that characterizes DKA appears to be absent in NHHS.

Diagnosis

DKA is readily diagnosed by history, clinical presentation, and the use of routine laboratory studies. From 70 to 80% of patients have a prior history of diabetes, most often type I. Symptoms include vomiting, polyuria, polydipsia, weight loss, generalized weakness, abdominal pain, muscle cramps, dyspnea, and lethargy. Often, there will be a history of infection or other precipitating illness. Symptoms generally precede presentation by several days. On examination, nearly one-third of patients will exhibit an altered level of consciousness from drowsiness to coma. Vital signs may reveal mild hypothermia, tachycardia, postural hypotension, or tachypnea. Kussmaul respirations may be present. The skin will have reduced turgor. Mucous membranes will be dry. An odor of acetone may be present on the breath. Abdominal tenderness and reduced bowel sounds are common. Hyperglycemia will be demonstrated on reagent strip testing for serum glucose. Classic laboratory findings include a serum glucose of >250 mg/dl, pH < 7.3, hypocapnea, bicarbonate <15 mEq/liter, and a positive nitroprusside reaction for serum ketones at a dilution of >1:2. The average serum glucose concentration is 500 mg/dl, but concentrations >1000 mg/dl occur. Serum osmolality may be elevated or normal. Azotemia is frequently evident. Up to one-third of patients will be hyperkalemic, whereas <5% have low serum potassium.

NHHS usually presents as coma. Patients predisposed to this condition are generally elderly type II diabetics. In one-third to one-half of cases, NHHS represents the initial manifestation of diabetes. Poor fluid intake often precedes clinical decompensation. The clinical picture is one of profound dehydration with dry mucous membranes, poor skin turgor, and shock. Laboratory criteria for the diagnosis include serum glucose >600 mg/dl, osmolality >330 mOsm/liter, bicarbonate >20 mEq/liter, pH >7.3, and a negative nitroprusside reaction for serum ketones at a 1:2 dilution. Glucose concentrations frequently exceed 1000 mg/dl and can reach 3000 mg/dl. Azotemia is common. Elevations of the anion gap, when present, usually reflect lactic acidosis from poor peripheral perfusion.

Indications for Treatment

Intravenous insulin therapy is indicated whenever a patient meets criteria for the diagnosis of DKA or NHHS. The mortality of DKA is 1 to 10%, constituting 16% of overall diabetes mortality and 50% of deaths in diabetic patients under 24 years of age. The mortality of NHHS is 40 to 60%. Poor outcomes will be avoided only by rapid diagnosis and early application of aggressive therapy with insulin, fluids, and potassium. Initial treatment for both conditions is correction of hypovolemia with isotonic intravenous fluids followed by insulin therapy. (See box.)

Discussion

Insulin therapy in DKA has evolved since the mid-1970s toward low-dose regimens utilizing continuous infusion. Earlier high-dose regimens (50 to 100 units IV or IM every 1 to 2 hours) had a significantly higher incidence of iatrogenic hypoglycemia and hypokalemia. Serum insulin levels required for maximum peripheral glucose utilization, inhibition of peripheral lipolysis and proteolysis, and suppression of hepatic ketogenesis and gluconeogenesis lie in the range of 20 to 200 microunits/ml. These levels are attainable with intravenous delivery rates of 4 to 10 units/hour in adults. Continuous infusion offers the advantages of being titratable, easily administered, and rapidly terminated as end-points are approached. Intravenous insulin reaches peak serum concentrations at 2 to 4 minutes, has a serum half-life of 3 to 6 minutes, and shows peak biologic effect at 20 minutes. Intravenous bolus therapy is useful primarily for the initiation of treatment during preparation of an insulin drip. Although the efficacy of intermittent intramuscular insulin is hampered by inconsistent absorption, delayed effect, and relative difficulty in titration, intramuscular therapy offers an option when an insulin drip is unavailable or impractical. Intramuscular insulin produces peak plasma levels 50 to 60 minutes after administration and a nadir in serum glucose at approximately 90 minutes. Although controlled studies have failed to demonstrate any significant differences in clinical response between human recombinant insulin

---

DRUG TREATMENT: DIABETIC KETOACIDOSIS AND NONKETOTIC HYPERGLYCEMIC HYPEROSMOLAR STATE

First-Line Therapy

Saline or Lactated Ringer's

Initial Dose	500–1000 ml/hour × 2 hours
Repeat Dose	250–500 ml/hour × 4–6 hours and reassess
End-Points	Repletion of intravascular volume
	Adequate urine output
	Signs of volume overload

AND

Regular Insulin (U-100)

Initial Dose	0.2–0.4 units/kg by IV push
Repeat Dose	0.2–0.4 units/kg by IV push. Repeat bolus dosing is indicated when serum glucose fails to fall by 75–100 mg/dl in the first hour of therapy.
Maintenance Dose	0.05–0.15 units/kg/hour continuous IV infusion
End-Points	Fall in serum glucose by 75–100 mg/dl/hour with a goal of 250–300 mg/dl
	Resolution of ketonemia and acidosis

and pork or beef preparations, human insulin is preferred because of reduced antigenicity. Only regular insulin is useful in the acute management of DKA. Insulin is adsorbed by glassware and plastic tubing, a problem that can be minimized by flushing 50 to 100 ml of the infusion solution through the line and discarding it.

Lipolysis and ketogenesis are inhibited at serum insulin concentrations lower than those required for suppression of hepatic glucose production and stimulation of peripheral glucose utilization. In spite of this, ketonemia and acidemia require longer to clear than does hyperglycemia. For this reason, continuous insulin infusion should continue after reaching the glycemic end-point (250 to 300 mg/dl) if serum ketones remain positive, serum bicarbonate is less than 15 mEq/liter, pH is less than 7.3, or the anion gap is elevated. Hypoglycemia can be avoided during this phase of therapy by decreasing the insulin drip to 0.05 units/kg/hour and adding 5 to 10% dextrose to the intravenous fluids. The amount of dextrose required to avoid hypoglycemia after target serum glucose levels are reached can be estimated by the following formulas:

$$\text{Volume of distribution of glucose (dl/kg)} \times \text{weight (kg)} = \text{glucose space (dl)}$$

1

$$\text{Glucose space (dl)} \times \text{rate of fall of serum glucose (mg/dl/hour)} = \text{amount of glucose consumed per hour (mg/hour)}$$

2

The volume of distribution of glucose is approximately 3.0 dl/kg. In a 70-kg man where the observed rate of fall of serum glucose is 50 mg/dl/hour, hourly glucose consumption would be 10.5 g/hour. Five percent dextrose contains 5 g of dextrose per deciliter. Thus, serum glucose could be maintained at target levels with intravenous solutions containing 5% dextrose infused at a rate of 200 ml/hour. The transition to subcutaneous insulin should overlap intravenous drip therapy by an hour once hyperglycemia, acidemia, and ketonemia have cleared.

Fluid deficits in DKA are commonly 100 to 150 ml/kg, with losses equally distributed between the intra- and extracellular fluid compartments. Lost fluid is hypotonic in composition and is approximated in sodium content by 0.5 to 0.75 normal saline. The goals of fluid therapy are to replace the deficit over 24 to 36 hours while covering maintenance requirements. Fifty percent of the deficit should be repleted in the first 8 to 12 hours. Although lost fluid is hypotonic, initial volume resuscitation is most appropriately accomplished with isotonic solutions. Replacement of circulating volume improves hemodynamics and peripheral perfusion, enhancing the actions of infused insulin. Support of adequate urine output facilitates the osmotic diuresis of glucose and the excretion of acids. Isotonic fluids are theoretically less likely to produce osmolar shifts of free water into cells of the central nervous system and thus minimize the possibility of cerebral edema.

Normal saline and lactated Ringer's are appropriate solutions for early fluid replacement. Lactated Ringer's is less likely to produce iatrogenic hyperchloremia than is saline. Once orthostatic hypotension and resting tachycardia have been eliminated, half-normal saline should be substituted. Five percent dextrose in half-normal saline is used once serum glucose reaches 250 to 300 mg/dl. Common fluid regimens give normal saline or lactated Ringer's at 500 to 1000 ml for 1 to 2 hours, then half-normal saline at 250 to 500 ml/hour for 4 to 6 hours. Five percent dextrose is added as indicated by serum glucose determinations. Replacement beyond this point is guided by clinical assessment and the calculated deficit. An exception to early repletion with isotonic fluids occurs when initial serum sodium exceeds 150 mEq/liter. In this setting, half-normal saline should be used from the outset. Rates of fluid replacement will require modification in patients with a history of congestive heart failure or renal insufficiency.

The use of alkali for the treatment of acidosis in DKA has lost favor since the publication of controlled studies that failed to demonstrate differences in outcome between patients treated with bicarbonate and those in whom bicarbonate was withheld. Theoretical advantages of alkali include reversal of the hemodynamic depression and ventilatory compromise that have been observed at low serum pH. Theoretical disadvantages of bicarbonate include the potential for induction of hypokalemia and paradoxical central nervous system (CNS) acidosis. In addition, bicarbonate therapy has the potential to decrease peripheral oxygen delivery by antagonizing the Bohr effect of oxyhemoglobin dissociation in the presence of reduced red cell 2,3-diphosphoglycerate (2,3-DPG). If bicarbonate is used at all, it should be reserved for patients with severe acidemia to maintain serum $pH \geq 7.1$. Efforts to return serum pH to normal levels using bicarbonate should be strictly avoided.

Total body potassium deficits of 3 to 5 mEq/kg occur commonly in DKA, and deficits as high as 10 mEq/liter can occur. Although serum determinations are a poor indicator of total body potassium status, patients with an initial serum potassium of <3.5 mEq/liter can be assumed to have severe deficits. Several factors contribute to potentially dangerous hypokalemia during therapy. Acidemia results in exchange of intracellular K^+ for extracellular H^+, permitting increased urinary potassium losses as renal perfusion is improved by restoration of intravascular volume. Volume replacement can also produce dilutional falls in serum potassium. Transmembrane shifts of serum potassium back into the intracellular compartment will accompany treatment with either insulin or bicarbonate. Thus, treatment of patients with DKA and low or normal serum potassium values poses the danger of inducing clinically significant hypokalemia if repletion is not initiated early. Serum potassium can be anticipated to fall by 0.5 mEq/liter/hour during conventional therapy for DKA. In the patient with measured hypokalemia or ventricular ectopy at presentation, potassium should be administered from the outset as 40 to 80 mEq/liter of intravenous fluid. When initial serum potassium is high or within the normal range, 20 to 40 mEq of potassium chloride should be added to each liter of intravenous fluid after intravascular volume expansion with 1 to 2 liters of isotonic fluid. The rapidity and duration of subsequent repletion should be guided by serum potassium determinations. Replacement of the total body potassium deficit will generally require days of combined intravenous and oral therapy.

Phosphate depletion in DKA is usually without clinical significance, although profound deficits can occur. Controlled studies comparing recovery from DKA in the presence and absence of early phosphate repletion have revealed no significant differences. Replacement of phosphate is suggested only in those patients with profound hypophosphatemia on presentation and in those with risk factors for total body phosphate depletion (alcoholism, malabsorption, malnutrition). Replacement solutions are available as potassium salts, containing 15 mmol of phosphate and 22 mEq of potassium per ampule. These can be added to intravenous fluids in exchange for an equivalent quantity of potassium as potassium chloride.

Insulin therapy for NHHS follows the same guidelines as for DKA. Although hyperglycemia is generally more severe in NHHS, reductions in serum glucose approaching 25% can be attained with hydration alone. For this reason, requirements for intravenous insulin are generally lower in NHHS than in DKA, and the duration of therapy with an insulin drip is often abbreviated. The majority of patients will reach glycemic end-points with a total insulin dosage of 25 to 50 units. Once serum glucose reaches 250 to 300 mg/dl, insulin infusion can be stopped. Patients without antecedent insulin requirements often can be maintained without additional insulin therapy at this time, and the need for intravenous dextrose is averted. Those with a prior history of insulin-requiring diabetes should undergo transition to subcutaneous insulin therapy, and 5% dextrose should be added to their intravenous fluids.

Fluid deficits in NHHS are more extreme than those in DKA and may be as high as 25% of total body water. Although free water is lost in excess of sodium, initial hydration should be with 1 to 2 liters of isotonic saline or lactated Ringer's when hypotension, tachycardia, or oliguria is present. Transition to half-normal saline should be made as soon as intravascular volume has been repleted and urine output is 30 to 50 ml/hour. One-half of the fluid deficit plus ongoing losses should be replaced in the first 12 hours, which usually requires 5 to 6 liters of fluid. The remainder of the fluid deficit is replaced in the second 12 to 24 hours of treatment. Because patients with NHHS are often elderly and have multiple medical problems, care should be taken to avoid precipitation of congestive heart failure. Monitoring of central venous pressure or pulmonary capillary wedge pressure may be required.

Potassium deficits in NHHS may be as high as 400 to 1000 mEq. Because severe acidemia is not a feature of NHHS, the transmembrane shift of serum potassium into intracellular fluid is unopposed when insulin is administered. Early replacement is paramount if life-threatening hypokalemia is to be avoided. Once renal failure and hyperkalemia are ruled out, potassium should be added to the intravenous fluids as potassium chloride, 20 to 40 mEq/liter. Arguments for the replacement of phosphate in NHHS are the same as in DKA. Bicarbonate has no place in the treatment of NHHS unless lactic acidosis is severe.

Phlebothrombosis is an uncommon but reported complication of DKA and NHHS and warrants prophylaxis with subcutaneous heparin when the patient has a history of deep venous thrombosis or significant risk factors for its development. An acute precipitant is identifiable in a significant proportion of presentations for both conditions. Evaluation of the patient should always include a search for infection or other physiologic stressors.

Hypercalcemia

Hypercalcemia is most frequently a consequence of either primary hyperparathyroidism or underlying malignant disease. Other causes of hypercalcemia, which are rare, include vitamin D toxicity, milk-alkali syndrome, Paget's disease of bone, immobilization, sarcoidosis, hyperthyroidism, adrenal insufficiency, acute renal failure, granulomatous lung disease, and certain medications (thiazides, lithium, estrogen).

Parathyroid hormone (PTH) is synthesized in the parathyroid glands. Release is stimulated by low levels of ionized calcium and high levels of phosphorus. PTH increases serum calcium by increasing osteoclastic bone resorption, enhancing gut absorption of calcium and increasing renal tubular reabsorption of calcium in the kidneys. Calcitonin inhibits the effect of PTH at the osteoclast. Vitamin D and magnesium are necessary cofactors for PTH to function.

Primary hyperparathyroidism is the autonomous overproduction of PTH by the parathyroids. This is due to a single adenoma in a vast majority of cases. Less commonly, hyperplasia of the parathyriods is the cause. Parathyroid carcinoma and multiple adenomas occur but are rare.

Secondary hyperparathyroidism is due to high levels of circulating phosphorus. This occurs most often as a result of renal failure and ensuing inability to excrete the phosphorus.

Malignancies that cause hypercalcemia have been associated with humoral agents that have functional similarities to PTH. These include lung, breast, pharynx/larynx, and gastrointestinal (GI) tract tumors. Multiple myeloma, in addition to causing "humoral hypercalcemia of malignancy," can also have direct osteolytic activity.

Diagnosis

The clinical presentation of hypercalcemia is usually a gradual progression of subtle nonspecific complaints. The signs and symptoms are proportional to the degree of hy-

---

DRUG TREATMENT: HYPERCALCEMIA

First-Line Drug
Saline

Initial Dose	200–500 ml/hour
Repeat Dose	200–500 ml/hour
End-Point	Lowering of serum calcium
	Brisk diuresis
	Congestive heart failure

Second-Line Drugs
Calcitonin-Salmon

Initial Dose	4 IU/kg IM or subcutaneously
Repeat Dose	4 IU/kg IM or subcutaneously every 12 hours
End-Points	Lowering of serum calcium
	Note: Patients should be skin tested before receiving IV calcitonin.

AND

Hydrocortisone Acetate

Initial Dose	100 mg IV
Repeat Dose	100 mg IV every 8 hours
End-Point	Lowering of serum calcium

Third-Line Drug
Plicamycin

Initial Dose	25 μg/kg IV infusion over 4 hours
Repeat Dose	25 μg/kg every day $\times$ 4 days
End-Point	Lowering of serum calcium over 48–72 hours

Fourth-Line Drug
Etidronate

Initial Dose	7.5 mg/kg in 250 ml saline over 2–4 hours
Repeat Dose	7.5 mg/kg infusion every 24 hour $\times$ 3
End-Point	Lowering of serum calcium

percalcemia as well as the rapidity of calcium elevation. The GI, cardiovascular, neurologic, and renal systems are the most frequently affected.

The most common complaints are GI symptoms of nausea, vomiting, constipation, and anorexia. Neurologic changes include fatigue, weakness, ataxia, behavioral changes, mental status changes (including coma), reduced muscle tone, and diminished deep tendon reflexes. Cardiovascular effects of hypercalcemia include mild hypertension, increased contractility, slowed conduction, dysrhythmias (bradycardia, heart block), and increased predilection to digoxin toxicity. Renal manifestations include polyuria, polydipsia, dehydration, nephrogenic diabetes insipidus, nephrocalcinosis, nephrolithiasis, and renal failure.

Hypercalcemia is diagnosed by the finding of an elevated serum calcium. Diagnosis of the underlying etiology of the hypercalcemia in the emergency setting is made moot by the universality of initial therapy and the length of time needed to obtain definitive test results. The ionized calcium is the active ion; however, total calcium is commonly the only test available acutely. When serum calcium is evaluated, the serum proteins (albumin, globulin, and total protein) to which the majority of calcium is bound should be evaluated simultaneously. A correction in calcium of 0.5 mg/dl should be made for every 1 g change in albumin or 0.8 mg/dl for every 1 g change in total protein.

Indications for Therapy

Emergency therapy is based on the serum calcium level and clinical status. Aggressive therapy is indicated for all patients with serum calcium levels >15 mg/100 ml and for any hypercalcemic patient with serious manifestations (e.g., cardiovascular impairment, neurologic involvement, etc.). (See box.)

Discussion

Calcium excretion is via a shared pathway with sodium. Accordingly, the mainstay of initial therapy is induction of natriuresis by means of administration of large volumes of saline to induce brisk diuresis. Although many patients may develop signs of heart failure and require loop diuretics such as furosemide, routine addition of a diuretic is not recommended. If a diuretic is needed, furosemide titrated to an adequate urine output

is a good choice. Patients often require invasive hemodynamic monitoring during saline infusion to prevent cardiovascular compromise. If diuretics are used, careful monitoring of serum electrolytes is essential.

If hypercalcemia is severe or saline hydration alone is not effective in lowering calcium, calcitonin is a reasonable second-line agent. Because it is a foreign protein, skin testing should be done prior to intravenous treatment. Intradermal injection of 1 IU should be observed for at least 15 minutes for a wheal and flare reaction. The hypocalcemic response to calcitonin may be potentiated by corticosteroids, and it is recommended that they be used concomitantly.

Plicamycin is also effective in lowering serum calcium and is more predictably successful than calcitonin. However, the calcium-lowering effects of plicamycin are delayed for at least 24 to 48 hours, and thus plicamycin is less useful if serum calcium must be lowered quickly. Nausea and vomiting are common with plicamycin, and antiemetic prophylaxis is probably indicated.

Diphosphonate compounds have shown great promise in treating hypercalcemia. These compounds may be second-line agents in the future in place of calcitonin and plicamycin. Etidronate is an approved diphosphonate for use in hypercalcemia.

If the patient has impaired renal function or is *in extremis,* acute hemodialysis against a low or zero calcium dialysate will quickly lower serum calcium. The calcium-lowering effect may be transient, and repeat dialysis may be required.

Acute Hypocalcemia

Calcium is the most abundant physiologic electrolyte, with a total body content of 15 to 20 g/kg of body weight. The vast majority occurs as relatively inert skeletal hydroxyapatite. Less than 0.1% is found in the extracellular fluid compartment, 0.03% as plasma calcium. Routine clinical determinations of serum calcium measure the total serum calcium. This is divisible into free (ionic), protein-bound, and chelated fractions. It is the ionic fraction that is physiologically active. Normal values for total serum calcium range from 8.5 to 10.5 mg/dl. Of this, 4.2 to 4.8 mg/dl is ionized. Ionization of serum calcium is influenced by plasma protein and free fatty acid content, plasma pH, and the concentration of organic anions and ionic phosphorus.

Homeostatic regulation of serum calcium is controlled through the actions of parathyroid hormone (PTH) and vitamin D. In response to low ionized serum calcium, PTH and the active metabolites of vitamin D facilitate the absorption of filtered calcium at the distal nephron, dietary calcium at the jejunal epithelium, and skeletal calcium at the bone–extracellular fluid interface. Processes that interfere with the production or action of PTH and vitamin D alter the equilibrium between free and bound or chelated calcium, or promote malabsorption or renal wasting of calcium independent of endocrine mechanisms can lead to hypocalcemia (Table 21–4). While calcium has a host of physiologic roles, those of clinical significance in acute hypocalcemia include involvement in impulse generation and conduction, membrane stability, and excitation–contraction coupling of muscle.

Diagnosis

The hallmark of acute hypocalcemia is enhanced neuromuscular irritability. This is manifested clinically as perioral or acral paresthesias, muscle cramps, carpopedal spasm, abdominal cramps, frank tetany, seizures, laryngospasm, and a variety of psychological disturbances. Latent tetany can be elicited

TABLE 21–4. Major Causes of Hypocalcemia

Hypoalbuminemia
Parathyroid gland or PTH insufficiency
   Surgery/neck trauma
   Infiltrative/idiopathic
   Hereditary
Calcitriol insufficiency (chronic)
   Nutritional/malabsorptive syndromes
   Severe hepatic insufficiency
   End-stage renal disease
   Anticonvulsant therapy
End-organ unresponsiveness
   Pseudohypoparathyroidism
   Acquired
Multifactorial
   Gram-negative sepsis
   Magnesium deficiency
   Pancreatitis
   Renal failure
Chelation of Ca^{++} (ionized hypocalcemia)
   Alkalosis
   Acute anion load (citrate, lactate, oxalate,
      bicarbonate, fluoride, phosphate, EDTA,
      radiographic contrast)
   Increased free fatty acids
   Albumin infusion

(Reproduced with permission from Olinger ML: Disorders of calcium and magnesium metabolism. Emerg Med Clin North Am 7:800, 1989.)

by tapping on the preauricular portion of the facial nerve (Chvostek's sign) or by inducing carpal spasm through occlusion of arterial flow to one arm with a blood pressure cuff (Trousseau's sign). Symptoms may worsen with hyperventilation. Generalized weakness is common. Steatorrhea may be evident. Rarely, cardiac conduction abnormalities and congestive heart failure occur. Evidence of preexisting chronic hypocalcemia includes brittle hair, ridged nails, scaly skin, pitted teeth, and cataracts. Patients with pseudohypoparathyroidism will exhibit consistent developmental abnormalities of the skeleton. A history of neck surgery, renal insufficiency, alcoholism, osteomalacia, malabsorption, and medication usage can be helpful (Table 21–5).

Laboratory evaluation includes determination of total and ionized serum calcium. Where direct measurement of ionized calcium is not possible, determination of serum protein allows its estimation by the following formula:

$$Ca^{2+} = Ca^{total} - (0.83 \times \text{total protein})$$
$$= Ca^{total} - [(1.1 \times \text{albumin}) + (0.2 \times \text{globulin})]$$

It is significant that ionic hypocalcemia can occur in the setting of normal total serum calcium. Measurement of serum magnesium, phosphorus, potassium, blood urea nitrogen, and creatinine can provide important clues to etiology and guide adjunctive treatment. Arterial blood gases may demonstrate alkalosis as a precipitating or exacerbating factor. Prolongation of the QT interval may be evident on electrocardiography. Determination of levels of immunoreactive PTH is essential for determining the ultimate cause of hypo-

TABLE 21–5. Drugs That Can Cause Hypocalcemia

Cimetidine	Norepinephrine
Phosphates (e.g., enemas, laxatives)	Citrate (blood)
	Mithramycin
Dilantin, phenobarbital	Calcitonin
Gentamicin, tobramycin	Loop diuretics
Cisplatin	Glucocorticoids
Heparin	Magnesium sulfate
Theophylline	Sodium nitroprusside
Protamine	
Glucagon	

(Reproduced with permission from Wilson RF: Fluid and electrolyte problems. In Tintiorelli JE, et al (eds): Emergency Medicine: A Comprehensive Study Guide. New York, McGraw-Hill, 1988, p 60.)

calcemia but is not useful in guiding emergent management.

Indications for Treatment

Due to the potential for laryngospasm and seizures, any patient with symptomatic hypocalcemia or evidence of latent tetany should be treated with intravenous calcium salts. Treatment must usually precede determination of the etiology of hypocalcemia. (See box.)

Discussion

Overly vigorous repletion of calcium can result in bradycardia, hypotension, syncope, or cardiac arrest. Cardiac rhythm and blood pressure should be monitored during therapy and the rates of infusion carefully followed. Calcium levels should be closely followed to avoid iatrogenic hypercalcemia. When hyperphosphatemia (>6 mg/dl) accompanies hypocalcemia, serum phosphorus must be reduced simultaneously to avoid

DRUG TREATMENT: ACUTE HYPOCALCEMIA

First-Line Therapy

Calcium Gluconate (10%)

Initial Dose	10–30 ml in 100 ml D$_5$W over 10–15 minutes (0.465 mEq/ml, 9.3 mg/ml elemental calcium)
Repeat Dose	As above 3–4 times per day, or continuous infusion at a rate of 0.05–0.1 mEq/kg/hour
	Dosages listed are for adults. The initial dosage for children is 0.5–0.7 mEq/kg. Rate of infusion should never exceed 0.7–1.5 mEq/min.
End-Points	Resolution of symptoms
	Maintenance of serum Ca^{total} at 7–9 mg/dl

OR

Calcium Chloride (10%)

Initial Dose	3–10 ml in 100 ml D$_5$W over 10–20 minutes (1.36 mEq/ml, 27.3 mg/ml elemental calcium)
Repeat Dose	As above 3–4 times per day, or continuous infusion at a rate of 0.05–0.1 mEq/kg/hour
	Dosages listed are for adults. The initial dosage for children is 0.5–0.7 mEq/kg. Rate of infusion should never exceed 0.7–1.5 mEq/min.
End-Points	Resolution of symptoms
	Maintenance of serum Ca^{total} at 7–9 mg/dl

OR

Calcium Gluceptate (22%)

Initial Dose	5–15 ml in 100 ml D$_5$W over 10–15 minutes (0.9 mEq/ml, 18.6 mg/ml elemental calcium)
Repeat Dose	As above 3–4 times per day, or continuous infusion at a rate of 0.05–0.1 mEq/kg/hour.
	Dosages listed are for adults. The initial dosage for children is 0.5–0.7 mEq/kg. Rate of infusion should never exceed 0.7–1.5 mEq/min.
End-Points	Resolution of symptoms
	Maintenance of serum Ca^{total} at 7–9 mg/dl

metastatic calcification with the administration of calcium salts. Serum phosphorus may be quickly brought down using intravenous 50% dextrose, insulin, and saline. Obvious precipitants, particularly hypomagnesemia and alkalosis, should be sought and corrected. Because calcium exacerbates the electrophysiologic effects of digitalis toxicity, digitalis should be given cautiously in these patients. The transition from parenteral to oral therapy can generally be accomplished over 24 to 48 hours. Oral therapy is instituted with 200 to 500 mg elemental calcium as gluconate or chloride salts every 2 hours while parenteral therapy is tapered. Effective enteral therapy may require supplementation of vitamin D or its active metabolites.

Of the parenteral calcium salts, calcium gluconate is considered the drug of choice for treatment of acute hypocalcemia. Calcium chloride is irritating to tissues and may cause necrosis and sloughing with extravasation, or thrombophlebitis if infused through a peripheral vein. Both calcium gluconate and gluceptate can be given intramuscularly when intravenous access is unobtainable. Intramuscular administration should be avoided in young children because of the potential for causing disfiguring sterile abscesses at the injection site.

Hypoglycemia

The most frequent acute cause of hypoglycemia is secondary to excess insulin administration in diabetics ("insulin reaction"). Other causes of hypoglycemia are relatively uncommon. There are two broad etiologic classifications of hypoglycemia based on temporal relation to food ingestion. The first category is labeled "fasting hypoglycemia" and the second class is designated as "reactive hypoglycemia." The majority of fasting hypoglycemias are the consequence of an underlying pathologic process that is often clinically apparent before the onset of hypoglycemia. There is no temporal relationship between the ingestion of food and the onset of symptoms. As mentioned above, the predominant etiology is hyperinsulinism. Aside from exogenous insulin, fasting hypoglycemia may be due to pancreatic tumors secreting insulin, nonpancreatic tumors that secrete insulin-like compounds, other drugs (e.g., aspirin, sulfonylureas, alcohol), end-stage liver or kidney disease, certain hormone deficiencies (e.g., growth hormone, glucocorticoid), cachexia, and certain congenital disorders of metabolism.

The reactive hypoglycemias do show a temporal relationship between the onset of symptoms and food ingestion. There are three subcategories in this category. The first is alimentary hypoglycemia, which is generally attributed to gastrectomy surgery, although it has been reported in persons without a history of surgery. The proposed pathophysiology is the rapid passage of carbohydrates into the small intestine, which leads to marked hyperglycemia 1 hour after a meal. Insulin levels rise markedly in response to the level of hyperglycemia; however, 2 hours after a meal there is relative insulin excess, resulting in hypoglycemia and the onset of symptoms.

A second subcategory of reactive hypoglycemia has been reported in non–insulin-dependent diabetics in whom symptoms occur 3 to 4 hours after meals. The final grouping is termed idiopathic reactive hypoglycemia with symptoms occurring late after meals (>4 hours).

Diagnosis

The patient's symptoms are, in part, an expression of the sympathetic adrenergic outflow that is triggered by hypoglycemia. These classically include anxiety, panic, tachycardia, palpitations, and cool, moist skin. The other associated symptoms are due to the glucose-deficient state of neurologic tissues. So many abnormalities of neurologic function have been reported as a consequence of hypoglycemia that the clinician should rule out hypoglycemia in all patients who present with a neurologic problem. A brief list of neurologic findings secondary to hypoglycemia includes behavioral changes, mental depression/coma, seizures, focal motor deficits, ataxia, visual changes, and paresthesias. The duration and severity of the hypoglycemic state appears to affect the degree and rate of neurologic recovery. Conversely, the adrenergic symptoms usually subside with correction of serum glucose.

The diagnosis of hypoglycemia rests on an accurate determination of serum glucose level. Rapid glucose tests using dipstick photometric methods may lack precision, but they are useful for ascertaining the extremes of hyperglycemia and severe hypoglycemia.

Indications for Treatment

It has become common practice in prehospital care settings to empirically treat patients with altered mental status with glucose. This is probably not necessary in the hospital setting since glucose determinations can be done photometrically in just over 1 minute. Patients with serious symptoms in whom a low or normal value is obtained should be given glucose immediately, whereas a hyperglycemic result would not support glucose administration.

Any symptomatic patient with a glucose level <60 mg/dl should be treated. Diabetic patients who routinely maintain elevated serum glucose levels may become symptomatic at "normal" levels and require treatment based on symptomatology and the finding of "relative hypoglycemia." (See box.)

Discussion

The oral administration of liquids containing glucose is effective, but the risk of aspiration in obtunded patients precludes the oral route for treatment in all but the mildest of cases. The preferred therapy for hypoglycemia is intravenous administration of 25 to 50 g of 50% dextrose solution. An immediate response after intravenous treatment is usually apparent, although a more gradual response would be expected in cases of prolonged hypoglycemia. An intravenous solution containing 5% dextrose should be continued. Frequent serial glucose determinations should be made initially and further replacement given as needed. Patients who fail to respond to intravenous dextrose should be checked for hypothermia, which may occur if hypoglycemia has been prolonged. After awakening, patients who have suffered an "insulin reaction" should be given something to eat to prevent a recurrence of hypoglycemia.

Patients who may be malnourished and vitamin deficient should always receive 50 to 100 mg thiamine IV prior to dextrose administration. Glucose administered without thiamine may precipitate acute Wernicke's encephalopathy in patients with severe thiamine deficiency.

If intravenous access is not immediately available, glucagon, 1 mg, may be given intramuscularly. Glucagon acts at the liver to stimulate glucose release. Liver glycogen stores are required for glucagon to be effective. Therefore, the onset of glucagon's action may be slow (20 minutes) and the effect negligible.

DRUG TREATMENT: HYPOGLYCEMIA

First-Line Drug

Dextrose

Initial Dose	25–50 ml of 50% dextrose solution by IV push (children: 2–4 ml/kg of 25% dextrose)
Repeat Dose	25–50 ml of 50% dextrose by IV push in 10–20 minutes or IV infusion of 10% dextrose solution
End-Points	Resolution of symptoms
	Return to normal blood sugar

Second-Line Drug

Note: Should be used only if IV dextrose unavailable

Glucagon

Initial Dose	1 mg IM
Repeat Dose	Not indicated
End-Points	Resolution of symptoms
	No response to 1-mg dose

Myasthenic Crisis

Myasthenia gravis is an autoimmune disorder in which antibodies are elaborated against components of the postsynaptic junctional folds of the motor end-plate. Neuromuscular transmission depends on the quantal release of acetylcholine (Ach) from presynaptic motor fibers and the subsequent interaction of Ach with conformationally specific acetylcholine receptors (AchR) on the postsynaptic membrane. At rest, baseline quantal release of Ach results in miniature end-plate potentials (MEPPs) in the postsynaptic junctional folds. With stimulation, Ach release is enhanced and an end-plate potential (EPP) is generated in the postsynaptic element. When the amplitude of the EPP reaches threshold there is generalized depolarization of the muscle fiber with subsequent contraction. The amplitude of the EPP depends on the number of quanta released from the presynaptic terminal and the amplitude of the postsynaptic MEPP. Reduction of the density of postsynaptic AchR results in diminution of the MEPP and interference with generation of an EPP sufficient to depolarize the fiber. Receptor deficiency is reflected clinically as muscle weakness, particularly with repetitive stimulation. In myasthenia gravis, complement-mediated destruction of AchR results in muscle weakness that is insidious in onset and periodic or fluctuant in nature. Weakness most commonly affects the bulbar musculature but may be generalized. Involvement of the muscles of deglutition and respiration results in frequent pulmonary infections and respiratory failure. Exacerbations of myasthenia gravis with respiratory compromise are termed *myasthenic crises*. Crisis occurs as a result of muscle weakness in approximately one-third of cases. In the remainder, aspiration, upper respiratory infection, or pneumonia represent the precipitants of crisis. Myasthenic crisis is not an inevitable occurrence in myasthenia gravis but may affect 16 to 53% of patients at some point in the course of the disease.

Therapy for myasthenia gravis is directed toward enhancing neuromuscular transmission by limiting the destruction of AchR and increasing the availability of Ach in the synaptic cleft. Toward the former end, patients have been treated with thymectomy, azathioprine, steroids, immunoglobulins, and plasmapheresis. Plasmapheresis and high-dose steroids have proven useful in the management of acute exacerbations. Acetylcholinesterases have been used both for chronic therapy and for myasthenic crisis. Frequently, positive-pressure ventilation is required during crisis. Occasionally, intubation and mechanical ventilation can be averted through the use of drugs. The goal of therapy in myasthenic crisis is to support the patient until the precipitant resolves.

Diagnosis

Myasthenic crisis as the initial manifestation of myasthenia gravis has not been reported; the patient will virtually always present with a history of established myasthenia. No firm criteria have been developed to define crisis. The diagnosis is clinical. The principal differential diagnosis is between myasthenic crisis and cholinergic excess secondary to overmedication with anticholinesterases. The distinction is critical, as therapy directed at one will exacerbate the other. Both conditions present with muscle weakness. In cholinergic excess, muscarinic symptoms may be prominent. Differentiation between myasthenic and cholinergic crises and the adequacy of anticholinesterase therapy can be assessed with the edrophonium challenge test. Edrophonium is a short-acting anticholinesterase that competitively inhibits the action of the enzyme on native Ach. This transiently increases the concentration of Ach in the synaptic cleft, potentiating the EPP and muscle fiber depolarization. In myasthenia gravis, edrophonium will briefly improve motor strength. In cholinergic crisis, edrophonium results in worsening muscle weakness or frank paralysis through potentiation of depolarizing neuromuscular blockade. Edrophonium challenge involves intravenous administration of 1 mg followed by observation of a repetitive motor task. If no response or adverse effects are noted within 1 minute, the dose can be repeated. Facilities for airway management must be available during edrophonium testing. Edrophonium can precipitate extreme muscarinic effects, which can be antagonized with atropine.

Determination of vital capacity, negative inspiratory force, and other respiratory parameters can assist in guiding appropriate treatment. Arterial blood gases are useful. Evidence for intercurrent pulmonary infection must be sought.

Indications for Treatment

Parenteral anticholinesterase therapy for myasthenic crisis is indicated whenever there is evidence of insufficient anticholinesterase treatment or when anticholinesterases have not yet been employed. Edrophonium challenge testing may demonstrate potential benefit from parenteral neostigmine or pyridostigmine in this setting. Steroids are indicated when optimal anticholin-

---

DRUG TREATMENT: MYASTHENIC CRISIS

Diagnostic Testing
Edrophonium Chloride (10 mg/ml)

For Diagnosis of Suspected Myasthenia Gravis

Initial Dose	2 mg by IV push over 15–30 seconds
Repeat Dose	8 mg by IV push over 15–30 seconds to be given 45–60 seconds after the initial dose if no response observed. The dosage for children <34 kg is 0.2 mg/kg divided as one-fifth for initial dosing and the remainder for repeat dosing. Infants can receive a total dose of 0.5 mg.
End-Point	Clear improvement in performance of a repetitive motor task

For Differentiation Between Myasthenic and Cholinergic Crises and Assessment of the Adequacy of Anticholinesterase Therapy

Initial Dose	1 mg by IV push over 15–30 seconds
Repeat Dose	1 mg by IV push over 15–30 seconds to be given 1 minute after the initial dose if no response observed
End-Points	Cholinergic crisis: increased respiratory motor weakness and oropharyngeal secretions
	Myasthenic crisis: improved respiratory motor performance
	Myasthenic crisis unresponsive to anticholinesterases: unchanged

First-Line Drugs
Pyridostigmine Bromide (1.0 mg/ml)

Dose	2.0 mg IM or by slow IV push every 2–3 hours
End-Points	Improvement in motor strength and respiratory performance without excessive muscarinic side effects

OR

Neostigmine Methylsulfate (0.25 mg/ml, 0.5 mg/ml, 1.0 mg/ml)

Dose	0.5–2.5 mg IM, subcutaneously, or by slow IV push every 2–6 hours
End-Points	Improvement in motor strength and respiratory performance without excessive muscarinic side effects

AND

Prednisone

Initial Dose	25–100 mg/day
Maintenance	Determined by individual patient response
End-Point	Objective improvement in muscle strength

esterase treatment and thymectomy are unable to control symptoms, or when thymectomy is not an option. Intubation and mechanical ventilation should not be delayed in favor of pharmacologic therapy when pulmonary status is marginal. (See box.)

Discussion

Chronic therapy with anticholinesterases can lead to a state of refractoriness to their effects, which is alleviated by temporary withdrawal of the drug. Myasthenic crisis may be precipitated by the development of refractoriness; obviously these patients will benefit little from increased dosages. Toxic effects of the anticholinesterases can also precipitate decompensation in myasthenia secondary to cholinergic crisis. This also requires withdrawal of the drug. These considerations have led some to recommend discontinuance of anticholinesterases in the setting of myasthenic crisis in favor of early intubation and mechanical ventilation. It is probable that therapy with parenteral neostigmine or pyridostigmine will be of benefit only in patients naive to these drugs or demonstrating clear evidence of improvement to edrophonium challenge testing. Among available anticholinesterase preparations, pyridostigmine is favored due to a lower incidence of muscarinic side effects and a greater duration of action. With both drugs, muscarinic effects may necessitate treatment with atropine. Neither preparation crosses the blood–brain barrier to a significant extent at conventional dosages, and central effects are minimal. Efforts have been directed at enhancing the affects of anticholinesterases with potassium chloride, ephedrine, and guanidine, but consistent benefit has not been demonstrated.

Prednisone shortens the duration of myasthenic crisis and induces long-term remission in a significant proportion of patients. However, initiation of therapy with prednisone transiently exacerbates weakness in up to 80% of those treated. This effect can persist up to 10 days, is dose related, and is more pronounced in patients on concurrent anticholinesterase therapy. As such, prednisone may adversely affect the early course of myasthenic crisis, necessitating aggressive airway management and mechanical ventilation.

Plasmapheresis can produce dramatic improvement during myasthenic crisis and in-duce temporary remissions lasting 4 to 6 weeks. This procedure requires four to six 3-liter plasma exchanges over a period of 2 to 5 weeks. It is generally reserved for patients who fail to respond to other therapeutic modalities and is impractical in the long-term management of myasthenia gravis.

Recent evidence suggests that intravenous immunoglobulin may be efficacious in the treatment of acute exacerbations of myasthenia and that beneficial effects can persist for up to 50 days. Transient worsening of muscle strength can occur with initial administration but appears to be less severe and shorter lived than that obtained with high-dose steroids. The rate of response to immunoglobulins is significantly lower than that obtained with prednisone therapy (75% versus 90%).

Although thymectomy and azathioprine therapy have proved useful in the management of chronic myasthenia gravis, they have no role in myasthenic crisis.

Myxedema Coma

Diagnosis

Hypothyroidism is a common clinical syndrome usually associated with suboptimal circulating levels of thyroid hormone. The onset is insidious, and the early signs and symptoms are nonspecific. The most common causes are autoimmune disease and thyroid ablation from either surgery or radioactive iodine treatment. Myxedema coma is the most severe manifestation of hypothyroidism and is fortunately rare. Elderly women are most frequently affected, and the disorder usually manifests in the winter months. Up to 50% of cases occur in patients hospitalized for other reasons. Precipitating factors include cold exposure, drugs, surgery, trauma, congestive heart failure, and stroke. The mortality rate approaches 50%.

The clinical presentation may vary depending on whether hypothyroidism is primary (thyroid failure), secondary (pituitary failure), or tertiary (hypothalamic failure). Over 90% of cases will be primary in nature. Hypothermia is a presenting finding in 80% of cases, and normal temperatures in myxedema suggest underlying infection. Other clinical manifestations include coma, bradycardia, hypoventilation, hypotension, hyponatremia, and hypoglycemia. The patient will usually have typical findings of long-standing hypothyroidism such as dry skin, puffy eyelids, hoarse voice, pseudomyotonic reflexes, nonpitting edema, thin eyebrows, pallor, and sparse pubic hair. Although coma is often present, patients may present with delirium (myxedema madness). Laboratory evaluation should include measures of thyroid function, arterial blood gases, electrolytes, glucose, and a complete blood count.

Indications for Treatment

Patients presenting with coma, hypothermia, shock, or delirium believed to be associated with hypothyroidism should be treated based on clinical findings. One should not await the results of thyroid function testing to begin treatment of patients with these severe manifestations. A single dose of levothyroxine is unlikely to have any detrimental effects in an euthyroid patient. (See box.)

Discussion

Because myxedema coma is a rare disorder, few studies exist that evaluate different treatment regimens. There is debate about the best form, route, and dosage for thyroid hormone replacement, but the regimen outlined below is generally recommended. The main risk with rapid replacement of thyroid hormone is cardiac arrhythmias. Hypercholesterolemia and coronary artery disease are common with hypothyroidism, and cardiac ischemia and arrhythmias may occur after rapid hormone replacement. For this reason, T_4 (levothyroxine) is probably safer than parenteral T_3 (triiodothyronine) because the onset of action is somewhat delayed (≈ 6 hours). If ischemia or arrhythmias occur, the dosage of thyroid hormone should be decreased.

Glucocorticoids are usually recommended for two reasons. The hypothalamic–pituitary axis may be depressed because of the severe stress of myxedema coma, and steroids may prevent the subsequent onset of addisonian crisis. In patients with secondary hypothyroidism, there will be coexistent adrenal failure.

Other treatment for myxedema is largely supportive. Hypothermia should be corrected by passive rewarming if possible. Hypoglycemia is treated with intravenous glucose and hypoventilation by mechanical ventilation. Although hyponatremia is usually not severe, it may on occasion require treatment with hypertonic saline rather than simple fluid restriction. If hypotension is present, careful volume expansion is indicated to avoid congestive heart failure. Although pericardial effusion is common, tamponade is rare. Large doses of corticosteroids should not be given because they will

---

DRUG TREATMENT: MYXEDEMA COMA

First-Line Drug

Levothyroxine

Initial Dose	300–500 µg IV over 10–15 minutes
Repeat Dose	50–100 µg/day IV or PO
End-Points	Normal thyroid function tests
	Resolution of symptoms
	Arrhythmias

Second-Line Drug

Hydrocortisone

Initial Dose	100 mg by IV push
Repeat Dose	50–100 mg by IV push every 6 hours
End-Point	Resolution of symptoms

interfere with the peripheral conversion of T_4 to T_3.

Thyroid Storm

Diagnosis

Thyroid hormones exert a multitude of effects. Their main role is in the regulation of growth, maturation, and metabolism. The exact mechanism by which these functions are effected remains unknown. The thyroid hormones are iodinated amino acids. The thyroid gland synthesizes mostly thyroxine (T_4) and a small amount of triiodothyronine (T_3). T_4 can be converted by deiodination to T_3, and this conversion usually occurs in peripheral tissues. Levels of T_3, the most potent form of the hormone, appear to be strictly controlled in normal individuals by negative feedback mechanisms.

Hyperthyroidism occurs with excess circulating levels of thyroid hormones. The most common cause is the autoimmune disorder, Graves disease. In Graves disease, an antibody to the thyroid-stimulating hormone (TSH) receptor on the thyroid cells is present. During the initial stages of the disease the thyroid responds to this antibody as if it were being stimulated by TSH. The excess hormones affect most organ systems, accelerating the rate of metabolism in most tissues.

Hyperthyroid patients will usually have an antecedent history of symptoms: anxiety, restlessness, fatigue, weight loss, heat intolerance, frequent bowel movements, or decreased menses. Signs of hyperthyroidism include tachycardia, atrial fibrillation, elevated systolic blood pressure with a resultant wide pulse pressure, thin moist skin and fine hair, fine tremor, decreased motor strength, lid lag, and increased deep tendon reflexes. An enlarged thyroid gland may be palpable. Findings in Graves disease include pretibial myxedema and ocular signs of ophthalmoplegia, periorbital edema, chemosis, or exophthalmos.

Thyroid storm is the most severe form of hyperthyroidism. It is characterized by the presence of cardiac failure, altered mental status or coma, and fever. Thyroid storm usually occurs as a consequence of an acute stressor in a hyperthyroid individual.

The diagnosis is made on the basis of history and physical examination, since results of confirmatory tests are not readily available.

Indications for Treatment

Thyroid storm requires emergent empiric therapy. Other suspected cases of hyperthyroidism can and should await results of confirmatory thyroid function testing prior to initiating specific therapy. (See box.)

Discussion

The treatment of thyroid storm includes supportive and specific therapy. Supportive measures include hemodynamic support (fluids, vasopressors, digoxin), standard measures to care for the comatose patient (airway protection, ventilatory support, etc.), and reduction of fever. The preferred antipyretic is acetaminophen. Aspirin has the potential to increase free hormone levels by interfering with thyroid hormone binding to serum protein carriers.

Specific therapy is aimed at reducing hormone synthesis, reducing the release of hormone from the thyroid, reducing peripheral conversion of T_4 to T_3, and blocking the effects of hormone at target organs.

The most important aspect of specific therapy is to block the peripheral effects of excess thyroid hormone. These effects are mediated by adrenergic catecholamines; therefore, the current treatment consists of beta-adrenergic blockade with propranolol. Initial treatment should be parenteral administration of propranolol, 1 to 2 mg IV. This may be repeated at 15-minute intervals until a desired effect is attained. Beta-adrenergic blockade can ameliorate a number of the signs and symptoms of hyperthyroidism, e.g., tachydysrhythmias, palpitations, agitation, tremor, and fever. The usual precautions and contraindications to the use of propranolol should be followed. A tachycardic patient in heart failure should probably receive inotropic support with digoxin initially, followed by the cautious use of propranolol if the cardiac failure is deemed to be rate related.

Propylthiouracil and methimazole are thionamides that inhibit hormone synthesis by preventing coupling of mono-iodotyrosenes and di-iodotyrosenes. Propylthiouracil is preferred because it has the advantage of inhibiting peripheral conversion of T_4 to T_3 at doses >800 mg/day. It is given orally or by nasogastric tube at a dose of 900 to 1200

DRUG TREATMENT: THYROID STORM

First-Line Drug
Propranolol

Initial Dose	1–2 mg IV
Repeat Dose	1 mg every 15 minutes to ameliorate symptoms
End-Points	Resolution of tachydysrhythmias, agitation, tremor

Second-Line Drugs
Propylthiouracil

Initial Dose	300 mg PO
Repeat Dose	300 mg PO every 6 hours
End-Point	Euthyroid state

OR

Methimazole

Initial Dose	30 mg PO
Repeat Dose	30 mg every 6 hours
End-Point	Euthyroid state

Third-Line Drug
Dexamethasone

Initial Dose	2 mg by IV push
Repeat Dose	2 mg IV every 6 hours
End-Point	Euthyroid state

Fourth-Line Drug
Lugol's Solution

Initial Dose	10 gtt PO
Repeat Dose	10 gtt every 8 hours
End-Point	Euthyroid state

Note: Iodine solutions should *not* be given until at least 1 hour after propylthiouracil or methimazole is given!

mg/day in divided doses every 6 or 8 hours. A parenteral form of propylthiouracil does not exist. Methimazole is administered at a dose of 90 to 120 mg/day in divided doses.

One hour after the thionamides are administered, iodine is given to prevent further secretion of hormone from the gland. The thionamide pretreatment is necessary to prevent the organification of the iodine. Iodine is given enterally either as Lugol's solution, 10 gtt, or potassium iodide (ssKI), 5 gtt every 8 hours. Alternatively, sodium iodide, 0.5 g every 8 hours, can be administered intravenously.

Peripheral conversion of T_4 to T_3 is most effectively inhibited by the administration of corticosteroids. Propranolol and propylthiouracil have the capability to inhibit this conversion, but clinically their efficacy is negligible. Dexamethasone, 2 mg every 6 hours, is the recommended corticosteroid. Other advantageous steroid effects include a decrease in hormone secretion by the thyroid and treatment of possible hyperthyroid-induced adrenal insufficiency.

SPECIFIC AGENTS

Calcitonin-Salmon (Calcimar)

Pharmacology

Distribution

The drug distribution is not yet fully determined. It does not cross the placenta. Passage through the blood–brain barrier and into breast milk is not known.

Elimination

Elimination is primarily by the kidneys. The drug is rapidly metabolized in the kidneys and in the blood.

Actions

Calcitonin-salmon lowers serum calcium and phosphate levels. It inhibits bone resorption activity by osteoclasts and osteocytes and increases excretion of calcium, phosphates, and sodium by the kidneys.

Indications

Symptomatic Paget's disease
Hypercalcemia
Postmenopausal osteoporosis

Cautions

Renal failure—no dosage adjustment necessary initially. Subsequent dosages may need to be adjusted.
Cardiac failure—no dosage adjustment necessary
Hepatic failure—no dosage adjustment necessary
Use in pregnancy—Category C. Its teratogenic risk is unknown as no clinical studies have been done. Low birth weight has been reported in rabbits.
Use in children—experience is limited.

Onset and Duration of Action

Dosage

Calcitonin-salmon, 4 Iu/kg subcutaneously or IM.

Although human calcitonin (Cibacalcin) is available, it is not indicated for the treatment of hypercalcemia.

Limits

Therapy of hypercalcemia should be guided by serial calcium determinations.

Repeat Dosing

Every 12 hours initially. Dosage can be increased to a maximum of 8 Iu/kg every 6 hours. Calcitonin resistance may develop after 2 to 3 days of therapy, requiring increased doses.

Toxicity

Drug Interactions

Corticosteroid/plicamycin—inhibit bone resorption

Specific Adverse Effects

Allergic reactions include anaphylaxis, local inflammatory reactions, nausea, and vomiting. Skin testing is advisable prior to parenteral use.

Treatment of Toxicity

Toxicologic data are not available.

Calcium Salts

Pharmacology

Distribution

Calcium is quickly distributed throughout the extracellular fluid compartment. Approximately 40% is bound to plasma proteins, 5 to 10% is chelated to organic anions such as citrate or to inorganic phosphorus, and the remainder is free or ionized. The degree of protein binding and chelation depends on the concentrations of anions, plasma proteins, and hydrogen ions. Calcium freely crosses the placenta.

Elimination

Ionic calcium is freely filtered at the glomerulus but largely reabsorbed in the distal nephron. The degree of reabsorption is affected by PTH, vitamin D, calcitonin, and diuretics. Calcium ions are also secreted in sweat, saliva, bile, pancreatic juices, and breast milk. Under normal circumstances, stool and urinary losses balance intestinal absorption.

Actions

In excitable tissues, calcium ions are involved in the maintenance of membrane stability and the generation of transmembrane potentials. Cardiac, skeletal and smooth muscle cells require calcium for excitation–contraction coupling. Calcium modulates the release of the secretory products of both endocrine and exocrine glands and is involved in the release of neurotransmitters at synaptic junctions. In cardiac tissue, calcium fluxes determine the rate of pacemaker discharge and the generation and maintenance of the plateau phase of the cardiac action potential. Cell-to-cell adhesion and the integrity of epithelial and endothelial membranes are dependent on the availability of ionic calcium.

Indications

Treatment of symptomatic hypocalcemia, asymptomatic hypocalcemia with latent tetany, and states of chronic hypocalcemia

Cautions

Hyperphosphatemia—correction of serum phosphate levels should be accomplished before, or coincident with, administration of calcium salts to prevent metastic soft-tissue calcification.

Digitalis use—calcium potentiates the electrophysiologic effects of digitalis and may exacerbate digitalis toxicity.

Use in pregnancy—calcium crosses placental membranes and is partitioned at higher concentrations in the fetal than in the maternal extracellular fluid. Whether significant clinical effects result from fetal calcium exposure is unknown. Risks versus benefits must be weighed in individual cases, although the potential for mortality in acute hypocalcemia generally mandates administration of calcium salts when this condition occurs during pregnancy.

Chronic lung disease/chronic renal failure—calcium chloride should be avoided in these settings due to the acidifying effect of chloride ions.

Cardiac failure—no dosage adjustment needed

Hepatic failure—no dosage adjustment needed

Use in children—may be used

Dosage

Initial dose: 100 to 300 mg elemental calcium IV over 10 to 15 minutes

Repeat dose: 100 to 300 mg elemental calcium every 6 to 8 hours, or continuous infusion of 1 to 2 mg/kg/hour

Toxicity

In the absence of iatrogenic hypercalcemia during therapy, calcium salts are without significant toxic effects except in the settings of hyperphosphatemia or digitalis toxicity. Hypercalcemia (serum total calcium exceeding 11 mg/dl) can present with weakness, lethargy, coma, nausea, vomiting, abdominal pain, or polyuria/polydipsia, although symptoms are seldom prominent when serum levels are less than 14 mg/dl. Rapid parenteral administration of calcium can result in bradycardia, hypotension, and syncope.

Colchicine

Pharmacology

Metabolism

Hepatic

Excretion

Primarily biliary; 10 to 20% renal. Elimination of drug may require up to 10 days because of high tissue uptake.

Half-Life

20 minutes for distribution and 60 minutes for elimination

Mechanism of Action

Decreases leukocyte mobility, phagocytosis, and lactic acid production with decrease in inflammatory response and deposition of uric acid crystals

Indications

Acute gouty arthritis
Familial Mediterranean fever
Pseudogout
Paget's disease

Cautions

Renal failure—when used chronically, doses may need to be decreased. Acute dosage is unchanged.

Hepatic failure—may accumulate excessive drug with chronic use. Acute dosage is unchanged.

Cardiac failure—may cause hypertension and vasocontriction. Use with caution.

Use in pregnancy—Category D. Should not be used. Excretion in breast milk is unknown.

Use in childhood—should not be used
Blood dyscrasias—may be exacerbated

Onset and Duration of Action

Dosage

Initial: 2 mg IV diluted in 20 ml of saline by slow IV push

Repeat Dose

0.5 to 1 mg every 4 to 6 hours until relief; not to exceed 4 to 5 mg daily

Toxicity

Drug Interactions

Alcohol—increased GI toxicity
Bone marrow depressants—additive toxicity
Vitamin B$_{12}$—absorption diminished

Adverse Reactions

Thrombophlebitis at injection site
Peripheral neuritis (chronic use)
Bone marrow depression (chronic use)
Nausea, vomiting
Stomach pain

Treatment of Toxicity

Discontinue drug.
Supportive care

Corticosteroids

Pharmacology

Distribution

About 90% of circulating hormone is protein bound to albumin and corticosteroid-binding protein. The free fraction of the hormone is biologically active. Steroid hormones freely enter cells.

Elimination

About 90% of circulating glucocorticoids are metabolized in the liver. The remainder are metabolized in peripheral tissues. Metabolites may retain some degree of biologic activity. Metabolites are primarily excreted in urine.

Actions

In sensitive tissues, glucocorticoids are bound by cytoplasmic receptors. Hormone–receptor complexes migrate to the nucleus, where they interact with nucleochromatin to promote the elaboration of specific messenger ribonucleic acids. These serve as templates for protein synthesis.

The glucocorticoids regulate intermediary metabolism, promoting hepatic gluconeogenesis and glycogen synthesis. Peripheral lipolysis and protein catabolism are stimulated, and peripheral glucose utilization is inhibited. As such, metabolic substrate for essential tissues is provided through the action of glucocorticoids. This is of particular importance in the setting of acute physiologic stress. Glucocorticoids also exert permissive effects on the actions of catecholamines on the cardiovascular system, allowing hemodynamic responses appropriate to the physiologic status of the organism.

Mineralocorticoids enhance sodium resorption in the distal nephron, promoting expansion of the extracellular fluid compartment. Excretion of hydrogen and potassium ions is facilitated by mineralocorticoids. Milligram for milligram, hydrocortisone has only one-four-hundredth of the mineralocorticoid activity of aldosterone. However, in stress doses hydrocortisone possesses adequate mineralocorticoid activity to facilitate reexpansion of intravascular volume in acute primary adrenal insufficiency.

Indications

Replacement therapy in acute or chronic adrenal insufficiency
Anti-inflammatory therapy of immunologically mediated diseases and neoplasms
Acute spinal cord injury

Cautions

Renal failure—no dosage adjustment necessary in acute management
Congestive heart failure—because of the potential for sodium and fluid retention secondary to mineralocorticoid effects, these drugs must be used cautiously in patients with cardiomyopathy.
Hepatic failure—no dosage adjustment is necessary in acute management, but chronic therapy may need to be modified to allow for reduced glucocorticoid metabolism in hepatic failure.
Use in pregnancy—no studies have specifically addressed the safety of glucocorticoids in pregnancy. There are reports of increased incidence of cleft lip and palate when used in the first trimester. Chronic exogenous maternal glucocorticoid therapy is a significant cause of neonatal functional hypoadrenalism. Risk versus benefit must be weighed in the use of these compounds during pregnancy.

Use during lactation—breast milk is known to contain a fraction of circulating levels of glucocorticoids. It is unknown whether exposure to exogenous steroids in breast milk is harmful when levels are maintained in the physiologic range.

Use in children—corticosteroids may be used in children. Complications are similar to those in adults and more related to chronic usage.

Dosage

Adrenal crisis: hydrocortisone sodium phosphate or sodium hemisuccinate, 100 mg by IV bolus, then continuous infusion of 100 mg every 6 to 8 hours

Chronic adrenal insufficiency: hydrocortisone, 20 to 40 mg PO every day, usually divided bid

Other: no firm dosage guidelines exist for the dosage of glucocorticoids in the treatment of immunologically mediated diseases or for adjunctive therapy of neoplasms.

Spinal cord injury: 30 mg/kg methylprednisolone IV over 1 hour, then 5.4 mg/kg/hour for 23 hours

No dosage limits have been determined.

Onset and Duration

Hydrocortisone is considered to be a short-acting glucocorticoid with an onset of action that is attained within 1 hour of intravenous dosing, and peak effects are attained at 4 to 6 hours. The half-life is 12 hours. Prednisone is intermediate-acting with a half-life of 12 to 36 hours. Long-acting preparations have a half-life of 36 to 72 hours and include dexamethasone.

Toxicity

Drug Interactions

Aspirin/nonsteroidal anti-inflammatory drugs (NSAIDs)—the risk of GI ulceration and bleeding is increased by concomitant use of exogenous glucocorticoids and NSAIDs. The metabolism of salicylates is induced by glucocorticoids, and lower salicylate levels can be expected.

Estrogens—estrogens potentiate the effects of hydrocortisone through enhanced protein binding and subsequent decreased availability for metabolic destruction.

Hepatic microsomal inducers—barbiturates, cimetidine, rifampin, phenytoin, and other drugs that induce hepatic microsomes stimulate metabolism of glucocorticoids and may alter dosing needs in chronic therapy.

Potassium-depleting drugs—diuretics or other drugs that promote renal excretion of potassium will enhance the potassium-wasting effects of glucocorticoids.

Anticoagulants—cortisone may increase the coagulability of blood, requiring increased dosage of oral anticoagulants.

Diabetic medications—glucocorticoids are diabetogenic due to effects on hepatic glucose handling and peripheral glucose utilization. Dosages of insulin or oral hypoglycemics may need to be increased during concomitant therapy with hydrocortisone.

Adverse Effects

Acute administration of even massive doses of glucocorticoids is usually well tolerated without significant side effects. Chronic administration can result in a variety of adverse reactions, many of which result from an exaggeration of the normal physiologic effect of the hormone.

Renal effects—sodium retention, volume overload, hypokalemic alkalosis, hypertension

Musculoskeletal effects—steroid myopathy, muscle wasting, generalized weakness, osteopenia

Gastrointestinal effects—peptic ulcers, GI bleeding, esophagitis, pancreatitis, nausea, vomiting, constipation, diarrhea, anorexia, or hyperphagia

Ocular effects—subcapsular cataracts, increased intraocular pressure

Endocrine effects—hypercorticism, amenorrhea, glucose intolerance or frank diabetes, functional adrenal insufficiency, adrenal crisis after abrupt withdrawal of therapy or physiologic stress

Neurologic effects—headache, mood swings, psychosis, vertigo, and seizures

Dermatologic effects—thinning and fragility of the skin, acneform rash, striae, hirsutism, and easy bruising

Immunologic effects—relative immunosuppression, increased susceptibility to infection, masked response to infection

Edrophonium Chloride (Tensilon)

Pharmacology

Distribution

An intravenous dose of edrophonium rapidly distributes throughout the extracellular fluid, interacting with Ach receptors on skeletal muscle within 30 seconds of administration. The drug is not protein bound. Edrophonium does not cross the blood–brain barrier to any clinically significant extent at normal dosages.

Elimination

The metabolism and excretory pathways for edrophonium have not been clarified.

Actions

Edrophonium reversibly binds to the anionic site of acetylcholinesterase, interfering with the hydrolytic destruction of Ach. This action enhances the interaction of Ach with postsynaptic receptors at autonomic ganglia and the neuromuscular junction. Cholinomimetic effects produce bronchial and ureteric constriction, increased secretion from exocrine glands, increased intestinal motility and tone, miosis, bradycardia, and enhanced neuromuscular transmission.

Indications

Edrophonium is the drug of choice for the diagnosis of myasthenia gravis. The drug may also be used to assess the adequacy of ongoing anticholinesterase therapy and to differentiate between myasthenic crisis and cholinergic crisis. Edrophonium can be used to antagonize neuromuscular blockade with the nondepolarizing neuromuscular blocking agents, although its short duration of action limits its usefulness for this purpose. Edrophonium has been used in the treatment of supraventricular tachycardias but is not approved for this purpose.

Contraindication

Known hypersensitivity

Cautions

Renal failure—no dosage adjustments are necessary.
Hepatic failure—no dosage adjustments are necessary.
Cardiac failure—carefully titrated dosing is indicated to avoid significant bradycardia. If bradycardia is present, the heart rate should be increased to >80 by pretreatment with atropine.
Use in pregnancy—Category C
Use in childhood—may be used in pediatric patients
Pulmonary disease—edrophonium is capable of inducing bronchospasm and should be used with caution in patients with asthma or chronic obstructive pulmonary disease.
Other—should be used with caution in patients with epilepsy, bradycardia, or other cardiac dysrhythmias

Dosage

For the diagnosis of myasthenia gravis, edrophonium is given as a 2-mg bolus over 15 to 30 seconds, with an additional 8 mg to follow if no response is observed within 1 minute. The intramuscular dosage is 10 mg. In children weighing less than 34 kg, the dose is 0.2 mg/kg IV with 20% given as the initial dose over 1 minute and the remainder to follow if no response is noted. The dosage in infants should not exceed 0.5 mg IV.

For the differentiation of myasthenic and cholinergic crises, 1 mg is given IV. This dose is repeated in 1 minute if no response is observed.

Toxicity

Drug Interactions

Edrophonium antagonizes the action of nondepolarizing neuromuscular blocking agents and also reverses phase II neuromuscular blockade with depolarizing agents. The brevity of these effects limits their clinical significance. In contrast, phase I depolarizing neuromuscular blockade is enhanced by edrophonium.

The actions of edrophonium on the cardiac conduction system are potentiated by digitalis glycosides, and high-grade atrioventricular block or asystole can result with concurrent use.

Use of edrophonium in patients on anticholinesterases can precipitate cholinergic crisis.

Specific Adverse Effects

Cardiac—bradycardia, atrioventricular block, asystole
Central nervous system—dysarthria, dysphonia, seizures

Respiratory—laryngospasm, increased secretions, bronchoconstriction, respiratory muscle paralysis

Gastrointestinal—salivation, increased gastric and intestinal secretion, nausea, vomiting, diarrhea, increased peristalsis, cramping

Ocular—lacrimation, miosis, diplopia, spasm of accommodation, conjunctival injection

Genitourinary—urinary frequency, incontinence

Skin—diaphoresis

Treatment of Toxicity

Discontinue drug.

Atropine antagonizes the muscarinic effects of edrophonium and is useful in treatment of these effects in edrophonium toxicity.

Etidronate Disodium (Didronel)

Pharmacology

Etidronate inhibits the formation and dissolution of bone hydroxyapatite crystals. The drug acts by direct chemisorption to calcium phosphate surfaces.

Distribution

Only 1 to 5% of an orally administered dose is adsorbed. The drug is rapidly distributed after intravenous administration and chemically adsorbed by bone, particularly in areas of active osteogenesis. The volume of distribution is 1370 ml/kg with a serum half-life of 6.0 hours after IV administration.

Elimination

Etidronate is not metabolized. Unadsorbed drug is excreted unchanged in the feces. About 50% of adsorbed or intravenously administered drug is excreted unchanged in the urine within 24 hours. Etidronate that has been adsorbed by bone is very gradually eliminated, unchanged, by the kidneys. The half-life of bone-adsorbed etidronate is 90 days.

Actions

The major pharmacologic action of etidronate is the reduction of bone resorption. This action results in a decrease in ionized serum calcium. Decreased resorption also results in increased serum phosphate concentrations.

Indications

Intravenous etidronate is indicated for the treatment of severe hypercalcemia of malignancy that cannot be controlled with hydration or dietary modification. Simultaneous saline hydration and loop diuretic administration are recommended.

Cautions

Renal failure—excess calcium is excreted by the kidneys after etidronate administration. The drug should not be administered to patients with high-grade renal impairment (serum creatinine >5.0 mg/dl). Some patients with preexisting renal disease will manifest elevations of blood urea nitrogen and serum creatinine in response to etidronate therapy. Since the drug is excreted unchanged by the kidney, a reduction of dosage should be considered in patients with serum creatinine >2.5 mg/dl and <5.0 mg/dl.

Cardiac failure—etidronate has no direct toxic effects on the myocardium. Saline hydration is required with etidronate therapy. Patients with congestive heart failure will require adequate diuretic administration during etidronate therapy.

Hepatic failure—no dosage adjustment required

Pregnancy—Category C. Long-term studies in rats have not shown any carcinogenic effects. Animal reproductive studies have not been performed.

Pediatric patients—safety and effectiveness in pediatric patients have not been established.

Dosage

The initial dose of intravenous etidronate is 7.5 mg/kg in 250 ml of normal saline over 2 to 4 hours. Infusion over less than 2 hours is associated with complications (see Toxicity).

Limits

Daily dosage should not exceed 7.5 mg/kg.

Repeat Dosing

The initial dose is usually repeated daily for 3 days. Treatment can be continued for up to 7 days, although hypocalcemia is more likely to occur with longer treatment. The 3-

day course of treatment may be repeated if hypercalcemia recurs or fails to respond to the initial course. At least 7 days should separate the initial course of treatment and repeat treatment intervals.

Toxicity

Adverse Effects

Approximately 10% of patients treated with this drug will develop elevated levels of serum creatinine and mild worsening of renal impairment. These changes are usually reversible after the end of a course of therapy. Renal function should be monitored during treatment. Patients with baseline serum creatinine >2.5 mg/dl should receive a reduced dosage. Patients with serum creatinine levels >5.0 mg/dl should not receive the drug.

Infusion of the drug at a rate faster than 7.5 mg/kg/2 hours is not recommended. Rapid intravenous infusion in animals has been associated with electrocardiographic abnormalities and bleeding problems. These adverse effects are most likely caused by rapid decreases in ionized serum calcium levels, probably due to direct chelation of calcium by the drug. Higher doses or faster rates of infusion may also impair renal function.

Treatment of Toxicity

Elevated serum creatinine and renal function usually revert to pretreatment levels after etidronate therapy is discontinued.

In animal studies, electrocardiographic abnormalities and bleeding problems associated with rapid intravenous infusion are rapidly reversed with calcium administration.

Indomethacin (Indocin, Novamethicin, Indocid)

Pharmacology

Mechanism Action

Inhibits cyclo-oxygenase, thereby decreasing prostaglandin production

Kinetics

Oral absorption rapid (90% within 4 hours)
Distribution half-life = 1 hour
Elimination half-life = 4.5 hours but subject to individual variation

Excretion

60% renal, 33% biliary
Excreted in breast milk
Not dialyzable

Indications

Arthritis
Gouty arthritis, pseudogout
Nonrheumatic inflammation
Treatment of patent ductus arteriosus

Cautions

Renal failure—may exacerbate or cause renal failure; should not be used in patients with chronic renal failure
Hepatic failure—increased incidence of renal failure
Cardiac failure—may cause renal failure in patient with marginal cardiac function
Use in pregnancy—should not be used
Use in childhood—toxicity is greater.
Peptic ulcer disease—may exacerbate and cause GI bleeding
Aspirin hypersensitivity—contraindicated
Systemic lupus—contraindicated

Dosage

The dosage for acute gouty arthritis is 100 mg initially, then 50 mg every 6 to 8 hours, not to exceed 300 mg/day. Dosage should be tapered as soon as pain relief is obtained.

Toxicity

Drug Interactions

NSAIDS, steroids—increased GI ulceration
Triamterene—may cause renal failure
Anticoagulants—increased GI bleeding
Lithium—increased lithium toxicity
Probenicid—increased indomethacin toxicity
Platelet inhibitors—increased GI bleeding

Adverse Reactions

Headache—>10%
Confusion, GI bleeding, fluid retention, depression, tinnitus—1%
Abdominal pain, diarrhea, hematuria, seizures, peripheral neuropathy, renal failure, hepatitis, decreased hearing—<1%

Treatment of Toxicity

Discontinue drug.
Supportive care

Insulin, Regular

Pharmacology

Absorption and Distribution

An intravenous dose of regular insulin rapidly distributes throughout the extracellular fluid compartment with peak plasma levels occurring 2 to 4 minutes after administration. Intramuscular dosage produces peak levels 50 to 60 minutes after injection, whereas subcutaneous insulin yields a plasma peak at 90 to 120 minutes. Absorption after subcutaneous dosage shows surprising variability within individuals (up to 25% difference in levels) and between patients (up to 50% difference in levels). Subcutaneous and intramuscular absorption is delayed by cigarette smoking, low ambient temperature, and the presence of anti-insulin antibodies. Absorption is facilitated by local massage, increased temperature, or exercise of the area injected. Subcutaneous absorption from the abdomen tends to be most rapid and reproducible.

Elimination

Insulin is metabolized primarily in the liver, with lesser sites of degradation in the kidney and in skeletal muscle. About 50% of insulin in portal blood undergoes first-pass hepatic metabolism. Insulin is freely filtered at the glomerulus; 98% of the filtered load is reabsorbed in the proximal tubule, and 60% of reabsorbed insulin is metabolized in the renal tubular epithelium. Renal degradation can partially compensate for reduced hepatic metabolism in the setting of liver disease.

Actions

Insulin binds to specific cell surface receptors and alters cellular metabolism through a mechanism that appears to involve cyclic nucleotides. Insulin inhibits adenylate cyclase and stimulates cyclic nucleotide phosphodiesterase, resulting in decreased intracellular cyclic adenosine monophosphate (cAMP) concentration. This effect is most pronounced when cAMP synthesis has been activated by the prior action of counterregulatory hormones. Glucose transport into hepatocytes, skeletal muscle cells, and adipocytes is enhanced by insulin, with stimulation of glycogen synthesis and inhibition of glycogenolysis and gluconeogenesis. Lipolysis is inhibited, and fat synthesis is promoted. Cellular uptake of amino acids and subsequent protein synthesis are increased. In addition to anabolic effects on intermediary metabolism, insulin results in shifts of K^+ and Mg^{2+} from extracellular fluid to the intracellular fluid compartment.

Indications

Type I diabetes mellitus
Type II diabetes when weight loss, diet, and oral hypoglycemic agents have failed to maintain glycemic control

Cautions

Cardiac failure—no dosage adjustments are necessary.
Hepatic failure—no dosage adjustments are necessary.
Renal failure—insulin half-life can be prolonged in renal failure and may necessitate dosage adjustment to avoid hypoglycemia.
Use in pregnancy—insulin has not been demonstrated to have teratogenic effects, and the benefits of use during pregnancy are considered to outweigh any risks to the fetus. Insulin does not cross the placental membrane.
Use in lactation—the extent of excretion of insulin in breast milk is unknown. Because insulin is destroyed by the action of proteolytic enzymes in the gut, it is unlikely that the insulin content of breast milk has any significant consequences for the nursing infant.
Use in children—may be used

Dosage

Maintenance dosing of subcutaneous insulin for the long-term management of diabetes requires titration to a desired level of control in the individual patient. Dosage recommendations below are for use in diabetic ketoacidosis or nonketotic hyperglycemic hyperosmolar state. Intravenous administration is preferred given the potential for erratic absorption of intramuscular insulin in the setting of hypovolemia and reduced peripheral perfusion. When available, recombinant human insulin should be used due to reduced immunogenic potential over purified animal insulins. The initial dose is 0.2 to 0.4 unit/kg regular insulin by IV push or IM. This may be repeated if serum glucose fails to fall by 80 to 100 mg/dl in the first hour of therapy. Infusion dosage is 0.1 to 0.15 unit/kg/hour by continuous IV infusion or every hour IM.

Toxicity

Drug Interactions

Enhanced hypoglycemic effect: oral hypoglycemics, ethanol, monoamine oxidase inhibitors, salicylate, anabolic steroids

Reduced hypoglycemic effect: cortisol, oral contraceptives, diazoxide, phenytoin, thiazides, loop diuretics, epinephrine, beta-blockers

Specific Adverse Effects

Cutaneous: local irritation, lipoatrophy

Immunologic: anaphylaxis, insulin resistance

Metabolic: hypoglycemia, rebound hyperglycemia

Levothyroxine (Levothyroid, Noroxine, Synthroid)

Pharmacology

Distribution

More than 99% is bound in the circulation to carrier proteins. The free hormone distributes to all tissues.

Elimination

Thyroxine is metabolized in the liver. There is enterohepatic circulation so only 20 to 40% of metabolized hormone is excreted in stool. Converting enzymes in the circulation result in inactive metabolites such as reverse T_3.

Actions

Levothyroxine binds to intracellular receptors to stimulate mRNA and protein synthesis. It acts on most tissues, notably the heart, liver, and kidneys, to stimulate a hyperdynamic, hypermetabolic state. Heat is generated as a consequence. Glucose utilization is increased but compensatory stimulation of GI glucose uptake, lipolysis, and gluconeogenesis occurs.

Indications

Supplemental therapy of thyroxine deficiency

Suppression of pituitary thyrotropin release

Diagnostic agent in thyroid suppression tests

Cautions

Renal failure—no dosage adjustment necessary. Nephrosis reduces plasma proteins, thus total T_4 may appear low.

Cardiac failure—caution should be used in cardiac disease as thyroxine increases oxygen demand and may exacerbate ischemic disease. However, the benefit of its use in heart failure due to hypothyroidism and myxedema coma far outweighs the risks.

Hepatic failure—no dosage adjustment necessary for initial emergent therapy. Maintenance therapy must be adjusted based on thyroid function testing.

Use in pregnancy—Category A. No dosage adjustment necessary. Thyroid hormone does not cross the placenta well. There are no adverse effects on the fetus in mothers on thyroxine. Women should not discontinue therapy during pregnancy.

Use in children—may be used

Onset and Duration of Action

Dosage

For myxedema coma, the dosage is 300 to 500 μg (100 μg/ml) IV. Clinical improvement is often delayed and may not be evident for 12 hours.

Limits

Determined by thyroid function testing or development of cardiac side effects

Repeat Dosing

Not necessary for 12 to 24 hours

Toxicity

Drug Interactions

Oral anticoagulants—T_4 may increase catabolism of vitamin K–dependent clotting factors. Protein binding decreased by dicumarol.

Insulin/oral hypoglycemic agents—may increase dosage requirement

Cholestyramine—binds T_4 and T_3

Estrogen/oral contraceptives—increase thyroxine-binding globulin

Salicylates—decrease protein binding

Specific Adverse Effects

Signs and symptoms of hyperthyroidism

Treatment of Toxicity

Reduce dosage. Treatment is supportive and symptomatic. Specific therapy for hyperthyroidism is rarely necessary.

Methimazole (Tapazole)

Pharmacology

Methimazole is a thioamide derivative similar to propylthiouracil (PTU). It inhibits synthesis of thyroid hormone by inhibiting incorporation of iodide into tyrosine and inhibiting coupling of iodotyrosines.

Elimination

Methimazole is metabolized in the liver and excreted in the urine. Only 7% is excreted as unchanged drug. Its half-life is 4 to 14 hours.

Indications

Treatment of hyperthyroidism and thyroid storm

Cautions

Pregnancy—Category D. Methimazole crosses the placenta and is known to cause adverse effects in the fetus.
Hepatic failure—may cause hepatotoxicity. Methimazole is more hepatotoxic than PTU and should probably not be used in patients with severe liver disease.
Renal failure—no dosage adjustment necessary
Cardiac failure—no dosage adjustment necessary
Use in childhood—may be used

Dosage

Severe hyperthyroidism: 60 mg/day at 8-hour intervals for 6 to 8 weeks
Thyroid storm: 30 mg every 6 hours for 1 day, then 20 mg every 8 hours for 6 to 8 weeks
Children: 0.4 mg/kg/day divided into 3 doses at 8-hour intervals

Toxicity

Drug Interactions

Anticoagulants (coumarin, heparin)—methimazole may enhance anticoagulant effects.
Bone marrow depressants—risk of agranulocytosis increased
Hepatotoxic medications—increased toxicity
Lithium, potassium iodide—hypothyroid effects enhanced

Adverse Effects

Agranulocytosis (incidence 0.2 to 1.6%)
Cholestatic hepatitis
Skin rash (incidence 3 to 5%)
Dizziness, loss of taste, nausea, peripheral neuropathy

Treatment of Toxicity

Discontinue drug.
Agranulocytosis and cholestatic hepatitis should resolve after drug discontinuation.

Neostigmine Methylsulfate (Prostigmin)

Pharmacology

Distribution

Neostigmine crosses the placental membrane and blood–brain barrier poorly due to its quaternary ammonium structure. However, high doses can produce central nervous system effects and result in measurable levels in the fetal circulation. Neostigmine is not secreted in breast milk. Approximately 15 to 20% of the drug is bound to plasma proteins.

Elimination

Neostigmine is hydrolyzed by serum cholinesterases, with lesser metabolism via the hepatic microsomal system. Both the parent drug and its metabolites are excreted in the urine. The elimination half-life is 45 to 60 minutes after intravenous or intramuscular dosing.

Actions

Neostigmine competitively inhibits the hydrolysis of acetylcholine at the neuromuscular junction and in autonomic ganglia, enhancing cholinergic transmission. At the motor end-plate, the amplitude of the MEPP is increased, with subsequent potentiation of the formation of the EPP and muscle action potential. This is reflected as improved motor strength for a given delivered stimulus. In autonomic ganglia, neostigmine produces muscarinic effects, resulting in miosis, bradycardia, and increased exocrine secretion, intestinal peristalsis, and bronchial muscle tone.

Indications

Control of symptoms of myasthenia gravis when oral therapy is insufficient or impractical

Differential diagnosis of myasthenia gravis when lengthy muscle strength testing is anticipated

Reversal of nondepolarizing neuromuscular blockade postoperatively

Treatment of postoperative urinary retention when obstructive causes have been ruled out

Contraindications

Known hypersensitivity, mechanical obstruction of the intestinal or urinary tracts, peritonitis

Cautions

Cardiac failure—carefully titrated dosing is indicated to avoid significant bradycardia. If bradycardia is present, the heart rate should be increased to >80 by pretreatment with atropine.

Use in pregnancy—Category C. In late pregnancy, neostigmine can precipitate premature labor. When neostigmine is used to enhance muscle strength during labor in myasthenic patients, transient weakness has been found in 10 to 20% of the delivered neonates.

Use in lactation—neostigmine has not been detected in breast milk. Use in lactation involves balancing potential risks to the infant with maternal benefit.

Use in childhood—safety has not been established, but neostigmine has been used in pediatric patients.

Pulmonary disease—neostigmine is capable of inducing bronchospasm and should be used with caution in patients with asthma or chronic obstructive pulmonary disease.

Other—should be used with caution in patients with epilepsy, bradycardia, or hyperthyroidism

Dosage

For parenteral therapy of adult myasthenia gravis, the dosage is 0.5 to 2.5 mg IM, by slow IV push, or subcutaneously. Dosage in children is 0.025 to 0.04 mg/kg IM. Neonatal dosage is 0.1 to 0.2 mg subcutaneously or 0.03 mg/kg IM. Dosing can be repeated every 2 to 6 hours as needed. During therapy, atropine should be available to antagonize muscarinic side effects. Pretreatment with 0.01 to 0.02 mg atropine sulfate is advocated by some authors when neostigmine is to be used intravenously.

Toxicity

Drug Interactions

Depolarizing neuromuscular blocking agents—neostigmine can prolong phase I of neuromuscular blockade with succinylcholine and decamethonium. Phase II neuromuscular blockade with these agents is antagonized.

Nondepolarizing neuromuscular blocking agents—neostigmine reverses neuromuscular blockade with gallamine and curare compounds.

Specific Adverse Effects

Central nervous system—seizures, headache, dizziness, decreased level of consciousness, dysarthria

Ocular—miosis, lacrimation, visual changes

Cardiovascular—bradycardia, high-grade atrioventricular block, asystole, syncope, hypotension

Respiratory—bronchospasm, dyspnea, respiratory arrest, increased oropharyngeal and bronchial secretions

Gastrointestinal—nausea, vomiting, increased peristalsis, abdominal cramps

Genitourinary—urinary frequency

Dermatologic—flushing, diaphoresis, rash, urticaria

Musculoskeletal—weakness, cramps, arthralgias, myalgias

Allergic—anaphylaxis

Treatment of Toxicity

Discontinue drug.

Atropine may be used to antagonize muscarinic effects.

Plicamycin (Mithramycin, Mithracin)

Pharmacology

Distribution

Greatest concentrations in liver, kidney tubules, and bone. No protein binding in blood. The drug crosses the blood–brain barrier.

Elimination

Cleared from blood within 2 hours. Renal excretion is also rapid: 67% in 4 hours, 75% in 8 hours, and 90% by 24 hours.

Actions

Plicamycin is a cytotoxic antibiotic that intercalates in deoxyribonucleic acid, inhibiting nucleic acid and protein synthesis, It also has a cytotoxic activity unrelated to DNA. It has direct action on osteoclastic function and response to PTH. It may inhibit vitamin D activity.

Indications

Symptomatic hypercalcemic or hypercalciuric patients
Treatment of disseminated testicular carcinomas

Contraindications

Thrombocytopenia
Coagulation disorders

Cautions

Renal failure—relative contraindication since nephrotoxic and clearance primarily by kidneys
Cardiac failure—no dosage adjustment necessary
Hepatic failure—relative contraindication since hepatotoxic
Use in pregnancy—Category X; contraindicated in pregnancy and breastfeeding
Use in children—contraindicated

Onset and Duration of Action

Dosage

Plicamycin, 25 μg/kg ideal body weight, diluted in 1 liter 5% dextrose or normal saline, administered by slow IV infusion over 4 to 6 hours.

Limits

Toxicity usually intervenes.

Repeat Dosing

Daily for 4 days for treatment of hypercalcemia

Toxicity

Drug Interactions

Antineoplastic agents—increased toxic potential
Anticoagulants/salicylates—bleeding diathesis

Adverse Effects

Hemorrhagic diathesis—impairs clotting factors
Bone marrow toxicity—pancytopenia
Hepatotoxic
Nephrotoxic
Electrolyte abnormalities—hypocalcemia, hypophosphatemia, hypokalemia

Treatment of Toxicity

Discontinue drug. Provide supportive measures for specific toxic side effects.

Propylthiouracil (Propyl-Thyracil)

Pharmacology

Distribution

The drug is present in serum 5 minutes after oral administration. Peak levels occur in approximately 1 hour. It is concentrated in the thyroid. The drug can cross the placenta and is found in breast milk.

Elimination

Majority of drug is excreted in the urine.

Actions

It inhibits peroxidase enzyme, thereby inhibiting the coupling of iodotyrosyl residues into iodotyronines (T_3, T_4). It interferes with iodination of tyrosyls and inhibits peripheral conversion of T_4 to T_3.

Indication

Hyperthyroidism

Cautions

Renal failure—no adjustment of initial dosage necessary. Subsequent doses may need to be adjusted.
Cardiac failure—no dosage adjustment necessary
Hepatic failure—may exacerbate hepatic dysfunction
Use in pregnancy—Category D. PTU

crosses the placenta and can cause fetal goiter and hypothyroidism. Breast milk concentration is approximately 10% of that of serum.

Use in children—may be used

Dosage

In thyroid storm, PTU should be given orally or by nasogastric tube at a dose of 600 to 900 mg/day divided in 3 or 4 doses. A parenteral form does not exist.

Toxicity

Drug Interactions

Bone marrow suppressants—may increase agranulocytosis

Specific Adverse Effects

Dizziness
Rash
Metallic taste in the mouth
Agranulocytosis
Cholestatic hepatitis
Nausea, vomiting

Treatment of Toxicity

Discontinue drug
Supportive care

Pyridostigmine Bromide (Mestinon)

Pharmacology

Distribution

Pyridostigmine crosses the placental membrane and blood–brain barrier poorly due to its quaternary ammonium structure. However, high doses can produce central nervous system effects and result in measurable levels in fetal circulation. Pyridostigmine is not secreted in breast milk.

Elimination

Pyridostigmine is hydrolyzed by serum cholinesterases, with lesser metabolism via the hepatic microsomal system. Metabolites are eliminated by renal tubular excretion.

Actions

Pyridostigmine competitively inhibits the hydrolysis of acetylcholine at the neuromuscular junction and in autonomic ganglia, enhancing cholinergic transmission. At the motor end-plate, the amplitude of the MEPP is increased, with subsequent potentiation of the formation of the EPP and muscle action potential. This is reflected as improved motor strength for a given delivered stimulus. In autonomic ganglia, pyridostigmine produces muscarinic effects, resulting in miosis, bradycardia, and increased exocrine secretion, intestinal peristalsis, and bronchial muscle tone. Muscarinic effects are generally less prominent with pyridostigmine than with neostigmine.

Indications

Control of symptoms of myasthenia gravis when oral therapy is insufficient or impractical
Reversal of nondepolarizing neuromuscular blockade postoperatively

Contraindications

Known hypersensitivity, mechanical obstruction of the intestinal or urinary tract, peritonitis

Cautions

Cardiac failure—carefully titrated dosing is indicated to avoid significant bradycardia. If bradycardia is present, the heart rate should be increased to >80 by pretreatment with atropine.
Use in pregnancy—Category C. In late pregnancy, pyridostigmine can precipitate premature labor. When pyridostigmine is used to enhance muscle strength during labor in myasthenics, transient weakness has been found in 10 to 20% of the delivered neonates.
Use in lactation—pyridostigmine has not been detected in breast milk. Use in lactation involves balancing potential risks to the infant with maternal benefit.
Use in childhood—safety has not been established, but pyridostigmine has been used in pediatric patients.
Pulmonary disease—pyridostigmine is capable of inducing bronchospasm and should be used with caution in patients with asthma or chronic obstructive pulmonary disease.
Other—should be used with caution in patients with epilepsy, bradycardia, and hyperthyroidism

Dosage

For parenteral therapy of adult myasthenia gravis, 2.0 mg IM or by slow IV push.

Dosing can be repeated every 2 to 3 hours as needed. In children, the parenteral dosage is one-thirtieth of the usual daily oral dose of 7 mg/kg divided every 2 to 3 hours. Neonatal dosage is 0.05 to 0.15 mg/kg IM every 4 to 6 hours. During therapy, atropine should be available to antagonize muscarinic side-effects. Pretreatment with atropine sulfate is advocated by some authors when pyridostigmine is used intravenously.

Toxicity

Drug Interactions

Depolarizing neuromuscular blocking agents—pyridostigmine can prolong phase I of neuromuscular blockade with succinylcholine and decamethonium. Phase II neuromuscular blockade with these agents is antagonized.

Nondepolarizing blocking agents—pyridostigmine reverses neuromuscular blockade with gallamine and curare compounds.

Specific Adverse Effects

Central nervous system—seizures, headache, dizziness, decreased level of consciousness, dysarthria

Ocular—miosis, lacrimation, visual changes

Cardiovascular—bradycardia, high-grade atrioventricular block, asystole, syncope, hypotension

Respiratory—bronchospasm, dyspnea, respiratory arrest, increased oropharyngeal and bronchial secretions

Gastrointestinal—nausea, vomiting, increased peristalsis, abdominal cramps

Genitourinary—urinary frequency

Dermatologic—flushing, diaphoresis, rash, urticaria

Musculoskeletal—weakness, cramps, arthralgias, myalgias

Allergic—anaphylaxis.

Peripheral vascular—thrombophlebitis after intravenous administration.

Treatment of Toxicity

Discontinue drug.

Atropine may be used to antagonize muscarinic effects.

REFERENCES

Arsura EL, et al: Effects of repeated doses of intravenous immunoglobulin in myasthenia gravis. Am J Med Sci 295:438–443.

Bagdade JD: Endocrine emergencies. Med Clin North Am 70:1115–1123, 1986.

Bayliss RIS: Adrenal cortex. Clin Endocrinol Metab 9:477–486, 1980.

Bergenstal RM: Diabetic ketoacidosis: How to treat and, when possible, prevent. Postgrad Med 77:151–161, 1985.

Braaten JT: Hyperosmolar nonketotic diabetic coma: Diagnosis and management. Geriatrics 42:83–92, 1987.

Burke CW: Adrenocortical insufficiency. Clin Endocrinol Metab 14:947–976, 1985.

Cohen MS, Younger D: Aspects of the natural history of myasthenia gravis: Crisis and death. Ann NY Acad Sci 670–677, 1983.

DeRosa G, et al: A clinical study of Addison's disease. Exp Clin Endocrinol 90:232–242, 1987.

Dorin RI, Kernes PJ: High output circulatory failure in acute adrenal insufficiency. Crit Care Med 16:296–297, 1988.

Drachman DB: Myasthenia gravis. I. N Engl J Med 298:136–142, 1978.

Drachman DB: Myasthenia gravis. II. N Engl J Med 298:186–193, 1978.

Fisher JN, Kitabchi AE: A randomized study of phosphate therapy in the treatment of diabetic ketoacidosis. J Clin Endocrinol Metab 57:177–180, 1983.

Foster DW, McGarry JD: The metabolic derangements and treatment of diabetic ketoacidosis. N Engl J Med 309:159–169, 1983.

Giouin PE, et al: Diabetic ketoacidosis: Outcome in a community hospital. South Medical J 78:941–943, 1985.

Grace TW: Hyperosmolar nonketotic diabetic coma. Am Fam Practitioner 32:119–125, 1985.

Haynes RC Jr, Murad F: Adrenocorticotropic hormone; adrenocortical steroids and their synthetic analogs; inhibitors of adrenocortical steroid biosynthesis. In Gilman RG, et al (eds): The Pharmacologic Basis of Therapeutics. New York, Macmillan, 1980, pp 1466–1550.

Heath DA: The emergency management of disorders of calcium and magnesium. Clin Endocrinol Metab 9:487–502, 1980.

Himathongkam T, et al: Acute adrenal insufficiency. JAMA 230:1317–1318, 1974.

Howard JF: Nonsteroidal immunosuppressive therapy for myasthenia gravis. Semin Neurol 2:265–269, 1982.

Janson CL: Fluid and electrolyte balance. In Rosen P, et al (eds): Emergency Medicine: Concepts and Clinical Practice. St Louis, CV Mosby, 1988, pp 1991–2003.

Johnston DG, Alberti KGMM: Diabetic emergencies: Practical aspects of the management of diabetic ketoacidosis and diabetes during surgery. Clin Endocrinol Metab 9:437–460, 1980.

Keller U: Diabetic ketoacidosis: Current views on pathogenesis and treatment. Diabetologica 29:71–77, 1986.

Kitabchi AE: Diabetic ketoacidosis and hyperosmolar hyperglycemia nonketotic coma. Med Clin North Am 72:1545–1563, 1988.

Kleerekoper M, Rao DS: Hypercalcemia and hypocalcemia. In Callahan ML (ed): Current Therapy in Emergency Medicine. Toronto BC Decker, 1987, pp 729–732.

Krane EJ: Diabetic ketoacidosis. Pediatr Clin North Am 34:935–960, 1987.

Kyner JL: Diabetic ketoacidosis. Crit Care Q 3:65–74, 1980.

Marx SJ, Bourdeau JE: Calcium metabolism. In Maxwell MH, et al (eds): Clinical Disorders of Fluid and Electrolyte Metabolism. New York, McGraw-Hill, 1987, pp 207–244.

Mier-Jedrzejowicz AK, et al: Respiratory muscle function in myasthenia gravis. Am Rev Respir Dis 138:867–873, 1988.

Morris LR, et al: Bicarbonate therapy in severe diabetic ketoacidosis. Ann Intern Med 105:836–840, 1986.

Moss JM: Diabetic ketoacidosis: Effective low-cost treatment in a community hospital. South Med J 80:875–881, 1987.

Moss JM: Treatment of diabetic ketoacidosis. Am Fam Practitioner 35:135–140, 1987.

Olinger ML: Disorders of calcium and magnesium metabolism. Emerg Med Clin North Am 7:795–824, 1989.

Pope DW, Dansky, D: Hyperosmolar hyperglycemic nonketotic coma. Emerg Med Clin North Am 7:849–871, 1989.

Potts JT Jr: Diseases of the parathyroid gland and other hyper- and hypocalcemic disorders. In Braunwald E, et al (eds): Harrison's Principles of Internal Medicine. New York, McGraw-Hill, 1987, pp 1870–1889.

Rusnak RA: Adrenal and pituitary emergencies. Emerg Med Clin North Am 7:908–915, 1989.

Sanson TH, Levine SN: Management of diabetic ketoacidosis. Drugs 38:289–300, 1989.

Schimke RN: Adrenal insufficiency. Crit Care Q 3:19–27, 1980.

Sellman MS, Mayer RF: Treatment of myasthenic crisis in late life. South Med J 78:1208–1210, 1985.

Skyler JS: Insulin pharmacology. Med Clin North Am 72:1337–1354, 1988.

Small M, et al: Diabetic hyperosmolar non-ketotic decompensation. Q J Med 66:251–257, 1988.

Snead OC III, et al: Plasmapheresis for myasthenic crisis in a young child. J Pediatr 110:740–742, 1987.

Sneid DS: Hyperosmolar hyperglycemic nonketotic coma. Crit Care Q 3:29–43, 1980.

Storms FEMG, et al: Comparison of the efficacy of human and porcine insulin in treatment of diabetic ketoacidosis. Diabetes Care 10:49–55, 1987.

Taylor P: Anticholinesterase agents. In Gilman AG, et al. (eds): The Pharmacological Basis of Therapeutics. New York, Macmillan, 1980, pp 100–119.

Wilson HK, et al: Phosphate therapy in diabetic ketoacidosis. Arch Intern Med 142:517–520, 1982.

CHAPTER 22

Antimicrobials

ALEXANDER TROTT, M.D.

INTRODUCTION

Although great progress has been made in recent decades in the treatment of infectious diseases, they still remain important life-threatening causes of acute illness. Recent epidemiologic data indicate that pneumonia and septicemia are the fifth and twelfth leading causes of death in the United States and are frequent causes of morbidity and mortality in noninfectious illnesses.

Emergency and critical care physicians make daily decisions concerning the appropriate use of antibiotics in critically ill patients. While airway and circulatory considerations take priority in the management of the severely ill infectious disease victim, reports indicate that rapid institution of antibiotics and the appropriate match of antibiotic choices to the likely causative microbiologic pathogen can reduce the incidence of both subsequent shock and mortality by up to 50% in patients with gram-negative bacteremia. This chapter provides the necessary clinical and pharmacologic information to make timely and effective choices of initial antimicrobial therapy for suspected life-threatening infectious diseases.

Numerous serious infectious diseases have the potential for causing morbidity and mortality. It is beyond the scope of this text to cover each in detail. Therefore, this chapter concentrates on the potentially rapidly fatal infectious diseases likely to be seen on a relatively frequent basis in emergency departments and in the early phases of critical care management. These diseases include acute meningitis and life-threatening infections (sepsis) of both known (pulmonary, urologic, and intra-abdominal) and unknown cause. Included in this discussion are the special considerations of pediatric age groups and the immunocompromised host, with attention to acquired immunodeficiency syndrome (AIDS) victims. Most of the discussion concerning antibiotic use is concentrated on empirical choices because, during initial care, culture results will be unknown and Gram's stain readings often are unreliable.

Epidemiologic and Pathophysiologic Considerations in Acute Meningitis

From a statistical vantage point, acute meningitis is largely a pediatric disease. The peak incidence of bacterial meningitis occurs between the ages of birth and 12 months, with an attack rate of between 63 and 99 cases per 100,000 population. This rate rapidly falls to 1 case per 100,000 by age 10 years and remains close to that figure throughout adolescence and adulthood.

A number of predisposing factors and conditions contribute to acquiring meningitis, but clearly the disease can strike the apparently healthy as well. Of the known risk determinants, cellular and immunologic factors

450

are well recognized. For example, histocompatibility leukocyte antigen (HLA-B12) is more common in children with *Hemophilus influenzae* bacterial meningitis than in noninfected children. Splenectomy and congenital asplenia, as well as sickle cell anemia and other hemoglobinopathies, lead to a greater susceptibility to both *H. influenzae* and *Streptococcus pneumoniae.* Meningococcal infections are seen more commonly in patients with alterations in the terminal components of complement (C5–C8).

Although there are several important pathophysiologic features in patients with meningitis, the role of the blood–brain barrier is useful to understand with regard to antibiotic effectiveness. Under normal conditions, the blood–brain barrier successfully excludes antibiotic penetration. Only 0.5% of the serum concentration of penicillin and 2 to 3% of that of ampicillin can be measured in the cerebrospinal fluid (CSF) after a single dose. In meningitis, penicillin penetration increases to 3% and ampicillin penetration to 15%. This phenomenon helps, in part, to explain why antibiotic doses in meningitis have to be so large. Additionally, it has also been demonstrated that, in order for a bacteria to be killed successfully, CSF concentrations have to be in excess of 10 to 100 times the minimum bactericidal concentration (MBC) of the blood. The reasons for this phenomenon are complex but include reduced immune response in the CSF, changes in CSF pH that can reduce effectiveness of antibiotics, protein binding in an inflammatory CSF, and *in vivo* (compared to *in vitro*) differences in bacterial growth curves that affect the bactericidal capability of antibiotics. Drugs that successfully penetrate the CSF and have good antibacterial activity in meningitis in appropriate doses include the penicillins, chloramphenicol, vancomycin, and selected cephalosporins such as cefuroxime, cefotaxime, ceftriaxone, ceftizoxime, moxalactam, and ceftazidime.

Epidemiologic and Pathophysiologic Considerations in Sepsis

Since the 1950s, cases of severe generalized infections, commonly referred to as *sepsis*, have increased in large part owing to the rise in infections caused by aerobic gram-negative rods. Sepsis has been estimated to

be present on admission or occurs during hospitalization in 1 of 100 patients. The sepsis syndrome represents the systemic response to infection. This syndrome must be recognized by its clinical presentation to allow early initiation of antibiotic therapy because delaying antibiotic treatment while awaiting culture results is associated with a higher morbidity and mortality. The clinical definition of the sepsis syndrome used by the Methylprednisolone Severe Sepsis Study Group (see Table 22–7) identifies a group of patients with a 45% incidence of bacteremia and a 59% incidence of septic shock (the sepsis syndrome plus hypotension to a systolic blood pressure less than 90 mmHg, or 40 mmHg less than the patient's usual baseline). Mortality can be expected to be 10 to 15% in the patients without shock and 30 to 50% in the patients with shock. Adult respiratory distress syndrome will occur in 25% of these patients. Thus, the sepsis syndrome represents a valid clinical entity that identifies a very high risk population who should immediately receive broad-spectrum antibiotic therapy, selected based on the patient's risk factors and presumed site of infection.

The pathophysiology of sepsis and septic shock is exceedingly complex, and the precise role of microorganisms has yet to be clearly defined. Bacteria, fungi, rickettsiae, and viruses have all been identified as potential initiators of the septic shock syndrome. For example, both exotoxins from *Staphylococcus aureus* and *Clostridium* species and endotoxins from aerobic gram-negative rods have been identified, purified, and shown to reproducibly cause shock in the laboratory setting. However, the same syndrome has been observed experimentally and clinically without any recoverable and identifiable toxin.

Once the septic process begins, a number of mediators initiate a series of biochemical and physiologic events that threaten the existence of the host. Complement is activated and can lead to release of toxic oxygen radicals. Activation of Hageman factor of the intrinsic coagulation system precipitates coagulation disorders including disseminated intravascular coagulation (DIC). Both the activation of these systems and the release of bradykinin, histamine, prostaglandins, and beta-endorphins can inappropriately cause capillary dilatation with excess permeability. The end result is temporary or permanent end-organ damage to the lung, kidney, liver, brain, and cardiovascular system. While appropriate antimicrobial therapy is an imperative in the management of these patients, airway management, ventilation, fluid therapy, and cardiovascular support are equally important in reversing this systemic multiorgan disaster.

CONDITIONS

Acute Meningitis

Acute bacterial meningitis can be one of the most rapidly fatal diseases from the onset of initial symptoms. It constitutes a "true" emergency and requires rapid and intense diagnostic and management efforts.

Microbiology

Hemophilus influenzae, Neisseria meningitidis, and *Streptococcus pneumoniae* cause approximately 90% of all cases of proved bacterial meningitis. In spite of these numbers, each age group has a different distribution and incidence of pathogens that must be accounted for in the empiric therapy of meningitis (Table 22–1). In the newborn, particularly under 7 days of age, most organisms that cause meningitis are acquired during delivery or in the nursery. The two main organisms are group B streptococcus and *Escherichia coli.* Other pathogens include group D streptococci (enterococci), gram-negative enteric bacilli (*Klebsiella, Enterobacter,* and *Serratia* species), and *Listeria monocytogenes.* Over the age of 7 days, particularly if the child has already been taken home, *H. influenzae* type B, *N. meningitidis,* and *S. pneumoniae* add to the list of potentially infecting agents.

From the ages of 3 months to 6 years, meningitis-causing bacteria are almost exclusively limited to *H. influenzae, N. meningitidis,* and *S. pneumoniae.* From 6 to 30 years of age, *H. influenzae* almost disappears as an important pathogen, with *N. meningitidis* and *S. pneumoniae* assuming predominance. It is important to note that there still is a risk of *H. influenzae* between the ages of 6 and 10 years, and some authorities feel that this possibility has to be recognized when selecting an antibiotic, especially in areas where there is not an active or effective vaccination program against that organism. From the ages of 30 to 60 years, *S. pneumoniae* becomes the most common organism; however, sporadic

TABLE 22–1. Bacterial Causes of Meningitis

Patient Group	Bacterial Pathogens
Age birth to 1 month	Groups B or D streptococci
	Escherichia coli
	Listeria monocytogenes
	Hemophilus influenzae
	Streptococcus pneumoniae
	Neisseria meningitidis
Age 1 to 3 months	*Hemophilus influenzae*
	Streptococcus pneumoniae
	Neisseria meningitidis
	Group B streptococci
Age 3 months to 6 years	*Hemophilus influenzae*
	Neisseria meningitidis
	Streptococcus pneumoniae
Age 6 to 30 years	*Neisseria meningitidis*
	Streptococcus pneumoniae
Age 30 to 60 years	*Streptococcus pneumoniae*
	Neisseria meningitidis
Age >60 or immunosuppressed	*Streptococcus pneumoniae*
	Gram-negative bacilli
	Pseudomonas species
	Listeria monocytogenes
	Hemophilus influenzae
Post trauma <4 days	*Streptococcus pneumoniae*
	Group A streptococci
Post trauma 4 or more days	Gram-negative bacilli
	Pseudomonas species
	Staphylococcus aureus
Post neurosurgical procedures	*Pseudomonas* species
	Staphylococcus aureus
	Gram-negative bacilli

cases of *N. meningitidis* occur throughout adulthood. Over the age of 60 years, *S. pneumoniae* is the most common cause of meningitis but there is a resurgence of gram-negative baccilli and *L. monocytogenes.* Table 22–1 lists the common bacteria likely to cause meningitis in head-injured and postoperative neurosurgical patient groups.

Clinical Recognition and Diagnosis of Acute Meningitis

The classic signs and symptoms of meningitis—headaches, lethargy, vomiting, and meningismus—occur in 80% of cases. Early recognition of the disease, therefore, can be difficult in some patients. The key to timely diagnosis is clinician sensitivity and suspicion. The Task Force on the Diagnosis and Management of Meningitis of the American Academy of Pediatrics recommends that lumbar puncture might be considered an appropriate action for a child in the midst of an apparent viral-like illness, who demonstrates a change in affect or alertness without yet manifesting specific signs of meningitis.

Neurologic changes are frequent in patients with meningitis. Only 20% of patients with bacterial meningitis present in a completely alert and oriented manner; 50% are irritable or lethargic; 20% are semicomatose; and 10% present in an outright coma. Approximately 20% of patients present with or have early onset of seizures, and 15% have focal neurologic deficits. Papilledema is rare at the outset of meningitis and should point the clinician to other intracranial pathology.

Rashes are common in cases of meningitis, and the petechial rash in meningococcal meningitis is most characteristic. The rash can be identified in 50% of patients with this form of meningitis, but it often starts as a maculopapular rash that is indistinguishable from that caused by viral meningitis. Other associated findings in patients with meningitis include otitis, sinusitis, and pneumonia.

Indications for Lumbar Puncture and Interpretation of Spinal Fluid

A lumbar puncture (LP) is indicated in any patient for whom the diagnostic suspicion, but no clinical proof, exists for meningitis. An old house staff adage, "if you think about it, do it," has merit. The consequences of missing the diagnosis or delaying appropriate therapy can be catastrophic.

The potential complications of LP have to be put into perspective so as not to unduly influence the clinician away from the procedure. The greatest fear is that of precipitating brain herniation following an LP. This fear originates from the days, before 1930, when LPs were done with large-bore, 12- to 16-gauge needles and large amounts of CSF were drained in an attempt to "treat" raised intracranial pressure. The actual incidence of herniation following LP using contemporary techniques, in cases with *proved* raised intracranial pressure, is only 2.5%. When these reported cases of herniation following LP are closely scrutinized, however, it cannot be said for certain if the progression of the disease process or the LP actually precipitated the herniation.

In spite of the minimal chance of herniation, the potential for that event still has to be respected. Current practice dictates that after a thorough examination, if any focal neurologic findings, papilledema, or other evidence of raised intracranial pressure exists, a computed tomographic (CT) scan should be performed prior to the LP (Fig. 22–1). However, antibiotic treatment is always initiated before transport to CT if men-

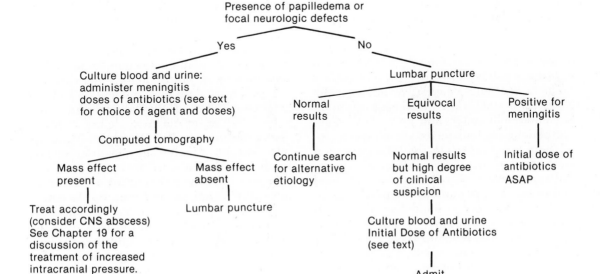

FIGURE 22–1. Treatment algorithm: initial approach to the patient with suspected meningitis. Note that empirical antibiotic therapy should be administered if lumbar puncture will be delayed to obtain computed tomography scans of the head.

ingitis is suspected. The delay to obtain a CT scan could potentially jeopardize the outcome of the patient if it interferes with the timely delivery of antimicrobial therapy.

Delivery of antimicrobial therapy to patients prior to LP does not significantly alter the clinician's ability to make the correct bacteriologic diagnosis. Approximately one-third of all patients with meningitis receive some form of antimicrobial therapy prior to seeking medical care. A number of studies have shown that prior antimicrobial therapy does not appreciably alter the pathologic changes in the CSF (cell count, glucose, protein, and culture results). By using Gram's stains, cultures, and rapid diagnostic antigen tests, the offending organism can be identified with almost the same accuracy as in patients who did not have antimicrobial therapy in approximately 90% of cases.

Interpretation of Spinal Fluid

Normal CSF is crystal-clear and colorless. With a patient in the proper lateral recumbent position, the opening pressure ranges between 50 and 200 mm of water, with a normal respiratory variation of 5 to 10 mm. A normal CSF can have a white blood cell count of 0 to 5 mononuclear cells. Even *one* polymorphonuclear leukocyte raises the suspicion of meningitis. It has also been well reported that patients with meningitis, particularly due to *N. meningitidis*, can initially have a normal CSF, and treatment has to be started empirically based on clinical suspicion alone. CSF glucose is usually 60 to 70% of serum glucose, or about 50 to 80 mg/dl in a fasting patient. Normal protein values range from 15 to 45 mg/dl. For neonates the range for normal white blood cells is 0 to 30 per cubic millimeter, and up to 60% polymorphonuclear leukocytes are allowed.

There is no way to clearly distinguish viral from bacterial meningitis early in the course. Both can have CSF with high white blood cell counts and predominately polymorphonuclear leukocytes on the differential count. Ninety percent of all cases of viral meningitis will convert to a predominately mononuclear cell differential within 8 to 12 hours after presentation. If this occurs, and the clinical status remains uncomplicated, the decision to withdraw antibiotic therapy can be considered. (See box.)

Discussion

Infectious disease authorities have stated that no more than *1* hour should pass be-

tween the presentation of patients with suspected meningitis and the initiation of specific treatment. Administering antibiotics to a patient who eventually proves not to have meningitis has to be considered less of a risk than the risk of any delay in treating the patient who is truly infected.

Selection of initial intravenous antibiotic therapy in the emergency department is largely empirical because the microbiologic diagnosis is uncertain. The most important factor to be considered in making this empirical choice is the age of the patient. Age determines the statistical likelihood of which organisms will predominate. Antibiotic coverage can be tailored to the specific cause when culture results are returned.

For newborns to the age of 3 months, current suggested empirical antibiotic therapy consists of ampicillin plus a third-generation cephalosporin such as cefotaxime. The alternative is ampicillin plus gentamicin. Ampicillin more effectively covers infection with enterococci and *L. monocytogenes* than the cephalosporins or aminoglycosides alone. A third-generation cephalosporin is chosen for its coverage of most enteric gram-negative organisms as well as the three predominant bacterial causes of meningitis. Combinations of certain antibiotics also act in a synergistic manner to eradicate the pathogen more effectively and rapidly. Third-generation cephalosporins are effective because (1) they adequately penetrate the CSF, (2) they achieve the required 10 to 100 times the blood MBC in the CSF, (3) they have greater killing power than gentamicin, and (4) they are effective against organisms that have developed resistance to ampillicin and chloramphenicol (i.e., *H. influenzae*). For neonates, cefotaxime is a good choice from this class of antibiotics. It is not secreted into the bile, thereby reducing any negative effect on the balance of the normal enteric flora. Cefotaxime, compared to ceftriaxone, also does not cause significant bilirubin displacement from serum protein in the young neonate.

From the age of 3 months to 10 years the antibiotic of choice is a third-generation cephalosporin alone. Of this generation, ceftriaxone has the advantage over cefotaxime of a less frequent dose schedule, twice a day, because of its long half-life of 6 to 8 hours. Cefotaxime, however, can be considered the alternative. Cefuroxime, the only second-generation cephalosporin active against the three main pathogens of meningitis, is another alternative choice, but there have

DRUG TREATMENT: SUSPECTED BACTERIAL MENINGITIS

Patient Group	Primary Treatment	Alternative Treatment
Age birth to 7 days	Ampicillin, 50 mg/kg q 8 hours plus Cefotaxime, 50 mg/kg q 12 hours	Ampicillin, 50 mg/kg q 8 hours plus Gentamicin, 2.5 mg/kg q 12 hours
Age 8 days to 1 month	Ampicillin, 50 mg/kg q 6 hours plus Cefotaxime, 50 mg/kg q 8 hours	Ampicillin, 50 mg/kg q 6 hours plus Gentamicin, 2.5 mg/kg q 8 hours
Age 1 month to 3 months	Ampicillin, 100 mg/kg q 6 hours plus Cefotaxime, 50 mg/kg q 6 hours	Ampicillin, 100 mg/kg q 6 hours plus Gentamicin, 2.5 mg/kg q 8 hours
Age 3 months to 10 years	Ceftriaxone, 50 mg/kg q 12 hours	Cefotaxime, 50 mg/kg q 6 hours
Immunocompetent adolescents	Penicillin G, 40,000 units/kg q 4 hours	Ceftriaxone, 50 mg/kg q 12 hours
Immunocompetent adults	Pencillin G, 4,000,000 units q 4 hours	Ceftriaxone, 2 g q 12 hours
Elderly or immunocompromised adults (alcoholics)	Ampicillin, 2 g q 4 hours plus Cefotaxime, 2 g q 4 hours	Ampicillin, 2 g q 4 hours plus Gentamicin, 2.5–3 mg/kg IV loading infusion over 30 minutes; subsequent doses based on individually measured pharmacokinetics
Post trauma <4 days or persistent CSF leak	Penicillin G, 4,000,000 units q 4 hours	Ceftriaxone, 2 g q 12 hours
Post neurosurgery, post trauma 4 days or more, or neutropenic patients	Vancomycin, 1 g q 12 hours plus Ceftazidime, 2 g q 8 hours plus Gentamicin, 2.5–3 mg/kg IV loading infusion over 30 minutes; subsequent doses based on individually measured pharmacokinetics	Vancomycin, 1 g q 12 hours plus Chloramphenicol, 2 g q 6 hours plus Gentamicin, 2.5–3 mg/kg IV loading infusion over 30 minutes; subsequent doses based on individually measured pharmacokinetics

been reports of delayed sterilization of the CSF with this antibiotic. For years, the standard of care has been ampicillin and chloramphenicol, but emerging resistance to chloramphenicol by *H. influenzae* makes this a less attractive alternative. In addition, chloramphenicol toxicity is becoming increasingly recognized, particularly in patients who are very ill and hemodynamically unstable.

For children older than 10 years, adolescents, and otherwise healthy adults, penicillin therapy is still the most effective regimen. In recent years, however, there has been a rise in the sporadic and geographical incidence of penicillin resistance in *S. pneumoniae*. Penicillin resistance, while very low nationwide, varies from community to community, and the clinician needs to be aware that it could exist. If resistance is locally evident, then a third-generation cephalosporin is recommended as the empirical antibiotic choice.

For immunocompromised patients and those over the age of 60, ampicillin plus a third-generation cephalosporin such as ceftriaxone, cefotaxime, or ceftazidime is recommended. An aminoglycoside is a reasonable substitution for the cephalosporins. Gram-negative organisms make a reappearance in these groups, as do enterococci and *L. monocytogenes*. The most common organism in the early post-trauma patient is *S. pneumoniae* (80%); therefore, penicillin or ceftriaxone can be used. Because *S. aureus* is a potential pathogen, in addition to a variety of gram-negative organisms, in the late (>4 days) post head injury and postoperative neurosurgical patient, coverage with a penicillinase-resistant penicillin is necessary in addition to an aminoglycoside. Ceftazidime provides additional coverage for *Pseudomonas aeruginosa*, which appears with some frequency in this setting.

Penicillin-Allergic Patients

Determining true penicillin allergy, particularly in the critical moments of a life-threatening illness, can be difficult, but the question occasionally arises. Cross-reactivity has been reported to be 2 to 15% between penicillin and the cephalosporins. Therefore, there is reluctance to administer the latter if a history of penicillin allergy is discovered. Most authorities agree that a reaction might occur only if the reported response to penicillin was anaphylactic in nature where profound urticaria, breathing difficulties, or hypotension were reported. For patients who suffered only skin rashes, cross-sensitivity with cephalosporins is unlikely. Under these latter circumstances, third-generation cephalosporins can be safely given as penicillin alternatives. An important consideration to remember is that the non–beta-lactam alternative drug of choice, chloramphenicol, is bacteriostatic, and some authorities feel that the needed bactericidal power of a third-generation cephalosporin outweighs the small risk of a cross-reaction in this major life-threatening illness. For clinicians who remain uncomfortable with this risk, chloramphenicol is the substitution of choice for beta-lactam antibiotics for all age groups after the neonatal period.

Sepsis of Unknown Source

Approximately 12 to 31% of patients with aerobic gram-negative bacteremia will have no proved source identified (Table 22–2). The diagnosis of suspected sepsis of unknown source is not uncommon in the emergency setting where the clinician is limited by time and the fact that adjunctive tests are often inconclusive. Before reaching that diagnostic conclusion, however, a careful history is taken and a physical examination is performed along with a chest x-ray, urinalysis, and appropriate Gram's stains. Occasionally a lumbar puncture is necessary to complete the emergency department search.

TABLE 22–2. Sources of Bacteremia and Fungemia

Source	Incidence (%)
Genitourinary	17
Respiratory	17
Gastrointestinal	16
Postsurgical	4
Skin	3
Intravenous catheter	3
Foley catheter	2
Central nervous system	1
Bone	0.5
Two or more sources	5.5
Source unknown	31
	100

(Adapted from Weinstein MP, Murphy JR, Reller LB, et al: The clinical significance of positive blood cultures. Rev Infect Dis 5:35, 1983. By permission of The University of Chicago Press.)

Even though a source may be later identified, it is important to start antibiotic therapy without delay, especially if the patient fulfills the criteria of the sepsis syndrome (see Table 22–7) before the patient leaves the emergency department, if that is the point of initial patient contact.

Microbiology

The range of microorganisms that can cause septicemia includes gram-positive and gram-negative bacteria, anaerobic bacteria, fungi, viruses, and rickettsiae. The initial empirical antimicrobial regimen should have a broad spectrum because of the possibility of a wide range of bacterial etiologies. Important modifiers of the bacterial range and therefore of the eventual choice of an antimicrobial are patient age and immune status.

Currently, the most common causes of neonatal septicemia are *Escherichia coli* and group B streptococci (Table 22–3). Other less common organisms include *Listeria monocytogenes*, anaerobic bacteria, group A streptococci, and group D streptococci (enterococci). An important concept to understand is that neonatal sepsis and meningitis are often considered as overlapping syndromes and the organisms are similar for each. As in most cases of septicemia in any age group, there are underlying factors that can predispose to this disease. Early onset of symptoms (less than 8 days after birth) has been associated with maternal perinatal infection, premature rupture of the membranes, prolonged labor, prematurity, low birth weight, and a low Apgar score. Late-

TABLE 22–3. Bacterial Causes of Neonatal Sepsis

Early Infection: <8 Days Postpartum
Group B streptococci
Escherichia coli
Group D streptococci (enterococci)
Klebsiella-Aerobacter
Listeria monocytogenes
Group A streptococci
Streptococcus pneumoniae
Hemophilus influenzae
Anaerobic species
Late Infection: >7 Days Postpartum
Staphylococcus aureus
Escherichia coli
Klebsiella-Aerobacter
Pseudomonas species
Staphylococcus epidermidis
Group D streptococci (enterococci)
Streptococcus pneumoniae
Hemophilus influenzae

onset neonatal sepsis (7 or more days after birth) is seen more often in patients with congenital anomalies, a prolonged intensive care stay, and the male sex.

Beyond the neonatal period, septicemia without a known source is an uncommon occurrence in childhood. Most serious infections have a definable source, and generalized infections usually accompany serious disease entities such as congenital abnormalities, immune defects, and malignancies. The risk of meningococcemia, however, must always be respected.

A special problem of childhood, from ages 3 to 24 months, is occult bacteremia. There is a direct correlation of bacteremia to the degree of fever. With fever below 38.9°C, less than 1% of patients have bacteremia; between 38.9°C and 39.4°C, the incidence is 4%; between 39.4°C and 41.1°C, the incidence rises to 8.9%; and in children who have fevers of greater than 41.1°C, up to a 26% incidence of bacteremia has been reported. The suspicion of bacteremia is supported if the fever is accompanied by a white blood cell count of ≥15,000 mm³ or an erythrocyte sedimentation rate (ESR) of greater than 30. In a study of 400 cases of bacteremia in children between the ages of 3 months and 2 years, 71% were due to *Streptococcus pneumoniae* and 23% were due to *Hemophilus influenzae* type B. Less common organisms in this setting include *Staphylococcus aureus* and *Neisseria meningitidis*. Most authorities recommend that a blood culture be drawn if the temperature exceeds

39.5°C and the white blood cell count is elevated.

With aging the risk of bacteremia and sepsis increases. Table 22–4 indicates the range of bacteria and other microorganisms of sepsis in adults. What is apparent from these data, and supported by other studies, is that a broad range of gram-positive, gram-negative, and anaerobic bacteria can cause sepsis, and the clinical distinction between them is often difficult. Therefore, any empirical choice of initial antibiotic therapy must be directed at the broad rather than narrow spectrum. Table 22–4 also shows a clear distinction in the distribution between hospital- and community-acquired bacteremia. *S. pneumoniae, Neisseria gonorrhoeae,* and *H. influenzae* are more commonly found in patients with community-acquired disease. As might be expected, the incidence of *S. aureus* and gram-negative organisms (including *Pseudomonas aeruginosa* and fungi) is more common in the hospital-acquired group.

One of the most important modifying factors in predicting the causes and outcome of sepsis is the underlying immune status of the patient. With effective regimens for cancer chemotherapy, increasingly successful transplantation of organs, widespread dialysis programs, and the use of parenteral nutrition, more patients will present in an immunocompromised state with suspicion for infection. The potential defects in the immune status of a patient are numerous. They range from the simple breakdown of the skin

TABLE 22–4. Microbiologic Causes of Adult Sepsis

Organism	Number (%) of Isolates in Indicated Category	
	Community Acquired	Hospital Acquired
Escherichia coli	48 (42)	65 (58)
Streptococcus pneumoniae	35 (81)	8 (19)
Staphylococcus aureus	27 (40)	41 (60)
Streptococcus species	33 (40)	49 (60)
Pseudomonas species	6 (17)	35 (83)
Other aerobic gram-negative bacilli	17 (40)	41 (60)
Anaerobic bacteria	38 (47)	43 (53)
Fungi	2 (4)	49 (96)
All	221 (35)	402 (65)

(Adapted from Weinstein MP, Murphy JR, Reller LB, et al: The clinical significance of positive blood cultures. Rev Infect Dis 5:35, 1983. By permission of The University of Chicago Press.)

(chronic dermatologic disorders, intravenous catheters, invasive monitoring lines, burns, and so forth) to specific disorders of the components of the immune defense network. Table 22–5 provides an overview of the specific defects, their likely causes, and the associated pathogenic microorganisms found with that immune defect. As is evident from this information, commonly noninfective organisms become pathogens. Organisms acquired early in life that become dormant can be reactivated to cause disease. Examples of these organisms include *Toxoplasma gondii*, herpes simplex, and *Mycobacterium tuberculosis*.

Because of the importance of phagocytosis as a defense against bacteria, granulocytopenia deserves special mention as an immune defect. There is a strong correlation between patient survival and the total granulocyte count in the setting of bacteremia and sepsis. This correlation is particularly true for aerobic gram-negative bacteria. For this reason antibiotic therapy has to be modified toward a broader spectrum of more potent antibiotics to ensure efficacy against the causative organisms. A specifically targeted organism in this setting is *P. aeruginosa*.

The most compelling example of a cellular immune dysfunction that predisposes to widespread infection is AIDS. This disorder is caused by the human immunodeficiency virus (HIV), which cripples the T-4 lymphocyte, an indispensable component of cellular immunity. Virtually any microorganism, bacterial, parasitic, fungal, or viral, can proliferate and thrive in patients afflicted with AIDS.

Clinical Recognition of Sepsis

The clinical recognition of sepsis, particularly when no source is revealed by history, physical examination, radiographic studies, appropriate Gram's stains, and blood analysis, can be troublesome in any age group. In the neonatal period, the signs of sepsis are often subtle. Poor feeding, unexplained vomiting, irritability, and lethargy are suspicious signs. Temperature instability, including hyperthermia or hypothermia, and respiratory distress are other findings. The erythrocyte sedimentation rate (ESR), with an abnormal value above 15 mm/hour, has been associated with neonatal sepsis. Neutropenia in the range of ≤ 2000 mm^3 or neutrophilia in the range of $\geq 16,000$ mm^3 may increase the sus-

picion of sepsis. Arterial blood gases may reveal an unexplained metabolic acidosis.

In adults, symptoms and signs of septicemia without a source can also be subtle. A high degree of suspicion is always necessary. For example, an early sign of sepsis in an elderly adult may be a slight alteration in mental status. Other early symptoms include fever, chills, and hyperventilation. While fever is the most common temperature change in these patients, hypothermia may be an important finding. In a study of 85 patients who presented primarily with hypothermia to the San Francisco General Hospital, 33 were found to have sepsis as the etiology. Blood pressure can remain normal in spite of early cardiovascular failure in the so-called warm phase of septic shock with a high cardiac output and accompanying vasodilation. The laboratory may be helpful in the diagnosis of early sepsis. Both leukocytosis and leukopenia can be present. In the patient who is tachypneic, respiratory alkalosis is an early abnormality detected by arterial blood gas analysis.

As sepsis progresses to cardiovascular failure and collapse, the signs and symptoms are more apparent. Tachycardia and hypotension are evident as the patient appears increasingly toxic. Hypoxemia and metabolic acidosis may be present on arterial blood gas analysis, and evidence for a coagulation disorder might appear. Finally, alterations of liver function tests have been described in sepsis.

Indications and Timing of Antibiotic Therapy

Early administration of antibiotics in patients with septicemia has been shown to decrease mortality. There is a commonly held principle that patients with meningitis should have antibiotics administered within 1 hour of seeking care at a medical facility. Because septicemia and meningitis are similarly life threatening, there is no reason for this time frame not to apply to both. For patients with suspected community-acquired sepsis who present to emergency care facilities, the work-up and treatment can be accomplished without delay.

There are no precise clinical or laboratory indications for the institution of antibiotics in sepsis. The decision to adminster them often rests on clinical suspicion. To wait for advanced clinical signs of sepsis and hypoten-

TABLE 22–5. Organisms Taking Advantage of Primary or Acquired Immune Defects

Immune Defect	Acquired Due to	Bacteria	Fungi	Parasites	Viruses

Phagocyte: Polymorphonuclear leukocyte (PMN)	Acute leukemia
	Chemotherapy
	Radiation therapy
	Other drugs
		Enteric bacilli
		  (*Pseudomonas,*
		  Escherichia coli,
		  Klebsiella)
		Staphylococcus aureus
			Candida species
			Aspergillus species
			Mucoraceae		

T-lymphocyte: Mononuclear phagocyte	Hodgkin's disease
	Lymphoma
	Chemotherapy
	Corticosteroids
	Viral infections
	AIDS
		Streptococcus pyogenes
		Listeria monocytogenes
		Salmonella species
		Mycobacterium species
		Legionella pneumophila
		Nocardia asteroides
			Cryptococcus
			  neoformans
			Candida species
			Histoplasma
			  capsulatum
			Coccidioides immitis
				Pneumocystis carinii
				Toxoplasma gondii
				Strongyloides
				  stercoralis
					Cytomegalovirus
					Herpes simplex
					Varicella-zoster
					Measles
					Adenovirus

Immunoglobulin	Multiple myeloma Chronic lymphocytic leukemia Chemotherapy Splenectomy	*Streptococcus pneumoniae* *Hemophilus influenzae* *Neisseria meningitidis* Enteric bacilli		*Pneumocystis carinii* *Giardia lamblia* *Babesia* species *Plasmodium* species	
Complement	Congenital deficiency	*Neisseria meningitidis* *Neisseria gonorrhoeae*			

(From Neese R, Douglas R: A Practical Approach to Infectious Diseases, 2nd ed. Boston, Little, Brown & Co, 1990; adapted from Armstrong D: Infections in patients with neoplastic disease. In Verhoef J, et al (eds): Infections in the Immunocompromised Host—Pathogenesis, Prevention, and Therapy. New York, Elsevier/North Holland, 1980, pp. 129–158.)

TABLE 22–6. Early Recognition of Sepsis

Predisposing Factors for Sepsis
Age >60 years
Serious underlying medical condition
Chronic-care institutionalization
Immunosuppressive therapy
Indwelling catheters—bladder or vascular
Recent major surgery
Mechanical ventilatory support

sion is possibly inviting disaster. Table 22–6 provides some guidelines to aid in the decision to institute antibiotic therapy. The key to making a decision concerning the administration of antibiotics rests, more often than not, on whether a serious underlying predisposing condition is present as well as on accompanying symptoms and signs of sepsis. If a patient should have suspected sepsis as indicated by the criteria listed in the Table 22–7, then the institution of major broad-spectrum antibiotic coverage can probably be justified. (See boxes, Drug Treatment: Suspected Neonatal Sepsis of Unknown Source and Drug Treatment: Suspected Childhood and Adult Sepsis of Unknown Source.)

Discussion

The most important goal of antimicrobial therapy is to eliminate bacteria from the bloodstream as rapidly as possible. Early achievement of this goal will reduce the incidence of shock, disseminated intravascular coagulation, and other end-organ dysfunction. Only after bacterial control or eradication will other support measures, such as ventilatory and hemodynamic support, be effective in restoring the normal physiologic state of the patient. The most important fac-

TABLE 22–7. The Sepsis Syndrome

1. Clinical evidence of an infectious focus
2. All of the following:
   Fever >101°F or hypothermia <96°F
   Tachycardia° >90 beats/min
   Tachypnea >20 breaths/min or need for
      mechanical ventilation
3. One of the following manifestations of inadequate
   perfusion:
   Deterioration in mental function
   Hypoxemia—PaO$_2$ <72 torr on 21% FiO$_2$
   Elevated plasma lactate
   Oliguria—urine output <0.5 ml/kg/hour

°Unless patient is receiving beta-blockers or has a pacemaker.

tor in the initial selection of antibiotics is the wide range of potential gram-positive, gram-negative, and anaerobic organisms that could be the actual cause of the septic state. There is no reliable way to accurately distinguish between these causes in the emergency department or initial intensive care unit setting. In recognition of this fact, any antimicrobials selected should be broad spectrum and have effective minimum bactericidal concentration against the likely pathogens.

It is important to note that the antibiotic recommendations reflect an attempt to achieve a broad consensus as to appropriate choices; however, there are many potential alternatives. Local patterns of bacterial activity and sensitivities significantly affect choices in given institutions. For example, in some institutions, bacterial resistance has caused a shift away from gentamicin as the primary aminoglycoside of choice to others such as amikacin. Vancomycin is often chosen over other penicillinase-resistant penicillins because of a high frequency of methicillin-resistant *Staphylococcus aureus*. In addition, initial diagnostic efforts, such as Gram's stains and x-rays, might provide good enough information to indicate a specific bacterial pathogen. In this case, antimicrobial therapy can be more specifically directed at that organism.

The choice of antibiotics in the newborn patient, when sepsis is suspected, reflects the fact that most cases are caused by group B streptococci and *E. coli*. It is important to note that *Staphylococcus aureus* and *Staphylococcus epidermidis* have become more frequent causes of neonatal sepsis in neonatal intensive care units. These organisms are usually associated with indwelling catheters or other invasive devices. In these cases, the addition of a penicillinase-resistant penicillin such as nafcillin or vancomycin might be considered to supplement the standard regimen.

The standard regimen for initial therapy in the newborn period continues to be a penicillin plus an aminoglycoside. Specifically, ampicillin is chosen because of its activity against enterococci and *Listeria monocytogenes*. Gentamicin is still selected as a good aminoglycoside because of its excellent spectrum against the gram-negative organisms. Cefotaxime, the alternative for the aminoglycoside, is an effective agent; however, it has a much greater capacity of producing fungal overgrowth than does an aminogly-

DRUG TREATMENT: SUSPECTED NEONATAL SEPSIS OF UNKNOWN SOURCE

Patient Group	Primary Treatment	Alternative Treatment
Age birth to 7 days	Ampicillin, 50 mg/kg q 8 hours *plus* Gentamicin, 2.5 mg/kg q 12 hours	Ampicillin, 50 mg/kg q 8 hours *plus* Cefotaxime, 50 mg/kg q 12 hours
Age 8 days to 3 months	Ampicillin, 50 mg/kg q 6 hours *plus* Gentamicin, 2.5 mg/kg q 8 hours	Ampicillin, 50 mg/kg 6 q hours *plus* Cefotaxime, 50 mg/kg q 8 hours

DRUG TREATMENT: SUSPECTED CHILDHOOD AND ADULT SEPSIS OF UNKNOWN SOURCE

Patient Group	Primary Treatment	Alternative Treatment
Child, not immunocompromised	Ceftriaxone, 50 mg/kg q 12 hours	Cefotaxime, 50 mg/kg q 6 hours
Child, neutropenic or immunocompromised	Nafcillin, 25 mg/kg q 6 hours *plus* Ceftazidime, 50 mg/kg q 8 hours	Vancomycin, 10 mg/kg q 6 hours *plus* Ticarcillin, 50 mg/kg q 4 hours *plus* Gentamicin, 2.5 mg/kg q 8 hours
Adult, not immunocompromised	Cefotaxime, 2 g q 6 hours	Ticarcillin plus clavulanate, 3.1 g q 4 hours
Adult, neutropenic or immunocompromised	Nafcillin, 2 g q 4 hours *plus* Ceftazidime, 2 g q 8 hours	Vancomycin, 1 g q 12 hours *plus* Ticarcillin, 3 g q 4 hours *plus* Gentamicin, 2.5–3 mg/kg loading dose IV over 30 minutes; subsequent doses based on individually measured pharmacokinetics

coside. Unless meningitis is highly suspected or confirmed by LP, the additional killing power of cefotaxime is unnecessary in the initial treatment of neonatal sepsis.

After the age of 3 months and throughout childhood, a third-generation cephalosporin will cover the major life-threatening infections of childhood. The third-generation cephalosporins are active against most of the common pathogens that cause serious, life-threatening infections in children. There are no clinical studies that show clear clinical superiority of one agent over another, but cefotaxime achieves minimal inhibitory concentrations in vitro at lower serum levels for gram-positive, gram-negative, and anaerobic bacteria than do the other agents. Ceftriaxone has the longest half-life and, therefore, the distinct advantage of a less frequent dosing interval. While a third-generation cephalosporin alone covers for most potential bacteria, it is less adequate when *S. aureus* is the infecting agent. The addition of a penicillinase-resistant penicillin is recommended if this organism is strongly suspected. If the infection is acquired in hospital, with the potential for multiply resistant organisms, then broader-spectrum coverage might be necessary, as discussed below for the immunocompromised patient.

For the immunocompromised or neutropenic child (less than 500 blood polymorphonuclear leukocytes/mm³), a pencillinase-resistant pencillin plus a third-generation cephalosporin is a good selection for initial treatment because this combination has a broader, and possibly more effective, spectrum against gram-positive and gram-negative organisms than do single agents. Ceftazidime is the third-generation cephalosporin of choice because of its good activity against *P. aeruginosa* as well as against the other gram-negative organisms. Clinical studies have confirmed the effectiveness of this agent in neutropenic patients. Some authorities prefer triple drug therapy to provide the widest possible coverage. The most commonly used triple drug regimen includes a penicillinase-resistant penicillin, an extended-spectrum penicillin, and an aminoglycoside. Vancomycin is substituted for the penicillinase-resistant penicillin, particularly if there is a possibility that methicillin-resistant *S. aureus* is an infecting agent.

For the adult with sepsis of unknown source, there are many potential antimicrobial selections. No studies show a clear effectiveness of one over the other in the nonimmunocompromised patient, either as single-agent therapy or multiple-agent combinations. The guiding principle is that, whatever the selection, it should have an effective, broad range of activity against both gram-positive and gram-negative aerobic and anaerobic organisms. A secondary guiding principle is that, as soon as culture and sensitivity results are available, modifications of therapy are carried out as necessary without delay. Currently, the third-generation cephalosporins enjoy widespread use and have demonstrated effectiveness as single agents in the treatment of sepsis, particularly of gram-negative aerobic origin. They are not as effective as other agents against gram-positive aerobes or anaerobic organisms but have sufficient range and killing power to serve as empirical first-line agents. An alternative choice is ticarcillin with clavulanate. It is very effective against gram-positive aerobes and anaerobic organisms but not equivalent in effectiveness to the third-generation cephalosporins for gram-negative aerobes. Its range and killing power against these latter organisms are sufficient, however, to make it a reasonable, empirical, single-agent alternative choice. Many authorities still recommend a penicillinase-resistant penicillin

in addition to an aminoglycoside, and this combination remains effective. There are few complications of therapy with the third-generation cephalosporins, and this fact has made the traditional usage of the aminoglycosides less attractive. The new agent imipenem has also been used successfully in this clinical setting.

In adult patients who are neutropenic or immunocompromised, broad-spectrum coverage is recommended against an even wider range of organisms. The addition of a penicillinase-resistant penicillin to ceftazidime makes a particularly good combination against the organisms likely to be present in this clinical setting. Clinical studies support the use of ceftazidime in this setting. Some authorities still recommend triple therapy with a penicillinase-resistant penicillin, an aminoglycoside, and an antipseudomonal penicillin to provide the broadest possible coverage. Vancomycin must be substituted for the penicillinase-resistant penicillin if methicillin-resistant *S. aureus* is suspected.

Penicillin-Allergic Patient

When a patient is truly allergic to penicillin (see discussion of penicillin allergy in the section on acute meningitis, earlier in this chapter), alternatives have to be considered. For the child, either immunocompetent or immunocompromised, chloramphenicol can be started if *H. influenzae* is the suspected organism or meningitis is suspected in spite of a normal LP. Otherwise, the combination of clindamycin and gentamicin can be started pending cultures. In adults, the combination of clindamycin and gentamicin is also a good starting treatment. Another alternative that has shown promise in recent studies is the use of the fluoroquinolone, ciprofloxacin, as a single agent.

Sepsis of Pulmonary Source

Despite the discovery and subsequent widespread use of antibiotics, pneumonia remains the most common cause of infectious disease death in the United States and is responsible for 10% of all hospital admissions. While bacterial pneumonia can afflict the apparently healthy, it is most commonly seen in individuals with underlying predisposing disorders that impair host defense mechanisms. These disorders and the degree to which they affect the host also account for the increased morbidity and mortality. As the population ages, with attendant chronic disabilities and the increased use of immunosuppressive therapies, pneumonia is likely to maintain its importance as a serious life threat.

Microbiology

While the traditional microbiologic causes of pneumonia are still important, there has been a gradual change in the spectrum of organisms isolated in various centers. *Hemophilus influenzae* has become an increasingly recognized cause of pneumonia and, because of its propensity to produce beta-lactamase, it is a more difficult bacteria to treat. *Branhamella catarrhalis*, once thought to be a harmless colonizer of the oropharynx, is now recognized as an important cause of otitis, sinusitis, and pneumonia. Legionella species, a relatively newly identified group of respiratory pathogens, have led to troublesome outbreaks, especially in health-care facilities. Finally, exogenous and endogenous suppression of the immune system (through cancer chemotherapy or AIDS) has opened the floodgate to a multitude of potential bacterial, viral, parasitic, and fungal respiratory pathogens.

Pneumonia in the neonatal period can be acquired intrapartum, nosocomially, or environmentally after discharge of the patient to the home environment (Table 22–8). Intrapartum pneumonia is usually caused by aspiration or acquisition of maternal organisms similar to those found in generalized sepsis, as discussed previously. The organisms of most concern during the first 7 days of life include group B streptococci and gram-negative organisms like *Escherichia coli*. If pneumonia develops after 7 days, it can be considered to be acquired nosocomially, and the spectrum of microorganisms broadens. In addition to the previously mentioned organisms, *Staphylococcus aureus* becomes an important pathogen, particularly in patients with invasive monitoring or therapeutic devices or in a neonatal intensive care unit. At this age, the child also becomes exposed to viral pathogens including respiratory syncytial virus, parainfluenzae 3 virus, influenzae virus, and enterovirus.

Of particular interest is *Chlamydia pneumoniae*. This organism can be acquired intrapartum but does not manifest itself for 4 to 8 weeks (up to 12 weeks in some cases). Approximately 10 to 20% of neonates exposed to infected mothers will develop pneumoni-

TABLE 22–8. Microbiologic Agents of Pneumonia in Children and Adults

Patient Group	Infecting Organism
Age birth to 7 days	Bacteria
	Group B *Streptococcus*
	Gram-negative bacilli
Age 7 days to 2 months	*Chlamydia*
	Viruses
	Bacteria
	Streptococcus pneumoniae
	Staphylococcus aureus
	Hemophilus influenzae
Age 2 months to 3 years	Viruses
	Bacteria
	S. pneumoniae
	H. influenzae
	S. aureus
Age 3 years to 12 years	Viruses
	Bacteria
	S. pneumoniae
	Mycoplasma pneumoniae
Age 13 years to 19 years	*M. pneumoniae*
	Viruses
	Bacteria
	S. pneumoniae
Age 19 years to 45 years	*M. pneumoniae*
	S. pneumoniae
	Viruses (during epidemics)
	S. aureus (associated with influenza A virus)
	Klebsiella pneumoniae
	H. influenzae
Age 45 years to 65 years	*S. pneumoniae*
	H. influenzae
	Legionella species
	Klebsiella pneumoniae
	Escherichia coli
	Branhamella catarrhalis
Hospital acquired	*Klebsiella* species
	Pseudomonas aeruginosa
	S. aureus
	E. coli
	Enterobacter species
	Proteus species
	S. pneumoniae
AIDS	*Pneumocystis carinii*
	Bacteria
	Viruses
	Fungi

tis. This pneumonia, however, causes few toxic problems and rarely is life threatening. Once the child grows to infancy (greater than 1 month of age), viruses predominate as the cause of pneumonitis. Encapsulated bacteria such as *Streptococcus pneumoniae* and *H. influenzae* type B as well as *Staphylococcus* species remain causes to be considered, particularly in the toxic-appearing patient. By age 5 years, in addition to viruses, *Mycoplasma pneumoniae* becomes the most common respiratory pathogen and causes up to

25% of all cases of childhood pneumonia. In early adulthood until the age of 45, *Mycoplasma* is probably the most common cause of pneumonia. The clinical syndrome caused by *M. pneumoniae* is usually not serious or life threatening. It is responsible for only 4% of patients hospitalized with pneumonia.

S. pneumoniae is still felt to be the most common community-acquired bacterial cause of pneumonia even late in life. As patients get older, however, particularly those who have chronic acquired respiratory disease, *H. influenzae* becomes increasingly common. *S. aureus* can occur in adults, but it is most commonly associated with epidemics of true type A influenza. Gram-negative species, as well as *Legionella* species, assume a greater importance in elderly and more debilitated patients.

Nosocomially acquired pneumonia is largely due to gram-negative organisms. Sixty percent of nosocomially acquired pneumonias are caused by aerobic gram-negative bacilli. The majority of these infections occur in intensive care or equivalent units, which harbor resistant organisms. Institutions in some geographical areas have had local outbreaks of *Legionella* pneumonia as well. Despite antibiotic therapy, the mortality rate has been reported to be as high as 50% in nosocomially acquired pneumonia. The virulence of these organisms and the severity of the underlying disease are significant factors that cause increased morbidity and mortality.

The range of etiologic agents in pneumonia in the immunocompromised patient is broad. These patients will often have combined or multiple etiologic agents, such as bacteria, viruses, and fungi. Approximately 80 to 90% of patients with AIDS will eventually acquire *Pneumocystis carinii* pneumonia. Of the bacterial organisms reported in AIDS patients, *H. influenzae*, *S. pneumoniae*, and group B streptococci have been reported in patients in whom the infection was acquired in the community.

Clinical and Laboratory Indicators Influencing Antibiotic Therapy

The clinical evaluation and subsequent findings in patients with pneumonia have a significant impact on the choice of antibiotic therapy. Age, predisposing conditions, radiologic picture, results of Gram's stain, and other adjunctive laboratory findings such as arterial blood gases and white blood cell count are important factors to consider. Patients who exhibit significant toxicity, respiratory distress with tachypnea, toxemia, and multiple lobe involvement are best managed in an intensive care setting.

Predisposing Conditions

Several predisposing conditions affect the management of the patient with pneumonia.

Alcohol. Alcoholism predisposes patients to pneumonia. In addition to *S. pneumoniae*, these patients are prone to pneumonia caused by aspiration, *H. influenzae*, *Klebsiella pneumoniae*, and *Mycobacterium tuberculosis*.

Aspiration. Aspiration occurs in patients with significant alterations in mental status, esophageal motility disorders, seizures, and poor dentition. In the community setting, these pneumonias are the result of aspirated mouth organisms, which are usually penicillin-sensitive anaerobes such as *Fusobacterium nucleatum*, *Bacteroides melaninogenicus*, and anaerobic gram-positive cocci. If the aspiration occurs in the hospital setting, gram-negative organisms that have colonized the oropharynx have to be suspected although it is very difficult to truly separate colonizers from actual infective agents. Aspiration is treated with antibiotics when there is accompanying fever and cough. The true therapeutic intervention, however, remains good pulmonary toilet.

Chronic Obstructive Pulmonary Disease. Patients with COPD have a high incidence of *H. influenzae* in addition to *S. pneumoniae* infections. Patients with cystic fibrosis are prone to staphylococcal infections as well as pneumonia caused by *Pseudomonas* species. These latter infections often arise just after administration of antibiotics.

Postinfluenza. Patients with true influenza can have primary viral or secondary bacterial pneumonia. The latter group of patients have the classic signs of influenza and a period of improvement. They then appear to have a relapse, with new onset of signs of pneumonia. *S. pneumoniae*, *H. influenzae*, and *S. aureus* have all been reported to occur in this setting. A high degree of suspicion has to be maintained for *S. aureus* because of its propensity for toxicity, morbidity, and mortality. In the setting of pneumonia associated with influenza, the Gram's stain is essential in attempting to diagnose that particular organism.

Hospitalized and Institutionalized Patients. These patients are a significant risk for pneumonias caused by aerobic gram-negative bacilli, especially *K. pneumoniae* and *Pseudo-monas aeruginosa.* In addition to these organisms, *E. coli* and *Proteus* species, as well as *S. aureus,* are frequently isolated. Of special note is *Legionella* species. Major outbreaks have occurred in hospital settings and have been traced to air-conditioning and water-evaporative devices. This pneumonia has been described in community settings as well as in pediatric age groups. While it can affect apparently healthy people, it has a stronger predilection for immunocompromised and dialysis patients, middle-aged and elderly males, and chronically debilitated patients.

Immunocompromised Host. Virtually any agent can cause pneumonia in the immunocompromised host. There are no clear clinical findings that definitely differentiate the organisms responsible for pneumonia. Laboratory findings are often nonspecific and unhelpful. Direct access to tissue through biopsy is often the only way to secure a diagnosis. It is important, however, to recognize that there are treatable organisms, and therapeutic strategies can be constructed to manage these infections. Of the bacteria, gram-negative aerobic organisms (*Klebsiella* species, *E. coli, Pseudomonas* species) are the most common pathogens. *S. aureus* has recently been reported, as well as *Legionella.*

Radiologic Evaluation

Although it is generally not possible to accurately predict the organism responsible for pneumonia by x-ray, knowledge of some of the patterns can be useful in selecting an antibiotic. Infiltrates in the upper lobes can occur in any pneumonia but are commonly found in *K. pneumoniae* and *M. tuberculosis.* If only the inferior segment of the right upper lobe or the apical segment of the right lower lobe is involved, aspiration can be suspected. In community-acquired pneumonia, a discrete lobar pattern is more common with *S. pneumoniae.* A bronchopneumonia pattern, patchy infiltrates without defined anatomic borders, can also occur with *S. pneumoniae* but is more common with *M. pneumoniae, Legionella* species, and *C. pneumoniae.* Unfortunately in the patient with underlying serious disease or immunosuppression, the patterns are even less reliable. The typical pattern of *P. carinii* pneumonia, often found in **AIDS** patients, is a diffuse bilateral infiltrate involving all lobes. Occasionally, however, this pattern can vary.

Gram's Stain

Every effort should be made to obtain an adequate sputum sample before initiating antibiotic therapy. Although transtracheal aspiration is rarely performed in an emergency department setting and has become less common in any setting, it can be considered under certain conditions: (1) in seriously ill patients who cannot raise their own sputum, (2) in cases of suspected anaerobic infections, and (3) for initial evaluation in the immunocompromised host.

An adequate sputum specimen for Gram's stain can be defined as a smear containing a predominance of polymorphonuclear leukocytes (usually greater than 25 per high-powered field) and less than 10 squamous cells per high-powered field. If classic gram-positive diplococci are seen as the predominant organism, then *S. pneumoniae* can be strongly suspected with an 85% specificity and 62% sensitivity. Although there are no clear statistical figures for *S. aureus,* bright clusters and tetrads of strongly gram-positive cocci that predominate in a Gram's specimen are highly suspicious for that organism. Small gram-negative diplococci are consistent with *H. influenzae* and gram-negative rods with gram-negative species. (See boxes, Drug Treatment: Suspected Neonatal and Childhood Sepsis of Pulmonary Source and Drug Treatment: Adult Sepsis of Pulmonary Source.)

Discussion

The choice of initial empirical antimicrobial therapy for patients with severe pneumonia is dependent on multiple factors. The four most important of these are age, the environment of the patient, his or her immune status, and the presence of underlying diseases. These factors are the most important general determinants of likely microbial etiology. It cannot be overemphasized that the most important clinical investigative factor is the result of Gram's stain. Every effort should be made to acquire an appropriate sputum specimen and examine it for likely microbial bacterial etiologies. Specifically, during a period of influenza, the discovery of grape-like clusters of gram-positive cocci on a Gram's stain will direct the clinician to institute therapy against *S. aureus.* This organism is particularly virulent and carries a high mortality rate. Early institution of antistaphylococcal therapy could be lifesaving.

In the newborn, the selection of antibiotics is similar to that for sepsis, since the organ-

DRUG TREATMENT: SUSPECTED NEONATAL AND CHILDHOOD SEPSIS OF PULMONARY SOURCE

Patient Group	Primary Treatment	Alternative Treatment
Age birth to 7 days	Ampicillin, 50 mg/kg q 8 hours *plus* Gentamicin, 2.5 mg/kg q 12 hours	Ampicillin, 50 mg/kg q 8 hours *plus* Cefotaxime, 50 mg/kg q 12 hours
Age 8 days to 1 month	Ampicillin, 50 mg/kg q 6 hours *plus* Gentamicin, 2.5 mg/kg q 8 hours	Ampicillin, 50 mg/kg q 6 hours *plus* Cefotaxime, 50 mg/kg q 8 hours
Age 1 month to 10 years	Ceftriaxone, 50 mg/kg q 12 hours	Cefuroxime, 50 mg/kg q 8 hours

DRUG TREATMENT: ADULT SEPSIS OF PULMONARY SOURCE

Patient Group	Primary Treatment	Alternative Treatment
Community acquired, no underlying conditions (lobar pneumonia)	Penicillin G, 1,000,000 units q 4 hours	Erythromycin, 1 g q 6 hours *plus* Cefazolin, 2 g q 4 hours
Community acquired, underlying diabetes, alcohol abuse or chronic obstructive pulmonary disease, or not lobar (bronchopneumonia)	Ticarcillin plus clavulanate, 3.1 g q 4 hours	Erythromycin, 1 g q 6 hours *plus* Cefotaxime, 2 g q 6 hours
Institutionally acquired (not immunocompromised or neutropenic)	Ticarcillin plus clavulanate, 3.1 g q 4 hours *plus* Gentamicin, 2.5–3 mg/kg loading dose IV over 30 minutes; subsequent doses based on individually measured pharmacokinetics	Imipenem, 1 g q 6 hours
Immunocompromised (steroids, lymphoma, neutropenic)	Erythromycin, 1 g q 6 hours *plus* Nafcillin, 2 g q 6 hours *plus* Cefotaxime, 2 g q 6 hours	Erythromycin, 1 g q 6 hours *plus* Imipenem, 1 g q 6 hours
HIV positive	Erythromycin, 1 g q 6 hours *plus* Trimethoprim/sulfamethoxazole, 5 mg/kg q 6 hours (based on trimethoprim dose)	
Aspiration pneumonia	Clindamycin, 900 mg q 8 hours	Ticarcillin plus clavulanate, 3.1 g q 4 hours

isms likely to cause infiltrates will be those responsible for sepsis. Ampicillin and an aminoglycoside, such as gentamicin, remain excellent choices. A third-generation cephalosporin, specifically cefotaxime, can be substituted for the aminoglycoside. After the neonatal period and through infancy and early childhood, viruses begin to predomi-nate as causes of pneumonia. However, in the seriously ill child, the bacteria *S. pneumoniae* and *H. influenzae* must be considered, with *S. aureus* being a less common but still an important organism. An initial empirical antibiotic can be the third-generation cephalosporin ceftriaxone. Ceftriaxone has good activity against the important pulmonary pathogens and the advantage of a less frequent dosing schedule than other second- and third-generation cephalosporins. Cefuroxime is a good alternative empirical choice for ceftriaxone. If *S. aureus* is suspected in any age group through either the Gram's stain or the typical pneumatocele appearance of the x-ray, a penicillinase-resistant penicillin must be added to the therapy.

Up to the age of 2 months, infants are at risk for pneumonia caused by *Chlamydia trachomatis*. However, these patients usually do not present in a seriously ill condition and are often afebrile. Initial empirical therapy is still directed at potential bacterial pathogens.

As the patient passes into adolescence and adulthood, the two most common organisms that cause pneumonia are *M. pneumoniae* and *S. pneumoniae*. During influenza epidemics, *S. aureus* is a serious cause of pneumonia. In the patient with community-acquired lobar pneumonia, without any underlying serious illnesses or immunosuppressive states, penicillin remains an excellent initial drug. In the more seriously ill and toxic-appearing patient, erythromycin plus a first-generation cephalosporin, such as cefazolin, is recommended because of its coverage of *S. pneumoniae*, *S. aureus*, *M. pneumoniae*, and *Legionella* species. For patients who have a community-acquired pneumonia and a serious underlying condition, such as diabetes, alcoholism, or chronic obstructive pulmonary disease, broader-spectrum antibiotic coverage to include organisms like *H. influenzae* and *K. pneumoniae* is necessary. In this case, the combination of ticarcillin plus clavulanate is recommended because of their excellent coverage of the gram-positive and gram-negative organisms likely to cause pneumonia under these circumstances. As an alternative, or if the possibility of *Legionella* pneumonia exists, erythromycin plus a third-generation cephalosporin provides even more extensive coverage.

For patients with institutionally acquired pneumonias (i.e., hospital, chronic-care facility), ticarcillin with clavulanate added to an aminoglycoside provides excellent coverage, particularly against the gram-negative organisms. One of the broadest possible single agents for coverage against pneumonia is imipenem. Imipenem has excellent activity against all bacterial causes of pneumonia and is a good alternative agent. It does not, however, cover methicillin-resistant *S. aureus*

and has recently been demonstrated to produce occasional resistance in *P. aeruginosa*.

For patients who are seriously immunocompromised (i.e., high-dose steroid therapy, lymphoma), coverage has to be extended to *S. aureus*, *Legionella* species, and a variety of aerobic gram-negative organisms. A good combination is a penicillinase-resistant penicillin plus erythromycin and an aminoglycoside. If methicillin-resistant *S. aureus* is suspected, then vancomycin can be substituted for the penicillinase-resistant penicillin. In addition, cefotaxime can be substituted for the aminoglycoside. As an alternative, imipenem plus erythromycin will cover most of the important organisms in this setting. If the patient has a clinical and radiographic picture of pneumonia and is HIV positive, erythromycin and trimethoprim-sulfamethoxazole are recommended.

In patients with acute gastric aspiration, initial antibiotic therapy has not been shown to prevent bacterial superinfection. Bronchoscopy for diagnosis and pulmonary toilet is recommended. If toxicity becomes evident (i.e., fever and leukocytosis), then clindamycin can be instituted. Cultures of any sputum should be done beforehand, however, because a wide range of gram-positive and gram-negative organisms, in addition to anaerobes, can infect the lung in this setting. Ticarcillin plus clavulanate is a good alternative empirical choice.

Penicillin-Allergic Patient

In patients who have had serious reactions to penicillin in the past and who could be cross-sensitive to cephalosporins (see discussion of penicillin allergy in the section on acute meningitis), erythromycin or clindamycin, in addition to an aminoglycoside, would be a good initial empirical choice in all age groups except neonates. Ciprofloxacin is a more recently developed non–beta-lactam antibiotic that could be used as a single agent in these circumstances. Ciprofloxacin, in the intravenous form, is expected to be approved for use in the United States in 1990. It is not, however, approved for pediatric patients.

Sepsis of Urinary Source

The urinary tract is the single most common source identified for serious life-threatening infections. Bacteriuria has been reported to occur in 3% of premature infants and 1% of full-term newborn infants. Bacteriuria has an incidence as high as 4.5% in preschool females but levels out to an incidence of 1 to 3% in the adult female. By age 65 years, the incidence of bacteriuria increases to 10% in males and to 20% in females. By this age, the dramatic increase in male bacteriuria drastically alters the 30:1 ratio of adult female to male bacteriuria. Indwelling catheters carry a special risk, with the incidence of bacteriuria rising by 5 to 10% per day that the catheter remains in place.

Microbiology

In the newborn period the common causes of urinary tract infections include *E. coli*, *Klebsiella* species, and enterococci. Other bacterial etiologies include *Streptococcus faecalis*, staphylococcal species, and other mixed infections. In childhood, *E. coli* is isolated in up to 80% of cases. By adulthood, uncomplicated urinary tract infections are overwhelmingly caused by *E. coli* (greater than 80%). Other organisms include *Proteus* species and *Staphylococcus saprophyticus*. In the patient at risk for life-threatening infection, however, the microbial spectrum broadens to include *Pseudomonas* species, *Klebsiella* species, other gram-negative bacilli, enterococci, and *S. aureus* (Table 22–9). These latter organisms are more likely to be acquired nosocomially in patients who are on urinary tract suppressive antibiotic therapy or as a result of complications of instrumentation. They are also seen more often in patients with preexisting renal calculi.

The presence of fungi in the urine presents a particularly difficult clinical dilemma. Fungi are most commonly found in diabetics, patients with catheters, previously instrumented patients, and those already receiving antibiotics. Colonization is usually the rule,

TABLE 22–9. Microbiologic Causes of Urinary Tract Infection

Escherichia coli
Proteus species
Klebsiella species
Enterobacter
Group D streptococci (enterococci)
Serratia species
Pseudomonas species
Staphylococcus aureus (stones, manipulation)
Staphylococcus saprophyticus
Chlamydia trachomatis (urethritis)

as opposed to true infection. However, distinction between colonization and true infection is very difficult and not likely to be accomplished during the initial evaluation of the patient.

Recognition of the Urinary Tract as a Source of Infection

Establishing the urinary tract as a source of life-threatening infection can be made both clinically and on laboratory grounds, and, therefore, specific antibiotic therapy can be directed toward the suspected uropathogens. On urinalysis, infection is suspected when 7 or more white blood cells are seen per high-powered microscopic field. Supportive evidence includes the presence of bacteria, nitrites, and leukocyte esterase.

For newborns and infants, a high degree of suspicion remains the key clinical indicator. Fever or hypothermia, failure to thrive, vomiting, and unexplained jaundice usually require a thorough search for infection, including the urinary tract. The investigative method of choice is suprapubic aspiration or catheterization, as opposed to obtaining a specimen using an adhesive plastic collection bag.

In older children and adults, the more classic signs of urinary tract infection become manifest, including abdominal pain, fever and chills, flank pain, urinary frequency, and urinary urgency. High fever and frequent shaking chills are especially indicative of upper urinary tract infection (pyelonephritis) and systemic toxicity. Other clinical findings that point toward the urinary tract as a source of infection include diabetes, neurologic disease, congenital urinary tract abnormalities, urinary tract obstruction (prostate, stones), and recent urinary tract instrumentation. (See box.)

Discussion

The initial management of the patient with sepsis from a suspected urinary tract source is directed primarily at gram-negative organisms. Through all age ranges, ampicillin plus an aminoglycoside is an excellent combination to initiate therapy pending the results of the culture. There are numerous alternatives to this regimen. The most common alternative is a third-generation cephalosporin, such as cefotaxime, to replace the aminoglycoside in the newborn period, or cefotaxime can be used as a single agent for older children and adults.

DRUG TREATMENT: SUSPECTED SEPSIS OF URINARY TRACT SOURCE

Patient Group	Primary Treatment	Alternative Treatment
Age birth to 7 days	Ampicillin, 50 mg/kg q 8 hours *plus* Gentamicin, 2.5 mg/kg q 12 hours	Ampicillin, 50 mg/kg q 8 hours *plus* Cefotaxime, 50 mg/kg q 12 hours
Age 8 days to 1 month	Ampicillin, 50 mg/kg q 6 hours *plus* Gentamicin, 2.5 mg/kg q 8 hours	Ampicillin, 50 mg/kg q 6 hours *plus* Cefotaxime, 50 mg/kg q 8 hours
Childhood	Ampicillin, 50 mg/kg q 6 hours *plus* Gentamicin, 2.5 mg/kg q 8 hours	Cefotaxime, 50 mg/kg q 6 hours
Adult	Ampicillin, 2 g q 6 hours *plus* Gentamicin, 2.5–3.0 mg/kg loading dose IV over 30 minutes; subsequent doses based on individually measured pharmacokinetics	Cefotaxime, 2 g q 6 hours

It is not uncommon for patients with severe urinary tract infections to present after having already been on suppressive oral antibiotic therapy. In this case, urine and blood cultures are essential. The choice of therapy should be directed toward organisms that are likely to be resistant. *P. aeruginosa, Klebsiella* species, *Enterobacter* species, and enterococci are possible infecting organisms. Ampicillin is specifically recommended when enterococci are suspected, usually in combination with an aminoglycoside or a third-generation cephalosporin. Other antibiotics to be considered in severe urinary tract infections include the antipseudomonal penicillins (ticarcillin, piperacillin) plus the third-generation cephalosporin ceftazidime, especially if *P. aeruginosa* is suspected as the infecting organism. The fluoroquinolones (ciprofloxacin), as single agents, are alternatives. Ciprofloxacin in the intravenous form is expected to be approved for use in the United States in 1990.

Penicillin-Allergic Patient

For children, gentamicin alone is the drug of choice for patients with serious pencillin allergy (see discussion of penicillin allergy in the section on acute meningitis, earlier in this chapter). In adults, an aminoglycoside or a fluoroquinolone (ciprofloxacin) can be used. Ciprofloxacin in the intravenous form is expected to be approved for use in the United States in 1990.

Sepsis of Abdominal Source

Intra-abdominal causes of life-threatening infection may present in several forms. Infection may be retroperitoneal or intraperitoneal and diffuse or localized. Specific entities to be discussed include primary and secondary peritonitis, intraperitoneal and visceral abscesses, and biliary tract sources.

Specific Conditions: Clinical and Microbiologic Considerations

Necrotizing enterocolitis is a severe and often fatal gastrointestinal disease that primarily affects premature neonates. The diagnosis is suspected when the infant demonstrates a high degree of distress and radiographs show intramural gas dissection or perforation with free air. See Table 22–10 for the associated microbiologic causes.

Spontaneous bacterial peritonitis can occur without any evidence of viscus perforation or contamination of the peritoneal cavity and has been described most commonly in patients under 10 years of age. The responsible organisms almost always are *S. pneumoniae* or group A streptococci (see Table 22–10). Often the diagnosis cannot be distinguished from acute appendicitis and is not ensured

TABLE 22–10. Microbiologic Causes of Intra-abdominal Sepsis

Necrotizing Enterocolitis
Salmonella species
Klebsiella species
Escherichia coli
Pseudomonas aeruginosa
Clostridium species
Viruses
Bacterial toxins
Peritonitis and Biliary Infections
Streptococcus pneumoniae
Group A streptococci
Staphylococcus species
Escherichia coli
Bacteroides species
Group D streptococci (enterococci)
Anaerobic streptococci
Fusobacterium
Clostridium species
Klebsiella species
Pelvic Peritonitis
Neisseria gonorrhoeae
Chlamydia trachomatis
Escherichia coli
Bacteroides species
Anaerobic streptococci

until a laparotomy is performed. These patients usually present with classic fever, chills, and signs of an acute abdomen such as guarding, rebound tenderness, and other peritoneal findings.

Spontaneous bacterial peritonitis can also be present in patients with underlying cirrhosis and nephrotic syndrome. These cases tend to be less acute with less frequent presence of peritoneal findings upon examination. Tenderness may be absent. The only clinical finding in these cases might be an unexplained fever in a patient with ascites. In this case, a paracentesis should be performed to rule out peritonitis. *E. coli* is the most common organism cultured in patients with bacterial peritonitis secondary to ascites (approximately 35% of cases), with *S. pneumoniae* recovered in 16%. Various other organisms, including alpha-hemolytic streptococci, *Pseudomonas* species, *Enterobacter*, *Klebsiella* species, and *Clostridium* species, have been recovered. The primary organism in peritonitis secondary to nephrotic syndrome is *S. pneumoniae*, presumably because of the massive urinary loss of gamma globulins that leads to a loss of protection against encapsulated organisms.

Secondary peritonitis can be due to a multitude of causes: rupture of a viscus, surgical postoperative leaks, pelvic inflammatory disease, rupture of an abscess, and peritoneal dialysis catheters. *E. coli* still predominates as the most common infecting organism in these cases, followed by enterococci. However, these infections are usually polymicrobial and include multiple anaerobic species such as *Bacteroides fragilis*, *Clostridium* species, and anaerobic streptococci. When gram-negative aerobes are involved, a more diffuse peritonitis results, with a higher mortality.

Intra-abdominal abscesses pose a serious diagnostic and therapeutic dilemma to clinicians. Hepatic, pancreatic, or retroperitoneal abscesses have a mortality ranging from 45 to 50%. In one large series, appendicitis accounted for 19% of the abscesses, pancreatitis for 12%, genitourinary causes for 18%, biliary tract for 8%, diverticuli for 7%, actinomycosis for 4%, perforating tumors for 3%, trauma for 3%, peptic ulceration for 2%, and recent surgical procedures for 2%. The great majority of patients have shaking chills and localized pain in the area of the abscess, which allows the clinician to direct specific diagnostic efforts such as ultrasound, gallium scanning, and computed tomography to make the diagnosis.

The organisms recovered in cases of intra-abdominal abscesses are commonly mixed and include *E. coli*, *S. aureus*, and a variety of anaerobic organisms including *B. fragilis*, anaerobic streptococci, and other aerobic gram-negative organisms such as *Klebsiella* species and *Enterobacter*.

Pelvic abscesses are often the sequelae of recurrent salpingitis, septic abortion, or puerperal infection. Unruptured abscesses can be difficult to diagnose clinically because they are not always palpable. They should be suspected in patients who have been treated appropriately for pelvic inflammatory disease but who are not improving clinically. Rupture of a tubo-ovarian abscess can be a sudden and dramatic event causing severe lower abdominal pain, peritoneal findings, and the rapid onset of hypotension and frank shock. Even with therapy, mortality has been reported to be about 50% in these cases. While *N. gonorrhoeae*, *C. trachomatis*, and *Mycoplasma* species can set the stage for the development of these abscesses, *E. coli*, aerobic and anaerobic streptococci, *B. fragilis*, and other *Bacteroides* species are the predominant pathogenic organisms.

Biliary disease does not always require antimicrobial therapy. Antibiotics are not usually needed in simple uncomplicated cholecystitis. There are no studies that demonstrate a definite advantage in their use. However, biliary gangrene and ascending cholangitis require the use of antibiotics.

Repeated chills, fever, and jaundice suggest ascending cholangitis in a patient with right upper quadrant pain. Untreated, this syndrome can progress to sepsis, shock, or liver abscess. The organisms responsible include *E. coli*, streptococci, enterococci, *Klebsiella* species, and *Proteus* species. In 41% of cases, anaerobic species such as *B. fragilis* and *Clostridium perfringens* can be recovered. (See box.)

Discussion

The range of organisms responsible for severe intra-abdominal infections is extremely broad. The organisms include a wide range of gram-positive and gram-negative organisms, both aerobic and anaerobic. Unlike other anatomic areas involved with severe infections, the anaerobic organisms assume a special prominence. For this reason, any antibiotic regimen selected for sepsis of abdominal source has to include coverage against these organisms.

Sepsis from an abdominal source in the newborn infant is likely to present as necrotizing enterocolitis. The currently recommended antibiotics include an antipseudomonal penicillin with the addition of an aminoglycoside. Mezlocillin, because of its greater efficacy against enterococci *in vitro*, is preferred by some authorities over ticarcillin. Mezlocillin also has fewer bleeding complications than other extended-spectrum penicillins. As an alternative, a third-generation cephalosporin can be substituted for the aminoglycoside.

There are two forms of peritonitis that can present in later childhood. One is primary peritonitis, which is caused most commonly by *S. pneumoniae* and group A streptococci. Other organisms have been implicated as well. The other form of peritonitis in childhood occurs secondary to rupture of the ap-

DRUG TREATMENT: SUSPECTED SEPSIS OF GASTROINTESTINAL SOURCE

Patient Group	Primary Treatment	Alternative Treatment
Newborn, necrotizing enterocolitis	Ticarcillin, 80 mg/kg q 8 hours *plus* Gentamicin, 2.5 mg/kg q 8 hours	Mezlocillin, 75 mg/kg q 8 hours *plus* Cefotaxime, 50 mg/kg q 8 hours
Peritonitis in childhood	Cefoxitin, 40 mg/kg q 6 hours *plus* Gentamicin, 2.5 mg/kg q 8 hours	Clindamycin, 10 mg/kg q 6 hours *plus* Gentamicin, 2.5 mg/kg q 8 hours
Peritonitis in adulthood	Cefoxitin, 2 g q 4 hours *plus* Gentamicin, 2.5–3.0 mg/kg loading dose IV over 30 minutes; subsequent doses based on individually measured pharmacokinetics	Metronidazole, 15 mg/kg loading dose and 7.5 mg/kg q 6 hours *plus* Gentamicin, 2.5–3.0 mg/kg loading dose IV over 30 minutes; subsequent doses based on individually measured pharmacokinetics
Gallbladder (biliary sepsis)	Cefoxitin, 2 g q 4 hours *plus* Gentamicin, 2.5–3.0 mg/kg loading dose IV over 30 minutes; subsequent doses based on individually measured pharmokinetics	Metronidazole, 15 mg/kg loading dose and 7.5 mg/kg q 6 hours *plus* Mezlocillin, 3 g q 4 hours
Pelvic peritonitis	Cefoxitin, 2 g q 6 hours *plus* Doxycycline, 100 mg q 12 hours	Clindamycin, 450 mg q 6 hours *plus* Gentamicin, 2.5–3.0 mg/kg loading dose IV over 30 minutes; subsequent doses based on individually measured pharmacokinetics

pendix or other hollow viscus. Because the distinction between these two entities might be difficult initially, it is recommended that broad antibiotic coverage be initially used in both cases. The second-generation cephalosporin cefoxitin plus an aminoglycoside will cover the important organisms responsible for peritonitis. Cefoxitin has the ability to provide good coverage against most gram-positive and gram-negative organisms as well as against the intestinal anaerobes, including *B. fragilis*. The aminoglycoside provides for more complete coverage against the gram-negative aerobes of the intestine. The proved alternative to cefoxitin is clindamycin.

Peritonitis in adults can be primary or secondary. Primary peritonitis can arise in patients with preexisting nephrotic syndrome or liver disease. Secondarily, it usually arises from perforation of the gastrointestinal tract. Appropriate initial antibiotic therapy in both groups of patients is a second-generation cephalosporin such as cefoxitin plus an aminoglycoside. An alternative regimen that has stood the test of time is metronidazole plus an aminoglycoside. Metronidazole, because of its excellent spectrum against anaerobes, has proved to be a good choice for intra-abdominal infections. Alternative therapies include third-generation cephalosporins, ticarcillin plus clavulanate, or imipenem used as single agents.

When biliary sepsis is suspected, the same combination of cefoxitin and an aminoglycoside can be given. More recently, an extended-spectrum penicillin, such as mezlocillin or piperacillin, in combination with metronidazole has been proved to be effective in this setting.

A separate form of peritonitis that is usually associated with infection of the pelvic organs is pelvic peritonitis. The selection of drugs in this case has to include those effective against both the intestinal organisms as well as the sexually transmitted diseases. The first combination choice is the second-generation cephalosporin cefoxitin plus doxycycline. This regimen will cover both the common bacterial causes *N. gonorrhoeae* and anaerobic organisms as well as *C. trachomatis*. An alternative initial antibiotic combination of choice is clindamycin and gentamicin. If, however, *C. trachomatis* remains a problem, doxycycline will have to be considered within a few days of initiation of this latter combination therapy.

Penicillin-Allergic Patients

Except for the newborn age group, the combination of clindamycin and gentamicin is the treatment of choice for patients of all ages who have had a serious reaction to penicillin in the past.

Other Potentially Life-Threatening Infections

In addition to the major infections that are often associated with sepsis, practitioners are confronted with several specific diseases for which there is an urgent need to administer antibiotics while performing other stabilizing procedures. These include epiglotittis, orbital cellulitis, acute frontal sinusitis, gas gangrene, facial cellulitis, septic arthritis, and toxic shock syndrome. (See box.)

SPECIFIC AGENTS

Aminoglycosides

Preparations for Intravenous Use

Gentamicin, tobramycin, netilmicin, and amikacin sulfates are the most commonly used aminoglycosides. Their use in a given institution is governed by several factors, including patterns of resistance, type of infection (community versus nosocomial), and ability to monitor serum levels. Gentamicin is historically the most commonly used agent, but the ultimate choice will be dependent on these factors.

Pharmacology

Mechanism of Action

Aminoglycosides are bactericidal in action. These drugs inhibit protein synthesis in susceptible bacteria by irreversibly binding certain ribosomal subunits. This binding leads to failure of bacterial protein synthesis.

Distribution

Aminoglycosides are widely distributed in body fluids and tissues. They diffuse poorly into the CSF, even in patients with meningeal inflammation. Gentamicin, tobramycin, and netilmicin have similar pharmacokinetics. Their half-lives and peak activity levels are similar. Amikacin, a kanamycin derivative, has a longer half-life and, therefore, more prolonged serum levels.

DRUG TREATMENT: SELECTED URGENT CONDITIONS

Condition	Primary Treatment	Alternative Treatment or Penicillin Allergy
Epiglottitis	Ceftriaxone, 50 mg/kg q 12 hours	Chloramphenicol, 20 mg/kg q 6 hours (Consult *Physician's Desk Reference*)
Orbital cellulitis		
Adult	Nafcillin, 2 g q 4 hours *plus* Gentamicin, 2.5–3.0 mg/kg loading dose IV over 30 minutes; subsequent doses based on individually measured pharmacokinetics	Vancomycin, 1 g q 12 hours *plus* Gentamicin, 2.5–3.0 mg/kg loading dose IV over 30 minutes; subsequent doses based on individually measured pharmacokinetics
Child	Nafcillin, 25 mg/kg q 6 hours *plus* Cefuroxime, 50 mg/kg q 8 hours	Chloramphenicol, 20 mg/kg q 6 hours (Consult *Physician's Desk Reference*)
Frontal or pansinusitis		
Adult	Cefuroxime, 1 g q 8 hours	Trimethoprim/sulfamethoxazole, 2 mg/kg q 6 hours (based on trimethoprim dose)
Child	Cefuroxime, 50 mg/kg q 8 hours	Trimethoprim/sulfamethoxazole, 2 mg/kg q 12 hours (based on trimethoprim dose)
Gas gangrene	Penicillin G, 2,000,000 units q 4 hours	Chloramphenicol, 20 mg/kg q 6 hours (Consult *Physician's Desk Reference*)
Facial cellulitis		
Adult	Cefazolin, 1 g q 4 hours	Vancomycin, 1 g q 12 hours
Child	Cefuroxime, 50 mg/kg q 8 hours	Chloramphenicol, 20 mg/kg q 6 hours (Consult *Physician's Desk Reference*)
Septic arthritis		
Adult	Imipenem, 1 g q 6 hours	Vancomycin, 1 g q 12 hours *plus* Gentamicin, 2.5–3.0 mg/kg loading dose IV over 30 minutes; subsequent doses based on individually measured pharmacokinetics
Child	Nafcillin, 25 mg/kg q 6 hours *plus* Cefuroxime, 50 mg/kg q 8 hours	Chloramphenicol, 20 mg/kg q 6 hours (Consult *Physician's Desk Reference*)
Toxic shock syndrome	Nafcillin, 2 g q 4 hours	Vancomycin, 1 g q 12 hours

Elimination

Aminoglycosides are not metabolized and are excreted unchanged in the urine. In patients with normal renal function, approximately 40 to 97% of a single intravenous dose is excreted in the urine within 24 hours. Because a small portion of each aminoglycoside dose accumulates in body tissues, complete recovery of a single dose requires approximately 10 to 20 days.

Indications

The aminoglycosides have some activity against gram-positive organisms, primarily staphylococci. There are some staphylococci, however, that are resistant to gentamicin but susceptible to amikacin. Aminoglycosides in combination with penicillin have the greatest activity of any antibiotics against enterococci. All four aminoglycosides have excellent bactericidal activity against most community-acquired gram-negative organisms. When the organism is susceptible to all four agents, the bactericidal ratio does differ. Tobramycin is 2 to 4 times more bactericidal than gentamicin or amikacin. If a particular gram-negative organism is resistant to at least one of the aminoglycosides, the other aminoglycosides will have varying ability to kill that organism. Of all the aminoglycosides, amikacin seems to be the most broadly effective against most gram-negative bacteria. None of the aminoglycosides is active against anaerobes or non-enterococcal streptococci. They are also not active against *Hemophilus* or *Neisseria* species.

It is important to note that the activity of individual aminoglycosides against bacteria can be community and institution specific. Before selecting an aminoglycoside, it is recommended that local sensitivity patterns be consulted.

Cautions

Hypersensitivity—because there is evidence of cross-sensitivity among aminoglycosides, a history of toxic or hypersensitivity reactions to one aminoglycoside preparation may contraindicate the use of any other aminoglycoside.

Renal disorders—renal function must be assessed prior to initiation of aminoglycoside therapy and be monitored at regular intervals (see Dosage and Administration, below).

Hearing loss—patients with preexisting tinnitus, vertigo, or subclinical hearing loss are susceptible to ototoxicity from aminoglycosides. Particularly, eighth cranial nerve function should be assessed, if possible, in geriatric patients or patients with prior hearing disorders. Function of this nerve should also be assessed in patients with renal impairment.

Neuromuscular disorders—aminoglycosides can aggravate conditions such as myasthenia gravis and Parkinson's disease.

Use in pregnancy and lactation—Category D. Aminoglycosides can cause fetal harm when administered to pregnant women. They have been shown to cross the placenta, and there have been several reports of total irreversible bilateral congenital deafness in children whose mothers received these agents during pregnancy. Aminoglycosides should be used in pregnancy only in life-threatening infections in which safer drugs cannot be used. Small amounts of aminoglycosides are distributed into breast milk. Because of the potential for serious adverse reactions to an aminoglycoside in nursing infants, the use of these drugs is generally discouraged in the nursing mother.

Use in pediatric patients—aminoglycosides should be used with caution in reduced doses in premature and full-term neonates younger than 6 weeks of age because of their renal immaturity and resulting prolongation of serum half-life of the drugs.

Dosage and Administration

The dosing ranges and intervals given below are very imprecise because of great individual variation in metabolism and volume of distribution. To immediately achieve therapeutic peak serum levels in acutely ill patients, it is necessary to give an initial loading dose of 2.5 to 3 mg/kg of gentamicin and tobramycin. This loading dose is given as a 30-minute intravenous infusion. Failure to load, especially in the critically ill patient with septic shock, has a high probability of delaying achievement of therapeutic levels, which is clearly related to a higher mortality in cases of gram-negative sepsis and pneumonia. It is recommended that aminoglycoside doses be individualized for each patient by directly measured pharmacokinetics using peak and trough levels or, better yet, a peak level drawn 30 minutes after the loading infusion and two additional levels at 4-hour intervals. Several computer programs are available that will translate these levels into specific dosing recommendations.

Monitoring of serum levels is particularly important in patients with renal disease, obesity, advanced age, or changing states of hydration. Patients with severe sepsis who require high volumes of fluid resuscitation are particularly at risk for having inadequate aminoglycoside levels at standard doses because they have an expanded volume of distribution.

Gentamicin Sulfate Dosing Ranges and Intervals

Neonates: 5 to 7.5 mg/kg/day divided q 8 to 12 hours

Children: 3 to 7.5 mg/kg/day divided q 8 hours

Adults: 3 to 5 mg/kg/day divided q 8 hours

Netilmicin Sulfate Dosing Ranges and Intervals

Neonates: 5 to 7.5 mg/kg/day divided q 8 to 12 hours

Children: 3 to 7.5 mg/kg/day divided q 8 hours

Adults: 4 to 6.5 mg/kg/day divided q 8 hours

Tobramycin Sulfate Dosing Ranges and Intervals

Neonates: 4 to 6 mg/kg/day divided q 8 to 12 hours

Children: 3 to 6 mg/kg/day divided q 8 hours

Adults: 3 to 5 mg/kg/day divided q 8 hours

Amikacin Sulfate Dosing Ranges and Intervals

Neonates: 15 to 30 mg/kg/day divided q 8 to 12 hours

Children: 15 to 30 mg/kg/day divided q 8 hours

Adults: 15 mg/kg/day divided q 8 to 12 hours

Toxicity

Drug Interactions

Neurotoxic, ototoxic, and nephrotoxic drugs—amphotericin, bacitracin, cephalosporins, colistin, cisplatin, methoxyflurane, polymyxin B, and vancomycin have toxic effects similar to those of the aminoglycosides. The combination of aminoglycosides with these drugs in a therapeutic regimen for patients has to be carefully considered because of potential additive effects.

Neuromuscular blocking agents—concurrent use of an aminoglycoside and neuromuscular blocking agents may potentiate neuromuscular blockade.

Anti-infective agents—penicillin can inactivate aminoglycosides *in vitro;* therefore, these drugs should not be administered simultaneously. Chloramphenicol, clindamycin, and tetracycline have been reported to antagonize the bactericidal activity of aminoglycosides *in vitro.* While synergism is a well-known characteristic of *in vivo* use of combined therapy with aminoglycosides and beta-lactam antibiotics, this synergism is less predictable with extended-spectrum penicillins.

Adverse Reactions

Hypersensitivity reactions—occasionally hypersensitivity reactions including rash, urticaria, stomatitis, and eosinophilia have occurred in patients receiving an aminoglycoside. Cross-allergenicity among the aminoglycosides has been demonstrated.

Renal—aminoglycosides can induce nephrotoxicity that is manifested by increases in blood urea nitrogen and serum creatinine. Renal toxicity is usually reversed following discontinuance of the drug.

Otic (auditory and vestibular)—eighth cranial nerve damage can occur with the use of aminoglycosides. This is manifested by hearing loss or vestibular symptoms such as dizziness, nystagmus, and vertigo.

Nervous system—aminoglycosides produce varying degrees of neuromuscular blockade. Although the blockade induced by an aminoglycoside is generally dose related and self-limited, it can rarely result in respiratory paralysis.

Other adverse effects—other less frequently reported effects of aminoglycosides include nausea and vomiting, anemia, leukopenia, thrombocytopenia, tachycardia, hepatomegaly, splenomegaly, myocarditis, and transient increases in the liver transaminases.

Cephalosporins

First-Generation Cephalosporins
Preparation for Intravenous Use

Cefazolin sodium, because it has a longer half-life and higher serum levels than other first-generation cephalosporins, is the preferred intravenous preparation.

Pharmacology

Mechanism of Action

Like other beta-lactam and penicillin antibiotics, first-generation cephalosporins interfere with several enzymes that are responsible for cell wall synthesis and division. They are bactericidal in action.

Distribution

Following absorption, first-generation cephalosporins are widely distributed to tissues and fluids throughout the body. Unlike second- and third-generation cephalosporins, they achieve therapeutic levels in the bile. First-generation cephalosporins achieve only low levels in CSF.

Elimination

Cefazolin is excreted unchanged in the urine. Approximately 60% of a single intravenous dose is excreted within 6 hours and 82 to 100% of the dose is excreted within 24 hours in adults with normal renal function.

Spectrum of Activity

First-generation cephalosporins are very active *in vitro* against gram-positive cocci including penicillinase-producing and non–penicillinase-producing *Staphylococcus aureus* and *S. epidermidis*. They are also active against beta-hemolytic streptococci, group B streptococci, and *Streptococcus pneumoniae*. First-generation cephalosporins have limited activity against gram-negative bacteria, although some strains of *Escherichia coli, Klebsiella pneumoniae, Proteus mirabilis,* and *Shigella* species are effectively inhibited *in vitro* by these drugs. They have limited activity against most anaerobes, and no activity against *Bacteroides fragilis*.

Cautions

Hypersensitivity—cephalosporins are contraindicated in patients with a history of allergic reactions to other cephalosporins. There is clinical and laboratory evidence of partial cross-allergenicity among cephalosporins and other beta-lactam antibiotics.

Renal disease—renal toxicity can occur in patients older than 50 years, patients with prior renal impairment, or patients receiving other nephrotoxic drugs. All cephalosporins should be administered with caution and in a reduced dosage in the presence of markedly impaired renal function (see Dosage and Administration, below).

Use in pregnancy and lactation—Category B. Although there have been no reports of adverse effects to the fetus to date, safe use of cephalosporins during pregnancy has not been definitely established. The drug should be used during pregnancy only when clearly indicated. Cephalosporins are distributed into breast milk; therefore, these drugs should be used with caution in nursing women.

Dosage and Administration

Cefazolin Sodium Dosage Ranges and Intervals

Children: 50 to 100 mg/kg/day divided q 8 hours

Adults: 6 to 12 g/day divided q 4 to 6 hours

Dosing in Renal Failure

Creatinine Clearance (ml/min)	Dose and Interval
>55	Full doses
30–55	Full doses q 8 hours
10–30	Half dose q 12 hours
<10	Half dose q 18 hours

Toxicity

Drug Interactions

Aminoglycosides—concurrent use of nephrotoxic agents such as aminoglycosides, colistin, polymyxin B, or vancomycin may increase the risk of renal toxicity with some cephalosporins. Caution has to be exercised when giving these drugs concurrently.

Adverse Reactions

Hypersensitivity reactions—hypersensitivity reactions have been reported to occur in 5% or less of patients receiving a cephalosporin. These reactions include urticaria, pruritus, rash, fever and chills, reactions resembling serum sickness, and other allergic-like symptoms. Anaphylaxis has occurred rarely.

Hematologic—positive direct and indirect Coombs' test results have been reported in 3% or more of patients receiving cephalosporins. Other adverse hematologic effects include rare, mild, and transient neutropenia, thrombocythemia or thrombocytopenia, and reversible leukopenia.

Renal—renal effects have occurred occasionally with administration of cephalosporin, including transient increases in blood urea nitrogen and creatinine concentrations.

Hepatic—transient increases in serum aminotransferases and alkaline phosphatase concentration have occurred occasionally with cephalosporin therapy.

Treatment of Toxicity

Hypersensitivity reactions are treated with basic airway and circulation support as necessary. Oxygen and intravenous fluid are administered for unstable patients. Antihistamines, epinephrine, and corticosteroids are administered as necessary.

Second-Generation Cephalosporins
Preparations for Intravenous Use

Of the second-generation cephalosporins, cefoxitin sodium and cefuroxime sodium are the most useful agents. Cefuroxime is useful for a wide variety of infections involving the meninges, skin, bone, lungs, and urinary tract. Cefoxitin has a more limited use but is frequently the drug of choice in intra-abdominal and pelvic infections.

Pharmacology

Mechanism of Action

Cefuroxime and cefoxitin, like other beta-lactam antibiotics, inhibit mucopeptide synthesis in the bacterial cell wall. They are bactericidal in action.

Distribution

Like other cephalosporins, the second-generation cephalosporins are widely distributed to tissues and fluids throughout the body. Of special note is that, of the second-generation cephalosporins, only cefuroxime will achieve therapeutic concentrations in the CSF under conditions where meninges are inflamed.

Elimination

Cefuroxime and cefoxitin undergo little metabolism in the liver and are primarily excreted by the kidneys. Excretion of these drugs is decreased in patients with renal failure, and doses have to be adjusted accordingly.

Indications

Cefuroxime is nearly as active *in vitro* as penicillin G against group A and B streptococci, *Streptococcus pneumoniae*, and *S. viridans*. It has good activity against penicillinase-producing *Staphylococcus aureus*. It is very active against a wide variety of gram-negative bacilli including *Escherichia coli*, *Proteus mirabilis*, *Klebsiella* species, *Salmonella*, *Shigella*, and *Yersinia* species. It is particularly active against penicillinase-producing *Hemophilus influenzae*. It also has excellent activity against *Neisseria meningitidis*. Other organisms for which it is effective include *N. gonorrhoeae* and *Pasteurella multocida*.

Cefoxitin is distinguished from cefuroxime by its increased activity against anaerobic organisms such as *Bacteroides fragilis*, although resistant strains have been reported. Cefoxitin is not as active as cefuroxime against gram-positive aerobic cocci. It does have a similar spectrum of activity against the gram-negative aerobic bacilli.

Cautions

Hypersensitivity—cephalosporins are contraindicated in patients with a history of allergic reaction to cephalosporin antibiotics. There is clinical and laboratory evidence of partial cross-allergenicity among cephalosporins and other beta-lactam antibiotics, including penicillin.

Renal failure—because second-generation cephalosporins are primarily excreted in the urine, adjustments of dosage have to be made under conditions of renal failure (see Dosage and Administration, below).

Use in pregnancy and lactation—Category B. Although there have been no reports of adverse effects to the fetus to date, safe use of cephalosporins during pregnancy has not been definitely established. Cephalosporins are distributed into the breast milk, and these drugs should be used with caution in nursing women.

Dosage and Administration

Cefuroxime Sodium Dosing Ranges and Intervals

Children: 75 to 250 mg/kg/day divided q 6 to 8 hours
Adults: 4.5 to 9 g/day divided q 8 hours

Cefoxitin Sodium Dosing Ranges and Intervals

Children: 80 to 160 mg/kg/day divided q 4 to 6 hours
Adults: 4 to 12 g/day divided q 4 to 6 hours

Dosing in Renal Failure

In patients with significant renal disease, the usual doses of cefuroxime can be given if the creatinine clearance is greater than 20 ml/min. In significant renal failure, if the creatinine clearance is between 10 and 20 ml/min, half the dose can be given every 12 hours. If the creatinine clearance is less than 10 ml/min, half the usual dose may be given every 24 hours.

In renal failure, the standard initial dose of cefoxitin is given. For a creatinine clearance of 30 to 50 ml/min, the usual dose is given every 8 to 12 hours. For creatinine clearances of between 10 and 30 ml/min, the dosing interval is increased to 12 to 24 hours. For creatinine clearances of less than 10 ml/min, half the usual dose is given every 18 to 24 hours after the initial loading dose.

Toxicity

Drug Interactions

Nephrotoxic drugs—concurrent use of nephrotoxic agents such as aminoglycosides, colistin, polymyxcin B, or vancomycin may increase the risk of nephrotoxicity with cephalosporins. Concurrent use should be carried out with caution.

Adverse Reactions

Hypersensitivity reactions—hypersensitivity reactions have been reported to occur in 5% or less of patients receiving a cephalosporin. These reactions include urticaria, pruritus, rash, fever and chills, and other allergic symptoms. Anaphylaxis has occurred rarely.

Hematologic—positive direct and indirect Coombs' test results have been reported in 3% or more of patients receiving second-generation cephalosporins. Other adverse hematologic effects of cephalosporins include rare, mild, and transient neutropenia, thrombocytopenia, and reversible leukopenia.

Renal—renal effects that have occurred occasionally with the administration of cephalosporins include a transient increase in blood urea nitrogen and serum creatinine concentrations. Nephrotoxicity is more likely to occur in patients older than 50 years of age, patients with prior renal impairment, or patients receiving other nephrotoxic drugs.

Treatment of Toxicity

Hypersensitivity reactions are treated with basic airway and circulatory support as necessary. Oxygen and intravenous fluids are administered for unstable patients. Antihistamines, epinephrine, and steroids are indicated for anaphylaxis.

Third-Generation Cephalosporins
Preparation for Intravenous Use

Of the many third-generation cephalosporins on the market, cefotaxime sodium, ceftriaxone sodium, and ceftazidime are the most efficacious for initial empirical use. Cefotaxime has the best overall record for effectiveness against serious gram-negative infections of all bacterial origins. Ceftriaxone has nearly an equal record and the additional advantage of twice-daily or, in some cases, once-daily dosing. Ceftazidime, while effective against a broad range of bacteria, has a particular utility in treating infections due to *Pseudomonas aeruginosa*.

Pharmacology

Mechanisms of Action

The antibacterial activity of third-generation cephalosporins, like other cephalosporins and beta-lactam antibiotics, results from inhibition of enzymes that are responsible for the synthesis of the bacterial cell wall. The target enzymes of beta-lactam antibiotics have been classified as penicillin-binding proteins. Third-generation cephalosporins have different affinities for these various penicillin-binding proteins, which appears to explain the differences between beta-lactam antibiotics and their antimicrobial activity against different bacteria.

Distribution

Third-generation cephalosporins are widely distributed to tissues and fluids throughout the body. Unlike first-generation and most second-generation cephalosporins, third-generation cephalosporins can reach therapeutic concentrations in the CSF, particularly under conditions of inflammation of the meninges.

Elimination

Depending on the particular agent, third-generation cephalosporins are metabolized and excreted by various mechanisms. Cefotaxime undergoes partial metabolism by the liver. Approximately 60 to 75% of cefotaxime is excreted unchanged in the urine. Ceftazidime undergoes no metabolism, and 100% is excreted in the urine unchanged. Ceftriaxone is excreted in both the urine and bile. Approximately 33 to 67% is excreted in the urine unchanged. The remainder is excreted in the bile. Because of this biliary excretion, use of ceftriaxone is usually avoided in newborns.

Spectrum of Activity

While third-generation cephalosporins have good activity against most gram-positive aerobic cocci, they offer no advantages over other cephalosporins. In fact, third-generation cephalosporins are less active against *Staphylococcus aureus* than are first-generation cephalosporins. Currently, they are not the drug of choice for any gram-positive coccal infection. The major advantage of third-generation cephalosporins is their excellent activity against gram-negative aerobic bacteria. Cefotaxime and ceftriaxone have similar activities against these bacteria. Ceftazidime, on the other hand, has a particularly good activity against *P. aeruginosa*. It must be emphasized, however, that no third-generation cephalosporin should be given alone when *Pseudomonas* species are the suspected pathogens. Third-generation cephalosporins have good activity *in vitro* against anaerobic organisms. They are, however, not indicated as the primary mode of therapy for anaerobic infections.

Cautions

Hypersensitivity—prior to the initiation of therapy with third-generation cephalosporins, careful inquiry should be made concerning previous hypersensitivity reactions to cephalosporins and penicillins. There is clinical and laboratory evidence of partial crossed-allergenicity among cephalosporins and other beta-lactam antibiotics. Some authorities feel that, unless the patient has exhibited a prior anaphylactic reaction to penicillin, third-generation cephalosporins can be considered an acceptable option for a patient with minor reactions (rash only) to penicillin. Because of the ability of these cephalosporins to achieve very high CSF concentrations, the small risk of reaction has to be balanced against the marked effectiveness in conditions such as meningitis.

Renal disorders—because the majority of third-generation cephalosporins or their metabolites are excreted in the urine, caution must be taken in patients with marked renal impairment (see Dosage and Administration, below).

Hepatic disorders—because cefotaxime is metabolized partially in the liver and ceftriaxone is excreted in the bile, precautions must be taken in administering high doses to patients with severe liver disease.

Use in pregnancy and lactation—Category B. Safe use of third-generation cephalosporins during pregnancy has not been clearly established. These drugs should only be used in pregnancy when clearly indicated. Third-generation cephalosporins are distributed into breast milk and should be used with caution in nursing women.

Use in pediatric patients—Ceftriaxone is contraindicated in children up to 1 to 2 months of age. Cefotaxime and ceftazidime have been used safely in all pediatric age groups.

Dosage and Administration

Cefotaxime Sodium Dosing Ranges and Intervals

Newborns: 100 to 150 mg/kg/day divided q 8 to 12 hours

Children: 100 to 200 mg/kg/day divided q 6 to 8 hours

Adults: 4 to 12 g/day divided q 4 to 6 hours

Ceftazidime Dosing Ranges and Intervals

Newborns: 100 to 150 mg/kg/day divided q 8 to 12 hours

Children: 100 to 150 mg/kg/day divided q 8 hours

Adult: 2 to 6 g/day divided q 8 to 12 hours

Ceftriaxone Sodium Dosing Ranges and Intervals

Children: 50 to 100 mg/kg/day divided q 12 to 24 hours

Adult: 1 to 4 g/day divided q 12 to 24 hours

Dosing in Renal or Hepatic Failure

Modification of the usual dose of cefotaxime is unnecessary for creatinine clearances of >20 ml/min. For creatinine clearances of less than 20 ml/min, half the usual dose is administered at the usual intervals.

For ceftazidime, the usual doses and intervals are observed for creatinine clearances >50 ml/min. For creatinine clearances of 31 to 50 ml/min, the usual dose is given every 12 hours; for clearances between 16 and 30 ml/min, the same dose is given every 24 hours; for clearances between 5 and 16 ml/min, half the dose is given every 24 hours; and for clearances <5 ml/min, half the dose is given every 48 hours.

Modification of the doses of ceftriaxone is unnecessary for renal or hepatic failure alone. It is recommended, however, that the total daily dose of ceftriaxone not exceed 2 g/day in patients when both organs are significantly impaired. In cases of either severe renal or hepatic failure, monitoring serum ceftriaxone levels to prevent excessive accumulation of the drug is also recommended.

Toxicity

Drug Interactions

Aminoglycosides—*in vitro*, cephalosporins and aminoglycosides can be incompatible when mixed. The aminoglycosides are inactivated. Inactivation does not occur *in vivo* when administration is separate. *In vivo*, a synergism can occur that increases the antibacterial effect of these agents.

Adverse Reactions

Hypersensitivity reactions—hypersensitivity reactions have been reported to occur with third-generation cephalosporins. Specifically, 2% of patients receiving cefotaxime and ceftriaxone can be expected to have a hypersensitivity reaction. Rash is the usual manifestation of these reactions, and anaphylaxis is rare.

Hematologic—a variety of hematologic effects can be observed in patients receiving third-generation cephalosporins. Ceftriaxone has the greatest effect on the hematologic system. Eosinophilia has been reported in 6% of patients. Thrombocytosis has occurred in 5% and leukopenia in 2% of patients receiving ceftriaxone. Transient leukopenia, neutropenia, and thrombocytopenia occur with the use of ceftazidine and cefotaxime but are uncommon.

Renal effects—elevations of blood urea nitrogen and creatinine concentration have been reported in patients using third-generation cephalosporins. Renal complications occur in approximately 1% of patients.

Hepatic effects—increased serum concentrations of liver aminotransferases have been reported to occur in patients receiving third-generation cephalosporins. This effect is most marked in patients receiving ceftriaxone, with approximately 3% of patients being affected.

Gastrointestinal effects—diarrhea, nausea, and vomiting have been reported to occur in 2% of patients receiving third-generation cephalosporins. Antibiotic-associated pseudomembranous colitis, caused by toxin-producing clostridia, may occur during or following the discontinuance of therapy with these agents.

Treatment of Toxicity

Severe hypersensitivity reactions, particularly anaphylaxis, are treated with basic airway and circulatory support as necessary. Oxygen and intravenous fluids are administered for unstable patients. Antihistamines, epinephrine, and steroids are indicated for anaphylaxis.

Chloramphenicol

Preparation for Intravenous Use

Chloramphenicol sodium succinate is the only preparation for intravenous use.

Pharmacology

Mechanism of Action

Chloramphenicol is considered a bacteriostatic agent but may be bactericidal in high concentrations or against highly susceptible organisms. Chloramphenicol inhibits protein synthesis by binding to specific ribosomal units. The primary effect is inhibition of peptide bond formation.

Distribution

Chloramphenicol is widely distributed throughout most body tissues and fluids. The concentration of chloramphenicol in CSF is reported to be 21 to 50% of concurrent plasma concentrations in patients with uninflamed meninges. This concentration rises to 45 to 89% under conditions of inflammation.

Elimination

Chloramphenicol is inactivated primarly in the liver. In adults with normal renal and hepatic function, approximately 30% of a single intravenous dose of chloramphenicol is excreted in the urine unchanged. In renal failure, the half-life of metabolically active chloramphenicol is not prolonged but it still should be used with caution under these conditions.

Spectrum of Activity

Most gram-positive cocci, both aerobic and anaerobic, are susceptible to chloramphenicol. Chloramphenicol is effective against *Neisseria meningitidis* and *Hemophilus influenzae*. It has variable activity against other gram-negative bacteria. It has excellent activity against gram-positive and gram-negative anaerobes, including *Bacteroides fragilis*. This agent is also effective against the rickettsial organisms. For the most part, chloramphenicol is reserved as an alternative for patients who are hypersensitive to beta-lactam antibiotics.

Cautions

Hypersensitivity—chloramphenicol is contraindicated in patients with a history of hypersensitivity or toxic reaction to this drug.

Hematologic disorders—serious, sometimes fatal reactions have been reported in patients who have received chloramphenicol. There is a narrow range between the therapeutic and toxic doses of chloramphenicol. Hematologic studies should be performed prior to and approximately every 2 days during chloramphenicol therapy. Where possible, chloramphenicol serum levels should be measured. They should be maintained between 5 and 20 μg/ml to ensure efficacy and avoid toxicity.

Hepatic and renal failure—patients with hepatic failure may not be able to conjugate chloramphenicol, and drug levels may rise to toxic concentrations under these conditions (see Dosage and Administration, below).

Use in pregnancy and lactation—Category D. Safe use of chloramphenicol during pregnancy has not been established. This drug crosses the placenta and is distributed into breast milk. In general, it is to be avoided in pregnant or nursing mothers.

Use in pediatric patients—chloramphenicol should be used with caution in infants and children with immature metabolic processes.

Dosage and Administration

Chloramphenicol Sodium Succinate Dosing Ranges and Intervals

Children and adults: 50 to 100 mg/kg/day divided q 6 hours (high doses should be reduced as soon as possible to prevent complications)

Dosing in Renal or Hepatic Failure

In patients with impaired renal or hepatic function, doses of chloramphenicol must be reduced in proportion to the degree of impairment and should be based on measured plasma chloramphenicol concentrations.

Toxicity

Drug Interactions

Phenobarbital—concurrent administration of chloramphenicol and phenobarbital may result in decreased plasma concentration of the antibiotic.

Anti-infective agents—chloramphenicol has been reported to antagonize the bactericidal activity of penicillins and aminoglycosides *in vitro*.

Myelosuppressive agents—concomitant administration of chloramphenicol with other drugs that cause bone marrow depression should be avoided.

Other drugs—chloramphenicol may interfere with the biotransformation of chlorpropamide, warfarin, phenytoin, and tolbutamide.

Adverse Reactions

Hypersensitivity reactions—hypersensitivity reactions have occurred and may be manifested by fever, macular and vesicular rashes, urticaria, and hemorrhage of the skin or mucous membranes. Anaphylactoid reactions have been reported.

Hematologic—one of the most serious adverse effects of chloramphenicol is bone marrow depression. Although rare, blood dyscrasias such as aplastic anemia, hypoplastic anemia, thrombocytopenia, and granulocytopenia have occurred during or following short-term or prolonged therapy with this agent. Two forms of bone marrow depression may occur with chloramphenicol. The first is an idiosyncratic, irreversible bone marrow depression causing aplastic anemia. Bone marrow aplasia may occur after a single dose of chloramphenicol and can occur weeks or months after the drug has been discontinued. The second and more common type of bone marrow depression is dose related and usually reversible on discontinuance of the drug. This type of bone marrow depression is characterized by anemia, reticulocytopenia, leukopenia, thrombocytopenia, and increased serum iron-binding capacity. Hemolysis may occur in patients with a severe deficiency of glucose-6-phosphate dehydrogenase.

Gray syndrome—gray syndrome, a form of circulatory collapse, has occurred in premature and newborn infants receiving chloramphenicol. This syndrome is characterized by abdominal distention, progressive pallor and cyanosis, and vasomotor collapse. This process may be reversible with early discontinuance of chloramphenicol. This syndrome has been attributed to high concentrations of the drug, which result from the inability of infants to conjugate chloramphenicol or to excrete the unconjugated drug.

Neuritis—optic and peripheral neuritis has been reported during chloramphenicol therapy.

Imipenem

Preparation for Intravenous Use

Imipenem with cilastatin is a preparation for intravenous use. This drug has one of the widest ranges of antimicrobial activity and inhibits 90% of all clinically important bacteria.

Pharmacology

Mechanism of Action

Imipenem is bactericidal in action. Like other beta-lactam antibiotics, the antibacterial action of imipenem results from inhibition of mucopeptide synthesis in the bacterial wall. Imipenem has an affinity for and binds most penicillin-binding proteins of susceptible organisms. There is no permeability barrier to imipenem in gram-negative bacteria. It has good stability against attack by beta-lactamases.

Distribution

Following intravenous administration, imipenem is widely distributed throughout the body fluids. Like most other beta-lactam antibiotics, diffusion into the CSF is inadequate under normal conditions. Meningeal inflammation does not appreciably increase CSF imipenem concentrations.

Elimination

When cilastatin is co-administered with imipenem, about 70% of imipenem is recovered in the urine. If imipenem is given alone, only 20% is recovered in the urine. Without cilastatin, imipenem is partially hydrolyzed in the kidneys by dihydropeptidase-1 to a microbiologically inactive metabolite. Imipenem is also metabolized to some extent by nonrenal mechanisms. Approximately 20 to 30% of imipenem is inactivated by nonspecific hydrolysis of the beta-lactam ring.

Spectrum of Activity

In vitro, imipenem has one of the widest spectrums of antimicrobial activity of any currently available beta-lactam antibiotic. Most gram-positive aerobes are very susceptible to this agent. These include Streptococcus pneumoniae (including penicillin-resistant species), group A and B streptococci, methicillin-susceptible Staphylococcus aureus, and S. saprophyticus. Methicillin-resistant S. aureus or coagulase-negative species are routinely resistant to imipenem. Imipenem has a broad spectrum against most gram-negative aerobic bacteria, including Neisseria meningitidis, N. gonorrhoeae and Hemophilus influenzae. It is also very active against the enteric pathogens such as Escherichia coli, Klebsiella species, Salmonella, and Shigella species. It has significant activity against Pseudomonas aeruginosa, although some Pseudomonas species are resistant. Imipenem should never be used as a single agent against suspected Pseudomonas infections. Imipenem also has excellent activity against most anaerobic organisms. It is the most active beta-lactam antibiotic against these pathogens. The most significant organism against which imipenem is inactive is the Legionella species.

Cautions

Hypersensitivity—there is clinical and laboratory evidence of partial cross-allergenicity among imipenem and other beta-lactam antibiotics. Therefore, this agent should be used with caution in patients with a history of hypersensitivity reaction to penicillins.

Renal, hepatic, and hematologic systems—because imipenem can have effects on these systems, routine testing of renal and hepatic function is recommended during high-dose imipenem therapy. Blood counts should also be obtained (see Dosage and Administration, below).

Use in pregnancy and lactation—Category C. Reproduction studies using rats and rabbits have not demonstrated evidence of harm to the fetus. Nevertheless, there are no adequate and controlled studies today using imipenem with cilastatin in pregnant women. The drug should be used with caution during pregnancy. Since imipenem is distributed into breast milk, the drug should be used with caution in nursing women.

Use in pediatric patients—imipenem and cilastatin use in children under the age of 12 years has not been clearly established. In limited studies of this agent in patients from 3 months to 13 years of age, it has been shown to have no unusual adverse effects.

Dosage and Administration

Imipenem and Cilastatin Sodium Dosage Range and Intervals

Adults: 2 to 4 g/day divided q 6 hours

Dosing in Renal Failure

Under conditions of renal impairment, imipenem plus cilastatin dosing needs to be modified. With a creatinine clearance of 30 to 70 ml/min, the dosing interval should increase to every 8 hours; for creatinine clearances between 20 to 30 ml/min, the dosing intervals increase to every 12 hours; under 20 ml/min, half the normal dose is given every 12 hours.

Toxicity

Drug Interactions

Beta-lactam antibiotics—*in vitro*, imipenem antagonizes the antibacterial activity of other beta-lactam antibiotics, including most cephalosporins and extended-spectrum penicillins.

Chloramphenicol—it has been reported that chloramphenicol can antagonize the bactericidal activity of imipenem *in vitro*.

Adverse Reactions

Hypersensitivity reactions—hypersensitivity reactions, including rash, fever, pruritus, and urticaria, have been reported in up to 3% of patients receiving imipenem and cilastatin.

Hematologic effects—eosinophilia has been reported in up to 4% of patients receiving imipenem and cilastatin. Transient leukopenia, neutropenia, thrombocytopenia, and thrombocytosis have been reported in 2% of patients.

CNS effects—adverse CNS effects have been reported in patients receiving this agent. Seizures have been reported in up to 1.5% of patients. Other reported symptoms include dizziness, somnolence, encephalopathy, confusion, myoclonus, and headache. Most adverse effects have been reported in patients with CNS disorders such as seizures, brain tumors, and head trauma.

Gastrointestinal—adverse gastrointestinal effects are among the most frequent reactions to imipenem and cilastatin sodium. Nausea, diarrhea, and vomiting have been reported in up to 4% of patients. Antibiotic-associated pseudomembranous colitis has occurred in 0.2% of patients receiving imipenem and cilastatin.

Renal—transient increases in blood-urea nitrogen and serum creatinine have been reported in up to 2% of patients.

Hepatic—transient increases in serum concentrations of aminotransferases and alkaline phosphatase have been reported in 2 to 6% of patients receiving imipenem and cilastatin.

Treatment of Toxicity

Hypersensitivity reactions are treated with basic airway and circulatory support as necessary. Oxygen and fluids are administered for unstable patients. Antihistamines, epinephrine, and steroids are indicated for anaphylactic reactions.

Lincosamides

Preparation for Intravenous Use

Clindamycin phosphate is the most commonly used lincosamide preparation.

Pharmacology

Mechanism of Action

Clindamycin may be bacteriostatic or bactericidal in action, depending on the concentration of the drug attained and susceptibility of the infecting organism. Clindamycin inhibits protein synthesis by binding to ribosomal units, and the effect of this binding is to inhibit peptide synthesis.

Distribution

Clindamycin is distributed widely to most body fluids and tissues. It does not penetrate the CSF well either in the uninflamed or inflamed state.

Elimination

Clindamycin is primarily metabolized in the liver to both active and inactive metabolites. The major active metabolites are excreted in the urine, bile, and feces. In severe hepatic insufficiency, the half-life of clindamycin is prolonged.

Spectrum of Activity

Clindamycin is effective against *Staphylococcus aureus* and group A streptococci. It has no useful activity against gram-negative aerobes. It is, however, very active against gram-positive and gram-negative anaerobes, including *Bacteroides fragilis* and *Clostridium perfringens*. The prime indication for clindamycin is for serious intra-abdominal and pelvic infections.

Cautions

Hypersensitivity—a history of hypersensitivity to this agent is a contraindication to its use.

Gastrointestinal disease—clindamycin should be used with caution in patients with a history of gastrointestinal disease, particularly colitis.

Hepatic or renal impairment—severe hepatic or renal disease is an indication to use clindamycin with caution. When possible, serum clindamycin concentrations should be monitored during high-dose therapy in these patients.

Use in pregnancy and lactation—Category C. Safe use of clindamycin in pregnant women has not been established. Clindamycin is distributed into breast milk. Because of the potential of serious adverse reactions from clindamycin in nursing infants, this drug should be avoided if possible.

Use in pediatric patients—When clindamycin is administered to neonates or infants, organ system function should be monitored. Particularly, the renal and hepatic functions need to be carefully observed.

Dosage and Administration

Clindamycin Phosphate Dosing Ranges and Intervals

Children: 25 to 40 mg/kg/day divided q 6 to 8 hours

Adults: 450 to 2700 mg/day divided q 8 hours

Dosing in Renal or Hepatic Failure

Changes in dosing of clindamycin in renal failure are unnecessary. In hepatic failure, doses should be reduced or alternative drugs should be chosen.

Drug Toxicity

Drug Interactions

Neuromuscular blocking agents—clindamycin has been shown to have neuromuscular blocking properties and may enhance the action of neuromuscular blocking agents.

Aminoglycosides—clindamycin can antagonize the bactericidal activity of aminoglycosides *in vitro*. These drugs should not be administered simultaneously in the same intravenous line.

Adverse Reactions

Gastrointestinal—the most serious adverse effect of clindamycin is gastrointestinal. This drug can cause nausea, vomiting, diarrhea, abdominal pain, and tenesmus. It also can cause potentially fatal antibiotic-associated pseudomembranous colitis.

Hypersensitivity and dermatologic reactions—a generalized morbilliform rash is the most frequently reported adverse reaction to clindamycin. Rarely, anaphylactoid reactions have occurred. Also rare reactions are erythema multiforme and Stevens-Johnson syndrome.

Local effects—thrombophlebitis and erythema have occurred with intravenous administration of clindamycin.

Other adverse effects—other reported effects of clindamycin include transient rises in serum bilirubin, alkaline phosphatase, and aminotransferases. Transient leukopenia, neutropenia, eosinophilia, and thrombocytopenia have occurred.

Treatment of Toxicity

Hypersensitivity reactions are treated with basic airway and circulatory support as necessary. Oxygen and intravenous fluids are administered to unstable patients. Antihistamines, epinephrine, and steroids are indicated for anaphylactic reactions.

Pseudomembranous colitis is treated by discontinuation of clindamycin.

Macrolides

Preparation for Intravenous Use

Erythromycin glucoheptonate and erythromycin lactobionate are the only currently available intravenous preparations of erythromycin.

Pharmacology

Mechanism of Action

Erythromycin is considered a bacteriostatic agent. It may, however, be bactericidal in high concentrations or against highly susceptible organisms. Erythromycin inhibits protein synthesis in susceptible organisms by inhibiting transfer ribonucleic acids, therefore inhibiting polypeptide synthesis. It is only effective against actively multiplying organisms.

Distribution

Erythromycin is widely distributed throughout most body tissues and fluids. Except within the brain, tissue concentrations of erythromycin are often higher and persist longer than in serum.

Elimination

Erythromycin is partially metabolized in the liver to inactive metabolites. It is mainly excreted unchanged in the bile. Only small amounts of erythromycin are excreted in the urine.

Indications

Erythromycin is considered the drug of choice for infections caused by *Mycoplasma pneumoniae, Legionella pneumophila, Chlamydia trachomatis* (pneumonia), *Bordetella pertussis, Campylobacter* infections, and *Corynebacterium diphtheriae*. It also is an alternative to penicillin in allergic patients with group A streptococcal and *Streptococcus pneumoniae* infections.

Cautions

Hypersensitivity—erythromycin is contraindicated in patients with a history of hypersensitivity to this drug.

Use in pregnancy—Category B. The safe use of intravenous erythromycin during pregnancy has not been clearly established. However, oral erythromycin has been used successfully to treat urogenital chlamydial infections in pregnant women.

Renal, hepatic, or cardiac failure—No dosage adjustments are necessary.

Dosage and Administration

Erythromycin Glucoheptonate and Erythromycin Lactobionate Dosing Ranges and Intervals

Children: 20 to 40 mg/kg/day divided q 6 hours
Adults: 1 to 9 g/day divided q 6 hours

Toxicity

Drug Interactions

Carbamazepine—concomitant use of erythromycin and carbamazepine in both adults and children can result in increased serum concentrations of carbamazepine. Ataxia, dizziness, drowziness, and vomiting can occur under these conditions.

Cyclosporine—the concentration of cyclosporine will rise substantially with the concomitant use of erythromycin.

Theophylline—elevated serum levels of theophylline will occur with concomitant use of erythromycin. Erythromycin will also prolong the serum half-life of this agent.

Oral anticoagulants—the initiation of erythromycin therapy in patients on warfarin can prolong the prothrombin and bleeding times.

Adverse Reactions

Local effects of venous irritation and thrombophlebitis occur commonly following intravenous administration of erythromycin lactobionate or glucoheptonate. Dilute solution should be administered over a minimum of 20 to 60 minutes. The large volumes of normal saline necessary for proper dilution of IV erythromycin may precipitate cardiac failure.

Metronidazole

Preparation for Intravenous Use

Metronidazole hydrochloride is the only drug with both antiparasitic and antibacterial properties used for acute, life-threatening bacterial infections.

Pharmacology

Mechanisms of Action

Metronidazole is bactericidal, amebicidal, and trichomonicidal in action. In susceptible organisms or cells, metronidazole is reduced by low–redox-potential electron transfer proteins. The reduction products appear to be responsible for the cytotoxic and antimicrobial effects of the drug. Their action is to disrupt deoxyribonucleic acid (DNA) and inhibit nucleic acid synthesis.

Distribution

Metronidazole is widely distributed into body tissues and fluids. Concentrations of metronidazole in the CSF are approximately half those of concurrent plasma concentrations.

Elimination

Approximately 30 to 60% of an oral or intravenous dose of metronidazole is metabolized in the liver. Some of its metabolites have antibacterial and antiprotozoal activity. Metronidazole is slowly excreted in the urine, and 77% of the dose can be recovered up to 5 days after administration. Urine may be dark or reddish brown in color following oral or intravenous administration of metronidazole because of the presence of water-soluble pigments, which are the result of the metabolism of this drug.

Spectrum of Activity

Metronidazole has parasiticidal activity against *Trichomonas vaginalis*, *Giardia lamblia*, and *Entamoeba histolytica*. It is active as an antibacterial against anaerobic bacteria including *Bacteroides fragilis* and other *Bacteroides* species, *Clostridium*, *Peptococcus*, and *Peptostreptococcus* species. It is somewhat less active against anaerobic gram-positive cocci. Metronidazole is not directly active against common aerobes, either gram-positive or gram-negative.

Cautions

Hypersensitivity—metronidazole is contraindicated in individuals with a history of hypersensitivity to this drug or other nitroimidazole derivatives.

Neurologic disease—metronidazole has to be cautiously administered to patients with known peripheral neuropathy. It can aggravate this condition.

Hematologic disorders—metronidazole is administered with caution to patients with a history of hematologic disorders. A total and differential leukocyte count should be performed before and during intravenous therapy with this agent.

Hepatic disorders—metronidazole should be used with caution and in reduced dosages in patients with severe hepatic impairment.

Cardiovascular—because 1 g of metronidazole contains 28 mEq of sodium, this fact should be taken into account when administering metronidazole to patients with cardiac failure.

Use in pregnancy and lactation—Category B. Reproduction studies in rats and rabbits using metronidazole have not revealed evidence of impaired fertility or harm to the fetus. However, they have shown mutagenic and carcinogenic potential in mice. The manufacturers recommend that this agent not be used during the first trimester of pregnancy. Because of the tumorigenic potential of metronidazole in mice and rats, it is not recommended for use in lactating women.

Use in pediatric patients—the safe use of intravenous metronidazole for any indication except amebiasis has not been established.

Dosage and Administration

Metronidazole Hydrochloride Dosing Range and Intervals

Adults: 15 mg/kg loading dose and 30 mg/ kg/day divided q 6 hours

Toxicity

Drug Interactions

Oral anticoagulants—metronidazole potentiates the effects of oral anticoagulants, and concurrent administration should be avoided if possible. If metronidazole is used in patients receiving an oral anticoagulant, prothrombin times should be monitored and dosage of the oral anticoagulant should be regularly monitored.

Alcohol—metronidazole appears to inhibit alcohol dehydrogenase. Disulfiram-like reactions, including flushing, headache, vomiting, and abdominal cramps, occur in some patients who ingest alcohol while receiving metronidazole.

Disulfiram—administration of disulfiram and metronidazole has been associated with acute psychoses and confusional states.

Phenobarbital—concomitant use of metronidazole and phenobarbital appears to decrease the serum half-life of metronidazole, presumably by increasing its metabolism.

Cimetidine—cimetidine reportedly increases the plasma half-life and decreases the total plasma clearance of metronidazole following single intravenous doses.

Adverse Reactions

Hypersensitivity reactions—erythematous reactions, including pruritus and urticaria, have been reported in patients receiving intravenous metronidazole.

Gastrointestinal—the most frequent adverse reactions to intravenous metronidazole are nausea, vomiting, abdominal discomfort, metallic taste in the mouth, and diarrhea. Antibiotic-associated pseudomembranous colitis has been reported with this agent.

Nervous system effects—peripheral neuropathy, characterized by numbness, tingling, or paresthesia of the extremity, and convulsive seizures have been reported rarely with intravenous metronidazole.

Hematologic effects—mild transient leukopenia has been reported rarely in patients receiving metronidazole. Bone marrow aplasia has also been reported.

Genitourinary effects—urine may be dark or reddish brown in color following intravenous administration of metronidazole because of the presence of water-soluble pigments.

Local effects—thrombophlebitis has been reported after intravenous infusion of metronidazole.

Penicillins

Aminopenicillins
Preparation for Intravenous Use

Of the aminopenicillins, ampicillin (aminobenzylpenicillin) is the only preparation for intravenous use.

Pharmacology

Mechanism of Action

Ampicillin has a mechanism of action similar to that of penicillin. In part because of the presence of a free amino group on the penicillin nucleus, ampicillin can penetrate the outer membrane of gram-negative bacteria more readily than can natural or penicillinase-resistant penicillins. Ampicillin is active against gram-negative bacteria that are resistant to the first- and second-generation penicillins.

Distribution

Ampicillin is widely distributed throughout the body after parenteral administration. Like the first- and second-generation penicillins, ampicillin attains only a minimal CSF concentration. Under conditions of meningitis, however, CSF concentrations range from 11 to 65% of simultaneous serum concentrations. Ampicillin is distributed into the bile, and its bile concentration may be 1 to 30 times greater than simultaneous serum concentrations.

Elimination

Of a single dose of ampicillin, 10 to 12% is metabolized by the liver to penicilloic acids. Ampicillin and its metabolites are rapidly secreted in the urine. Small amounts of ampicillin are also secreted by feces and bile. From 73 to 90% of a single intravenous dose of ampicillin is excreted unchanged in urine.

Spectrum of Activity

Ampicillin has similar activity as penicillin G for gram-positive cocci. However, it has an expanded spectrum that includes *Hemophilus influenzae*, *Escherichia coli*, *Proteus mirabilis*, and several *Salmonella* species. Of particular notice is that ampicillin is active against enterococcus and *Listeria monocytogenes,* two important pathogens responsible for neonatal infections and infections in the immunocompromised host or patient with advanced age.

Cautions

Hypersensitivity—hypersensitivity reactions reported with ampicillin are similar to those reported with other penicillins and beta-lactam antibiotics such as the cephalosporins. Although rare, anaphylaxis has been reported.

Hematologic disorders—ampicillin has been reported to have adverse hematologic effects, and a complete blood count should be obtained periodically during therapy with high-dose ampicillin.

Renal disorders—because acute interstitial nephritis has been reported with ampicillin, renal function should be determined prior to and during high-dose ampicillin therapy (see Dosage and Administration, below).

Use in pregnancy and lactation—Category B. Safe use of ampicillin during pregnancy has not definitely been established. However, ampicillin has been administered during pregnancy, especially in the treatment of urinary tract infections, without evidence of adverse effects on the fetus. Ampicillin is distributed into breast milk and should be used cautiously in nursing women.

Dosage and Administration

Ampicillin Dosing Ranges and Intervals

Neonates: 100 to 200 mg/kg/day divided q 6 to 12 hours

Children: 100 to 400 mg/kg/day divided q 4 to 6 hours

Adults: 6 to 12 g/day divided q 4 to 6 hours

Dosing in Renal Failure

When the creatinine clearance is <30 ml/min, it is suggested that the usual doses be delivered but that the dosing interval be increased to 8 to 12 hours.

Toxicity

Drug Interactions

Aminoglycosides—like other penicillins, ampicillin is incompatible with amino-glycosides when mixed *in vitro.* There is synergism, however, when each drug is administered separately.

Allopurinol—an increased incidence of rash reportedly occurs in patients with hyperuricemia who are receiving allopurinol and ampicillin.

Adverse Reactions

Hypersensitivity reactions—hypersensitivity reactions similar to those of other penicillins have been reported with ampicillin. Urticaria, exfoliative dermatitis, and erythema multiforme have been reported. Occasionally anaphylaxis occurs.

Hematologic—ampicillin has been reported to cause eosinophilia and hemolytic anemia. It has also been reported to cause anemia, leukopenia, neutropenia, agranulocytosis, and thrombocytopenia.

Gastrointestinal—nausea and diarrhea have been reported in up to 3% of patients receiving intravenous ampicillin.

Renal—acute interstitial nephritis has been reported rarely with ampicillin.

Hepatic—a moderate increase in serum concentrations of aminotransferases has been reported.

Nervous system—myoclonic seizures have been reported rarely following intravenous administration of high doses of ampicillin, especially in patients with impaired renal function.

Treatment of Toxicity

Hypersensitivity reactions are treated with basic airway and circulatory support as necessary. Oxygen and intravenous fluids are administered for unstable patients. Antihistamines, epinephrine, and corticosteroids are administered if required.

Extended-Spectrum Penicillins
Preparations for Intravenous Use

Ticarcillin disodium (with and without clavulanate), mezlocillin sodium, and piperacillin sodium are intravenous preparations of extended-spectrum penicillins. These drugs as single agents are not usually considered for first-line empirical therapy of serious infections. They are most commonly used in combination with the aminoglycosides against serious gram-negative infections. Ticarcillin with the beta-lactamase inhibitor clavulanate, however, has great potential as a first-line empirical choice.

Pharmacology

Mechanism of Action

Extended-spectrum penicillins have a mechanism of action similar to that of other penicillins. Extended-spectrum penicillins, however, are more active than natural penicillins, penicillinase-resistant penicillins, and third-generation penicillins against gram-negative bacilli. They more readily penetrate the outer membranes of these organisms.

Distribution

Extended-spectrum penicillins are widely distributed following absorption from parenteral injection sites. Like other penicillins, low concentrations of extended-spectrum penicillins are generally obtained in the CSF. Higher CSF concentrations may be attained when the meninges are inflamed.

Elimination

Extended-spectrum penicillins are metabolized in the liver to varying extents. These drugs and their metabolites are rapidly excreted in the urine by tubular secretion and glomerular filtration. Following intravenous administration, approximately 40 to 90% of piperacillin and 80 to 93% of ticarcillin are excreted in the urine unchanged within 24 hours.

Spectrum of Activity

Extended-spectrum penicillins, in general, are reserved for patients with serious gram-negative bacterial infections. Specifically, when *Pseudomonas aeruginosa* is suspected, these drugs, often in combination with aminoglycosides, are usually effective. Piperacillin and mezlocillin have a greater activity than ticarcillin. They are more effective against gram-negative organisms, particularly *P. aeruginosa,* and have a wider spectrum of activity against gram-positive cocci and a variety of anaerobes. When clavulanate is added to ticarcillin, it provides remarkably broad coverage. It is very effective against gram-positive organisms including streptococci and *Staphylococcus aureus* (including penicillinase-producing strains), a broad range of gram-negative aerobic rods, and many species of anaerobes, including *Bacteroides fragilis.*

Cautions

Hypersensitivity—hypersensitivity reactions reported with extended-spectrum penicillins are similar to those reported for other penicillins. Severe hypersensitivity has been reported less frequently with these penicillins than with natural penicillins. Caution must be exercised in administering these drugs in patients sensitive to penicillin and other beta-lactam antibiotics such as the cephalosporins.

Hematologic disorders—extended-spectrum penicillins can cause varying degrees of cell line suppression in the bone marrow. Caution should be exercised in deliverying these drugs in high doses to patients with hematologic disorders.

Renal and electrolyte disorders—extended-spectrum penicillins have been known to cause interstitial nephritis. Hypokalemia, sometimes associated with metabolic alkalosis, has been reported with these drugs as well. Hypernatremia can occur with the administration of ticarcillin. This effect is less often seen with the administration of mezlocillin and piperacillin.

Use in pregnancy and lactation—mezlocillin—Category B; piperacillin—Category B; ticarcillin—Category B. Safe use of mezlocillin, piperacillin, or ticarcillin during pregnancy has not been definitely established. Reproduction studies in mice and rats using azlocillin and mezlocillin doses up to twice the usual human dose or piperacillin doses up to four times the usual human dose have not revealed any evidence of impaired fertility or harm to the fetus. However, ticarcillin has been shown to be teratogenic in mice when given in doses equivalent to the usual human dose. These drugs should be used in pregnancy only when clearly needed. They are distributed into breast milk, and caution should be used in nursing mothers. Clavulanate is also distributed into breast milk.

Use in pediatric patients—while ticarcillin can be safely used in pediatric patients, safe doses of this agent plus clavulanate have not been established for patients under the age of 12 years. Safe dosages for piperacillin have not been established for children under 12 years of age.

Dosage and Administration

For dosing of mezlocillin and piperacillin, please refer to standard sources such as the *Physician's Desk Reference.*

Ticarcillin dosing range and intervals in children: 200 to 300 mg/kg/day divided q 4 to 6 hours

Ticarcillin dosing range and intervals in adults: 18 g/day divided q 4 hours

Ticarcillin plus clavulanate dosing range and interval in adults: 12.4 to 18.6 g/day divided q 4 to 6 hours

Dosing in Renal Failure

Schedule for ticarcillin with and without clavulanate

Creatinine Clearance (ml/min)	Dose and Interval
30–60	2 g q 4 hours
10–30	2 g q 8 hours
<10	2 g q 12 hours

Toxicity

Drug Interaction

Aminoglycosides—*in vitro,* extended-spectrum penicillins and aminoglycosides are incompatible when mixed. The aminoglycosides are inactivated. Inactivation does not occur *in vivo* when administration is separate. *In vivo* synergism usually occurs.

Adverse Reactions

Hypersensitivity reactions—hypersensitivity reactions to extended-spectrum penicillins are usually manifested by rash, fever, and eosinophilia. Rarely exfoliative dermatitis and serum sickness occur. Anaphylaxis is also a rare event.

Hematologic effects—eosinophilia, thrombocytosis, leukopenia, and neutropenia have been reported with the use of extended-spectrum penicillins.

Gastrointestinal effects—diarrhea and loose stools have been reported in 1% of patients using these drugs.

Renal and electrolyte effects—hyperkalemia, hypokalemia, and interstitial nephritis have been reported rarely with the use of extended-spectrum penicillins.

Hepatic effects—transient increases in serum concentrations of aminotransferases and alkaline phosphatase have been reported.

Nervous system effects—headaches, blurred vision, mental deterioration, hallucinations, and seizures have rarely been reported.

Treatment of Toxicity

Hypersensitivity reactions are treated with basic airway and circulatory support as necessary. Oxygen and intravenous fluids are administered for unstable patients. Antihistamines, epinephrine, and corticosteroids are given as necessary.

Natural Penicillins

Preparations for Intravenous Use

Penicillin G potassium and Penicillin G sodium are available for intravenous use. Penicillin G potassium is the preparation usually preferred for patients with normal renal function because the sodium preparation contains 2 mEq of sodium per 1,000,000 units. The potassium preparation contains 1.7 mEq potassium per 1,000,000 units of penicillin, which must be taken into consideration in patients with severe renal failure.

Pharmacology

Mechanism of Action

While the true and complete mechanism of action of penicillin has not been fully elucidated, penicillin-like antibiotics bind to several enzymes in the bacterial cytoplasmic membrane necessary for cell wall synthesis and division. The target enzymes of penicillin are called penicillin-binding proteins (PBPs) and vary with the penicillin or beta-lactam drug being administered. This interference results in the formation of bacterial cell walls that are incapable of sustaining bacterial life. Penicillin and other beta-lactam antibiotics are considered bactericidal.

Distribution

Penicillin G is widely distributed following intravenous administration. Under normal conditions, only 0 to 10% of concurrent serum concentrations of penicillin will be found in the CSF. Penicillin more readily penetrates an inflamed meninges. The combination of an inflamed meninges and very high doses of penicillin is necessary to reach effective antibacterial concentrations in the CSF.

Elimination

Approximately 15 to 30% of penicillin G is metabolized by the liver to penicilloic acid, and 4 to 5% is excreted in the bile. The majority of penicillin G and its metabolites are excreted through the kidneys by tubular secretion.

Spectrum of Activity

Penicillin G is active against the gram-positive aerobic cocci including *Streptococcus pneumoniae*, groups A, B, C, G, and H beta-hemolytic streptococci, *Streptococcus viridans*, and penicillin-sensitive *Staphylococcus aureus*. It has some activity against enterococci (group D streptococci). Of the gram-negative aerobes, it is most active against *Neisseria meningitidis*, *Neisseria gonorrhoeae*, and *Pasteurella multocida*. It is very effective against anaerobic cocci and *Clostridium* species, but it is ineffective in treating infections due to *Bacteroides fragilis*. It has no place in the treatment of gram-negative aerobic enteric organisms.

Cautions

Hypersensitivity—a history of hypersensitivity is a contraindication to the administration of penicillin G. Patients with a history of asthma should be questioned carefully concerning the possibility of allergy to penicillin prior to administration of that antibiotic. There is a reported 10 to 15% cross-allergenicity between penicillin and other beta-lactam antibiotics such as the cephalosporins.

Hematologic disorders—high-dose penicillin can cause transient neutropenia, leukopenia, and thrombocytopenia. Caution should be exercised in administering high doses of penicillin in patients with hematologic abnormalities.

Renal failure, cardiac failure, or electrolyte imbalance—as discussed earlier, penicillin G potassium is the preferred preparation for intravenous use. Patients with significant renal failure and potassium intolerance should not receive high doses of the potassium preparation of penicillin G (see Dosage and Administration, below). Caution should also be exercised in delivering the high sodium load to patients with significant myocardial depression.

Use in pregnancy and lactation—Category B. Safe use of penicillin G during pregnancy has not been definitively established. There are no controlled studies using natural penicillin in pregnant women, and the drug should be used in pregnancy only when clearly indicated. Penicillin G, however, has been administered to pregnant women without evidence of any unusual adverse effect on the fetus. Since penicillin G is distributed into breast milk, the drug should be administered with caution in nursing women.

Dosage and Administration

Penicillin G Dosing Ranges and Intervals

Children: 100,000 to 250,000 units/kg/day divided q 4 to 6 hours

Adults: 12 to 30,000,000 units/day divided q 4 hours

Dosing in Renal Failure*

Creatinine Clearance (ml/min)	Dose (Units) and Interval
60	2,000,000 q 4 hours
40	1,400,000 q 4 hours
20	1,000,000 q 4 hours
10	800,000 q 6 hours
<10	600,000 q 6 hours

Toxicity

Drug Interactions

Aminoglycosides—*in vitro*, penicillins and aminoglycosides are incompatible when mixed. The aminoglycosides are inactivated. Inactivation does not occur *in vivo* when administration is separate. *In vivo*, a synergism usually occurs that increases the antibacterial effectiveness of each agent.

Potassium-sparing diuretics—the concomitant use of potassium-sparing diuretics and penicillin G potassium can lead to hyperkalemia.

Adverse Reactions

Hypersensitivity reactions—allergic responses range from skin rashes and urticaria to exfoliative dermatitis. Occasion-

---

*These doses are calculated to be equivalent to 20,000,000 units per day in the adult patient with normal renal function. A loading dose of 1,000,000 units is suggested for a creatinine clearance of 20 ml/min or less. Otherwise, the initial dose can be equivalent to that administered to the patient with normal renal function.

ally, severe or fatal anaphylaxis can occur.

Hematologic—hemolytic anemia, leukopenia, and thrombocytopenia have been reported.

Neurologic—hyperreflexia, seizures, and coma have been observed with high intravenous doses given to seriously ill patients.

Treatment of Toxicity

Hypersensitivity reactions are treated with basic airway and circulatory support as necessary. Oxygen and intravenous fluids are administered to unstable patients. Antihistamines, epinephrine, and steroids are indicated for anaphylactic reactions.

Penicillinase-Resistant Penicillins
Preparation for Intravenous Use

Nafcillin sodium is usually chosen over other penicillinase-resistant penicillins because it has a lower incidence of adverse effects and a greater volume of distribution than either methicillin or oxacillin.

Pharmacology

Mechanism of Action

Penicillinase-resistant penicillins have a mechanism of action that is similar to that of other penicillins (see discussion under Natural Penicillins.) In addition, they resist the action of penicillinase.

Distribution

Penicillinase-resistant penicillins are widely distributed throughout the body following absorption. Nafcillin has a somewhat greater volume of distribution than do other penicillinase-resistant penicillins because it is sequestered in the liver. Unlike natural penicillins, therapeutic concentrations of penicillinase-resistant penicillins may be obtained in bone following intravenous administration. Like natural penicillins, however, only minimal concentrations of penicillinase-resistant penicillins are observed in the CSF following intravenous dosing. Slightly higher concentrations are observed in the CSF under conditions of inflammation of the meninges.

Elimination

Nafcillin has a slightly longer serum half-life than the other penicillinase-resistant penicillins. Of all these agents, nafcillin is the most extensively metabolized by the liver. Only a small amount of nafcillin is excreted in the urine, and the majority is eliminated via the bile and undergoes enterohepatic circulation.

Spectrum of Activity

The main indication for penicillinase-resistant penicillins is infection suspected to be due to *Staphylococcus aureus.* Penicillinase-resistant penicillins are also active against *Streptococcus pneumoniae* and *Staphylococcus pyogenes* but are not as effective as natural penicillins. They are also active against *Steptococcus viridans* but are not the drugs of choice for this bacteria. Penicillinase-resistant penicillins have some activity against anaerobic organisms but, again, are less active than the natural penicillins. These agents are not effective against gram-negative bacteria.

Cautions

Hypersensitivity—nafcillin is similar to the naturally occurring penicillins with regard to its potential for hypersensitivity reactions.

Hematologic disorders—penicillinase-resistant penicillins have been observed to have adverse hematologic effects such as reduction of total white blood cell count. It is recommended that periodic complete blood counts be done during high-dose intravenous therapy with penicillinase-resistant penicillins.

Renal disorders—penicillinase-resistant penicillins have been observed to cause acute interstitial nephritis. Renal function should be monitored during high-dose therapy.

Hepatic dysfunction—hepatic dysfunction resembling hepatitis or intrahepatic cholestasis occurs occasionally during therapy with penicillinase-resistant penicillins. Aminotransferases should be measured prior to institution of, and periodically during, therapy.

Use in pregnancy and lactation—Category B. Safe use of nafcillin during pregnancy has not been definitely established. However, clinical experience with nafcillin during pregnancy has not revealed evidence of adverse effects on the fetus. Nafcillin should be used cautiously during pregnancy. Penicillinase-resistant penicillins are distributed into breast milk and should be used with caution in nursing women.

Use in pediatric patients—only limited data are available concerning the intravenous administration of nafcillin in neonates and infants. Nafcillin is primarily metabolized by the liver, which may be immature in the newborn. In general, nafcillin is not recommended for pediatric patients under the age of 1 month. More commonly, methicillin is the drug of choice for *Staphylococcus aureus* infections in neonates. Methicillin is not recommended for adult use.

Dosage and Administration

Nafcillin Sodium Dose Ranges and Intervals

Children: 100 to 200 mg/kg/day divided q 6 hours

Adults: 6 to 12 g/day divided q 6 hours

Dosing in Renal and Hepatic Failure

Modification of doses of nafcillin is unnecessary in either renal or hepatic failure alone. Some downward adjustments should be considered if both renal and hepatic failure exist concurrently.

Toxicity

Drug Interactions

Aminoglycosides—like other penicillins, penicillinase-resistant penicillins are incompatible *in vitro* with aminoglycosides. The aminoglycosides can be inactivated. These drugs, however, are synergistic *in vivo* when administered separately.

Oral anticoagulants—high-dose nafcillin has been observed to decrease the hypoprothrombinemic effect of warfarin. The prothrombin time should be monitored carefully when high-dose nafcillin is being administered.

Adverse Reactions

Hypersensitivity reactions—hypersensitivity reactions reported with penicillinase-resistant penicillins are similar to those with other penicillins; however, severe hypersensitivity reactions have been reported less frequently with penicillinase-resistant penicillins. Rashes, including maculopapular and urticarial types, have been reported. Fever, eosinophilia, pruritus, and serum sickness–like reactions have also been reported.

Hematologic—in addition to eosinophilia and hemolytic anemia, other adverse hematologic effects include transient neutropenia, leukopenia, granulocytopenia, and thrombocytopenia.

Renal—acute interstitial nephritis as manifested by fever, rash, eosinophilia, microscopic hematuria, azotemia, and oliguria has been reported with the use of penicillinase-resistant penicillins.

Hepatic—hepatitis or intrahepatic cholestasis has been reported with penicillinase-resistant penicillins.

Local reactions—intravenous administration of penicillinase-resistant penicillins occasionally results in phlebitis or thrombophlebitis, especially in the older age group of patients.

Treatment of Toxicity

Severe hypersensitivity reactions are treated with basic airway and circulatory support as necessary. Oxygen and intravenous fluids are administered for unstable patients. Antihistamines, epinephrine, and corticosteroids are given as necessary.

Quinolones

Preparations for Intravenous Use

Ciprofloxacin is the only currently available intravenous fluoroquinolone preparation. It is scheduled for approval, as an intravenous preparation, in the United States in 1990.

Pharmacology

Mechanism of Action

The quinolones inhibit bacterial DNA gyrase, an enzyme that nicks and seals DNA in the process of transcription and reduces the intracellular size of DNA. These agents are biochemically related to nalidixic acid. The fluoroquinolones are bactericidal agents.

Distribution

The fluoroquinolones are widely distributed throughout body tissues and fluids. They have a small molecular size, a structure that promotes exceptional tissue penetration, especially for ciprofloxacin.

Elimination

Ciprofloxacin is excreted by the liver. In patients with renal failure, the half-life of the fluoroquinolones is increased. In patients with hepatic failure, ciprofloxacin may accumulate because of reduced metabolism and reduced biliary excretion.

Spectrum of Activity

Ciprofloxacin is effective against a wide range of microbial pathogens. Gram-negative aerobic bacilli are highly susceptible to the quinolones. These include *Escherichia coli, Klebsiella pneumoniae, Enterobacter* species, *Salmonella* species, *Shigella* species, and *Campylobacter. Pseudomonas aeruginosa* is susceptible to ciprofloxacin, but other species of *Pseudomonas* have shown resistance. While ciprofloxacin has good activity against a wide range of gram-positive organisms, including *Streptococcus pyogenes, Staphylococcus aureus*, and *Streptococcus pneumoniae*, it is not considered a first-line choice against these organisms. Ciprofloxacin is active against *Clostridium* species, anaerobic cocci, *Bacteroides fragilis*, and other *Bacteroides* species. It is also active against *Chlamydia trachomatis*.

Cautions

Hypersensitivity—patients who have known hypersensitivity to the quinolones should not receive these agents.

Seizures disorders—convulsions and central nervous system toxicity may occur when high doses are administered. Caution should be exercised in administering these agents to patients with preexisting central nervous system disease.

Use in pregnancy and lactation and in pediatric patients—Category C. The quinolones accumulate in and damage joint cartilage in developing experimental animals. Consequently, they are not recommended for use in children (patients under the age of 18 years) or in pregnant or nursing women.

Dosage adjustments in hepatic failure—see Dosage and Administration, below.

Dosage adjustment in renal failure—no dosage adjustment is necessary.

Dosage and Administration

Ciprofloxacin Hydrochloride Dosing Range and Intervals

Adults: 500 to 1500 mg/day divided q 12 hours (final recommended dose to be determined by the FDA before release in the United States)

Dosing in Hepatic Failure

In patients with significant hepatic impairment, the half-life of ciprofloxacin is significantly increased. Dosage adjustments have to be made based on the severity of the hepatic damage.

Toxicity

Drug Interactions

Theophylline—the fluoroquinolones appear to increase the serum levels of concomitantly administered theophylline. Theophylline levels should be monitored frequently during therapy with these agents.

Oral anticoagulants—the fluoroquinolones may interfere with the hepatic metabolism of warfarin, thereby increasing the serum concentration of this drug.

Adverse Reactions

Hypersensitivity reactions—hypersensitivity reactions have been seen in less than 1% of patients receiving these agents.

Cartilage toxicity—the quinolones can produce cartilage erosion in young animals. Therefore, there is some concern if these agents are used in pediatric age groups.

Gastrointestinal symptoms—nausea, vomiting, and anorexia are the most common side effects, occurring in 4% of patients. They are, however, usually not severe enough to necessitate discontinuing therapy.

Central nervous system symptoms—headaches and dizziness have been reported to occur.

Laboratory effects—mild leukopenia and abnormal liver function tests have been reported.

Tetracyclines

Preparation for Intravenous Use

Doxycycline hyclate

The main use of the tetracycline doxycycline in potentially life-threatening infections is for pelvic infections, in combination with a cephalosporin.

Pharmacology

Mechanism of Action

Tetracyclines are considered to be bacteriostatic in action. They inhibit protein synthesis in susceptible organisms by inhibiting the action of transfer ribonucleic acid.

Distribution

Tetracyclines are widely distributed into body tissues and fluids. Only small amounts diffuse into the CSF. All tetracyclines are concentrated in the liver and distributed into the bile, and they undergo some enterohepatic circulation. Concentration of tetracycline agents in the bile may be 2 to 32 times higher than concurrent serum levels.

Elimination

Twenty percent of doxycycline is eliminated via the kidneys and the rest is excreted into the gastrointestinal tract via bile and by nonbiliary routes, where it becomes bound to fecal materials.

Spectrum of Activity

Tetracyclines are the drugs of choice for infections caused by rickettsiae, *Mycoplasma, Chlamydia trachomatis, Brucella,* and the organisms responsible for granuloma inguinale, cholera, and relapsing fever.

Cautions

Hypersensitivity—tetracyclines are contraindicated in patients who are hypersensitive to these agents.

Hepatic and renal impairment—liver and renal function tests should be performed prior to and during high-dose intravenous therapy. Other potential hepatotoxic drugs should not be administered concomitantly.

Use in pregnancy and lactation—Category D. Tetracycline should not be used in women during the second half of pregnancy. Use of the drug in pregnant women has resulted in retardation of skeletal development and bone growth in the fetus and child. Tetracyclines are distributed into the breast milk. Because of the potential for serious adverse reactions from tetracycline in nursing infants, this drug should not be used in nursing mothers.

Use in pediatric patients—tetracyclines are not recommended in children under the age of 8 years unless other appropriate drugs are ineffective or contraindicated. Tetracyclines localize in dentin and enamel of developing teeth, and use of these drugs may cause enamel hyperplasia and discoloration.

Dosage and Administration

Doxycycline hyclate adult dose and intervals: 100 to 200 mg/day divided q 12 to 24 hours

Dosing in Renal Failure

Unlike other currently available tetracycline derivatives, the usual doses of doxycycline may be used in patients with impaired renal function.

Toxicity

Drug Interactions

Oral anticoagulants—tetracyclines may potentiate the effects of oral anticoagulants. Prothrombin time should be monitored more frequently than usual in patients receiving these agents.

Anti-infective agents—tetracyclines have been reported to antagonize the bactericidal activities of aminoglycosides and penicillins *in vitro.*

Other drugs—barbiturates, phenytoin, and carbamazepine decrease the serum half-life and serum concentrations of doxycycline. Preoperative or postoperative administration of tetracyclines to patients undergoing methoxyflurane anesthesia can produce fatal nephrotoxicity. These drugs should be avoided in combination with this anesthetic agent.

Adverse Reactions

Hypersensitivity reactions—hypersensitivity reactions have been reported rarely with tetracyclines but include maculopapular, morbilliform, and erythematous rashes. Exfoliative dermatitis and anaphylaxis have also been reported.

Renal toxicity—increased urinary excretion of nitrogen and increased blood urea nitrogen concentrations have been reported rarely during tetracycline therapy.

Hepatotoxicity—hepatotoxicity has rarely been reported with tetracyclines. Fatalities have occurred because of irreversible deterioration of pancreatic, hepatic, and renal functions. Liver toxicity has been reported most frequently following intravenous administration of large doses (more than 2 g daily) of tetracycline hydrochloride.

Hematologic effects—leukocytosis, neutropenia, leukopenia, hemolytic anemia, and thrombocytopenia have occurred with long-term tetracycline therapy.

Jarisch-Herxheimer reaction—Jarisch-Herxheimer reaction has occurred occasionally when tetracyclines were used to treat brucellosis or spirochetal infections, including syphilis.

Nervous system effects—tetracyclines have been reported to cause benign intracranial hypertension.

Local effects—intravenous administration of tetracycline frequently causes thrombophlebitis.

Trimethoprim-Sulfamethoxazole

Preparations for Intravenous Use

Trimethoprim-sulfamethoxazole (TMP-SMX), also known as co-trimoxazole, is the only intravenous preparation of this combination of antimicrobials.

Pharmacology

Mechanism of Action

Co-trimoxazole is usually bactericidal in action. Of its components, sulfamethoxazole is bacteriostatic and trimethoprim is slowly bactericidal. Co-trimoxazole acts by sequentially inhibiting enzymes of the folic acid pathway. For most organisms, optimum synergistic antibacterial action occurs at a trimethoprim:sulfamethoxazole blood ratio of 1:20.

Distribution

Co-trimoxazole is widely distributed into body fluids and tissues. It achieves good levels in the CSF, approximately 40 to 50% of concurrent serum concentrations.

Elimination

Co-trimoxazole is partially metabolized by the liver but is primarily excreted in the urine via glomerular filtration and tubular secretion.

Indications

Co-trimoxazole has a wide spectrum of activity against gram-positive and gram-negative bacteria. It is active against the majority of *Staphylococcus aureus, Staphylococcus epidermidis, Streptococcus pneumoniae,* and *Streptococcus pyogenes,* as well as *Streptococcus viridans.* It is active against many gram-negative aerobic bacteria including *Escherichia coli, Proteus* species, and *Klebsiella* species. It is also active against *Salmonella, Shigella, Hemophilus influenzae,* and *Pneumocystis carinii.* Co-trimoxazole is not active against *Pseudomonas aeruginosa* or enterococci. It is not very effective against anaerobic bacteria.

Cautions

Hypersensitivity—co-trimoxazole is contraindicated in patients with known hypersensitivity to trimethoprim or sulfonamides.

Hematologic disorders—co-trimoxazole should be used with caution in patients with hematologic disorders. These include glucose-6-phosphate dehydrogenase deficiency and megaloblastic anemia secondary to folate deficiency.

AIDS—patients with AIDS who receive co-trimoxazole should be carefully monitored, since they appear to have a particularly high incidence of adverse reactions to this drug (fever and adverse dermatologic and hematologic reactions).

Use in pregnancy and lactation—Category C. Trimethoprim and sulfamethoxazole, alone or in combination, have been documented to produce teratogenic effects. In general, this drug should be avoided in pregnant or lactating women.

Use in pediatric patients—safety and efficacy of co-trimoxazole in infants younger than 2 months of age have not been established, and it is not recommended for use in this age group.

Dosage and Administration

Co-trimoxazole Dosing Ranges and Intervals

Children: 6 to 12 mg/kg trimethoprim/30 to 60 mg/kg sulfamethoxazole divided q 12 hours (increase dose to 20 mg/kg trimethoprim/100 mg/kg sulfamethoxazole for *Pneumocystis carinii* pneumonia divided q 6 hours)

Adults: 8 to 10 mg/kg trimethoprim/40 to 50 mg/kg sulfamethoxazole divided q 12 hours (increase to 20 mg/kg trimethoprim/100 mg/kg sulfamethoxazole divided q 6 hours for *Pneumocystis carinii* pneumonia)

Toxicity

Drug Interactions

Oral anticogulants—co-trimoxazole may prolong the prothrombin time of patients receiving concomitant warfarin.

Other drugs—because co-trimoxazole possesses antifolate properties, the drug could theoretically increase the incidence of folate deficiencies induced by other drugs such as phenytoin. Co-trimoxazole should also be used cautiously in patients receiving methotrexate.

Adverse Reactions

Hypersensitivity reactions—hypersensitivity reactions are the most common adverse effects of co-trimoxazole. They occur, however, in less than 2.5% of patients. Fatal reactions (Stevens-Johnson syndrome), erythema multiforme, epidermal necrolysis, exfoliative dermatitis, serum sickness, and allergic myocarditis have also been reported.

Hematologic—hematologic toxicity has rarely been manifested by aplastic anemia or agranulocytosis. Leukopenia, neutropenia, thrombocytopenia, eosinophilia, megaloblastic anemia, methemoglobinemia, and hypoprothrombinemia have been reported. Hematologic toxicity may occur with increased frequency in folate-deficient patients, particularly those who are malnourished or alcoholic. Geriatic patients are also more sensitive to this agent.

Hepatic—hepatocellular necrosis and cholestatic jaundice have rarely been reported with the use of co-trimoxazole.

Treatment of Toxicity

Hypersensitivity reactions are treated with basic airway and circulatory support if necessary. Oxygen and intravenous fluids are administered to unstable patients. Antihistamines, epinephrine, and steroids are used as necessary.

Vancomycin

Preparation for Intravenous Use

Vancomycin hydrochloride is available for intravenous use. This drug is unrelated to other classes of antibiotics and, to some extent, this fact makes it a useful agent, particularly for life-threatening infections caused by multiply-resistant strains of *Staphylococcus aureus*.

Pharmacology

Mechanism of Action

Vancomycin is bactericidal. It binds to the cell wall and inhibits glycopeptide synthesis. This effect produces immediate inhibition of cell wall synthesis and cytoplasmic membrane damage. The importance of this mechanism is that it occurs at a different binding site than penicillin binding sites.

Distribution

Vancomycin is widely distributed to most body tissues with the exception of the brain. Low concentrations are achieved in the CSF under conditions of inflammation.

Elimination

Vancomycin is primarily excreted by glomerular filtration. Of a single intravenous dose, 80% can be recovered in the urine in 24 hours.

Spectrum of Activity

Vancomycin is only effective against gram-positive aerobic bacteria. It is bactericidal against penicillin-susceptible and penicillin-resistant *Staphylococcus aureus, S. epidermidis*, group A streptococci, *Streptococcus pneumoniae, S. viridans, Corynebacterium diphtheriae,* and *Clostridia* species. Its most important activity is against methicillin-resistant *S. aureus* and *S. epidermidis*. It is also active against enterococci. The main clinical use of vancomycin is for serious infections in the penicillin-allergic patient or the patient with multiply-resistant organisms such as *S. aureus*.

Cautions

Hypersensitivity—vancomycin is contraindicated in patients with known hypersensitivity to the drug.

Renal failure—vancomycin is nephrotoxic and must be used with caution in patients with renal disease (see Dosage and Administration, below).

Hearing loss—vancomycin can aggravate previous hearing loss, and auditory function tests are recommended, if possible, prior to institution of therapy in these patients.

Use in pregnancy and lactation—Category C. Animal reproduction studies have not been done with vancomycin. It is not known whether this drug is harmful to the fetus. It should only be used in pregnant women when it is clearly needed. It is also not known whether vancomycin is distributed into breast milk, and it therefore should be used with caution in nursing mothers.

Use in pediatric patients—because of its potential for nephrotoxicity, vancomycin should be used with caution in premature and young infants. Concomitant use of vancomycin and anesthetic agents can cause histamine-like flushing reactions in children.

Dosage and Administration

Vancomycin Hydrochloride Dosing Ranges and Intervals

Children: 40 to 60 mg/kg/day divided q 6 hours
Adults: 2 g/day divided q 12 hours

Dosing in Renal Failure

In renal failure, vancomycin doses must be carefully reduced after the administration of a normal initial dose. Some authorities recommend that vancomycin, in normal doses, can be given every 12 hours in patients with serum creatinines of <1.5 mg/dl. The dosing intervals are increased to every 3 to 6 days for serum creatinines between 1.5 and 5 mg/dl. If the serum creatinine is greater than 5 mg/dl, the intervals stretch out to every 12 to 14 days. When possible, peak and trough levels of vancomycin should be measured to aid dosing. Nomograms and more specific dosing schedules have been published and can be consulted during vancomycin therapy.

Toxicity

Drug Interactions

Nephrotoxic and ototoxic drugs—because of the possibility of additive toxicity, the concurrent administration of these drugs should be avoided.

Adverse Reactions

Hypersensitivity reactions—rashes have been reported to occur in 5% of patients receiving vancomycin.

Nephrotoxicity—although a serious adverse reaction, nephrotoxicity is now felt to be uncommon if standard dosing regimens are adhered to and if appropriate reduced dosing is used in renal failure patients.

Ototoxicity—this is a major side effect and appears to occur more commonly if serum levels of vancomycin rise above 80 μg/ml.

Hematologic effects—neutropenia has been reported to occur in patients receiving vancomycin.

Local effects—phlebitis can occur if the drug is not appropriately diluted prior to and during infusion.

REFERENCES

Bohr V, Hansen B, Jessen O, et al: Eight hundred and seventy-five cases of bacterial meningitis. Part I of a three-part series: Clinical data, prognosis, and the role of specialised hospital departments. J Infect 7:21–30, 1983.

Bone RC, Fisher CJ, Clemmer TP, et al: The sepsis syndrome: A valid clinical entity. Crit Care Med 17:389–393, 1989.

Bush LM, Calmon J, John CC: Newer penicillins and beta-lactamase inhibitors. Infect Dis Clin North Am 3(3):571–593, 1989.

Chase RA, Trenholme GM: Overwhelming pneumonia. Med Clin North Am 70:945–960, 1986.

Chelluri L, Warren J, Jastremski MS: Pharmacokinetics of a 3 mg/kg body weight loading dose of gentamicin or tobramycin in critically ill patients. Chest 95:1295–1297, 1989.

Cherubin CE, Eng RHK: Experience with the use of cefotaxime in the treatment of bacterial meningitis. Am J Med 80:398–404, 1986.

Cockerill FR, Edson R: Trimethoprim-sulfamethoxazole. Mayo Clin Proc 62:921–929, 1987.

Donowitz GR: Third generation cephalosporins. Infect Dis Clin North Am 3(3):595–612, 1989.

Edson RS, Terrell CL: The aminoglycosides: Streptomycin, kanamycin, gentamicin, tobramycin, amikacin, netilmicin, and sisomicin. Mayo Clin Proc 62:916–920, 1987.

Ellrodt AG: Sepsis and septic shock. Emerg Med Clin North Am 4:809–840, 1986.

Glatt AE, Chirgwin K, Landesman SH: Current concepts: Treatment of infections associated with human immunodeficiency virus. N Engl J Med 318:1439–1445, 1988.

Haddy RI, Klimberg S, Epting RJ: A two-center review of bacteremia in the community hospital. J Fam Prac 24:253–259, 1987.

Hermans PE, Wilhelm MP: Vancomycin. Mayo Clin Proc 62:901–905, 1987.

Klein JO, Feigin RD, McCracken GH: Report of the task force on diagnosis and management of meningitis. Pediatrics 78:959–982, 1986.

Korein J, Cravioto H, Leicach M: Reevaluation of lumbar puncture: A study of 129 patients with papilledema or intracranial hypertension. Neurology 9:290–297, 1959.

Kreger BE, Craven DE, Carling PC, et al: Gram-negative bacteremia: Reassessment of etiology, epidemiology and ecology in 612 patients. Am J Med 68:332–343, 1980.

Kreger BE, Craven DE, Carling PC, et al: Gram-negative bacteremia: Re-evaluation of clinical features and treatment in 612 patients. Am J Med 68:344–355, 1980.

Linton DM, Aitchison JM, Potgieter PD: Evaluation of the efficacy and tolerance of intravenously administered imipenem/cilastatin in the treatment of septicaemia. S Afr Med J 75:529–531, 1989.

Lode H: Initial therapy in pneumonia: Clinical, radiographic, and laboratory data important for the choice. Am J Med 80:70–74, 1986.

Mann MJ, Fuhs DW, Awang R, et al: Altered aminoglycoside pharmacokinetics in critically ill patients with sepsis. Clin Pharmacol 6:148–153, 1987.

McGravey A, Wise PH: Evaluation of the febrile child under 2 years of age. J Emerg Med 1:299–305, 1984.

Mitchell F: Adults with community-acquired bacteremias in two suburban hospitals: Factors predicting outcome. J Gen Intern Med 2:36–39, 1987.

Morris DL, Chambers HF, Morris MG, et al: Hemodynamic characteristics of patients with hypothermia due to occult infection and other causes. Ann Intern Med 102:153–157, 1985.

Nelson JD (ed): 1987–1988 Pocketbook of Pediatric Antimicrobial Therapy, 7th ed. Baltimore, Williams & Wilkins, 1987.

Neu HC: New antibiotics: Areas of appropriate use. J Infect Dis 155:403–417, 1987.

Ng PK: Determining aminoglycoside dosage and blood levels using a programable calculator. Am J Hosp Pharm 37:225–231, 1980.

Polsky B, Gold JWM, Whimbey E, et al: Bacterial pneumonia in patients with the acquired immunodeficiency syndrome. Ann Intern Med 104:38–41, 1986.

Quagliarello VJ, Scheld WM: Review: Recent advances in the pathogenesis and pathophysiology of bacterial meningitis. Am J Med Sci 292:306–309, 1986.

Rhodes KH, Johnson CM: Antibiotic therapy for severe infections in infants and children. Mayo Clin Proc 62:1018–1024, 1987.

Sanford JP (ed): Guide to Antimicrobial Therapy. Bethesda, MD, 1989.

Simmons DH, Nicoloff J, Guze LB: Hyperventilation and respiratory alkalosis as signs of gram-negative bacteremia. JAMA 174:2196–2199, 1960.

Sobel JD: Imipenem and aztreonam. Infect Dis Clin North Am 3(3):613, 1989.

Starr SE: Antimicrobial therapy of bacterial sepsis in the newborn infant. J Pediatr 106:1043–1048, 1985.

Tally FP: Factors affecting the choice of antibiotics in mixed infections. J Antimicrob Chemother 22(Suppl A):87–100, 1988.

Walker RC, Wright AJ: The quinolones. Mayo Clin Proc 62:1007–1012, 1987.

Weinstein MP, Murphy JR, Reller LB, et al: The clinical significance of positive blood cultures: A comprehensive analysis of 500 episodes of bacteremia and fungemia in adults. I. Laboratory and epidemiologic observations. Rev Infect Dis 5:35–53, 1983.

Weinstein MP, Murphy JR, Reller LB, et al: The clinical significance of positive blood cultures: A comprehensive analysis of 500 episodes of bacteremia and fungemia in adults. II. Clinical observations, with special reference to factors influencing prognosis. Rev Infect Dis 5:54–70, 1983.

Wilkowske CJ, Hermans PE: Symposium on antimicrobial agents. Part I: General principles of antimicrobial therapy. Mayo Clin Proc 62:789–798, 1987.

Wilson WR, Cockerill FR: Tetracyclines, chloramphenicol, erythromycin, and clindamycin. Mayo Clin Proc 62:906–915, 1987.

Wright AJ, Wilkowske CJ: The penicillins. Mayo Clin Proc 62:806–820, 1987.

CHAPTER 23

Obstetric and Gynecologic Emergency Drug Therapy

LYNNETTE DOAN-WIGGINS, M.D.

INTRODUCTION

Premature delivery complicates from 5% to 10% of all births in the United States, and prematurity continues to be the single greatest cause of neonatal morbidity and mortality. A wide variety of treatments for the inhibition of preterm labor have been advocated, including bed rest and prophylactic administration of progesterone, ethanol, prostaglandin inhibitors, magnesium sulfate, and, most recently, beta-mimetic agents such as terbutaline and ritodrine. Efficacy of each of these regimens is difficult to establish because of a paucity of well-controlled clinical studies and inconsistently defined indications for the use of tocolytic therapy.

Uterine contractions and therefore labor are the result of the interaction of the uterine smooth muscle filaments actin and myosin sliding upon one another, thereby shortening the uterine smooth muscle cell. This interaction depends on a transient phosphor-ylation of myosin by the enzyme myosin light-chain kinase. The activation of this kinase is, in turn, dependent on a relatively high level of intracellular calcium ions (Ca^{++}). Intracellular Ca^{++} concentration is dependent on the intracellular concentration of cyclic adenosine monophosphate (cAMP), which acts to lower intracellular Ca^{++} concentration by a variety of mechanisms. Uterine activity is therefore increased by the presence of a high concentration of Ca^{++} and a low concentration of cAMP. cAMP is produced from adenosine triphosphate (ATP) at the cell membrane by the enzyme adenyl cyclase; cAMP is destroyed within the cell by the enzyme phosphodiesterase. Adenyl cyclase inhibits uterine activity through the production of cAMP; phosphodiesterase promotes uterine activity by counteracting the effects of adenyl cyclase and lowering the level of intracellular cAMP.

Currently, the cornerstone of pharmacologic management of preterm labor is the use of beta-adrenergic receptor agonists and magnesium sulfate. The mechanism of action of the beta agonists involves the attachment of the drug to the beta$_2$-adrenergic receptors with subsequent activation of adenyl cyclase. The resultant increase in cAMP decreases myosin light-chain kinase activity, thereby interfering with the actin–myosin interaction. Although the exact mechanism by which magnesium sulfate reduces uterine activity is unknown, it is postulated that magnesium competes with the calcium ion, thereby inhibiting the actin–myosin interaction.

CONDITIONS

Premature Labor

Diagnosis

During the third trimester of normal pregnancy the gravid uterus, which is relatively quiescent throughout the first half of gestation, begins to increase its muscular activity. As the mother becomes aware of this activity, she begins to experience so-called false labor or Braxton-Hicks contractions. Irregular and periodic at first, Braxton-Hicks contractions gradually become the contractions of true labor, by definition those that result in progressive effacement and dilatation of the cervix. Frequently a gravida may experience multiple, brief episodes of regular and somewhat painful uterine contractions that cease spontaneously without producing cervical change. The clinical differentiation between true and false labor before the detection of cervical change is therefore difficult. Because successful treatment of preterm labor must be implemented early and the effectiveness of tocolytic therapy diminishes as labor advances, the decision of when to initiate tocolytic therapy is often difficult.

The criteria for defining preterm labor vary among authors, and, as mentioned earlier, this contributes to the difficulty in accurately assessing the efficacy of therapy. In the woman who is between 20 and 37 weeks of gestation, a presumptive diagnosis of premature labor may be based on the following: (1) the presence of regular uterine contractions occurring at intervals of 10 minutes or less and lasting at least 30 seconds, (2) progressive cervical effacement and dilatation during a period of observation, or (3) a cervix that is well effaced and at least 2 cm di-

lated when the patient is admitted to the hospital. Because rupture of the membranes frequently means that delivery is imminent, uterine contractions accompanied by membrane rupture may also be used to establish the diagnosis. External monitoring devices, when available, can be helpful in providing objective evidence of the character of uterine contractions as well as the condition of the fetus. Extended observation is undesirable because the effectiveness of tocolytic therapy diminishes as labor advances.

Indications for Treatment*

Ideally, when preterm labor is suspected, obstetric consultation should be obtained and the patient transferred immediately to the labor and delivery area for monitoring and determination of fetal maturity. When transfer is delayed or appropriate obstetric facilities are not available, attempts to arrest labor should be initiated at the earliest feasible time. Because uterine hypoxia may induce uterine contractions, supplemental oxygen, rapid intravenous infusion of 500 to 1000 ml of lactated Ringer's solution, and positioning of the patient in the left lateral decubitus position should be tried in an attempt to improve uterine perfusion. If contractions persist despite these maneuvers, obstetric consultation and tocolytic therapy may be indicated.

Tocolytic therapy should be considered in all women between 20 and 36 weeks of gestation in whom the diagnosis of preterm labor is suspected. Indications for tocolysis include (1) an apparently healthy fetus, (2) gestational age between 20 and 36 weeks, (3) cervical dilatation of 4 cm or less, and (4) intact fetal membranes. The latter criteria may be waived in occasional cases when time is required to accelerate fetal lung maturity with corticosteroid therapy. Tocolysis is generally contraindicated in the presence of (1) gestation less than 20 weeks or greater than 36 weeks, (2) maternal disease that would become increasingly severe if pregnancy continued (e.g., preeclampsia-eclampsia and severe cardiovascular or renal disease), (3) uncorrected fetal distress, (4) obstetric complications requiring early delivery (e.g., abruptio placentae, placenta previa with major hemorrhage, severe preeclampsia-eclampsia, hemolytic disease, or hydramnios), and (5) chorioamnionitis as indicated by the presence of ruptured membranes and fever. Tocolytic therapy in advanced labor as evidenced by cervical dilatation of greater than 4 cm or bulging membranes is ill-advised because it is generally unsuccessful.

Criteria for selecting patients for tocolytic therapy are listed in Table 23–1. (See box.)

Discussion

About half the patients suspected of being in premature labor will respond to bed rest, the avoidance of pelvic examinations, and basic attempts to improve uterine perfusion (i.e., intravenous fluids, supplemental oxygen, and positioning in the left lateral decubitus position). When tocolytic therapy is indicated, the selective beta$_2$-adrenergic agents and magnesium sulfate have been proved effective in the treatment of premature labor and are commonly found in most hospital formularies.

TABLE 23–1. Criteria for Selecting Patients for Tocolytic Therapy

Indications
Gestational age 20–36 weeks
An apparently healthy fetus
Regular uterine contractions
Cervical dilatation 4 cm or less
Intact fetal membranes (This criterion may be waived occasionally when time is required to accelerate fetal lung maturity with corticosteroid therapy.)
Contraindications
Gestational age <20 weeks or >36 weeks
Known fetal lung maturity
Uncorrected fetal distress or fetal death
Severe fetal disease or malformation, e.g., hemolytic disease or hydramnios
Abruptio placentae or placenta previa with major hemorrhage
Chorioamnionitis
Severe preeclampsia-eclampsia
Severe maternal disease such as untreated hyperthyroidism or cardiac or renal disease

---

DRUG TREATMENT: PREMATURE LABOR

First-Line Drugs: Beta-Adrenergic Agents
Ritodrine

Preparation	Add 150 mg ritodrine per 500 ml 5% dextrose in water (D$_5$W) yielding final concentration of 0.3 mg/ml
Initial Dose	0.1 mg/min (0.33 ml/min) IV infusion
Repeat Dose	Increase by 0.05 mg/min (0.17 ml/min) every 10 minutes.
End-Points	Maximum dose of 0.35 mg/min
Adverse maternal side effects
Cessation of contractions

OR

Terbutaline

Initial Dose	0.25 mg subcutaneously
or
0.01 mg/min by IV infusion
Repeat Dose	0.25 mg subcutaneously every 1–6 hours or may increase IV infusion by 0.005 mg/min every 10 minutes to maximum dose of 0.025 mg/min
End-Points	Maximum dose inherent in dosage schedule
Adverse maternal effects
Cessation of uterine contractions

Second-Line Drug
Magnesium Sulfate (MgSO$_4$)

Initial Dose	4–8 g IV over 20 minutes
Maintenance Dose	1–3 g/hour IV infusion
End-Points	Cessation of uterine contractions
Clinical evidence of magnesium toxicity

The *beta-adrenergic agents* act directly on beta$_2$-receptors to relax the uterus and uterine vessels. Their use is limited by dose-related major cardiovascular side effects related to residual beta$_1$-activity, including fetal and maternal tachycardia, elevated systolic and reduced diastolic blood pressure, and pulmonary edema. Maternal metabolic side effects include a decrease in serum potassium and an increase in blood glucose and lactic acid. Maternal medical contraindications to the use of beta-adrenergic agents include cardiac disease, hyperthyroidism, uncontrolled diabetes, and chronic hepatic or renal disease. Commonly observed side effects during intravenous administration are palpitations, tremors, nervousness, and restlessness.

In the United States, ritodrine is the only beta$_2$-agonist that has received approval by the Food and Drug Administration for the treatment of preterm labor. Although not approved in the United States, terbutaline has been used elsewhere as a tocolytic agent, has documented efficacy in inhibiting labor, and is frequently more available to non-obstetricians than is ritodrine. Other beta-mimetic agents such as salbutamol, fenoterol, hexoprenaline, and isoxsuprine are not currently approved as tocolytics, appear to offer no advantage over ritodrine and terbutaline, and are therefore not commonly recommended for tocolysis.

Magnesium sulfate has not been approved in the United States for use as a tocolytic agent. Although apparently less effective than ritodrine and terbutaline, magnesium sulfate is less likely to cause serious side effects and is the best alternative if beta-mimetic drugs are contraindicated or toxic. The major side effect of magnesium sulfate therapy is impairment of the muscles of respiration with subsequent respiratory arrest, an effect usually seen at serum magnesium levels above 10 mEq/liter. The first sign of impending toxicity is loss of the patellar reflex, which occurs at plasma levels between 7 and 10 mEq/liter. The presence of the patellar reflex and respiratory status must therefore be monitored throughout therapy. Because magnesium is almost totally eliminated by the kidneys, renal function and urinary output should also be monitored. If respiratory depression develops, calcium gluconate, 10 to 20 ml of a 20% solution, is an effective antidote.

Other therapies have been tried in an attempt to arrest premature labor but are not currently recommended. Ethanol, used as a tocolytic following favorable reports published in 1967, is no longer used because of the necessity for prolonged administration and many undesirable side effects associated with its use. The prostaglandin inhibitors, although effective tocolytics, may be associated with major cardiovascular changes in the fetus, including premature closure of the fetal ductus arteriosus, and are currently not recommended for the acute management of preterm labor. The calcium antagonists, most notably verapamil and nifedipine, are potential tocolytic agents still under study. Although their use appears promising, they are not yet recommended for routine clinical use.

Postpartum Hemorrhage

Postpartum hemorrhage, defined as maternal blood loss greater than 500 ml following delivery of the fetus, is estimated to occur in 5 to 8% of all pregnancies. It accounts for up to 25% of obstetric deaths resulting from hemorrhage and is conventionally divided into immediate hemorrhage (within 24 hours of delivery) and delayed hemorrhage (more than 24 hours after delivery). The majority of cases of *immediate postpartum hemorrhage* are due to uterine atony and occur when the myometrium fails to contract, thereby failing to effect compression and tamponade of uterine vessels. *Delayed postpartum hemorrhage* typically occurs 7 to 14 days after delivery and most commonly involves retention of placental tissue and subinvolution of the placental site. When retained placental tissue or necrotic debris sloughs off the endometrium, open blood vessels are exposed. Because there is no stiumlus for contraction and therefore no means to tamponade the exposed vessels, hemorrhage ensues. Medical therapy for both immediate and delayed postpartum hemorrhage is aimed at inducing uterine contraction to produce tamponade of bleeding uterine vessels through the use of the hormone oxytocin, the ergot alkaloids ergonovine and methylergonovine, and the prostaglandin $F_{2\alpha}$ ($PGF_{2\alpha}$).

Diagnosis

Immediate postpartum hemorrhage occurs within 24 hours of delivery and is frequently characterized by steady, moderate bleeding, rather than sudden massive bleeding, and may cause serious hypovolemia. Between 75 and 90% of cases of immediate postpartum hemorrhage are due to uterine atony. The diagnosis is made when pelvic examination reveals a soft, boggy uterus. The uterus may contract with manual massage, only to relax and resume bleeding when massaging stops. Although retained placental tissue and abnormal placental insertion are not common, they should always be considered as a cause of uterine atony, and the placenta should be inspected carefully for missing tissue and anatomic abnormalities. Other causes of immediate postpartum hemorrhage include lacerations to the perineum, vagina, and cervix and, less commonly, coagulopathies, uterine rupture, and inversion of the uterus.

Delayed postpartum hemorrhage most commonly occurs 7 to 14 days after delivery and typically presents with sudden, brisk, painless vaginal bleeding that may have been preceded by intermittent spotting or complaints of a foul-smelling lochia. Abdominal examination usually reveals a large, nontender, boggy uterus. Pelvic examination reveals bleeding through the cervical os, and bimanual examination confirms the findings of the abdominal examination. The presence of fever, purulent discharge, or uterine tenderness suggests endoparametritis as the cause of bleeding.

Indications for Treatment

The initial management of *immediate postpartum hemorrhage* due to uterine atony consists of manual massage of the uterine fundus. Oxytocics should be administered in conjunction with massage and may be given intravenously or intramuscularly. Because of the danger of entrapping the placenta or a second twin in a contracting uterus, oxytocics should not be administered prior to delivery of the placenta.

Similarly, the initial management of patients with *delayed postpartum hemorrhage* consists of administration of oxytocic drugs, either oxytocin or one of the ergot alkaloids. Response to initial therapy will dictate further treatment as outlined below. When uterine infection is suspected as the cause of bleeding, antibiotic therapy should be added to the treatment regimen. (See box.)

Discussion

In addition to adequate volume replacement, the initial management of *immediate postpartum hemorrhage* due to uterine atony consists of manual massage of the uterine fundus plus administration of the hormone *oxytocin*. Because the onset of action of intravenously administered oxytocin is rapid, uterine contractions and therefore slowing of hemorrhage should be observed within minutes of administration. If bleeding persists and the uterus remains boggy despite oxytocin therapy, an *ergotamine preparation* such as methylergonovine (Methergine) or ergonovine (Ergotrate) should be given intramuscularly to help stimulate uterine contraction. Typically uterine contractions occur within minutes of ergot administration and persist for several hours. If bleeding persists, the use of *prostaglandin* therapy should be considered. Injection of 0.5 to 1 mg of prostaglandin ($PGF_{2\alpha}$) transabdominally or transvaginally into the myometrium has been reported to control postpartum hemorrhage refractory to other therapy. Recently a 15-methyl analogue of $PGF_{2\alpha}$ with higher potency and longer duration of action has also been shown to be effective; it may be given as an intramuscular injection and may be repeated. It should be noted that the use of prostaglandin compounds for the purpose of arresting postpartum hemorrhage due to uterine atony has not yet been approved by the Food and Drug Administration. They may be used as a last resort, however, to help control life-threatening hemorrhage unresponsive to more traditional therapies.

When vaginal bleeding persists despite the presence of a firm, contracted uterus and appropriate therapy for uterine atony, the vagina and cervix should be inspected for lacerations. Management of refractory postpartum hemorrhage frequently requires the expertise of the obstetrician and operative intervention.

In the majority of cases, *delayed postpartum hemorrhage* results from subinvolution of the placental implantation site due to retained placental tissue or infection. Initial treatment consists of administration of either intravenous oxytocin or, alternatively, intramuscular methylergonovine or ergonovine. If bleeding is initially mild and stops with oxytocic therapy, the patient may be discharged home on methylergonovine or ergonovine (0.2 mg PO every 6 to 8 hours). In such cases, necrotic placental tissue is usually carried away with the onset of bleeding, and curettage is not necessary. If bleeding is initially severe or fails to respond to oxytocic therapy, an excessive amount of retained placental tissue should be suspected, in

DRUG TREATMENT: POSTPARTUM HEMORRHAGE

First-Line Drug

Oxytocin

Preparation	Add 20 to 40 units to 1000 ml Ringer's lactate or normal saline
Dosage	200 to 500 ml/hour IV infusion (If intravenous access is unavailable, 10 units of oxytocin may by given intramuscularly.)
End-Points	Contraction of uterus Cessation of bleeding

Second-Line Drug

Ergot Alkaloids (Methylergonovine, Ergonovine)

Initial Dose	0.2 mg IM
Repeat Dose	If bleeding resolves, 0.2 mg PO every 6–8 hours
End-Points	Contraction of uterus Cessation of bleeding

Third-Line Drugs (Immediate Pospartum Hemorrhage)

15-Methyl Prostaglandin $F_{2\alpha}$

Initial Dose	0.25 mg IM
Repeat Dose	0.25 mg IM every 2 hours
End-Points	Contraction of uterus Cessation of bleeding

OR

Prostaglandin $F_{2\alpha}$ ($PGF_{2\alpha}$)

Initial Dose	0.5–1 mg injected directly into the myometrium
Repeat Dose	None
End-Points	Contraction of uterus Cessation of bleeding

which case curettage is usually necessary. When uterine infection is suspected as the cause of subinvolution, antibiotic therapy should be added to the treatment regimen.

When administered rapidly, oxytocin may cause transient hypotension, which typically resolves following discontinuation of the drug. Because of this hypotensive effect, oxytocin should never be given intravenously as a large bolus. In addition to its cardiovascular effects, oxytocin has intrinsic antidiuretic hormone activity, which may occur when the drug is administered at a rate of 20 mU/min or greater. This antidiuretic effect must be considered when monitoring urinary output as an indication of renal perfusion and hemodynamic status.

The most common serious side effect of the ergot preparations is their tendency to cause vasoconstriction and severe hypertension. Ergot preparations should therefore be avoided in women who are known to be hypertensive. In addition, nausea and vomiting occur in approximately 20% of patients receiving parenteral ergots; muscle weakness is another troublesome side effect.

The most common side effects of prostaglandin therapy include nausea, vomiting, and diarrhea, which occur in less than half of the patients. Less commonly a mild, transient temperature elevation or a moderate but transient elevation of blood pressure may occur. Prostaglandins are contraindicated in patients with known hypersensitivity to the compound or asthma.

Pregnancy-Induced Hypertension

Pregnancy-induced hypertension occurs in 5 to 10% of all pregnancies and, despite recent advances in perinatal care, continues to be one of the principal contributors to maternal and fetal morbidity and mortality. It represents an area of medical practice marked by substantial controversy concerning cause, pathophysiology, and treatment.

Pregnancy-induced hypertension may be divided into three categories: (l) hypertension alone, (2) preeclampsia, and (3) eclampsia. Preeclampsia refers to the development of pregnancy-induced hypertension plus generalized edema or proteinuria, or both. Untreated or in its severe forms, preeclampsia can rapidly progress to eclampsia, which is manifested by grand mal seizures, one of the most dramatic and life-threatening complications of pregnancy.

Hypotheses concerning the etiology and pathogenesis of pregnancy-induced hypertension abound and are confounded by lack of a suitable animal model in which to study the disease. Essential to the development of the disease is the presence of chorionic villi, although these need not support a fetus nor be located within the uterus. Recent interest has focused on an immunologic cause of preeclampsia, and a growing body of evidence suggests failure of the maternal immune response as the underlying mechanism.

Vasospasm, principally of the arterioles, is the primary disease process of pregnancy-induced hypertension. Vasoconstriction raises systemic vascular resistance by imposing a resistance to blood flow and leads to the development of arterial hypertension. In addition, vasospasm probably exerts an adverse effect on the blood vessels themselves by impairing circulation to the vasa vasorum and leading to damage of the vascular walls. Together with local hypoxia of the surrounding tissues, these vascular changes lead to hemorrhage, necrosis, and the other organ disturbances observed in severe pre-eclampsia.

The etiology of eclamptic convulsions is poorly understood. Seizures are generally attributed to platelet thrombi that obstruct the cerebral microcirculation or to intense, sometimes localized, vasoconstriction. Although seizures correlate with the severity of hypertension, they may also arise when blood pressure elevations are mild or blood pressure differs little from that recorded during the previous 24 hours.

Uteroplacental blood flow decreases two- to threefold in pre-eclampsia and is almost certainly a major factor in the increased incidence of fetal loss, intrauterine growth retardation, and small-for-date infants associated with the disease. Limited data from human studies suggest that acute reductions in maternal blood pressure may decrease uteroplacental perfusion even further and compromise fetal well-being.

The treatment of preeclampsia/eclampsia is aimed at (1) the prevention or control of convulsions, (2) control of markedly elevated blood pressure, and (3) steps to bring about the delivery of the infant once the maternal condition has stabilized. It must be emphasized that the only cure for preeclampsia/eclampsia is removal of the trophoblastic tissue; once delivery is accomplished, the pathologic changes of eclampsia begin to resolve. Drug therapy is principally aimed at the prevention or control of convulsions and the control of hypertension.

Diagnosis

Clinically the diagnosis of pregnancy-induced hypertension is easily established and is defined as a blood pressure of 140/90 mmHg or greater in a gravid patient in whom previous blood pressure is unknown or as an increase in systolic pressure of 30 mmHg or diastolic pressure of 15 mmHg in a patient whose blood pressure has been previously documented. Preeclampsia typically refers to the presence of hypertension plus generalized edema or proteinuria, or both. Edema, even of the hands and face, is a common finding during normal pregnancy. Therefore, to be useful in the diagnosis of preeclampsia, edema must involve the hands and face and be present in the morning after rising. Proteinuria, an important but late sign to develop in preeclampsia, is defined as the presence of 300 mg or more of protein in a 24-hour urine collection (usually 1+ or 2+

on dipstick). It should be noted that the degree of proteinuria may fluctuate widely in the same person over any 24-hour period. Therefore, even in severe cases a single random sample may fail to detect significant proteinuria; conversely, mild proteinuria alone may be physiologic and, without associated hypertension, has little influence on the outcome of the pregnancy.

The differentiation of mild preeclampsia from *severe preeclampsia* is somewhat artificial, and even an apparently mild case of preeclampsia can rapidly become severe. Blood pressure alone is not always a reliable indicator of the severity of pregnancy-induced hypertension; other signs and symptoms such as headache, visual disturbances, hyperreflexia, and abdominal pain indicate severe disease and typically precede the development of eclampsia (Table 23–2). Hyperreflexia may be absent in up to 20% of cases.

Eclampsia is an acute disorder characterized by tonic–clonic convulsions superimposed on preeclampsia. Eclampsia usually occurs in the last trimester of pregnancy and becomes increasingly frequent as term approaches; it may occasionally occur during the first 48 hours following delivery. In general, until the diagnosis can be excluded, all pregnant women with convulsions should be considered to have eclampsia and be initially treated for the disease.

Indications for Treatment

Hospitalization is indicated for most if not all women presenting with new-onset preeclampsia and in all women with preeclampsia in whom the systolic blood pressure is 140 mmHg or greater or diastolic pressure is 90 mmHg or greater. Bed rest throughout

TABLE 23–2. Indicators of Severe Preeclampsia

Clinical Signs
Diastolic blood presure ≥110 mmHg
Headache
Visual disturbances
Hyperreflexia
Upper abdominal pain
Seizures
Oliguria
Laboratory Abnormalities
Proteinuria persistently ≥2+
Elevated serum creatinine
Significant elevation of SGOT
Hyperbilirubinemia
Thrombocytopenia

most of the day is beneficial. The role of volume expansion in the management of preeclampsia and eclampsia is controversial. Oral sodium and fluid intake should be neither restricted nor forced. When intravenous therapy is initiated, it is prudent to use a solution of Ringer's lactate with 5% dextrose at a rate of 60 to 150 ml/hour unless fluid requirements are increased by vomiting, diarrhea, or blood loss at delivery.

Drug therapy should be initiated in any woman with eclampsia and in those demonstrating signs and symptoms of severe preeclampsia, as outlined in Table 23–2. Because seizures are more likely to develop during labor, many authorities recommend that all women suspected of having pregnancy-induced hypertension be treated with magnesium sulfate during labor and the early puerperium. Drug therapy is aimed at the prevention and control of convulsions and control of hypertension and is typically divided into anticonvulsant and antihypertensive agents. (See box.)

Discussion
Antihypertensives

Treatment of hypertension in the preeclamptic and eclamptic patient is indicated when the diastolic blood pressure is greater than 110 mmHg after treatment with magnesium sulfate. The goal of therapy is to gradually lower the diastolic pressure to 90 to 100 mmHg, a level that will reduce the likelihood of intracranial bleeding without compromising placental blood flow.

Hydralazine has long been considered the drug of choice for the acute management of pregnancy-induced hypertension. Acting by directly reducing peripheral vascular resistance, it is thought to have a beneficial effect on cardiac output and renal blood flow. Its effect on uteroplacental blood flow is less clear. In preeclamptic women, treatment with hydralazine appears to increase uterine blood flow, but in chronically hypertensive women it appears to reduce placental blood flow. Ominous decelerations in fetal heart rate have been reported in women treated with hydralazine, but this effect appears to be limited to patients in whom diastolic pressure drops below 90 mmHg. Clinical experience with the drug has yielded favorable outcomes. Maternal side effects are common and consist of headaches, anxiety, restlessness, nausea, vomiting, and epigastric pain.

DRUG TREATMENT: SEVERE PREECLAMPSIA AND ECLAMPSIA

Antihypertensives

First-Line Drug

Hydralazine

Initial Dose	5 mg IV
Repeat Dose	5–10 mg IV at 15- to 20-minute intervals
End-Point	Diastolic pressure of 90–100 mmHg

Second-Line Drug

Diazoxide

Dose	30-mg bolus repeated every 1–2 minutes, or IV infusion of 15 mg/min to total dose of 5 mg/kg body weight
End-Point	Diastolic pressure of 90–100 mmHg

Anticonvulsants

First-Line Drug

Magnesium Sulfate

Initial Dose	4 g (20% solution) by IV push at a rate of 1 g/min
Repeat Dose	Up to 2 g (20% solution) by IV push within 20 minutes at a rate of 1 g/min if needed
Maintenance Dose	IV infusion (25 g in 500 ml D₅W) of 1–3 g/hour
	or
	When IV access is unavailable: 10 g (20 ml of a 50% solution) IM, one-half in each buttock, followed by 5 g IM every 4 hours thereafter
End-Point	Continue until 24 hours after delivery or clinical evidence of magnesium toxicity.

Second-Line Drug

Sodium Amobarbital

Dose	50-mg increments by slow IV push to a total dose of 250 mg given over 3 minutes
End-Points	Cessation of convulsions Respiratory depression

Diazoxide, another rapidly acting parenteral antihypertensive agent, exerts its hypotensive effect by a relatively selective reduction in arteriolar tone and a decrease in peripheral vascular resistance. Although it is effective in reducing blood pressure in the preeclamptic/eclamptic patient, diazoxide has resulted in episodes of profound maternal hypotension, fetal distress, and maternal and neonatal hyperglycemia when given as the standard 300-mg dose. Diazoxide should therefore be reserved for cases of hypertension resistant to hydralazine and should be administered in small doses, as described earlier (Chapter 12). Although diazoxide causes relaxation of the myometrium, which may inhibit labor, it does not block the effects of oxytocin on the uterine musculature.

The use of *nitroprusside* during pregnancy remains controversial. Nitroprusside causes relaxation of arterial and venous smooth muscle, but in therapeutic doses it has no effect on myocardial or uterine contractility. Nitroprusside readily crosses the placenta, and its metabolic products may accumulate, causing cyanide toxicity in the fetus. However, clinlical evidence suggests that in short-term use, maternal and fetal toxicity may not be a serious problem. As a general rule, nitroprusside should not be considered the drug of choice to control severe hypertension during pregnancy and should be reserved for hypertensive emergencies refractory to other therapy.

Experience with the calcium channel blocker *nifedipine* is limited. Preliminary evidence indicates that it produces a rapid therapeutic fall in blood pressure without adverse fetal effects. Like diazoxide, nifedipine relaxes the myometrium; its effect on uteroplacental blood flow has not yet been defined. More detailed evaluation is required before its use during pregnancy can be recommended.

The use of *diuretics* in the treatment of preeclampsia/eclampsia is condemned by most authorities because of the relative hypovolemia accompanying the disease. Diuretics increase the risk of compromising uteroplacental and renal perfusion and increase the susceptibility of some women to intrapartal hypotension and puerperal vascular collapse.

Anticonvulsants

Magnesium sulfate (MgSO₄) is the initial drug of choice for the prophylaxis and control of seizures secondary to preeclampsia. Its mechanism of action has not been fully elucidated. High concentrations of the magnesium ion are known to decrease the release of acetylcholine at the neuromuscular junction, thereby decreasing motor endplate excitability. In addition, magnesium seems to have a primary effect on the central nervous system, suppressing neuronal burst firing and interictal electro-encephalographic spike generation in subhuman primates. Although an antihypertensive action has long been ascribed to the drug when administered intravenously, its antihypertensive effect is minimal and results from a brief and transient fall in peripheral vascular resistance, which resolves after discontinuation of the drug. Because parenterally administered magnesium is cleared almost totally by renal excretion, renal function must be continually monitored throughout therapy.

Although magnesium crosses the placenta readily, fetal magnesium toxicity is usually not a problem. The major maternal side effect of magnesium therapy is impairment of the muscles of respiration with subsequent respiratory arrest, an effect usually seen at serum magnesium levels above 10 mEq/liter. The first warning sign of impending toxicity is loss of the patellar reflex, which occurs at plasma levels between 7 and 10 mEq/liter. Magnesium toxicity can be avoided by continually ensuring that an active patellar reflex is present, urine output is at least 35 ml/hour, and there is no respiratory depression. Calcium gluconate, 10 to 20 ml of a 10% solution injected slowly over 3 minutes, is an effective antidote to magnesium-induced respiratory depression.

Because neurologic irritability usually responds to magnesium sulfate therapy, the use of other anticonvulsants is infrequently necessary. The rapid-acting *barbiturates*, most notably sodium amobarbital, are very effective in controlling eclamptic seizures. Although they cross the placenta and may cause neonatal depression, they are indicated as second-line therapy for seizures not controlled by magnesium sulfate. Although the widely used anticonvulsant *diazepam* is effective in treating eclamptic convulsions, its effect on the fetus limits its use. Diazepam readily crosses the placenta and is metabolized slowly by the infant. Newborns of mothers treated with large doses of diazepam have been noted to have low Apgar scores, apnea several hours after birth, drowsiness, hypotonia, and an impaired metabolic response to cooling.

Prevention of Pregnancy Following Sexual Assault

Sexual assault is a crime reported with increasing frequency in the United States. During 1981, 81,536 rapes were reported, and it is estimated that ten times that number occurred. The incidence of pregnancy following sexual assault is low, probably between 1 and 5%.

Estrogen compounds have been the most commonly used postcoital contraceptives. Although many theories have been proposed to explain the antifertility effect of high-dose estrogens, it is generally accepted that they act by preventing implantation of the fertilized ovum through alteration of the endometrial lining. Due to a complex feedback mechanism involving estrogens, progester-

DRUG TREATMENT: POSTCOITAL PREGNANCY PREVENTION

First-Line Drug
Ovral
   Dose   2 tablets PO followed by 2 tablets PO in 12 hours

Second-Line Drug
Conjugated Estrogens (Premarin)
   Dose   25 mg PO every day for 5 days or 50 mg IV over 5 minutes

one, luteinizing hormone, and human chorionic gonadotropin (HCG), it is felt that postcoital estrogens may be unsuccessful in preventing pregnancy if administered in the presence of an implanted ovum and that those women who delay treatment until after implantation has occurred will remain pregnant. The high-dose estrogen regimens are therefore only effective if instituted within 72 hours of intercourse.

Diagosis and Indications for Treatment

There is no absolute indication for the use of postcoital contraceptives in the emergency management of the sexual assault victim. Postcoital contraception should be offered as an option to every fertile, unprotected female rape victim if she is seen within 72 hours of the assault and if the assailant's penis penetrated her vaginally. Although failure to find motile sperm in the vaginal aspirate or noting that the patient is near her menses may diminish the risk of pregnancy, these conditions do not eliminate the risk. The decision of whether to initiate treatment should be made by the patient in conjunction with her physician and is based on the patient's desire to prevent or terminate a pregnancy that may result from the sexual assault. Consideration should be given to alternative methods of pregnancy termination, including abortion, as well as to the possible short- and long-term effects of each of the methods considered. In all cases, preexisting pregnancy must be ruled out by history, physical examination, and laboratory analysis. (See box.)

Discussion

Hormonal therapy must be started within 72 hours of intercourse to be effective. Because the most common side effects of estrogens are nausea and vomiting, an antiemetic should be prescribed in conjunction with the drug. Relative contraindications to the administration of estrogens should be noted and include a history of thrombophlebitis, pulmonary embolism, estrogen-dependent tumor, and cardiovascular or liver disease.

The current postcoital contraceptive of choice is the birth control pill Ovral. Each tablet contains 0.5 mg of the synthetic progestin, norgestrol, and 0.05 mg of the synthetic estrogen, ethinyl estradiol. Two Ovral tablets are effective and infrequently cause nausea and vomiting. The two most commonly used abortives in the past, diethylstilbestrol (DES) and Premarin, both cause significant nausea and vomiting. In addition, DES can no longer be recommended because of the risk of developing clear-cell carcinoma of the cervix or vagina in female fetuses should conception occur despite DES prophylaxis. Other nonhormonal options for pregnancy interruption include insertion of an intrauterine device and elective abortion.

$Rh_0(D)$ Incompatibility

Isoimmune hemolytic disease of the newborn is the result of destruction of the red blood cells of the fetus and neonate by maternal antibodies to a blood group factor on the red cells of the fetus. The disorder occurs in approximately 1.5% of all pregnancies; it arises when the fetus inherits a blood group antigen from the father that is not possessed by the mother and the mother either has, or forms, the corresponding antibody against that particular fetal blood group antigen. This results in the destruction of fetal red blood cells, which clinically manifests as neonatal jaundice, anemia, and death. Although incompatibilities among the ABO blood group antigens and several other blood group factors may all result in hemolytic disease of the newborn, the most important incompatibility involves the Rh system, specifically the D antigen, and occurs when an $Rh_o(D)$-negative mother carries an $Rh_o(D)$-positive fetus. Fetal antigens may be introduced into the maternal circulation in a variety of ways but usually results from fetomaternal transfusion of antigen-positive red blood cells during the current or a prior pregnancy (Table 23–3). In rare instances, an Rh-negative woman may have been sensitized in utero by Rh-positive cells from her mother via maternal-to-fetal transfusion.

The obstetric patient may be exposed to red blood cells from her Rh-positive fetus via fetomaternal transfusion during the normal course of pregnancy; as a consequence of abdominal trauma, amniocentesis, or abortion; or at delivery. If the mother is Rh negative and the infant is Rh positive, there is a 5 to 13% chance that maternal sensitization to $Rh_o(D)$ will occur. Although the risk of maternal sensitization rises with the volume of fetal transplacental hemorrhage, it is estimated that as little as 1 ml of fetal red cells entering the maternal circulation may elicit the antibody response.

The perinatal mortality rate from Rh hemolytic disease is 25 to 30%. In recent years, the number of perinatal deaths has dropped markedly owing to improved methods of identification of mothers who possess antibody to $Rh_o(D)$ antigens, improved identification and treatment of sensitized fetuses, and, most importantly, the development and release in 1968 of $Rh_o(D)$ immune globulin (RhIG) for the prevention of maternal isosensitization.

TABLE 23–3. Causes of Maternal $Rh_o(D)$ Sensitization

Previous pregnancy, $Rh_o(D)$-positive fetus
    No or insufficient $Rh_o(D)$ immunization
    Fetomaternal hemorrhage with maternal
      isoimmunization during gestation
Current pregnancy, $Rh_o(D)$-positive fetus
    Spontaneous fetomaternal hemorrhage
    Fetomaternal hemorrhage due to trauma
    Amniocentesis
    Spontaneous or induced abortion
    Ectopic pregnancy
Previous transfusion of $Rh_o(D)$-positive blood
Sensitization in utero from Rh-positive mother via
    maternal–fetal transfusion

Passively administered RhIG acts by suppressing the immune response of Rh-negative individuals to Rh-positive red blood cells. RhIG attaches to the fetal $Rh_o(D)$-positive red blood cells that have entered the maternal circulation. The antibody-coated red cells are then trapped in the maternal spleen, where they take up more antibody from the circulating plasma. This stimulates immunosuppression by suppressor cells and/or the production of anti-idiotypic antibody, the result of which is the effective suppression of maternal antibody production.

Diagnosis and Indications for Treatment

The injection of RhIG will prevent isoimmunization of Rh-negative women who have had fetal-to-maternal transfusion of Rh-positive red cells. Therefore, Rh immunization should be considered for all Rh-negative women (1) following delivery of an Rh-positive infant, (2) following spontaneous or therapeutic abortion or ectopic pregnancy, (3) when fetomaternal hemorrhage is suspected such as following trauma, (4) after accidental or inadvertent transfusion of Rh-positive blood, and (5) following amniocentesis.

Because the highest risk for Rh immunization occurs at the time of *delivery*, the Rh-negative, antibody-negative mother should receive RhIG within 72 hours after delivery of an Rh-positive infant or when the Rh type of the infant is unknown (e.g., stillborn) and the father is not known to be Rh negative. Maternal and, when available, cord blood should be sent to the blood bank for antigen typing and Rh antibody screening immediately following delivery. Administration of RhIG will subsequently be based on the results of these tests.

About 2 to 5% of Rh-negative women who abort spontaneously or therapeutically will become sensitized to Rh-positve antigen. RhIG should therefore be given to all Rh-negative, antibody-negative women who undergo elective or therapeutic *abortion* or have an *ectopic pregnancy*. Because of the small fetal blood volume during early gestation, patients who abort or terminate an ectopic pregnancy before 12 weeks of gestation may receive the microdose of RhIG; after 12 weeks of gestation the regular dose of RhIG is required.

Fetomaternal hemorrhage as a result of trauma has only recently been described, and the true incidence of this hemorrhage is unknown. Although it is more commonly of concern following blunt abdominal trauma during the latter half of pregnancy, neither the nature of the trauma nor the gestational age of the infant is a reliable predictor of either the frequency or volume of hemorrhage. Fetomaternal hemorrhage can be detected by the Kleihauer-Betke test, in which maternal blood is subjected to acid and then stained. Fetal cells contain hemoglobin resistant to acid and will remain dark. Maternal hemoglobin is eluted by the acid, causing maternal cells to appear as ghosts. A careful differential count of the cells will serve to approximate closely the percentage of fetal cells in the maternal blood, and the volume of fetal hemorrhage may be calculated by the following formula:

$$\frac{\text{Number of fetal cells} \times \text{maternal blood volume}}{\text{Number of maternal cells}} = \frac{\text{Volume of}}{\text{fetal maternal hemorrhage}}$$

Maternal blood volume, i.e., the apparent volume of distribution of red cells in the intravascular compartment, will average approximately 5 liters before delivery and 4 liters shortly afterward. The amount of RhIG required to neutralize the Rh antigen is then calculated as described below.

Accidental or inadvertent transfusion of Rh-positive red blood cells to an Rh-negative woman of childbearing age may occur and will cause isoimmunization in 70 to 80% of those receiving such a transfusion. Platelet and leukocyte concentrates may also contain variable amounts of red blood cells and also cause isoimmunization. RhIG is indicated in all Rh-negative women who receive Rh-positive blood or blood products. (See box.)

Discussion

One vial or 300 μg of RhIG is the dose usually employed for the majority of obstetric situations, including delivery of an Rh-positive infant and abortion or termination of ectopic pregnancy at or beyond 13 weeks of gestation. For abortions or termination of pregnancies up to and including 12 weeks' gestation, a microdose containing approximately 50 μg of RhIG may be used. The microdose of RhIG has the advantages of reduced cost and administration without cross-matching. Full-dose RhIG must be cross-matched with the patient's blood.

When *fetomaternal hemorrhage* has occurred, the actual volume of hemorrhage must be determined by a quantitative test such as the Kleihauer-Betke test, described earlier; and a 300-μg dose of RhIG administered for every 15 ml (or fraction thereof) of fetal red blood cells calculated to be in the maternal circulation. IgG has a half-life of 23 to 26 days. Therefore, when RhIG has been administered more than 3 weeks antepartum, the patient will require a repeat dose of RhIG within 72 hours of delivery if the infant is Rh positive.

The amount of RhIG required for the treatment of *transfusion "accidents"* is also calculated and is based on the total volume of red cells transfused. A 300-μg dose of RhIG should be administered for every 15 ml of Rh-positive red blood cells transfused, whether as red blood cells, in whole blood, or in components such as granulocytes or platelets prepared from Rh-positve blood.

RhIG is of no benefit once a person has been actively immunized and has formed anti-D. If anti-D is identified in the potential recipient, administration of RhIG is not indicated unless it can be shown that the presence of anti-D is due to the previous administration of RhIG.

RhIG is not indicated for the mother if the infant is found to be $Rh_o(D)$ negative. Since it is usually impossible to determine Rh status of the fetus in abortions, stillbirths, and ectopic pregnancies, RhIG should be administered in these circumstances unless the father is known *with certainty* to be $Rh_o(D)$ negative. RhIG is not to be given to the newborn infant.

In the United States, the standard vial of RhIG contains sufficient anti-D to protect against 15 ml of Rh-positive red blood cells entering the maternal circulation. Although the standardization in the United States is not based on micrograms, the regular dose vial is equivalent to 300 μg of World Health Organization (WHO) reference material, and for convenience this terminology is used.

RhIG prepared by the Cohn fractionation technique may be injected intramuscularly only. Intravenous injections can cause severe anaphylactic reactions. The entire calculated dose of RhIG should be administered within 72 hours of delivery or transfusion, since all of the clinical studies to date use this time span. Because it is unknown how much delay would still allow complete protection, RhIG

DRUG TREATMENT: Rh₀(D) INCOMPATIBILITY

First-Line Drug

Rh₀(D) Immune Globulin

> **Dose**   Usual dose = 300 μg (1 vial) IM
> Dose is variable and dependent on the clinical situation as described below.
>
> **End-Point**   Neutralization of all Rh-positive antigen present in maternal circulation;
> neutralization is based on clinical situation and calculations described below.

---

should be given even if administration is delayed beyond 72 hours. When large doses of RhIG are required, it may be administered in multiple doses at different times and at different sites, provided the total dose is administered within 72 hours of delivery, transfusion, or receipt of red blood cells.

Systemic reactions associated with the administration of RhIG are uncommon. Fever occurs occasionally; severe anaphylactic reactions are rare. Local reactions are frequent and most commonly consist of discomfort at the injection site. RhIG has been reported to contain antibody to both hepatitis A and B and thus may cause false-positive hepatitis serology. Although transmission of non-A and non-B hepatitis has recently been reported following *intravenous* administration of RhIG, other viral diseases including the acquired autoimmune deficiency syndrome have not been transmitted.

SPECIFIC AGENTS

Beta-Adrenergic Receptor Agonists: Ritodrine and Terbutaline

Ritodrine (Yutopar)

Pharmacology

Distribution

Ritodrine is probably widely distributed. When administered orally, ritodrine has a bioavailability of approximately 30% when compared to intravenous administration. Approximately 32% of the drug is bound to albumin. Although ritodrine and its inactive conjugates readily pass the placental barrier, drug levels found in cord blood are about 20% of those found in the maternal circulation.

Elimination

Ritodrine is partially metabolized in the liver and is eliminated primarily in the urine (71 to 93%). Maximum excretion occurs 1 hour after oral administration. Ninety percent of the drug is excreted within 24 hours, the majority in the form of inactive metabolites.

Actions

Ritodrine hydrochloride is a beta-adrenergic agonist with preferential affinity for beta₂-receptors such as those in the uterine smooth muscle; it is a weak beta₁-agonist and has no alpha-sympathomimetic effects. Ritodrine relaxes uterine smooth musculature via its effects on cAMP and intracellular Ca^{++}.

Indications

Ritodrine is indicated for the treatment of preterm labor. Specific indications and contraindications are listed in Table 23–1.

Cautions

Renal failure—no dosage adjustment
Cardiac disease—because cardiovascular effects such as a rise in pulse rate and blood pressure are common, ritodrine should be used with caution in patients with cardiac disease. Before instituting therapy a baseline electrocardiogram is recommended to rule out occult heart disease.
Hepatic failure—no dosage adjustment
Use in pregnancy—Category B. Ritodrine has not been shown to have adverse permanent fetal effects in either clinical or animal studies; however, the possibility of such effects cannot be excluded with certainty. Ritodrine should therefore be used only when clearly indicated. Because there are no adequate well-controlled studies on ritodrine administered

to women of less than 20 weeks of gestation, it should not be used before the 20th week of pregnancy.

Other—relatively contraindicated in patients with hyperthyroidism or hypertension

Onset and Duration of Action

Dosage

Ritodrine is administered by intravenous infusion beginning at 100 μg/min (0.1 mg/min), which may be increased by 50 μg/min (0.05 mg/min) every 10 minutes. When administered as an intravenous infusion for 1 hour, ritodrine has a distribution half-life of 6 to 9 minutes and an effective half-life of 1.7 to 2.6 hours.

Limits

Limits are cessation of uterine contractions, development of unacceptable side effects, or maximum dose of 350 μg/min (0.35 mg/min). If unacceptable side effects develop the infusion should be progressively reduced to a tolerable level. If contractions persist despite the maximum dose of ritodrine, the infusion should be stopped.

Repeat Dosing

If labor is successfully arrested, intravenous therapy should be continued for at least 12 hours after contractions cease. Oral therapy is begun 30 minutes before discontinuing the intravenous infusion and usually initially consists of 10 mg every 2 hours.

Toxicity

Drug Interactions

Anesthetics—may increase cardiac arrhythmias and hypotensive effects

Beta-adrenergic blockers—may inhibit action of ritodrine

Corticosteroids—may lead to pulmonary edema, additive diabetogenic effects

Parasympatholytics—may aggravate systemic hypertension

Sympathomimetics—may increase toxicity

Magnesium sulfate, meperidine, diazoxide—may potentiate cardiovascular effects, especially arrhythmias and hypotension

Specific Adverse Effects

Maternal cardiovascular effects with intravenous ritodrine typically include a dose-related increase in heart rate, a widening of pulse pressure, and a slight increase in cardiac output. Fetal heart rate also increases slightly and should be monitored. Infrequent side effects such as maternal hypertension, vomiting, chest discomfort, and shortness of breath are more commonly observed when the infusion rate of ritodrine is being increased. Pulmonary edema has been reported in women who were also receiving steroids, usually when excessive fluid was administered intravenously. Because cardiovascular effects are common and more pronounced during intravenous therapy, maternal pulse rate and blood pressure and fetal heart rate should be closely monitored. Maternal metabolic effects during ritodrine therapy include transient increases in glucose, free fatty acids, lactic acid, and insulin and a moderate decrease in potassium and calcium. Unpleasant but probably physiologically insignificant side effects include tremor (10 to 15%), palpitations (33%), and nervousness or restlessness (5 to 10%). There have been no reports in which ritodrine has been associated with post-term pregnancy, abnormal labor, postpartum uterine atony, or increased neonatal morbidity.

Treatment of Toxicity

Side effects are usually self-limited and resolve with dosage reduction or discontinuation of the drug. Treatment of the majority of side effects is supportive. Severe cardiovascular effects may be treated with cardioselective beta-blocking agents.

Terbutaline (Brethine, Bricanyl)
Pharmacology

Distribution

Terbutaline is probably widely distributed. It is well absorbed when administered subcutaneously or intravenously. Orally administered terbutaline sulfate is 30 to 70% absorbed in the gastrointestinal tract. Terbutaline crosses the placenta; cord blood levels range from 11 to 48% of maternal blood levels.

Elimination

Terbutaline is partially metabolized in the liver to an inactive sulfate conjugate. Excretion is primarily renal.

Actions

Terbutaline is a direct-acting sympatho-mimetic agent. Although animal studies have shown it to exert a preferential effect on beta$_2$-adrenergic receptors, controlled clinical studies of orally and subcutaneously administered terbutaline demonstrate cardiovascular effects consistent with beta$_1$ activity. Terbutaline relaxes uterine smooth musculature via its effects on cAMP and intracellular Ca^{++}

Indications

Treatment of preterm labor is an indication for terbutaline use. Specific indications and contraindications are listed in Table 23–1. Although clinical studies have demonstrated terbutaline's effectiveness in halting premature labor, it is *not* currently approved by the Food and Drug Administration for this use.

Cautions

Renal failure—no dosage adjustment

Cardiac disease—because cardiovascular effects such as a rise in pulse rate and blood pressure are common, terbutaline should be used with caution in patients with cardiac disease.

Hepatic failure—no dosage adjustment

Use in pregnancy—Category B; terbutaline has not been shown to have adverse effects on the fetus in experimental animals. Well-controlled studies in pregnant women, however, are lacking.

Other—relatively contraindicated in patients with hyperthyroidism or hypertension

Onset and Duration of Action

Dosage

Subcutaneous: 0.25 mg, which may be repeated at intervals of 1 to 6 hours. Terbutaline is absorbed very rapidly after subcutaneous administration with an absorption half-life of 7 minutes; peak plasma concentration is reached in 15 to 30 minutes.

Intravenous: 10 μg/min (0.01 mg/min), which may be increased by 5 μg/min (0.005 mg/min) every 10 minutes

Limits

Terbutaline administration should be stopped when contractions cease, intolerable maternal side effects develop, or, when administered intravenously, a maximum dose of 25 μg/min (0.025 mg/min) is reached.

Repeat Dosing

When tocolysis is successfully achieved with these regimens, maintenance therapy is started with 0.25 mg terbutaline subcutaneously every 4 hours or 0.25 to 0.5 mg orally every 4 hours.

Toxicity

Drug interactions

Beta-adrenergic blockers—may inhibit action of terbutaline

Monoamide oxidase inhibitors, tricyclics—may potentiate vascular effects

Sympathomimetics—may increase toxicity

Specific Adverse Effects

Side effects are similar to those seen with ritodrine and include an increase in maternal and fetal heart rate, an increase in systolic blood pressure and pulse pressure, and mild elevations in serum glucose. There have been isolated reports of pulmonary edema occurring in women treated simultaneously with terbutaline and steroids to enhance fetal lung maturity. Orally administered terbutaline produces no significant maternal biochemical or biophysical changes or any side effects on the fetus.

Treatment of Toxicity

Side effects usually resolve with reduction in drug dosage. Severe cardiovascular effects may be treated with cardioselective beta-adrenergic blocking agents.

Ergot Alkaloids: Methylergonovine Maleate (Methergine) and Ergonovine Maleate (Ergotrate)

Pharmacology

Distribution

Ergot alkaloids may be administered orally, intramuscularly, or intravenously. After administration, ergots are rapidly distributed from plasma to the peripheral tissues, with an alpha phase half-life of 2 to 3 minutes or less.

Elimination

The ergot alkaloids are detoxified in the liver and eliminated in the urine.

Actions

Ergonovine and methylergonovine act directly on uterine smooth muscle. They increase the tone, rate, and amplitude of rhythmic myometrial contractions and produce a rapid and sustained tetanic uterotonic effect that may persist for hours. Uterine responsiveness to ergot stimulation increases steadily as gestation progresses. The most significant nonuterine effect is vasoconstriction from direct smooth muscle stimulation.

Indications

Treatment of postpartum or postabortion uterine hemorrhage

Cautions

Renal failure—use with caution.
Cardiac disease—use with caution.
Hepatic failure—use with caution.
Use in pregnancy—Category C; contraindicated owing to induction of nonphysiologic uterine contractions; animal studies have not been conducted.
Use in lactation—at oral dosage levels, a small quantity of drug appears in breast milk. Although adverse effects have not been described, caution should be used.
Other—caution in patients with obliterative vascular disease; relatively contraindicated in patients with hypertension

Onset and Duration of Action

Dosage

Intramuscular: 0.2 mg, which may be repeated in 2 to 4 hours
Intravenous: 0.2 mg *slowly* over at least 60 seconds with careful monitoring of blood pressure

Because intravenous administration may precipitate sudden and severe hypertension, it should only be used as a lifesaving measure.
Onset of action after intravenous administration is 40 seconds; after intramuscular administration, 2 to 7 minutes; and after oral administration, 5 to 10 minutes. Clinical effects persist for several hours.

Limits

Cessation of uterine bleeding
Limit inherent in dosage schedule

Repeat Dosing

If bleeding resolves, oral therapy may be started using 0.2 mg every 6 to 8 hours for a maximum duration of 1 week.

Toxicity

Drug Interactions

Other ergot alkaloids—use with caution.
Vasoconstrictors—use with caution.

Specific Adverse Effects

The most common side effect is hypertension occasionally accompanied by seizures or headache. Hypotension has been reported, and nausea and vomiting have occurred occasionally. Rarely observed reactions include transient chest pain, palpitations, dyspnea, hematuria, and thrombophlebitis.

Treatment of Toxicity

Supportive

Magnesium Sulfate

Pharmacology

Distribution

In the normal adult, approximately 50% of total body magnesium is found in bone, approximately 45% exists as an intracellular cation, and 5% is found in the extracellular fluid. The normal concentration of magnesium in the plasma is 1.5 to 2.2 mEq/liter, with about two-thirds existing as free cation and one-third bound to plasma proteins. When given intravenously, magnesium sulfate rapidly distributes in the plasma of both the mother and the fetus, and fetal blood levels approach those of the mother. A dose of 4 g of magnesium sulfate administered intravenously over a 3- to 4-minute period causes an increase in maternal plasma concentration to about 7 to 9 mEq/liter. This level falls to approximately 4 to 5 mEq/liter over the next 45 minutes. This fall in serum magnesium level is due to both renal excretion and rapid movement of the cation from the circulation into the extracellular compartment and from there into bone and to a lesser degree into cells.

Elimination

Excretion of magnesium is primarily renal. Magnesium not bound to protein is filtered by the glomeruli and variably reabsorbed by the proximal tubule. As serum magnesium concentration increases, the fraction of filtered magnesium reabsorbed decreases and renal clearance of the ion increases. Although renal excretion is the major pathway for loss of parenterally administered magnesium, a fraction of injected magnesium is reversibly deposited in surface bone.

Actions

PREECLAMPSIA AND ECLAMPSIA. The mechanism by which magnesium decreases the neurogenic irritability of preeclampsia and eclampsia is not fully understood. High concentrations of magnesium ions decrease the release of acetylcholine at the neuromuscular junction, thereby decreasing motor endplate excitability and producing neuromuscular blockade. A primary effect on the central nervous system is also postulated as an underlying mechanism for magnesium's anticonvulsant action. When magnesium is administered intravenously, a mild antihypertensive effect is observed, which results from a brief and transient fall in peripheral vascular resistance that resolves after discontinuation of the drug. Magnesium may also benefit the fetus by increasing uterine blood flow.

TOCOLYSIS. Magnesium ions in high concentration suppress uterine activity. Although the exact mechanism of this action is speculative, it is probable that magnesium ions compete with calcium ions at the cellular level, thereby inhibiting the actin/myosin interaction. The inhibition of uterine contractions by magnesium is dose related; serum concentrations of 4 to 8 mEq/liter should effectively reduce uterine contractions.

Indications

Primary anticonvulsant agent for the treatment of severe preeclampsia and eclampsia

Second-line therapy for inhibition of preterm labor

Cautions

Renal failure—relatively contraindicated; measure serum magnesium levels frequently.

Cardiac failure—no dosage adjustment necessary

Hepatic failure—no dosage adjustment necessary

Use in pregnancy—maternal administration of magnesium sulfate usually does not compromise the neonate. Magnesium crosses the placenta promptly by active diffusion and can produce fetal serum concentrations that are comparable to those of the mother. Isolated cases of neonatal depression have been reported. Apgar scores do not relate to concentrations of magnesium in cord blood.

Other—contraindicated in myasthenia gravis

Onset and Duration of Action

Preeclampsia and Eclampsia

DOSAGE

Initial: 4 g IV at a rate not to exceed 1 g/min

Repeat dose: if seizure activity persists, an additional dose of up to 2g may be administered at the same rate within 20 minutes.

Maintenance: IV infusion of 1 to 3 g/hour

LIMITS

Cessation of seizure activity
Clinical signs of toxicity

(Because intramuscular administration may be associated with unpredictable absorption, it is not recommended when intravenous access is available.)

Tocolysis

DOSAGE

Initial: 4 to 8 g IV over 20 minutes
Maintenance: IV infusion of 1 to 3 g/hour. Infusion rates of 2 to 3 g/hour are usually required for tocolysis.

LIMITS

Cessation of uterine contractions
Clinical signs of toxicity

Toxicity

Drug interactions

Calcium—antagonizes neuromuscular effects of magnesium

Diuretics—may increase renal excretion of magnesium

Neuromuscular blocking agents (d-tubocurarine, decamethonium, succinylcholine)—magnesium potentiates neuromuscular blockade.

Specific Adverse Effects

The major maternal toxic effects of magnesium are related to neuromuscular blockade and impairment of the muscles of respiration, with toxicity directly related to elevation of serum magnesium concentration. Magnesium levels up to 7 mEq/liter are not accompanied by evidence of toxicity. Loss of the patellar reflex, the first sign of toxicity, occurs at plasma concentrations between 7 and 10 mEq/liter. Respiratory depression develops at levels above 10 mEq/liter and respiratory arrest occurs at levels of 12 mEq/liter or greater.

High concentrations of magnesium (10 to 15 mEq/liter) may cause increased cardiac conduction time with lengthened PR and QRS intervals on the electrocardiogram. Although rare, isolated cases of pulmonary edema have been reported when magnesium sulfate was used for tocolysis.

Treatment of Toxicity

Calcium gluconate, 10 to 20 ml of a 10% solution IV over 3 minutes

For severe respiratory depression, prompt endotracheal intubation and ventilation

Oxytocin (Pitocin, Syntocinon)

Pharmacology

Distribution

When administered parenterally, oxytocin is distributed throughout the extracellular fluid. Although it crosses the placenta, the extent of this passage is unknown and probably only small amounts of the drug reach the fetal circulation.

Elimination

Removal of oxytocin from the plasma is accomplished largely by the kidneys and liver. Only small amounts of the hormone are excreted unchanged in the urine.

Actions

Oxytocin exerts a selective action on uterine smooth muscle, stimulating rhythmic contractions of the uterus, increasing the frequency of existing contractions, and raising the tone of the uterine musculature. The exact mechanism by which oxytocin stimulates myometrial activity is unknown but is felt to be related to the binding of oxytocin to receptors on myometrial cell membranes where cyclic adenosine 5'-monophosphate (cAMP) is eventually formed and by increasing intracellular Ca^{++}. The effect of oxytocin on the uterine musculature increases throughout pregnancy, with the greatest increase in uterine responsiveness occurring during the last 9 weeks of gestation.

Indications

Oxytocin is used to produce uterine contractions during the third stage of labor and for the control of postpartum hemorrhage. When used for the latter purpose, oxytocin should be administered in conjunction with uterine massage. Due to the danger of entrapping the placenta or a second twin in a contracting uterus, oxytocin should not be administered prior to delivery of the placenta.

Oxytocin is also used extensively in obstetrics for the augmentation of uterine contractions in term and preterm labor and during the intrapartum period.

Cautions

Renal failure—no dosage adjustment
Cardiac disease—no dosage adjustment
Hepatic failure—no dosage adjustment
Use in pregnancy—there have been no animal reproduction studies conducted with oxytocin. There are no known indications for its use in the first trimester of pregnancy other than that associated with spontaneous or induced abortion. Based on wide experience with this drug and its chemical structure and pharmacologic properties, it would not be expected to present a risk of fetal abnormalities when used as indicated.

Onset and Duration of Action

Dosage (Postpartum Indications)

Intravenous: 20 to 40 units in 1 liter of crystalloid or dextrose solution, with infusion rate adjusted to sustain uterine contractions and control uterine hemorrhage.

Intramuscular (when intravenous access not available): 10 units IM

Oxytocin has a half-life of 12 to 17 minutes. Following intravenous administration, uterine response occurs almost immediately and subsides within 1 hour. Oxytocin should not be administered rapidly as an intravenous bolus.

Administered intramuscularly, uterine response occurs within 3 to 5 minutes and persists for 2 to 3 hours.

Limits

Sustained uterine contractions
Control of uterine hemorrhage

Repeat Dosing

Inherent in dosage schedule

Toxicity

Drug Interactions

Cyclopropane anesthesia—unexpected hypotension, maternal bradycardia with atrioventricular block

Vasoconstrictors—severe hypertension reported when oxytocin was given 3 to 4 hours after vasoconstrictors were administered in conjunction with caudal block

Specific Adverse Effects

When used to control postpartum hemorrhage, the side effects from oxytocin are principally related to its effect on the cardiovascular system and its structural similarity to antidiuretic hormone (ADH).

When administered rapidly in large doses, oxytocin causes a marked but transient relaxation of vascular smooth muscle, which results in a decrease in systolic and diastolic blood pressure, flushing, and reflex tachycardia.

When large doses (40 to 50 mU/min) are infused for long periods, particularly when administered in conjunction with large volumes of intravenous or oral fluids, water intoxication with convulsions or coma may occur. This effect can be minimized by infusing the drug in a balanced electrolyte solution.

Infrequently anaphylaxis, cardiac arrhythmias including premature ventricular contractions, nausea and vomiting, and transient hypertension may occur.

Treatment of Toxicity

Discontinuation of the drug plus symptomatic and supportive care

Prostaglandins: Carboprost Tromethamine (Prostin/15M) and Dinoprost Tromethamine (Prostin F2 Alpha)

Pharmacology

Distribution

Prostaglandins are considered local hormones because, with few exceptions, they exert their effects and are inactivated principally in the tissues and organs in which they are synthesized.

Elimination

Elimination is usually rapid since many tissues are capable of utilizing and converting these compounds. Metabolites are considered to be biologically inactive.

Actions

The prostaglandins stimulate uterine smooth muscle contraction by acting on specific cell receptors to alter or inhibit the action of adenylcyclase, thereby inhibiting the formation of cAMP and promoting myometrial activity. An effect on calcium release has also been postulated. Although prostaglandins can affect uterine contractions at any stage of pregnancy, as with oxytocin, the sensitivity of the uterus to these compounds increases as gestation progresses.

Indications

The prostaglandins are indicated in management of postpartum hemorrhage in women who have failed to respond to treatment with oxytocin and the ergot alkaloids.

In obstetrics, prostaglandins are generally used to stimulate uterine contractions for pregnancy termination, most notably in pregnancies complicated by intrauterine fetal demise, nonmetastatic gestational trophoblastic disease, and therapeutic abortion between the 12th and 27th weeks of gestation.

Cautions

Renal failure—use with caution.
Cardiac failure—use with caution.
Hepatic failure—use with caution.
Other—contraindicated in patients with pelvic inflammatory disease, asthma, or active pulmonary disease. Caution should be used in patients with hypertension, anemia, jaundice, diabetes, or epilepsy.

Onset and Duration of Action

Carboprost (15 Methyl PGF$_{2\alpha}$)

Dosage: 0.25 mg IM
Limits: cessation of bleeding, contraction of uterus
Repeat dosing: 0.25 mg at intervals of 2 hours or greater

Dinoprost (PGF$_{2\alpha}$)

Dosage: 0.5 to 1 mg injected transabdominally directly into the myometrium
Limits: inherent in dosage schedule
Repeat dosing: none

Toxicity

Specific Adverse Effects

Side effects, although common, are usually mild and self-limited. Nausea, vomiting, and diarrhea occur in over 60% of patients; transient fever occurs in greater than 10%. Hypertension following large doses of prostaglandins has been reported.

Treatment of Toxicity

Supportive
Antiemetic and antidiarrheal agents may be used.

Rh$_o$(D) Immune Globulin (RhoGAM, MICRhoGAM, Gamulin Rh, Mini-Gamulin Rh, HypRho-D, HypRho-D Mini Dose)

Pharmacology

Distribution

IgG compounds distribute in the circulation and eventually equilibrate in the extravascular space. A regular single-dose vial of RhIG contains sufficient immune globulin to protect against 15 ml of Rh-positive packed red blood cells and is approximately equivalent to 300 μg of the WHO RhIG reference material. The microdose vial contains sufficient anti-Rh$_o$(D) to neutralize approximately 2.5 ml of packed red blood cells and is the approximate equivalent of 50 μg of WHO reference material.

Elimination

Passively administered IgG has a half-life of 23 to 26 days.

Actions

RhIG acts by suppressing the specific immune response of Rh-negative individuals to Rh-positive red blood cells. Although the mechanism of action is unclear, it is believed that passively administered RhIG attaches to fetal Rh$_o$(D)-positive red blood cells in the maternal circulation. The antibody-coated red cells are then trapped in the maternal spleen, stimulating immune suppression.

Indications

RhIG is indicated to prevent Rh-hemolytic disease of the newborn (erythroblastosis fetalis) whenever it is known or suspected that fetal red blood cells have entered the circulation of an Rh$_o$(D)-negative woman, unless the fetus or the father can be shown conclusively to be Rh$_o$(D) negative. RhIG should therefore be administered to all nonimmunized Rh$_o$(D)-negative women within 72 hours following the birth of an Rh$_o$(D)-positive infant, after abortion or ectopic pregnancy, and after amniocentesis or other abdominal trauma that allows fetal cells to enter the maternal circulation. When there is any doubt as to the patient's or fetus's Rh$_o$(D) type, RhIG should be administered. RhIG is also indicated in all Rh-negative premenopausal females following transfusion of Rh-positive red blood cells or blood components prepared from blood containing such cells.

Cautions

Renal failure—none
Cardiac disease—none
Hepatic failure—none
Use in pregnancy—Category C. Animal reproduction studies have not been conducted with RhIG. It is not known whether RhIG can cause fetal harm when administered to a pregnant woman or affect reproductive capacity. Use of full doses of Rh antibody during the third trimester, however, has not been reported to produce evidence of hemolysis in the infant. RhIG should be given to a pregnant woman only when clearly indicated.
Other—RhIG is contraindicated in Rh-positive patients, in Rh-negative patients who have already developed Rh antibodies, and in individuals who have had anaphylactic or severe systemic reactions to human globulin. RhIG should not be given intravenously nor injected into the neonate.

Onset and Duration of Action

Dosage

Postpartum and miscarriage, abortion, or ectopic pregnancy at or beyond 13 weeks' gestation: 1 vial of standard dose (300 µg) IM within 72 hours of event*

Miscarriage, abortion, or ectopic pregnancy up to 12 weeks' gestation: 1 vial of microdose preparation (50 µg) IM within 72 hours of the termination of pregnancy

Transfusion accident or fetomaternal hemorrhage: 1 vial of the standard dose (300 µg) given IM for each 15 ml of Rh-positive red blood cells calculated to have entered the maternal circulation. For transfusion accidents using whole blood, the volume of red blood cells may be calculated by multiplying the total volume of whole blood transfused by the hematocrit of the donor; alternatively, the volume may be approximated by multiplying the total volume by 0.45. When fetomaternal hemorrhage has occurred, the volume of hemorrhage should be quantitated using an approved laboratory assay such as the Kleihauer-Betke test, described earlier in this chapter, and a single vial of RhIG administered for every 15 ml of fetal red cells calculated to be in the maternal circulation.

Limits

The limit is inherent in the dosage schedule. Although the entire dose of RhIG should be administered within 72 hours of transfusion of Rh-positive cells, if greater time has elapsed, RhIG should still be given.

Repeat Dosing

In rare instances a patient may be encountered who has had prior antepartum administration of RhIG. Because IgG has a half-life of 23 to 26 days, when RhIG has been administered during the antepartum period more than 3 weeks prior to the present event, the patient will require a repeat dose of RhIG within 72 hours of the event.

Toxicity

Drug Interactions

Immunizations—may interfere with the response to live vaccines; live vaccines should not be given within 3 months following immunization with RhIG.

*Standard dose RhIG must be crossmatched with the patient's blood.

Specific Adverse Effects

These are infrequent and most commonly consist of soreness at the site of injection and slight temperature elevation. When multiple doses have been given to treat mismatched transfusions, fever, myalgias, and lethargy have occurred as well as occasional elevations of bilirubin.

Treatment of Toxicity

Symptomatic and supportive

REFERENCES

General

Benson RC (ed): Current Obstetric and Gynecologic Diagnosis and Treatment. Los Altos, CA, Lange, 1984.

Drug Evaluations, 6th ed. Prepared by the American Medical Association Department of Drugs, Division of Drugs and Technology. Philadelphia, WB Saunders, 1986.

Farrell RG (ed): OB/GYN Emergencies: The First 60 Minutes. Rockville, MD, Aspen, 1986.

Gilman AG, Goodman LS, Rall TW, Murad F (eds): Goodman and Gilman's Pharmacological Basis of Therapeutics, 7th ed. New York, Macmillan, 1985.

Physicians' Desk Reference. Oradell, NJ, Medical Economics, 1988.

Pritchard JA, MacDonald PC, Gant NF (eds): Williams Obstetrics, 17th ed. Norwalk, CT, Appleton-Century-Crofts, 1985.

Rayburn WF, Zuspan FP (eds): Drug Therapy in Obstetrics and Gynecology. Norwalk, CT, Appleton-Century-Crofts, 1986.

Preterm Labor

Andersson KE, Forman A, Ulmsten U: Pharmacology of labor. Clin Obstet Gynecol 26:56, 1983.

Barden TP, Peter JB, Merkatz IR: Ritodrine hydrochloride: A beta-mimetic agent for use in preterm labor. Obstet Gynecol 56:1, 1980.

Caritis SN, Darby MJ, Chan L: Pharmacologic treatment of preterm labor. Clin Obstet Gynecol 31:635, 1988.

Cotton DB, Strassner HT, Hill LM, et al: Comparison of magnesium sulfate, terbutaline and a placebo for inhibition of preterm labor. J Reprod Med 29:92, 1984.

Eggleston MK: Management of preterm labor and delivery. Clin Obstet Gynecol 29:230, 1986.

Elliott JP: Magnesium sulfate as a tocolytic agent. Am J Obstet Gynecol 147:277, 1983.

Ferguson JE, Hensleigh PA, Kredenster D: Adjunctive use of magnesium sulfate with ritodrine for preterm labor tocolysis. Am J Obstet Gynecol 148:166, 1984.

Gonik B, Creasy RK: Preterm labor: Its diagnosis and management. Am J Obstet Gynecol 154:3, 1986.

Hollander DI, Nagey DA, Pupkin MJ: Magnesium sulfate and ritodrine hydrochloride: A randomized comparison. Am J Obstet Gynecol 156:631, 1987.

Huddleston JF: Preterm labor. Clin Obstet Gynecol 25:123, 1982.

Huszar G, Naftolin F: The myometrium and uterine cervix in normal and preterm labor. N Engl J Med 311:571, 1984.

Miller JM, Keane MWD, Horger EO: A comparison of magnesium sulfate and terbutaline for the arrest of premature labor. J Reprod Med 27:348, 1982.

Spisso KR, Harbert GM, Thiagarajah S: The use of magnesium sulfate as the primary tocolytic agent to prevent premature delivery. Am J Obstet Gynecol 142:840, 1982.

Stubblefield PG, Heyl PS: Treatment of premature labor with subcutaneous terbutaline. Obstet Gynecol 59:457, 1982.

Postpartum Hemorrhage

Hayashi RH, Castillo MS, Noah ML: Management of severe postpartum hemorrhage due to uterine atony using an analogue of prostaglandin $F_{2\alpha}$. Obstet Gynecol 58:426, 1981.

Herbert WNP: Complications of the immediate puerperium. Clin Obstet Gynecol 25:219, 1982.

Herbert WNP, Cefalo RC: Management of postpartum hemorrhage. Clin Obstet Gynecol 27:139, 1984.

Toppozada M, El-Bossaty M, El-Rahman HA, El-Din AHS: Control of intractable atonic postpartum hemorrhage by 15-methyl prostaglandin $F_{2\alpha}$. Obstet Gynecol 58:327, 1981.

Watson P: Postpartum hemorrhage and shock. Clin Obstet Gynecol 23:985, 1980.

Pregnancy-Induced Hypertension

Bourgeois FJ, Thiagarajah S, Harbert GM, DiFazio C: Profound hypotension complicating magnesium therapy. Am J Obstet Gynecol 154:919, 1986.

Gant, NF, Pritchard JA: Pregnancy-induced hypertension: 1984. Semin Nephrol 4:260, 1984.

Lindheimer MD, Katz AI: Hypertension in pregnancy. N Engl J Med 313:675, 1985.

Lindheimer MD, Katz AI: Pathophysiology of preeclampsia. Ann Rev Med 32:273, 1981.

Pritchard JA: Management of preeclampsia and eclampsia. Kidney Int 18:259, 1980.

Pritchard JA: The use of magnesium sulfate in preeclampsia-eclampsia. J Reprod Med 23:107, 1979.

Pritchard JA, Cunningham G, Pritchard SA: The Parkland Memorial Hospital protocol for treatment of eclampsia: Evaluation of 254 cases. Am J Obstet Gynecol 148:951, 1984.

Redman CWG: The management of hypertension in pregnancy. Semin Nephrol 4:270, 1984.

Sibai BM, Lipshitz J, Anderson GD, Diltz PV: Reassessment of intravenous magnesium $MgSO_4$ therapy in preeclampsia-eclampsia. Obstet Gynecol 57:199, 1981.

Pregnancy Prevention Following Sexual Assault

Cook CL, Wiist LJ, Kraft SL: Pregnancy prophylaxis: Parenteral postcoital estrogen. Obstet Gynecol 67:331, 1986.

Glover D, Gerety M, Bromberg S, et al: Diethylstilbesrol in the treatment of rape victims. West J Med 125:331, 1976.

Kobernick ME, Seifert S, Sanders AB: Emergency department management of the sexual assault victim. J Emerg Med 2:205, 1985.

Soules MR, Stewart SK, Brown KM, Pollard AA: The spectrum of alleged rape. J Reprod Med 20:33, 1978.

$Rh_o(D)$ Incompatibility

Farrell RG, Stonington DT, Ridgeway RA: Incomplete and inevitable abortion: Treatment by suction curettage in the emergency department. Ann Emerg Med 11:652, 1982.

Hensleigh PA, Leslie W, Dixon E, et al: Reduced dose of $Rh_o(D)$ immune globulin following induced first-trimester abortion. Am J Obstet Gynecol 129:413, 1977.

Rose PG, Strohm PL, Zuspan FP: Fetomaternal hemorrhage following trauma. Am J Obstet Gynecol 153:844, 1985.

Stewart FH, Burnhill MS, Bozorgi N: Reduced dose of Rh immunoglobulin following first trimester pregnancy termination. Obstet Gynecol 51:318, 1978.

CHAPTER 24

Anticoagulants and Thrombolytics

MARK S. SMITH, M.D.
WILLIAM G. BARSAN, M.D.

INTRODUCTION

Overview of Clot Structure

A blood clot is composed of a mixture of red blood cells, white blood cells, platelets, and fibrin. The relative proportions of these constituents are determined by the location of the clot and by the characteristics of blood flow in the region. The "white clot" that is formed in a high-flow arterial area is predominantly composed of alternating layers of platelets and fibrin. The "red clot" that develops in the low-flow venous system is primarily made up of red blood cells embedded in a scant fibrin meshwork.

Thrombus may be classified as pathologic (e.g., in a coronary artery or iliofemoral vein) or physiologic (e.g., overlying a duodenal ulcer) and as either acute, subacute, or chronic. The damage caused by a pathologic thrombus is a function of its location (arterial or venous) and of the characteristics of the tissues served by the involved vessel.

Arterial thrombi cause problems because they produce ischemia or serve as a source of emboli that break off and travel distally. For most tissues, cell death from ischemia does not occur instantaneously but progresses over time and space. The time course may be less than 1 hour (for brain neurons),

several hours (for myocardial tissue), or up to 24 hours (for extremity tissue). The time limit of viability of ischemic tissue is further complicated by the concept of an "ischemic penumbra" or zone of reversibly ischemic tissue, which may regain viability if reperfusion is achieved in a timely fashion.

Pathologic venous thrombi cause problems because they disrupt the function of the involved organ and serve as sources of pulmonary emboli. Disruption of normal pressure relationships by pathologic clot can result in a debilitating postphlebitic syndrome in the lower extremities, cor pulmonale if clot lodges in the pulmonary arterial system, portal hypertension if clot occurs in the portal vein, and an effort-fatigue syndrome if clot is in the subclavian or axillary veins.

Clot Formation

The hemostatic equilibrium of circulating blood is maintained by complex interactions among five components: the blood vessel itself, blood flow, platelets, coagulation factors, and the fibrinolytic system. The cross-sectional geometry of the blood vessel and the presence of exposed nonendothelial tissue determine blood flow turbulence and set up the initial conditions for clot nidus formation. Platelets *adhere* to a damaged vessel wall; *secrete* (release) their granules, which contain various biochemical mediators; and *aggregate* with additional platelets. Aspirin interferes with platelet release (and thus secondary aggregation) by permanently acetylating and inactivating the enzyme cyclooxygenase. This prevents thromboxane A_2 formation, a molecule that is critical to the process of platelet granule release. The platelet plug that forms is the initial defense against bleeding, and this process is termed *primary hemostasis*. This plug is supplemented and stabilized by the addition of fibrin clot, which is produced by initiation of the coagulation factor cascade, a process termed *secondary hemostasis*. The interaction among the vessel wall, platelets, and the coagulation cascade is complex and nonlinear.

The coagulation and fibrinolytic systems comprise the fluid phase of clot formation and lysis. The members of these systems (Factors XII, XI, IX, X, VIII, VII, and V and thrombin, fibrinogen, Factor XIII, plasminogen, antithrombin III, protein C, and antiplasmin) interact in a complex balance of inhibition and feedback. Each individual factor may enhance coagulation, oppose coagulation, enhance fibrinolysis, oppose fibrinolysis, or exert several (sometimes seemingly contradictory) effects simultaneously.

In general, most coagulation factors circulate as inactive forms (zymogens) in concentrations many times that which is physiologically required for coagulation. Activation occurs by one of two mechanisms:

1. Proteolytic cleavage of a small peptide piece by a serine protease enzyme (XIIa on XI, XIa on IX, IXa on X, Xa on prothrombin, VIIa on X, thrombin on fibrinogen; an "a" after a factor number indicates the activated form of the factor)
2. Introduction of three-dimensional conformational change in a target molecule (Va on Xa, VIIc on IXa)

The end product of the coagulation cascade is fibrin clot, a result of thrombin-induced cleavage of fibrinogen. In the presence of Factor XIII (whose activation is also caused by thrombin), fibrin monomer is polymerized and stabilized into an insoluble polymer that is relatively resistant to dissolution.

Thrombin is the central molecule in the clotting cascade and has several important functions:

1. Formation of fibrin (by catalyzing fibrinogen to fibrin)
2. Polymerization of fibrin (through activation of Factor XIII)
3. Aggregation of platelets
4. Activation of Factors V and VIII (the former, in turn, helps to activate thrombin)
5. Activation of protein C

Thrombin is created from its procoagulant prothrombin by activated Factor X in the presence of activated Factor V and calcium. Activation of Factor X is the common final end product of both the extrinsic and the intrinsic coagulation pathways.

The extrinsic pathway is initiated by the release of tissue factor (thromboplastin) into the circulation from damaged tissue (e.g., a torn vessel wall). Tissue thromboplastin, which is ordinarily "extrinsic" to the circulating pool of clotting factors, activates Factor VII, the vitamin K–dependent clotting factor with the shortest half-life (4 to 6 hours). Activated Factor VII in turn activates Factor X, which in turn activates thrombin. The integrity and functionality of the extrinsic pathway are measured by the prothrombin time.

The intrinsic pathway is initiated by the activation of Factor XII through contact with disrupted vascular surface; no substance extrinsic to the already circulating procoagulant is necessary for its activation. The intrinsic pathway proceeds through a cascade of activations: XIIa on XI, XIa on IX, and IXa on X. The integrity of this pathway is measured by the partial thromboplastin time.

There are two key inhibitors of the coagulation cascade: antithrombin III and protein C. Antithrombin III neutralizes the serine proteases thrombin, XIIa, XIa, IXa, and Xa. The activity of antithrombin III is enhanced 1000-fold by heparin, thus explaining the mechanism of heparin's action as an anticoagulant; its effect initially results in a prolonged thromboplastin time, but in large quantities it also prolongs prothrombin time because of its effect on thrombin and Xa.

Protein C, which requires thrombin for its activation, neutralizes the conformational Factors V and VIII. In addition to its anticoagulant role, protein C exerts a pro-fibrinolytic effect by causing the release of plasminogen activator from blood vessel walls. Like Factors VII, IX, and X and thrombin, protein C is dependent on vitamin K for its synthesis. An additional protein, protein S, complexes with activated protein C to form the physiologically active C:S complex. Genetic deficiencies of antithrombin III, protein C, and protein S cause a predisposition to spontaneous venous thrombosis. In addition, patients with genetically mediated deficiencies of protein C may develop skin necrosis with warfarin therapy.

Once formed, most clot undergoes some degree of physiologic lysis by endogenous plasmin, a nonspecific serine protease that lyses clot by degrading fibrinogen and fibrin. The fibrin(ogen) degradation products (also called fibrin[ogen] split products) that result are themselves potent inhibitors of fibrin polymerization and of platelet aggregation and thus provide a negative feedback for clot formation. In addition to its action on fibrin and fibrinogen, plasmin degrades and depletes Factors V, VII, and VIII. Thus, plasmin acts not only as a fibrinolytic but also as a primary anticoagulant.

Plasmin is converted from its inactive precursor plasminogen by plasminogen activator, a substance that exists in both a tissue-bound and a circulating form. Plasmin activity is maintained in equilibrium by the circulating alpha-2 antiplasmin, which complexes with the catalytic site of circulating plasmin and interferes with its fibrinolytic function. Plasmin that is already bound to fibrin cannot be degraded by alpha-2 antiplasmin. The pharmacologic agent aminocaproic acid inhibits fibrinolysis by preventing the binding of plasmin to the fibrin substrate.

Thrombolytic Agents

All thrombolytic agents lyse clot by the same mechanism: they all produce plasmin from its inactive precursor plasminogen. The thrombolytic agents commercially available are streptokinase, urokinase, tissue plasminogen activator (alteplase), and anisoylated streptokinase plasminogen activator complex (APSAC or anistreplase). Single-chain urokinase plasminogen activator (scu-PA or pro-urokinase) will probably be approved for use soon.

Thrombolytic agents may be compared along the following dimensions: site of plasmin production (i.e., how much of the plasmin generated is fibrin-bound versus how much circulates freely), degree of specificity for degrading fibrin as opposed to fibrinogen, efficacy at lysing clots (both success rate and speed), half-life, nonhematologic side effects, tendency to cause bleeding complications, incidence of reocclusion after successful lysis, duration of infusion, and cost.

Thrombolytic agents differ in the extent to which they degrade circulating fibrinogen. The earliest thrombolytic agents—streptokinase and urokinase—exert a nonspecific lytic effect; their success at clot lysis is associated with fibrinogen depletion and the creation of a "systemic lytic state." Tissue plasminogen activator (t-PA) requires the presence of a fibrin substrate for its activation and thus is a more fibrin-specific agent. Fibrinogen levels decline less with t-PA than they do with streptokinase and urokinase for the same degree of clot lysis, although the actual degree of fibrin selectivity varies with the dose used. Under standard therapeutic regimens, streptokinase and urokinase cause fibrinogen to decline by 50 to 80% from pretreatment levels, whereas t-PA causes decreases of fibrinogen of 30 to 40%. The extent of fibrinogen depletion by anistreplase is intermediate between that of streptokinase and t-PA.

It was hoped that the more fibrin-selective agents would be safer in terms of having fewer bleeding complications, but this does not seem to be the case, probably because fibrin-selective agents are as effective at lysing clots as are the nonselective agents and because no agent can distinguish pathologic clot from physiologic clot.

CONDITIONS

Deep Venous Thrombosis

Thrombus in the deep veins of the legs, arms, or pelvis may embolize to the lungs or may cause local dysfunction producing pain, discomfort, or loss of function. In the subacute state, deep venous thrombosis may destroy the venous valvular system and leave the patient with chronic venous insufficiency. As a clinical entity with potentially life-threatening consequences, acute deep venous thrombosis is part of the differential diagnosis in any patient who presents emergently with a painful or swollen leg.

Phlegmasia cerulea dolens is the most severe form of deep venous thrombosis, usually occurring in the lower extremity. Near-total occlusion of the venous system results in a syndrome of "ischemic thrombophlebitis," whose clinical manifestations are massive edema, cyanosis (hence the descriptor "cerulea"), loss of pulses, and excruciating pain. The condition is usually preceded by the more typical manifestations of deep venous thrombosis. Untreated, phlegmasia cerulea dolens progresses to venous gangrene with loss of limb and a systemic shock state.

Diagnosis

Symptoms of deep venous thrombosis of the lower extremity are swelling, pain, and heaviness; signs are tenderness, differential size, and a host of eponymic signs (Homans sign, etc.) Many cases of deep venous thrombosis, especially those in the iliofemoral and pelvic veins, are clinically silent.

Clinical conditions that may masquerade as deep venous thrombosis of the lower extremity are ruptured Baker's cyst, leg cellulitis, muscle strain or rupture, muscle hematoma, and superficial thrombophlebitis. The diagnosis of deep venous thrombosis by clinical criteria alone is inaccurate. Diagnosis must be based on objective laboratory tests if potent pharmacologic therapy is to be used.

Standard diagnostic modalities are Doppler ultrasonography, impedance plethysmography, radionuclide imaging (using tagged fibrinogen), B-mode ultrasound scanning (duplex ultrasonography), and ascending contrast venography.

Both Doppler ultrasonography and impedance plethysmography provide measures of venous hemodynamics that are then extrapolated to conclusions about venous anatomy. Doppler ultrasonography measures the speed with which blood leaves the veins of the legs and depends on detecting normal phasic variations that occur during breathing and heart contraction. It is relatively insensitive to calf vein thrombosis and dependent on operator skill.

Impedance plethysmography is based on the principle that electrical resistance is a function of blood volume and that venous outflow obstruction prevents expected variations in resistance from occurring. It is an excellent technique for detecting clot at the level of the thigh, although it is relatively insensitive for detecting calf-only clot. A normal impedance plethysmogram effectively excludes thrombosis of the femoral veins.

Radiofibrinogen imaging is more sensitive for calf or distal thrombus than for proximal thrombus but requires 24 hours for a reading.

B-mode ultrasonic imaging has been described by some observers as having the same positive and negative predictive values as ascending contrast venography and in some institutions has replaced contrast venography as the standard imaging modality.

Ascending contrast venography is the "gold standard" for diagnosis of deep venous thrombosis, although it is an invasive procedure that is uncomfortable and may precipitate a chemical phlebitis in 1 to 4% of patients. Interobserver variability among radiologists in reading venograms is as high as 10%.

Indications for Treatment

Any acute deep venous thrombosis of the lower extremity that is proximal to the calf and is documented by laboratory studies should be treated with pharmacologic therapy.

The purpose of therapy for deep venous thrombosis of the lower extremity is threefold: relief from local swelling and pain, prevention of pulmonary emboli, and avoidance of the long-term sequelae of the postphlebitic syndrome. Therapy of deep venous thrombosis is judged by how well it corrects or prevents the occurrence of acute complications (pulmonary embolism, limb dysfunction) and how well it prevents the occurrence of chronic sequelae.

If untreated, patients with proximal deep venous thrombosis have approximately a 50% incidence of pulmonary emboli. If the thrombosis is localized to the calf only, the incidence of pulmonary emboli is low, although proximal extension does occur in about 20% of cases. The proper management strategy for calf-only thrombosis is not fully resolved and may include serial noninvasive testing with plethysmography to detect if and when proximal extension occurs or immediate full anticoagulation. (See box.)

Discussion

Standard therapy for deep venous thrombosis is heparin followed by 4 to 6 months of warfarin anticoagulation. This therapeutic regimen is successful in preventing pulmonary emboli from occurring because it stops

DRUG TREATMENT: LOWER EXTREMITY DEEP VENOUS THROMBOSIS

First-Line Drug

Heparin

Initial Dose	5,000–10,000 units IV (100 units/kg)
Continuous Infusion	1,000–1,500 units/hour
End-Points	Infusion rate titrated to maintain activated partial thromboplastin time (APTT) at 1.5–2 times the control value; APTT should be assayed 4 hours after initiation of therapy.
	Heparin anticoagulation may be terminated when warfarin anticoagulation reaches therapeutic end-point (see below), usually by day 4–6.

Second-Line Drug

Streptokinase

Initial Dose	250,000 IU over 30 minutes
Continuous Infusion	100,000 IU/hour
End-Points	Improvement in venous flows
	Therapy usually continued for 24–96 hours

OR

Urokinase

Initial Dose	4,400 IU/kg over 30–60 minutes
Continuous Infusion	4,400 IU/hour
End-Points	Improvement in venous flows
	Therapy usually continued for 24–96 hours

the formation of new friable clot, the type of clot that has a tendency to embolize. Thrombus that had formed prior to initiation of the anticoagulant therapy undergoes adherence, organization, fibrosis, and eventually recanalization. Unfortunately, recanalization occurs at the expense of destroyed or incompetent venous valvular structures, which in turn results in sustained high pressure in the veins and the consequent postphlebitic syndrome: problems of edema, ulceration, varicosities, pain, and skin abnormalities.

Several small controlled clinical trials have demonstrated the superiority of lytic therapy over heparin therapy in two ways. Lytic therapy seems to be more effective than heparin anticoagulation in restoring a patent venous passage; lytic agents succeed in lysing the clot approximately 50 to 70% of the time in the lower limbs, whereas acute lysis oc-

curs only 20 to 30% of the time in patients treated with heparin therapy.

With thrombolytic therapy, venous hemodynamics become more normal, valves remain more competent, and the incidence of postphlebitic syndrome is lower. Disagreement exists as to the proper time window within which lytic therapy is most effective at maintaining venous architectural integrity. Various authors suggest that if the vein can be treated with lytic therapy within 36 hours, the venous valvular system will emerge unscathed; other authors cite 72 hours as the time window after which streptokinase therapy loses its superiority to heparin therapy in ensuring preservation of venous valves. How long preservation of vascular integrity persists is not known.

Oral therapy with warfarin should begin concomitantly with heparin therapy. After thrombolytic therapy, heparin/warfarin may begin after the prothrombin time has returned to less than twice normal.

Pulmonary Embolism

In the United States, approximately 70,000 patients per year sustain acute pulmonary emboli. While many of these occur in hospitalized patients who have predisposing stasis from bedrest and operative manipulation, pulmonary emboli occur in many outpatients as well.

The short-term sequelae of pulmonary embolism are pain, hypoxemia, acute pulmonary hypertension, and, if the embolus is large enough, circulatory collapse and death. Small pulmonary emboli tend to lodge peripherally and produce symptoms of respirophasic pain and dyspnea. Massive (greater than 50% occlusion of pulmonary artery) and submassive emboli that lodge in the central pulmonary arterial circulation cause primarily cardiovascular manifestations: hypotension, syncope, right heart strain, decreased cardiac output, and elevated central venous pressure. Repeated pulmonary emboli can cause chronic pulmonary hypertension.

Diagnosis

The risk factors for pulmonary embolus are prolonged immobilization, obesity, congestive heart failure, malignancy, pregnancy, oral contraceptives, polycythemia, deep venous thrombosis, previous history of pulmonary embolus, and family history of pulmonary embolus (suggesting an inherited deficiency of an endogenous anticoagulant such as antithrombin III or protein C).

The clinical diagnosis of pulmonary embolism is notoriously inaccurate. Laboratory tests that may be helpful in supporting the diagnosis are the electrocardiogram, arterial blood gases, and chest x-ray film. The standard for diagnosis is radionuclide perfusion lung scanning (with ventilation scanning if any perfusion defects are detected) and pulmonary angiography in those cases where the radionuclide scan is not definitive and clinical suspicion is high. Documentation of deep venous thrombosis by plethysmography in patients suspected of having a pulmonary embolus is tantamount to confirmation of the diagnosis of pulmonary embolus, but approximately 20% of patients with pulmonary emboli have no demonstrable deep venous clot.

The symptoms and signs of pulmonary embolus are not specific. They may vary depending on the size of the embolus and whether or not it lodges far enough peripherally to cause infarction. Patients with massive or submassive pulmonary emboli obstructing lobar or segmental flow present primarily with cardiovascular symptoms and signs (syncope, hypotension, elevated central venous pressure), whereas patients with smaller pulmonary emboli that lodge in the periphery of the lung present with pulmonary symptomatology (dyspnea, pleuritic pain, cough) and tachycardia. The four most prevalent symptoms in the Urokinase Pulmonary Embolism Trial of 215 patients were dyspnea, pleuritic pain, apprehension, and cough.

Physical signs of pulmonary emboli are also nonspecific. The most important abnormalities are those of the vital signs. Patients often exhibit tachycardia and tachypnea. Massive embolus may cause hypotension. Fever may be present. Pulmonary emboli sufficiently large to affect the cardiovascular system may manifest as right-sided heart strain with elevated central venous pressure and a loud pulmonic component of the second heart sound. In cases of pulmonary infarction, a pleural friction rub may be present. The neurohumoral factors released during platelet aggregation may cause bronchospasm. A nonprecordial peripheral pulmonary artery systolic murmur best heard in the interscapular, subclavicular, and right anterior axillary area of the chest has been described; it is thought to be secondary to pulmonary arterial flow through a partially obstructed lumen or secondary to increased bronchial artery collateral flow.

Because of the high incidence of deep venous thrombosis of the lower extremities as a cause of pulmonary emboli, a careful physical assessment of the lower extremities is mandatory. In general, with the exception of elevation of the respiratory rate and pulse, the patient's physical examination will usually be normal.

In order for pulmonary infarction to occur, the embolus must be small enough to lodge peripherally where the secondary bronchial circulation is inadequate to sustain parenchymal viability. Pulmonary infarctions present with pleuritic pain, hemoptysis, a pleural friction rub, pleural effusion, and a wedge-shaped infiltrate on a chest radiograph.

The list of differential diagnoses in patients with pulmonary embolism is usually long. The other diagnoses can be conveniently categorized by the presenting symptomatology that they share with the different types of pulmonary emboli—massive, peripheral, or infarction-causing (Table 24–1).

Diagnosis

Laboratory data serve primarily to rule out competing diagnoses. The two most useful laboratory tests are the *chest x-ray* and the *electrocardiogram*. The chest x-ray may be completely normal in cases of pulmonary emboli, although a great number of nonspecific signs have been described. Some of the specific signs to look for are

Unilateral or segmental oligemia secondary to decreased pulmonary blood circulation because of the embolus

Basilar atelectasis and elevated hemidiaphragm secondary to volume loss from pain-induced splinting and from the neurohumoral factors released

Pleural-based, wedge-shaped density with associated pleural effusion that is associated with pulmonary infarction

TABLE 24–1. Differential Diagnosis of Pulmonary Embolism

Differential Diagnosis	Signs and Symptoms
Pleuritis	Respirophasic pain, fever, ±dyspnea
Pericarditis	Respirophasic pain, tachycardia, fever
Pneumonia	Dyspnea, shortness of breath, fever, tachycardia, tachypnea
Hyperventilation syndrome	Shortness of breath, tachycardia, tachypnea
Costochondritis/ musculoskeletal chest pain	Respirophasic pain, ±shortness of breath
Pneumothorax	Respirophasic pain, dyspnea, shortness of breath
Bronchitis	Dyspnea, shortness of breath
Bronchospastic disease	Shortness of breath, tachypnea, tachycardia
Myocardial infarction	Syncope, hypotension, shock, chest pain
Pericardial tamponade	Hypotension, shock, elevated central venous pressure, tachycardia
Aortic dissection	Hypotension, shock, chest pain
Intra-abdominal castastrophe	Hypotension, shock

The main use of the electrocardiogram is to rule out a myocardial infarction or pericarditis. Electrocardiographic changes in pulmonary emboli are tachycardia, nonspecific T wave inversions and ST segment abnormalities, and signs of right heart strain (right precordial T wave inversions, rightward axis, and the S_1-Q_3-T_3 pattern, which indicates acute cor pulmonale and is very uncommon).

An *arterial blood gas* determination is helpful in confirming the clinical impression that the patient is genuinely hypoxemic, although pulse oximetry delivers similar information in a noninvasive manner. The pCO_2 of an arterial blood gas may be used in conjunction with the pO_2 to calculate the alveolar-arterial (A-a) oxygen gradient (on room air, at sea level, the A-a gradient is equal to the $150 - [1.25 \times pCO_2] - p_aO_2$). The normal A-a gradient is 3 to 6 mmHg on room air, although it does increase with age ($2.5 + 0.21 \times age$).

The diagnostic standard for ruling out a pulmonary embolus is the *ventilation-perfusion lung scan*. The perfusion scan is a remarkably sensitive procedure for detecting abnormalities in pulmonary blood flow. A normal perfusion scan effectively eliminates the possibility of a pulmonary embolus. Perfusion scans are safe in pregnancy.

Unfortunately many clinical conditions other than pulmonary embolus cause abnormal pulmonary blood flow and an abnormal perfusion scan. These include infection, bronchospasm, tumor, and a host of other inflammatory conditions. The specificity of perfusion scan can be enhanced by the addition of a xenon-133 ventilation scan. Because pulmonary embolus should not affect airway caliber, the classic ventilation-perfusion (VQ) lung scan pattern for pulmonary embolus is ventilation-perfusion mismatch, i.e., multiple perfusion defects with a normal ventilation scan. Perfusion defects are described as lobar, segmental, or subsegmental; as single or multiple; and as matched or mismatched to ventilation defects. Perfusion defects that occur in the same area as an abnormality on chest x-ray are labeled indeterminate. A ventilation-perfusion lung scan is classified as high probability, intermediate probability, low probability, or indeterminate probability for pulmonary embolus by the size of the perfusion defect(s), the number of perfusion defects, and the extent of match or mismatch with ventilation defects and chest radiographic abnormalities. Lung scans are not as sensitive for small pulmonary emboli as they are for large ones.

A normal perfusion scan rules out a pulmonary embolus. A markedly positive high probability scan (e.g., multiple segmental defects on perfusion scan with a normal ventilation scan) in a patient in whom clinical suspicion for pulmonary embolus is high constitutes enough evidence of the presence of a pulmonary embolus to initiate treatment. A low probability scan in the face of a strong clinical suspicion or an intermediate probability scan mandates the next diagnostic step: pulmonary arteriography. Pulmonary embolus can be present in a disturbingly high percentage (25 to 40%) of ventilation-perfusion scans that are "low probability" for pulmonary embolus, although legitimate questions have been raised about the clinical significance of those pulmonary emboli.

Pulmonary arteriography is the gold standard for the diagnosis of pulmonary embolus. It is an invasive procedure with a reported 1 to 4% morbidity rate and a 0.1 to 0.4% mortality rate; complications occur because of the injection of hypertonic contrast material and the mechanical problems caused by the presence of a catheter in the heart. In experienced hands it is a safe procedure whose risks must be balanced against the risks of not having the information it provides. Patients with chronic pulmonary hypertension (right ventricular end-diastolic pressure greater than 20 mmHg) or severe cardiac or respiratory decompensation have a higher incidence of complications.

Pulmonary arteriography is both extremely sensitive and specific for diagnosing pulmonary embolus. Because it is the "gold standard," there is no higher authority with which to compare it; however, patients with suspected pulmonary emboli who have negative pulmonary arteriograms, generally have no further clinical evidence of embolism. Radiographic criteria for a "positive" pulmonary arteriogram are presence of either an intravascular filling defect or an abrupt arterial cut-off. Second-tier criteria are pruning of blood vessels, retardation of blood flow, and alteration of blood vessel caliber. Blood vessels to a 2-mm size may be visualized by pulmonary arteriography.

Indications for Treatment

Any case of documented acute pulmonary embolism should be treated with pharmaco-logic therapy. Because heparin anticoagulation and thrombolytic therapy have risks, the diagnosis of pulmonary embolism should usually be made by diagnostic imaging. If the appropriate laboratory test, such as lung scan, is not immediately available, and if the index of clinical suspicion is appropriately high, it is acceptable to initiate pharmacologic therapy and to continue it pending the outcome of the test.

Pulmonary embolus carries an untreated mortality rate of 20 to 30%; with treatment, the mortality rate is reduced to less than 10%. The purpose of therapy is prevention of recurrent pulmonary emboli, resolution of the thrombus source, prevention of propagation of the embolus in the pulmonary vasculature, clearing of thromboemboli from the pulmonary vasculature, restoration of normal pulmonary hemodynamics, prevention of chronic recurrent venous thromboembolism, and prevention of chronic venous insufficiency. (See box.)

Discussion

Heparin is the standard therapy for pulmonary emboli. Its role is to prevent recurrent emboli by preventing fresh clots from forming and by permitting the old clot to organize or be dissolved by the body's endogenous fibrinolytic system. Heparin may also limit the deleterious effects of neurohumoral release from platelets.

A difficult question is when to initiate heparin therapy: when pulmonary embolus is first suspected on the basis of clinical presentation or when it is confirmed by lung scan or pulmonary arteriography? In patients with neither absolute nor relative contraindications to heparin therapy and in whom there will be a delay in obtaining the appropriate diagnostic test, heparin therapy should be begun immediately. If the diagnosis is equivocal on the basis of the clinical presentation, if the diagnostic test is imminent, or if relative contraindications to heparin use are present, heparin therapy should be withheld until the diagnosis of pulmonary embolus is firmly established.

In contrast to the abundant clinical trial data comparing thrombolytic therapy to standard therapy in acute myocardial infarction, there is little data on efficacy of lytic therapy in acute pulmonary embolism.

The gold standard of controlled clinical trials of lytic therapy in pulmonary embolism is the 1973 Urokinase in Pulmonary Embolism Trial (UPET). Its 160 patients were random-

DRUG TREATMENT: PULMONARY EMBOLISM

First-Line Drug
Heparin

Initial Dose	5,000–10,000 units IV (100 units/kg)
Continuous Infusion	1,000–1,500 units/hour
End-Points	Infusion rate titrated to maintain activated partial thromboplastin time (APTT) at 1.5–2 times the control value; APTT should be assayed at hour 4 after initiation of therapy.
	Heparin anticoagulation may be terminated when warfarin anticoagulation reaches therapeutic end-point, usually by day 4–6.

Second-Line Drug

(But considered first-line drug in cases of massive or submassive pulmonary embolism or in cases of severe hemodynamic compromise [systolic blood pressure < 90 mmHg] or severe hypoxemia [pO_2 <60 mmHg with supplemental oxygen])

Urokinase

Initial Dose	4,400 IU/kg IV over 30–60 minutes
Alternative Dose	1,000,000 IU by IV bolus over 10 minutes followed by 2,000,000 units over remaining 2 hours
Continuous Infusion	4,400 IU/kg/hour
End-Points	Bleeding complications
	Therapy usually continued for 12–24 hours

OR

Tissue Plasminogen Activator (t-PA)

Initial Dose/Continuous Infusion	50–100 mg over 2 hours
End-Points	Bleeding complications
	100 mg t-PA

OR

Streptokinase

Initial Dose	250,000 IU IV over 30 minutes
Continuous Infusion	100,000 IU/hour
End-Points	Bleeding complications
	Therapy usually continued for 24–96 hours

ized to receive 12 hours of a peripheral urokinase infusion or standard intravenous heparin therapy. Because of the relatively small size of the trial and because the incidence of mortality from pulmonary embolism is low, the outcome measure of the clinical trial was not mortality but rather the speed and completeness with which the radiographic, hemodynamic, and clinical abnormalities resolved. The UPET demonstrated that lytic therapy results in greater resolution of hemodynamic abnormalities and earlier and more complete resolution of imaging abnormalities (angiographic filling defects and radionuclide scan perfusion defects) than does standard heparin therapy, but the UPET did not demonstrate a long-term benefit of lytic therapy over heparin therapy.

The search for the best thrombolytic agent and treatment regimen for pulmonary emboli is the subject of intense clinical investigation. Phase II of the UPET study compared three different infusion regimens: 12 hours of urokinase, 24 hours of urokinase, and 24 hours of streptokinase. Although all three regimens were more effective than heparin therapy alone, urokinase was a more effective lytic agent than streptokinase.

A study of intravenous t-PA showed an 83% incidence of marked or moderate clot lysis at 1 to 6 hours after the start of infusion. Clot lysis was accompanied by resolution of echocardiographic signs of right heart failure. A comparison of a 2-hour infusion of intravenous t-PA (100 mg over 2 hours) with the 24-hour regimen of intravenous urokinase demonstrated that t-PA was nearly twice as effective at lysing clot at 2 hours, had a much lower incidence of bleeding complications, and had an identical effect on the lung scan at 24 hours. There seems to be equal efficacy of t-PA whether it is administered directly into the pulmonary artery or intravenously.

The precise role of thrombolytic therapy in reducing mortality and improving pulmonary hemodynamics is unknown at this point. It does seem clear that decreased pulmonary capillary blood flow is more pronounced in those patients treated with heparin therapy alone. Clinical data support the use of thrombolytic therapy in massive pulmonary embolus, submassive pulmonary embolus with hemodynamic compromise (as might occur in a patient with preexistent cardiopulmonary disease), and in submassive pulmonary embolus not responsive to conventional heparin management. Other authorities recommend lytic therapy for any case of pulmonary embolism with pulmonary vascular obstruction of one lobar or three segmental arteries. Furthermore, the larger the deep venous thrombosis in the lower extremity, the greater the indication for thrombolytic therapy.

Experience with surgical embolectomy has in general been poor. Mortality is high (up to 50%). The usually cited indications for embolectomy are shock (blood pressure less than 90 mmHg; urine output less than 20 ml/hour) and hypoxemia (pO_2 less than 60 mmHg). Results with lytic therapy in the same population of patients suggest that lytic therapy is as efficacious as surgical embolectomy for these patients. Embolectomy is usually reserved for those patients who fail to respond to a lytic drug or who have an absolute contraindication to its administration.

Patients with pulmonary emboli who have absolute contraindications to the use of heparin and lytic agents require interruption of the inferior vena cava, usually by percutaneous insertion of an umbrella device that serves as a barrier to embolus migration. One such device is the Greenfield filter, which reduces the recurrence rate of pulmonary emboli to 5%. Vena cava barriers are also indicated in patients who experience the recurrent pulmonary emboli while therapeutically anticoagulated.

Myocardial Infarction

Thrombolytic therapy, in conjunction with heparin, provides a physiologically sound treatment for the precipitating cause of most myocardial infarctions—coronary artery thrombus. Properly administered, thrombolytic therapy salvages myocardium that is at risk for necrosis, reducing mortality by up to 80%, and substantially decreases the expected post-myocardial infarction decrement of left ventricular function.

The benefit obtained by thrombolytic therapy is greater (1) the earlier after onset of symptoms that thrombolytic medication is administered and (2) the larger the amount of myocardium served by the infarct-related artery. The greatest benefits accrue if thrombolytic therapy is administered within 2 hours of the onset of symptoms in a large anterior wall myocardial infarction. The time window for therapeutic efficacy is at least 6 hours, although some data suggest that thrombolytic therapy may be beneficial even up to 24 hours after symptom onset (Second International Study of Infarct Survival [ISIS-2 trial]). Patients with inferior wall myocardial infarction also benefit from thrombolytic therapy. Thrombolytic therapy is clearly beneficial in ST segment elevation infarctions. The role of thrombolytic therapy in unstable angina, in non–ST segment elevation infarctions, and in patients whose onset of symptoms is greater than 6 hours prior to emergency department presentation is not yet well delineated.

The general principles underpinning the application of thrombolytic therapy in myocardial infarction are as follows:

1. The precipitating/sustaining cause of an acute myocardial infarction is thrombus occluding the coronary ar-

tery, occurring at the site of a preexistent atherosclerotic plaque.

2. Myocardial cell death in the region served by the infarct-related artery is neither instantaneous nor simultaneous but occurs as a wave front of necrosis, progressing from endocardium to epicardium over a period of 4 to 6 hours, and affects different myocardial tissue differentially.
3. The reestablishment of perfusion in the infarct-related artery within that 4- to 6-hour time window may salvage myocardium that is at risk for necrosis.
4. The most important factor determining whether reperfusion succeeds in salvaging myocardium is *time* between onset of symptoms and administration of thrombolytic agent.

Diagnosis

The emergency diagnosis of acute myocardial infarction is made by factoring the compatibility of the clinical presentation with the presence of diagnostic electrocardiographic abnormalities. Presenting symptoms may be chest pain, chest heaviness or discomfort, neck or arm pain, epigastric discomfort, nausea or vomiting, diaphoresis, syncope or near-syncope, and extreme weakness or lassitude. A history of ischemic heart disease by either symptoms (e.g., angina) or laboratory documentation (e.g., exercise testing, coronary arteriography, history of myocardial infarction) constitutes important background information. In the absence of such a history, the presence of risk factors for coronary artery disease (i.e., hypertension, diabetes, hypercholesterolemia, smoking, and positive family history) may be helpful in raising the physician's index of suspicion, although the precise role of risk factors in determining the probability that a particular patient has sustained a myocardial infarction is uncertain. The electrocardiographic abnormality diagnostic for acute myocardial infarction is ST segment elevation. Other ST segment and T wave abnormalities (ST depression, T wave inversion) are less diagnostic.

The in-hospital diagnosis of myocardial infarction is made by demonstrating a sequential rise in the MB fraction of serum creatine kinase or by characteristic evolution of the electrocardiogram. Imaging techniques such as thallium scanning and echocardiography may reveal dyskinetic areas of myocardium. Additional diagnostic strategies (e.g., early sequential creatine kinase MB testing or echocardiography) may become standards for acute diagnosis in the future.

Patients presenting acutely with myocardial infarction symptoms who require hospital admission may be divided into two groups: those in whom the diagnosis of acute myocardial infarction is nearly certain because of diagnostic ST segment elevations on the electrocardiogram, and those who lack a diagnostic electrocardiogram but in whom the clinical presentation raises the index of suspicion to a level high enough to warrant admission. Because of the high morbidity that can occur if the diagnosis of myocardial infarction is missed, many patients who are appropriately admitted to the hospital to "rule out myocardial infarction" turn out to have neither a myocardial infarction nor even coronary artery disease.

Indications for Treatment

The current indications for administration of thrombolytic therapy for myocardial infarction are straightforward, although they will probably evolve substantially during the 1990s. Thrombolytic therapy is beneficial in those patients who have

1. A presentation compatible with myocardial infarction, that is, a prolonged (greater than 20 minutes) episode of chest discomfort or a chest discomfort equivalent such as neck pain, epigastric pain, diaphoresis, arm pain, or jaw pain
2. An electrocardiogram that demonstrates ST segment elevation of at least 1 mm in two or more contiguous leads
3. Symptomatology and ST segment elevation that do not normalize with nitroglycerin (this criterion is designed to eliminate cases of coronary artery spasm)
4. Presentation within 6 hours of the onset of symptoms
5. Absence of contraindications

These are strict criteria, which are fulfilled by substantially less than half of the patients who have sustained a myocardial infarction diagnosed by serial creatine kinase MB assay. The electrocardiographic criterion of ST segment elevation is based on evidence that coronary artery thrombus plays a much larger causative role in transmural myocardial infarction, manifested by ST segment elevation, than it does in subendocardial infarction, manifested by ST segment depression and T wave inversion. Although the benefit of thrombolytic therapy for infarction with ST segment depression is an open question, and although subgroup analysis of clinical trial data is fraught with danger, in both the GISSI trial and the ISIS-2 trial such patients did worse or no better with thrombolytic therapy than with placebo.

The issues around "late" (i.e., more than 6 hours since symptom onset) administration of thrombolytic agents are complex. Data from several trials indicate the independent benefit to mortality from having a patent infarct-related artery, even if that patency occurs after myocardial salvage could be expected to occur. These data not withstanding, the routine use of thrombolytic therapy for myocardial infarction should be limited to patients falling within the 6-hour time window at this time.

The decision to employ thrombolytic therapy is a risk-benefit decision that balances the statistical benefit likely to accrue to the patient with the chance for harm from hemorrhage. In general, patients benefit more if they are treated earlier and have a larger amount of myocardium at risk (anterior wall myocardial infarctions demonstrate more measurable salvage with thrombolysis than inferior wall myocardial infarctions), and they are at less risk if they are without any of the relative contraindications to therapy. (See box.)

Discussion

Presently, only t-PA, streptokinase, and anistreplase are approved by the Food and Drug Administration for treatment of acute myocardial infarction. Urokinase, although it may be more effective than streptokinase in clot lysis, has not enjoyed widespread use in the management of acute myocardial infarction. Prourokinase is likely to be approved for routine use in myocardial infarction in the future. APSAC, because it is converted to its active form in the body, can be administered as a single bolus.

In general, heparin is coadministered with the thrombolytic agent in order to prevent reocclusion of the successfully recanalized artery. A study by Topol documented no difference in recanalization rates if heparin administration is withheld until alteplase therapy has terminated or if it is begun at the onset of thrombolytic therapy.

Intravenous thrombolytic therapy results in successful recanalization of the infarct-related artery approximately 40 to 80% of the time. Initial clinical investigation of streptokinase utilized an intracoronary route of administration with coronary artery patency resulting approximately 75% of the time. However, intracoronary administration of a thrombolytic agent has four serious drawbacks: its applicability is limited to tertiary care facilities, it requires the constant availability of an interventional cardiologist, it carries a higher incidence of bleeding complications because of the invasiveness of the procedure, and the onset of thrombolysis is delayed by the time needed to mobilize the catheterization team. Consequently, the intravenous administration of thrombolytic agents has completely replaced the intracoronary route as the initial treatment for acute myocardial infarction. Intravenous streptokinase is approximately 30% less effective than intracoronary streptokinase in obtaining recanalization, but intravenous alteplase seems to be as effective as any intracoronary agent, with patency rates of 70 to 80%. Anistreplase is equivalent or slightly superior to streptokinase in effecting reperfusion.

Successful reperfusion of the infarct-related artery may be marked by relief of presenting symptoms, appearance of reperfusion dysrhythmias (ventricular tachycardia, idioventricular rhythm), and resolution of ST segment elevation. However, no bedside marker of reperfusion has enough predictive value to constitute a test of infarct-related artery patency. The usual time course for coronary artery recanalization is that one-third of the patients who will recanalize will do so within the first 30 minutes, one-third from minutes 30 to 60 after administration of the lytic agent, and one-third from minutes 60 to 90. How to detect the approximately 25% of patients who do not successfully recanalize constitutes one of the unsolved problems of thrombolytic therapy.

The role and timing of percutaneous angioplasty in acute myocardial infarction have been well studied. Immediate or routine angioplasty in acute myocardial infarction provides no benefit in mortality, left ventricular function, or recurrence of myocardial infarction. Angioplasty should be considered for those patients who are clinically unstable (e.g., cardiogenic shock) or who manifest reocclusion or recurrent ischemia. Routine late angioplasty may increase left ventricular function following exercise.

DRUG TREATMENT: ACUTE MYOCARDIAL INFARCTION

First-Line Drug

Tissue Plasminogen Activator

Loading Dose	6–10 mg bolus IV
Followed by	54–50 mg (60 mg—bolus dose) over first hour; 20 mg/hour for hours 2 and 3
	Alternative dose for patients less than 65 kg: 1.25 mg/kg with 60% administered in first hour (with 6–10 mg bolus) and remaining 40% administered over subsequent 2 hours
End-Point	Successful reperfusion (see Discussion, below)

OR

Streptokinase

Loading Dose	1,500,000 IU IV* over 30–60 minutes
End-Point	Successful reperfusion (see Discussion, below)

OR

Anistreplase

Initial Dose	30 units IV push over 2–5 minutes
Repeat Dose	None
End-Point	Successful reperfusion (see Discussion, below)

AND

Heparin

Loading Dose	5,000–10,000 units
Constant Infusion	1,000–2,000 units/hour
End-Points	Partial thromboplastin time titrated to 1.5–2 times control
	Heparin infusion continued for 24–48 hours

AND

Aspirin

Initial Dose	160 mg PO
Repeat Dose	160 mg/day
End-Points	Bleeding complications

*Note that streptokinase may also be administered as an intracoronary infusion at 4,000 IU/min.

Arterial Occlusion

Arterial occlusion may occur from either arterial embolus or arterial thrombosis. It is important to distinguish the two because the management strategies differ greatly. Embolic occlusion is treated surgically with balloon removal of the embolus; thrombotic occlusion is treated with anticoagulation and surgical revascularization if necessary. Thrombolytic therapy may play a role in both embolic and thrombotic occlusion.

Diagnosis

The initial symptoms of arterial occlusion in the extremity are pain and paresthesia (delicate sensory nerves are most sensitive to hypoxia), followed by paresis, pallor, coolness, pulselessness, and mottling.

Distinguishing embolic from thrombotic occlusion is not always easy. Most embolic occlusions have a cardiac source, either thrombus in the left atrium (from atrial fibrillation) or a mural thrombus of the left ventricle (from a hypokinetic or dyskinetic segment of myocardium). The embolus may also originate from atherosclerotic debris in the abdominal aorta. Arterial emboli tend to cause symptoms of abrupt onset, that is, if the extremity in question is the leg, then a previous history of claudication is absent and the contralateral leg will possess normal pulses. In contrast, arterial thrombosis occurs on a background of longstanding symptomatic peripheral vascular disease, with the final thrombotic event usually occurring in well-defined areas (e.g., Hunter's canal in the superficial femoral artery).

The ultimate diagnostic test is arteriography. Arteriography may show emboli lodged at arterial bifurcations with absence of hemodynamically significant stenoses or the characteristic angiographic signature of thrombosis: vessels damaged by atherosclerosis circumvented by well-formed collateral circulation.

DRUG TREATMENT: ARTERIAL OCCLUSION

First-Line Drug
Heparin

Initial Dose	5,000–10,000 units IV (100 units/kg)
Continuous Infusion	1,000–1,500 units/hour
End-Points	Infusion rate titrated to maintain activated partial thromboplastin time (APTT) at 1.5–2 times the control value; APTT should be assayed at hour 4 after initiation of therapy.
	Heparin anticogulation may be terminated when warfarin anticoagulation reaches therapeutic end-point (see below) usually by day 4–6.

Second-Line Drug: Thrombolytic Agent
Urokinase

Initial Dose	4,000 IU/min directly into clot
Subsequent Dose	1,000–2,000 IU/min once antegrade flow established
End-Point	Successful clot lysis or less than 10% progress after 500,000 IU in increments

OR

Streptokinase

Initial Dose	5,000–100,000 IU/hour directly into the clot
Subsequent Dose	5,000–100,000 IU/hour
End-Point	Successful clot lysis may require 24–96 hours.

OR

Tissue Plasminogen Activator

Initial Dose	0.05–0.1 mg/kg/min directly into the clot
Subsequent Dose	Continuous infusion at 0.05–0.1 mg/kg/min
End-Point	Successful clot lysis (usually within 1–8 hours)

Indications for Treatment

The treatment of arterial embolization is usually surgical embolectomy, particularly if there is limb-threatening ischemia. Usually, the lesion is defined by arteriography prior to therapy.

Acute arterial thrombosis occurring on a background of atherosclerotic vascular disease may be successfully treated with thrombolytic therapy and heparin anticoagulation. Arteriography should be obtained with a goal of defining the anatomy for eventual surgical reconstruction. Thrombolytic therapy has been most effective when delivered locally into the thrombus through the arteriography catheter. (See box.)

Discussion

The initial treatment for both arterial embolus and thrombosis is full-dose heparinization. Acute embolic occlusion of extremity arteries may be treated by balloon embolectomy. Lytic therapy has been used to lyse peripheral arterial clots in arteries not accessible to catheter embolectomy. Some studies indicate that for local administration of streptokinase to be successful at lysing clot, it must be delivered in quantities sufficient to cause systemic effects on the coagulation system (i.e., decreased fibrinogen and increased fibrin degradation products). Other studies indicate that for the same degree of systemic depletion of fibrinogen, local instillation is more efficient at embolus lysis than is systemic therapy. Efficacy of local instillation of thrombolytic agents improves if the infusion catheter is pushed directly into the clot. Femoropopliteal or aortoiliac occlusions respond better to lytic therapy than does tibioperoneal thrombosis.

A high success rate (81%) of clot lysis of peripheral artery clots has been achieved with a high-dose urokinase regimen (4,000 IU/min initially, tapered to 1,000 IU/min administered directly into the clot). Mean infusion time with this regimen was 18 hours. Most successful recanalizations occur within 2 hours of starting the infusion. High-dose urokinase utilizing a technique of infusion directly into the clot is almost twice as effective as a low-dose streptokinase regimen, has a much lower incidence of side effects and complications, and requires less than 50% of the infusion time. Successful lysis can result in showering of emboli peripherally; in general, these are successfully treated with continued infusion of the lytic agent. Concomitant heparinization may help to prevent the formation of thrombus around the catheter.

One study of t-PA in patients with native peripheral arterial occlusions of bypass graft thrombosis reported successful thrombolysis in 93%. Major complications occurred in only four patients. Another study comparing t-PA with surgical thrombectomy for thrombosed arterial bypass grafts showed a 100% successful lysis rate in t-PA patients. Patients undergoing surgical thrombectomy had a three-times greater chance of amputation than those receiving t-PA.

Femoral artery or iliac artery thrombosis secondary to indwelling arterial catheters for purposes of infusion of chemotherapeutic agents or hepatic embolization has been successfully treated with low-dose infusions of streptokinase (5,000 IU/hour) or urokinase (35,000 IU/hour) for 24 to 96 hours.

Subclavian Vein Thrombosis

Axillary-subclavian vein thrombosis is an uncommon condition of the upper extremity that constitutes a diagnostic and therapeutic challenge for the clinician. It is usually classified into those cases for which there is a clear precipitating cause (an indwelling catheter, a mediastinal mass obstructing venous outflow, or an anatomic abnormality at the thoracic outlet) and those for which no precipitating cause can be identified other than effort or repetitive motion (e.g., swinging a tennis racket).

Diagnosis

The symptoms of axillary-subclavian vein thrombosis are upper extremity swelling, pain, heaviness, limb dysfunction, achiness, fatigue, and paresthesias. Physical examination signs are an objectively swollen extremity and a prominent surface venous pattern. Because of its relative rarity, the diagnosis of axillary-subclavian vein thrombosis is often missed at first presentation.

The definitive diagnosis of axillary-subclavian vein thrombosis is made by contrast venography. An indwelling plastic intravenous catheter is inserted in the affected extremity and radiopaque contrast material is injected.

Indications for Treatment

All patients with axillary-subclavian vein thrombosis require pharmacologic treatment. (See box.)

DRUG TREATMENT: AXILLARY-SUBCLAVIAN VEIN THROMBOSIS

First-Line Drug
Heparin

Initial Dose	5,000–10,000 units IV (100 units/kg)
Continuous Infusion	1,000–1,500 units/hour
End-Points	Infusion rate titrated to maintain activated partial thromboplastin time (APTT) at 1.5–2 times the control value; APTT should be assayed at hour 4 after initiation of therapy.

OR

Urokinase

Initial Dose	4,000 IU/min directly into clot
Subsequent Dose	1,000–2,000 IU/min once antegrade flow established
End-Point	Successful clot lysis

OR

Streptokinase

Initial Dose	5,000–100,000 IU/hour directly into the clot
Subsequent Dose	5,000–100,000 IU/hour
End-Point	Successful clot lysis may require 24–96 hours.

Discussion

The traditional management of axillary-subclavian vein thrombosis consists of rest and heparin followed by warfarin. Results with this regimen are poor; more than 50% of the patients develop a chronic form of the syndrome that consists of symptoms similar to those of the acute presentation.

Although no controlled trials exist comparing lytic therapy with the standard management approach, the medical literature is replete with reports of successful lysis of clot by infusion of thrombolytic agents. The lytic agent may be infused directly into the clot through a venography catheter located just proximal to the clot or systemically through a vein on the other extremity. The first rib may need to be resected in order to help prevent a recurrence.

Ischemic Stroke

Stroke remains one of the leading causes of death and disability in the United States each year. Approximately 80% of all strokes are ischemic in nature. Nearly all ischemic strokes are caused by embolus or thrombus. Despite advances in understanding the pathophysiology of acute brain ischemia, no effective treatment has been developed for patients with acute ischemic stroke. Ongoing trials evaluating the effects of thrombolytic agents, calcium channel blockers, hemodilution, and other agents appear promising, but none is recommended for general use at this time. Anticoagulation for stroke syndromes has been evaluated extensively in the past. In particular, anticoagulation has been studied in transient ischemic attacks (TIAs), evolving or progressing stroke, cardioembolic stroke, and partial stroke.

Diagnosis

TIAs are an important warning sign for acute cerebral infarction. As many as 20% of patients with TIAs who go on to have a stroke do so within one month of the initial event. Anterior circulation TIAs may be characterized by amaurosis fugax, aphasia or unilateral paresis, numbness, or paresthesias of the face, arm, or leg. Posterior or vertebrobasilar TIAs may consist of unilateral or bilateral paresis or paresthesias, ataxia, dysarthria, vertigo, diplopia, or binocular visual symptoms. Although most TIAs resolve within 30 minutes, the duration can be longer. Three or more TIAs occurring within 72 hours may be termed *crescendo TIAs*.

In progressing stroke, focal ischemia shows a pattern of worsening, which may occur over minutes or hours. It has been stated that 20% of anterior circulation and 40% of posterior circulation strokes will show progression. Posterior circulation strokes may progress over 2 to 3 days. There is evidence to suggest that propagation of thrombus may be the causative agent in progressing stroke.

Partial acute stroke is one in which patients have an acute stroke with relatively mild neurologic deficits. There is the possibility that such strokes, which are minor initially, may progress over time and lead to severe disability or death.

Cardioembolic strokes are caused by embolization from damaged valves or from ventricular or atrial mural thrombus. Patients will typically have a history of valvular heart disease, atrial fibrillation, or previous myocardial infarction. The risk of cardioembolic stroke in patients with nonvalvular atrial fibrillation is not well defined.

Indications for Treatment

Heparin anticoagulation has not been proved to be of benefit in promoting *neurologic recovery* in any of the above stroke syndromes, but data are controversial, particularly in progressing stroke and crescendo TIAs. Some authorities recommend treating patients with crescendo TIAs or progressing stroke with immediate heparin anticoagulation.

In cardioembolic stroke, anticoagulation has been shown to be beneficial in reducing the incidence of further embolization. Anticoagulation may be initiated after a computed tomography scan is obtained 24 to 48 hours after the onset of symptoms to rule out hemorrhage. If hemorrhage is not detected, anticoagulation can proceed at that time. (See box.)

Discussion

Heparin anticoagulation for any stroke syndrome should not proceed until a computed tomography scan has demonstrated the absence of hemorrhage. Detecting hemorrhage on clinical grounds is unreliable even for experts. Once heparin treatment has been started, the dosage should be adjusted on the basis of the APTT. The first APTT should be obtained within 4 to 6 hours of initiating therapy. Oral warfarin should be started shortly after heparin initiation if long-term anticoagulation is desired.

A caveat in the use of anticoagulants for stroke concerns the presence of hypertension. If there is sustained systolic (>180 mmHg) or diastolic (>110 mmHg) hypertension, anticoagulation may increase the risk of hemorrhage. Blood pressure should be adequately controlled before anticoagulation is initiated. However, overzealous administration of antihypertensives should be avoided since hypertension with acute stroke may be transient and excessive lowering of the blood pressure may worsen ischemic stroke. Anticoagulation will also increase the risk of hemorrhage in patients with massive thrombotic infarcts.

DRUG TREATMENT: CARDIOEMBOLIC STROKE

First-Line Drug

Heparin

Initial Dose	5,000–10,000 units IV (100 units/kg)
Continuous Infusion	1,000–1,500 units/hour
End-Point	Infusion rate titrated to maintain activated partial thromboplastin time (APTT) at 1.5–2 times the control value; APTT should be assayed at hour 4 after initiation of therapy.

Other Clots

Acute *renal vein thrombosis* presents with flank discomfort and a decreased creatinine clearance, usually in the setting of underlying renal disease (membranous glomerulonephritis and nephrotic syndrome). Pulmonary embolus is a common complication. Standard treatment is heparin followed by warfarin anticoagulation, but this results in slow resolution of both the symptoms and the renal dysfunction. Several case reports of systemic and local lytic therapy have documented clot lysis, resolution of symptoms, and lowering of serum creatinine.

The *Budd-Chiari syndrome* of hepatic vein thrombosis presents with right upper quadrant pain, ascites, and abnormalities of liver transaminases. Diagnosis is suggested by computed tomography scan and made by inferior vena cava venography. Localized instillation of urokinase has been reported to be successful in lysing the occluding clot.

Paroxysmal nocturnal hemoglobinuria is an unusual hematologic disorder of stem cell dysfunction manifested by red blood cell hemolysis and hemoglobinuria, thrombocytopenia, leukopenia, and a tendency toward thromboses. Most patients experience intra-abdominal thrombosis for which standard heparin therapy usually is unsuccessful. Several case reports have documented the clinical benefits of streptokinase infusion.

Several case reports have documented the benefit of thrombolytic therapy for *prosthetic valve thrombosis,* which presents with absent prosthetic valve sounds and hemodynamic compromise. Diagnosis may be made on echocardiogram or at cardiac catheterization. Thrombolytic agents may be administered through a right atrial line (for right-sided valves) or through a peripheral vein. The major complication in management of prosthetic valve thrombosis with thrombolytic therapy is not bleeding but embolism, which occurs with a moderate incidence (15%) in cases of left-sided valves, resulting in TIAs, splenic infarcts, and upper arm ischemia.

Left ventricular thrombi that result from myocardial infarction may be successfully lysed with lytic therapy. In one case series, lytic therapy was successful in lysing mural thrombi in 60% of cases. Newer thrombi (within 4 weeks of myocardial infarction) and absence of ventricular aneurysm seem to enhance the likelihood of successful lysis.

A controlled clinical trial of streptokinase in *central retinal vein* occlusion yielded disappointing results: although there was some improvement in visual acuity and a decrease in post-thrombotic glaucoma, there were several cases of vitreous hemorrhage that were probably a direct result of the thrombolytic therapy.

Rarely, *thoracic outlet syndrome* may be manifested by occlusion of the subclavian artery with distal vascular symptomatology. One such case was successfully treated with an intra-arterial infusion of urokinase at 60,000 IU/hour for 72 hours through a catheter embedded in the clot. Distal emboli also resolved with the infusion.

Specific Agents

Anistreplase (Eminase)

Chemical Structure

Anistreplase is an inactive complex of human lys-plasminogen, streptokinase, and an anisoyl group.

Pharmacology

Pharmacokinetics

The duration of fibrinolytic activity is controlled by deacylation of the activator complex, with a half-life of 2 hours. The half-life of fibrinolytic activity is 70 to 120 minutes (mean = 94 minutes).

Actions

Anistreplase converts plasminogen to plasmin both at the site of the clot and systemically. Anistreplase contains fibrin binding sites that allow for clot attachment, in addition to a catalytic center that is responsible for the conversion of plasminogen to plasmin.

Indication

Acute ST segment elevation myocardial infarction

Cautions

Renal failure—anistreplase should be used with caution because of the defect in platelet function associated with uremia.

Hepatic failure—anistreplase may contribute to hemorrhage if a coagulopathy is present.

Cardiac failure—no alteration in dosage needed

Use in pregnancy—Category C. Anistreplase should be used only if clearly indicated.

Use in pediatric patients—the safety and effectiveness of anistreplase have not been established. Avoid its use in children.

Onset and Duration of Action

Dosage

The dosage of anistreplase is 30 units IVP over 2 to 5 minutes. Each unit of anistreplase is approximately 1 mg and contains 36,000 IU of streptokinase. The potency of anistreplase is expressed in units specific for anistreplase only.

Repeat Dosing

Because anistreplase has a long half-life, repeat dosing is not necessary.

Toxicity

Drug Interactions

The risk of hemorrhage may be exacerbated by concurrent use of heparin, aspirin, or oral anticoagulants.

Adverse Effects

The major risk of anistreplase therapy is hemorrhage. Most studies place the risk of intracerebral hemorrhage at 0.5% and the risk of serious gastrointestinal bleeds at 3 to 7%. Many serious hemorrhagic episodes can be avoided by careful screening for contraindications and proper patient handling. Female patients and patients with diabetes seem to have a higher incidence of serious bleeding complications. Techniques to minimize bleeding complications are shown in Table 24–2. The following are other adverse effects specific to anistreplase:

Allergic reaction: because of its origin as a bacterial protein, anistreplase is antigenic and causes an allergic reaction in 1 to 5% of cases; manifestations may include bronchospasm, angioedema, urticaria, flushing, nausea, pruritus, and headache.

Fever: This occurs somewhat more frequently than allergic reactions and is due to the pyrogenic nature of anistreplase.

Treatment of Toxicity

Minor hemorrhagic complications can be controlled by local measures. Blood volume

TABLE 24–2. Avoidance of Bleeding Complications

1. Peripheral lines should be utilized whenever possible, not central lines. If central lines must be used, compressibility should be the site-selection criterion: femoral, internal jugular, and subclavian veins should be utilized in that order.
2. Blood should be drawn from indwelling catheters, not by venous sticks. No vascular hole should be left unfilled; a heparin lock or arterial line is a useful site for drawing blood while the thrombolytic agent is infusing.
3. Nasotracheal intubation should be avoided; orotracheal intubation should be used if intubation is necessary.
4. An external pacemaker should be used if pacing is required; if a transvenous pacemaker is necessary, it should be placed under fluoroscopic control through a femoral approach.
5. Nasogastric tubes should be avoided if possible or placed through the mouth if needed.

should be maintained with infusion of crystalloid or packed red blood cells. The anistreplase-induced hemostatic defect can be corrected by administration of fresh-frozen plasma or cryoprecipitate, both of which are rich in fibrinogen. The use of aminocaproic acid to reverse the lytic state is theoretically sound, but clinical experience is minimal; the dose is a load of 5 g IV or PO followed by 1 g/hour for 2 to 4 hours.

Allergic reactions may be managed by antihistamine and corticosteroid therapy. Some practitioners routinely pretreat their patients with both agents; most reserve such use only for cases of an actual allergic reaction. Severe allergic reactions require cessation of anistreplase and the usual therapeutic regimens for anaphylaxis.

Fever should be managed with acetaminophen, not with aspirin.

Hypotension is usually transient and self-limited. It can be managed with the usual regimen of crystalloid therapy and Trendelenburg position. Bradycardia (Bezold-Jarisch reflex) during infusion for inferior infarction can be managed with atropine.

Antistreptococcal antibodies render some patients "anistreplase resistant." For those patients, either much higher doses or, preferably, switching to another thrombolytic agent is indicated.

Heparin

Pharmacology

Heparin is not a single specific molecule but rather a heterogeneous collection of polymer mucopolysaccharides (glycosaminoglycans) whose core disaccharide unit is either D-glucosamine-L-iduronic acid or D-glucosamine-D-glucuronic acid. Most heparin consists of 8 to 15 units of each disaccharide and has a molecular weight of 10,000 to 16,000 daltons; the lower molecular weight heparins (5,000 to 9,000 daltons) with fewer disaccharide units have a more specific effect on Factor Xa and less of an effect on platelets and thrombin than do the higher molecular weight units. Heparin is a strongly acidic compound. Sodium is attached to the carboxylic acid and sulfate groups of each mucopolysaccharide unit, and hence the term sodium heparin.

Commercial heparin is derived from pig intestine and cow lung. Porcine heparin has greater anti-Factor Xa potency, less effect on platelets, and greater lipolytic activity than bovine heparin. Synthetic heparins are available.

Distribution

Because of the large size of its molecules, heparin is not absorbed from the gastrointestinal tract, does not cross the placenta, and is not absorbed sublingually. Heparin exerts its effects directly in the circulating blood.

Elimination

After uptake by the reticuloendothelial cells, heparin is metabolized in the liver by heparinase. Heparin is excreted intact in the urine only if large doses are administered. The half-life of heparin is better measured as the half-life of its anticoagulant function, which generally obeys first-order kinetics, is dose dependent, and at standard doses ranges from 60 to 100 minutes, so that inadvertent excess anticoagulation with heparin should clear by itself in a short time. The half-life of heparin effect is significantly prolonged in patients with cirrhosis or renal failure; patients with pulmonary embolism clear heparin more rapidly than normal.

Actions

Heparin induces a conformational change in anti-thrombin III that enhances its inhibition of Factors IIa (thrombin), Xa, IXa, XIa, and XIIa. Because most of these factors appear on the intrinsic arm of the coagulation cascade, heparin administration disproportionately lengthens the activated partial thromboplastin time more than the prothrombin time; however, in large doses, heparin prolongs both the prothrombin and partial thromboplastin time. Heparin also catalyzes the inhibition of thrombin by heparin cofactor II, an effect that may be of importance during the period of high serum heparin levels that occurs after an intravenous bolus.

In addition to its effect on the fluid phase of coagulation, heparin inhibits the neurohumoral release from platelet-thrombin interaction that may affect airway size and gas exchange, and heparin releases lipoprotein lipase, which results in clearing of lipemic serum.

Primary Indications

Deep venous thrombosis
Pulmonary embolus
Acute myocardial infarction

The main use of heparin in emergency situations is for deep venous thrombosis, pulmonary embolism, and acute myocardial infarction (the latter in conjunction with thrombolytic therapy). Heparin should be employed in cases of peripheral arterial thrombosis. The role of heparin in the management of neurologic emergencies—stroke, stroke in evolution, transient ischemic attacks—is not yet well delineated.

Cautions

Renal failure—heparin dosage should be carefully titrated in renal failure. Renal failure patients are routinely anticoagulated for hemodialysis. The renal failure–induced platelet dysfunction may increase the risk of heparin therapy.
Cardiac failure—no dosage adjustment necessary
Hepatic failure—heparin dose should be decreased and titrated to partial thromboplastin time (PTT).
Use in pregnancy—Category C. Heparin is considered safe in pregnancy because it does not cross the placenta.
Use in pediatric patients—heparin is safe in all age groups. Dosage must be modified (loading dose, 50 units/kg).

General Contraindications

Heparin is contraindicated in patients who are at risk for hemorrhage. The list of contraindications is essentially identical to the contraindications to thrombolytic therapy: patients actively bleeding; patients with recent intracranial, eye, or intraspinal surgery; patients undergoing a spinal tap; patients with severe hypertension; patients with bleeding tendencies (hemophilia, thrombocytopenia); patients with possibility of cerebral metastases; patients with endocarditis; patients with bleeding lesions of the gastrointestinal tract.

Lack of Antithrombin III

Because heparin action depends on the presence of antithrombin III, resistance to heparin occurs in conditions in which there is a quantitative or qualitative defect in antithrombin III. In addition to genetic absence of antithrombin III (which predisposes to thromboembolism), decreased amounts of antithrombin III occur in massive venous thromboembolism, disseminated intravascular coagulation, and severe liver failure. In these situations, in order for heparin therapy to be effective, it has to be supplemented by antithrombin III–containing fresh-frozen plasma.

Onset and Duration of Action

Dosage

Loading dose: 5,000 to 10,000 units (50 to 100 units/kg)

Maintenance dose: 1,000 to 1,500 units/hour (10 to 20 units/kg/hour; 30,000 to 40,000 units/24 hours)

Intravenous administration can be by either continuous infusion or intermittent bolus. The incidence of bleeding complications is lower with continuous infusion than with bolus therapy (1 to 5% versus 10 to 12%), and the prolongation of clotting time is more even. If intermittent intravenous bolus doses are administered, they should be given as 5,000 to 10,000 units every 4 to 6 hours. Low-dose subcutaneous heparin for prophylaxis against thrombosis is administered as 5,000 to 10,000 units every 12 hours. Full-dose subcutaneous heparin therapy is initiated as one-third of the daily intravenous dose every 12 hours.

Limits

Full-dose heparin therapy has no fixed dose; its use is guided by the level of anticoagulation achieved. As a general rule, the APTT should be kept at $1\frac{1}{2}$ to 2 times the control value so as to ensure adequate anticoagulation effect without an undue risk of increased bleeding. Failure to achieve an adequate anticoagulant response is associated with a high rate of recurrent venous throm-

boembolism (10 to 25%). In cases of administration of excessive heparin, elevations of prothrombin time will also occur because of the effect of antithrombin III on Factor Xa and on thrombin. Initially, a 4- to 6-hour and then daily APTT assays should be obtained when full-dose heparinization is employed. Low-dose heparin therapy is not monitored with laboratory tests. Because of the potential for heparin-induced thrombocytopenia, heparin therapy should be monitored with platelet counts.

Repeat Dosing

Heparin may be maintained as a continuous infusion for weeks, although usually patients are switched to oral anticoagulants within one week. Careful attention must be paid to thrombocytopenia, especially after 1 week of therapy when immune-mediated thrombocytopenia is most common.

Toxicity

Drug Interactions

The tendency for heparin to cause bleeding is enhanced by concomitant or preceding administration of antiplatelet drugs such as aspirin.

Adverse Effects

Heparin is a drug with major side effects, the most serious being *bleeding*. Most large-scale reviews identify a 1 to 5% incidence of serious bleeding with heparin therapy.

Heparin exerts two different effects on platelets. Heparin-induced platelet aggregation may cause mild *thrombocytopenia* in 25% of patients. A more severe thrombocytopenia occurs via an immunologic mechanism in up to 5% of patients usually between day 6 and day 12 of therapy. An anti-heparin antibody interacts with the heparin-platelet complex to cause platelet release, platelet aggregation, and thrombocytopenia. This process has the characteristics of a consumptive coagulopathy with elevated fibrin degradation products and reductions in plasma fibrinogen. It occurs most often in the arterial circulation, may manifest itself as thrombocytopenia with a worsening of the underlying thromboembolic disease, and is usually very difficult to diagnose. In rare instances, serious arterial thrombotic events may occur, resulting in stroke, limb amputation, or myocardial infarction. Porcine heparin may cause less immune thrombocytopenia than beef heparin.

Heparin may cause *local skin necrosis*, usually at the site of subcutaneous injection. This phenomenon is probably also due to heparin-induced thrombosis and is treated in the identical manner as heparin-induced thrombocytopenia.

Because heparin is derived from animal tissue, *hypersensitivity reactions* do occur, manifested by fever, urticaria, and anaphylaxis. Prolonged use of heparin can result in myalgias, bone pain, and osteoporosis.

Treatment of Toxicity

Because of heparin's short half-life, most cases of "overheparinization" can be treated by discontinuing the heparin infusion.

In cases of heparin overdose with serious clinical hemorrhage, protamine sulfate may be used to counter the effects of the heparin. Protamine is a strongly basic compound that complexes with and inactivates heparin (see Chap. 16).

The diagnosis of heparin-induced consumptive thrombocytopenia should be suspected when platelet counts drop to less than 50,000/mm^3 and concomitant thrombosis develops. The treatment is to discontinue heparin. Dextran, dipyridamole, or aspirin may be administered for its antiplatelet function. Most serious cases of heparin-induced thrombocytopenia can be avoided by beginning oral anticoagulation concomitant with the start of heparin therapy and thereby limiting the heparin therapy to a maximum of 7 days.

Streptokinase (Kabikinase, Streptase)

Pharmacology

Streptokinase is a nonenzymatic protein derived from group C beta-hemolytic streptococci.

Streptokinase activity is specified in international units (IU). One IU is the amount of streptokinase necessary to activate enough plasminogen to lyse a standard fibrin clot in 10 minutes *in vitro.*

Distribution

Streptokinase is rapidly protein-bound. No assay other than activity exists, so exact distribution is unknown.

Elimination

Streptokinase is inactivated by antibody combination and reticuloendothelial system uptake. There are two half-lives: a "fast" half-life of 18 minutes that results from antibody complexing and a longer half-life of 83 minutes that occurs without antibody assistance. The plasmin-mediated reduction in clotting factor concentration that is produced by streptokinase persists after the streptokinase has disappeared from the circulation and lasts until new clotting factor manufacture has occurred in the liver.

Actions

Streptokinase combines with plasminogen to form a complex that has protease activity and that converts free plasminogen to plasmin; streptokinase is thus an indirect activator of plasminogen. Because the streptokinase-plasminogen complex circulates freely in the plasma, streptokinase is not fibrin-specific in its lytic action; circulating fibrinogen is broken down to fibrinogen degradation products. Streptokinase has a rheologic effect of decreasing blood viscosity and slightly reducing peripheral resistance. The therapeutic benefit of these effects is not known.

Indications

Acute ST segment elevation myocardial infarction
Acute massive pulmonary embolism
Acute deep venous thrombosis
Acute arterial thrombosis and embolism
Occluded arteriovenous cannulas

Cautions

Renal failure—streptokinase should be used with caution in renal failure because of the defect in platelet function associated with uremia.
Liver failure—streptokinase should be used with caution in liver failure because of the coagulopathy that may exist with that condition.
Cardiac failure—no contraindication exists to using streptokinase in cardiac failure
Use in pregnancy—streptokinase should not be used during the first 18 weeks of pregnancy because of the risk of abruptio placentae. The use of streptokinase after 20 weeks of gestation should be done with great caution and only if no alternatives exist.
Use in pediatric patients—safety and efficacy in children are not known.

Onset and Duration of Action

Dosage

The dose and duration of streptokinase therapy depend on the clinical condition for which it is being used. Because of the presence of anti-streptococcal antibodies which inactivate streptokinase, a high initial dose is typically employed.

Myocardial infarction: 1.5 million IU over 1 hour

Pulmonary embolism: 250,000 IU load over 30 minutes, followed by 100,000 units per hour for 24 hours

Deep venous thrombosis: same as pulmonary embolism except infusion continued for 72 hours

Arterial embolism and thrombosis: 5,000 to 100,000 IU/hour for 24 to 96 hours

Occluded cannulas: 250,000 IU diluted to 2 ml and injected into cannulas by pump for 30 minutes, 2-hour dwell, and then aspirated

Limits

Streptokinase may be administered by continuous infusion for up to 96 hours; laboratory monitoring is usually not indicated: thrombin time should be prolonged to twice normal as evidence of efficacy and may be checked after 3 to 4 hours. Streptokinase causes prolongation of all coagulation time tests—prothrombin time, partial thromboplastin time, thrombin time—which begin to return toward normal 4 hours after discontinuation of therapy.

Repeat Dosing

Because of the appearance of anti-streptokinase antibodies and the consequent risks of allergic reactions and resistance, a full course of streptokinase should not be repeated for 6 months.

Toxicity

Drug Interactions

The risk of hemorrhage may be exacerbated by concomitant administration of heparin, aspirin, or oral anticoagulants. Nevertheless, many therapeutic regimens call for just such combinations of clot-retardant drugs. The relative benefits of simultaneous versus sequential therapy with heparin for acute myocardial infarction have not been fully elucidated. There is probably no difference in recanalization efficacy if the heparin

is begun after streptokinase therapy is completed. The standard therapeutic regimen for pulmonary emboli uses heparin after streptokinase infusion is completed and after the thrombin time or prothrombin time has returned to less than twice control.

Adverse Effects

The major risk of streptokinase therapy is hemorrhage. Most studies place the risk of intracerebral hemorrhage at 0.5% and the risk of gastrointestinal bleeds at 3 to 7%. Many serious hemorrhagic episodes can be avoided by careful screening for contraindications and proper patient handling. Female patients and patients with diabetes seem to have a higher incidence of serious bleeding complications. Techniques to minimize bleeding complications are shown in Table 24–2.

The following are other adverse effects specific to streptokinase:

Allergic reaction: because of its orgin as a bacterial protein, streptokinase is antigenic and causes an allergic reaction 1 to 5% of the time; manifestations may include bronchospasm, angioedema, urticaria, flushing, nausea, pruritus, and headache.

Fever: this occurs somewhat more frequently (10 to 15%) than allergic reactions and is due to the pyrogenic nature of streptokinase.

Hypotension: in the ISIS-2 trial of 8,592 patients suspected of acute myocardial infarction who received a 1.5 million IU bolus of intravenous streptokinase, the excess incidence of hypotension over those patients receiving placebo was 7.9%.

Treatment of Toxicity

Minor hemorrhagic complications can be controlled by local measures. If serious bleeding occurs, streptokinase infusion should be terminated. Blood volume should be maintained with crystalloid or packed red blood cells. The streptokinase-induced hemostatic defect can be corrected by administration of fresh-frozen plasma or cryoprecipitate, both of which are rich in fibrinogen. The use of aminocaproic acid to reverse the lytic state is theoretically sound, but clinical experience is minimal; the dose is a load of 5 g IV or PO followed by 1 g/hour for 2 to 4 hours.

Allergic reactions may be managed by antihistamine and corticosteroid therapy. Some practitioners routinely pretreat their patients with both agents; most reserve such use only for cases of an actual allergic reaction. Severe allergic reactions require cessation of streptokinase and the usual therapeutic regimens for anaphylaxis.

Fever should be managed with acetaminophen, not with aspirin.

Hypotension is usually transient and self-limited. It can be managed with the usual regimen of crystalloid therapy and Trendelenburg position. Bradycardia (Bezold-Jarisch reflex) during infusion for inferior infarction can be managed with atropine.

Antistreptococcal antibodies render some patients "streptokinase resistant." For those patients, either much higher doses or, preferably, switching to another thrombolytic agent is indicated.

Tissue Plasminogen Activator—Alteplase (Activase)

Pharmacology

Alteplase is the synthetic form of the human enzyme tissue plasminogen activator (t-PA) that is derived from recombinant deoxyribonucleic acid synthesis. t-PA is a two-chain polypeptide molecule of 562 amino acids.

Distribution

The volume of distribution is 30 to 50 liters; therefore, alteplase seems to distribute in total body water. The extent of penetration into the placenta, cerebrospinal fluid, and milk is unknown.

Elimination

Alteplase is cleared by the liver and excreted by the kidney. The half-life of distribution from the plasma is very short—3 to 4 minutes. Eighty percent of the drug is cleared from the plasma within 10 minutes. The half-life of elimination from the body is approximately 30 minutes.

Actions

Alteplase is a fibrin-specific plasminogen activator. Its affinity for plasminogen is greatly increased after binding to fibrin, although this clot selectivity is relative rather than absolute, and some dose-related decrement in circulating fibrinogen does occur.

Indications

Alteplase is indicated in the acute management of ST segment elevation myocardial infarction and pulmonary embolus. Alteplase has been used in acute deep venous thrombosis, arterial occlusion, and mesenteric or subclavian vein occlusion, although none of these other uses currently have Food and Drug Administration approval.

Cautions

Renal failure—alteplase should be used with caution in renal failure because of the hemorrhagic diathesis of uremia-induced platelet dysfunction.

Liver failure—the dosage of alteplase may need to be decreased.

Cardiac failure—no modification of dosage

Use in pregnancy—Category C. No evidence that alteplase is teratogenic; increased risk of hemorrhage puts fetus at risk; unknown whether or not alteplase is secreted into breast milk

Use in pediatric patients—safety of alteplase in children is not known.

Onset and Duration of Action

Dosage

For myocardial infarction, alteplase is usually administered as 100 mg over 3 hours, with an initial dose in the first hour of 60 mg (with the initial 6 to 10 mg as a bolus) and the remaining 40 mg given as 20 mg/hour during the second and third hours. The efficacy of more compressed regimens (e.g., 100 mg over 90 minutes) is under investigation.

The mg/kg dosing is 1.25 mg/kg, of which 60% should be administered in the first hour (with 6 to 10 mg administered as an immediate bolus) and the remaining 40% over the subsequent 2 hours. This weight-adjusted dosage is used for patients whose body weight is less than 65 kg.

The dosage regimen that has been employed for pulmonary embolus is 50 to 100 mg IV over 2 hours.

Limits

In the absence of hemorrhagic complications, all patients receive alteplase in a standard dosing regimen.

Repeat Dosing

Alteplase may be repeated after several hours either in its initial dosage or at half dose.

Toxicity

Drug Interactions

The risk of hemorrhage may be exacerbated by concomitant administration of heparin, aspirin, or oral anticoagulants. Nevertheless, the therapeutic regimen for acute myocardial infarction calls for just such a combination of clot-retardant drugs. The relative benefits of simultaneous versus sequential therapy with heparin for acute myocardial infarction have not been fully elucidated, but there is probably no difference in recanalization efficacy if the heparin is begun after alteplase therapy is completed.

Adverse Effects

The primary adverse effect of alteplase is hemorrhage. The incidence of intracerebral hemorrhage is approximately 0.5% with a 100-mg dose of alteplase. A higher incidence occurred when a 150-mg dose was used.

Risk of hemorrhage can be minimized if standard precautions and patient selection criteria are employed.

Unlike with streptokinase, there is no appreciable incidence of allergic reactions, fever, or hypotension.

Treatment of Toxicity

Minor hemorrhagic complications can be controlled by local measures. If serious bleeding occurs, alteplase infusion should be terminated. Blood volume should be maintained with crystalloid or packed red blood cells. The hemostatic defect can be corrected by administration of fresh-frozen plasma or cryoprecipitate, both of which are rich in fibrinogen. The use of aminocaproic acid to reverse the lytic state is theoretically sound, but clinical experience is minimal; the dose is a load of 5 g IV or PO, followed by 1 g/hour for 2 to 4 hours. Because of the short half-life of alteplase, cessation of the infusion is very effective if serious hemorrhage results.

Urokinase (Abbokinase)

Pharmacology

Urokinase is an enzyme produced in the kidney and excreted in the urine. It is isolated from human kidney tissue culture or extracted from human urine.

Distribution

Urokinase is measured by its activity; its exact distribution is unknown.

Elimination

Elimination occurs primarily by metabolism in the liver and excretion in the kidney. The plasma half-life is 10 to 20 minutes.

Actions

Urokinase is a direct activator of plasminogen. Urokinase is not specific for clot-bound fibrin; circulating fibrinogen is degraded as well. Although the direct effects of urokinase therapy disappear after several hours, decreased levels of fibrinogen and plasminogen, increased levels of fibrin and fibrinogen degradation products, and prolongation of thrombin time, prothrombin time, and partial thromboplastin time can persist for 12 hours.

Indications

Acute massive pulmonary emboli
Acute deep venous thrombosis
Peripheral arterial occlusion
Occluded central venous catheters

Urokinase has been used for acute myocardial infarction but is not nearly as well studied as streptokinase or tissue plasminogen activator. Urokinase has been used for peripheral arterial occlusion and occluded central venous catheters.

Cautions

Renal failure—urokinase should be used with caution in renal failure because of the defect in platelet function associated with uremia.

Liver failure—urokinase should be used with caution in liver failure because of the coagulopathy that may exist with that condition.

Cardiac failure—no contraindication exists to using urokinase in cardiac failure.

Use in pregnancy—Category B. It is not known if urokinase is safe in pregnancy, nor is it known if urokinase is secreted during lactation. A case report exists in which urokinase has been administered without problems to a pregnant patient. Use in pediatric patients—safety and efficacy in children are not known.

Onset and Duration of Action

Dosage

For pulmonary embolism, deep venous thrombosis, and other large vessel clot, the loading dose is 4400 IU/kg, followed by 4400 IU/kg/hour for 12 to 72 hours. The UPET study demonstrated that 12 hours constitutes sufficient therapy for pulmonary emboli. An alternative dosage regimen for pulmonary embolism is to administer 3,000,000 IU IV over 2 hours, with a 1,000,000-IU loading dose delivered over the first 10 minutes.

Urokinase has not been well studied for intravenous use in acute myocardial infarction; intracoronary dosage is 6,000 IU/min for up to 2 hours.

For occluded intravenous catheters, a syringe containing 5,000 IU of urokinase should be injected in a volume equal to the volume of the catheter; aspiration may be attempted every 5 minutes; the urokinase may be allowed to dwell for 30 to 60 minutes before a second round of drug is attempted.

Limits

Urokinase may be administered for up to 96 hours. Laboratory monitoring of coagulation parameters is not required, but the infusion should be stopped if serious bleeding develops. Urokinase causes prolongation of all coagulation time tests—prothrombin time, partial thromboplastin time, thrombin time—which begin to return toward normal 4 hours after discontinuation of therapy.

Toxicity

Drug Interactions

The risk of hemorrhage may be exacerbated by concomitant administration of heparin, aspirin, or oral anticoagulants. The standard therapeutic regimen for pulmonary emboli uses heparin after urokinase infusion has been terminated and the thrombin time or prothrombin time has returned to less than twice control.

Adverse Effects

The major risk of urokinase therapy is hemorrhage. Most studies place the risk of intracerebral hemorrhage at 0.5% and the risk of gastrointestinal bleeds at 3 to 7%. Many serious hemorrhagic episodes can be avoided by careful screening for contraindications and by proper patient handling. Female patients and patients with diabetes seem to have a higher incidence of serious bleeding complications. Unlike with streptokinase, urokinase administration does not result in allergic reactions, fever, or hypotension.

Treatment of Toxicity

Minor hemorrhagic complications can be controlled by local measures. If serious bleeding occurs, urokinase infusion should be terminated. Blood volume should be maintained with crystalloid or packed red blood cells. The hemostatic defect can be corrected by administration of fresh-frozen plasma or cryoprecipitate, both of which are rich in fibrinogen. The use of aminocaproic acid to reverse the lytic state is theoretically sound but clinical experience is minimal; the dose is a load of 5 g IV or PO followed by 1 g/hour for 2 to 4 hours.

REFERENCES

Amery A, DeLoof W, Vermylen J, Verstraete M: Outcome of recent thromboembolic occlusions of limb arteries treated with streptokinase. Br Med J 4:639–644, 1970.

Ansari A: Acute and chronic pulmonary thromboembolism: Current perspectives. (8 parts.) Clin Cardiol 9:398–402, 449–456, 512–524, 567–572, 614–620, 1986; 10:40–43, 124–126, 181–188, 1987.

Ansell AE: Handbook of Hemostasis and Thrombosis. Boston, Little, Brown & Co., 1986.

Arnesen H, Hoiseth A, Ly B: Streptokinase or heparin in the treatment of deep venous thrombosis. Acta Med Scand 211:65–68, 1982.

Arnesen H, Hoiseth A, Ly B: Streptokinase or heparin in the treatment of deep vein thrombosis. Acta Med Scand 203:457–463, 1978.

Camerota AJ, Rubin RN, Tyson RR, et al: Intra-arterial thrombolytic therapy in peripheral vascular disease. Surg Gynecol Obstet 165 (1):1–8, 1986.

Common HH, Seaman AJ, Rosch J, et al: Deep vein thrombosis treated with streptokinase or heparin: Follow-up of a randomized study. Angiology 27(11):645–654, 1976

Duckert F, Muller G, Nyman D, et al: Treatment of deep vein thrombosis with streptokinase. Br Med J 1:479–481, 1975.

Elliot MS, Immelman EJ, Jeffrey P, et al: A comparative randomized trial of heparin versus streptokinase in the treatment of acute proximal vein thrombosis. Br J Surg 66:838–843, 1979.

Elliot MS, Immelman EJ, Jeffrey P, et al: The role of thrombolytic therapy in the management of phlegmasia cerulea dolens. Br J Surg 66:422–424, 1979.

Gagnon RM, Beaudet R, Leumire J, et al: Streptokinase

thrombolysis of a chronically thrombosed mitral prosethetic valve. Cathet Cardiovasc Diagn 10:5–10, 1984.

GISSI (Gruppo Italiano per lo studio della streptochinasi nell'infarto miocardico): Long-term effects of intravenous thrombolysis in acute myocardial infarction: Final report of the GISSI study. Lancet 2:871–874, 1987.

Goldhaber SZ, Kessler CM, Heit J, et al: Randomized controlled trial of recombinant tissue plasminogen activator versus urokinase in the treatment of acute pulmonary embolism. Lancet 2:293–298, 1988.

Goldhaber SZ, Meyerovitz MF, Markis JE, et al: Thrombolytic therapy of acute pulmonary embolism: Current status and future potential. J Am Coll Cardiol 10(5):96B–104B, 1987.

Greenwood LH, Yrizarry JM, Hallett JW, Scoville GS: Urokinase treatment of Budd Chiari syndrome. AJR 141:1057–1059, 1983.

ISIS-2 (Second International Study of Infarct Survival) Collaborative Group: Randomized trial of intravenous streptokinase, oral aspirin, both, or neither, among 17,817 cases of suspected acute myocardial infarction: ISIS-2. Lancet 2:350–360, 1988.

Kakkar VV, Lawrence D: Hemodynamic and clinical assessment after therapy for acute deep vein thrombosis. Am J Surg 150(4):54–63, 1965.

Kakkar VV, Howe CT, Laws JW, Flanc C: Late results of treatment of deep venous thrombosis. Br Med J 1:810–811, 1969.

Kohner EM, Petit JE, Hamilton AM, et al: Streptokinase in central retinal vein occlusion: A controlled clinical trial. Br Med J 1:550–553, 1976.

Koults RL, Kuehner ME, Swanson MK, et al: Local intraarterial streptokinase therapy for acute peripheral arterial occlusions. Am Surg 51(7):381–382, 1985.

Kudo S, Chuang VP, Wallace S, et al: Transcatheter thrombolysis in cancer patients. Cardiovasc Intervent Radiol 8:1–7, 1985.

Kremer P, Fiebig RM, Tilsner V, et al: Lysis of left ventricular thrombi with urokinase. Circulation 72(1):112–118, 1985.

Kurzrok S, Singh AK, Most AS, Williams DO: Thrombolytic therapy for prosthetic cardiac valve thrombosis. J Am Coll Cardiol 9(3):592–598, 1987.

Landercasper J, Gall W, Fischer M, et al: Thrombolytic therapy of axillary-subclavian venous thrombosis. Arch Surg 122:1072–1075, 1987.

Marder VJ: Relevance of changes in blood fibrinolytic and coagulation parameters during thrombolytic therapy. Am J Med 83(Suppl 2A):15–19, 1987.

Marder VJ Rothbard RL, Fitzpatrick PG, Francis CW: Rapid lysis of coronary artery thrombi with anisoylated plasminogen streptokinase activator complex. Ann Intern Med 104:304–310, 1986.

McNamara TO, Fischer JR: Thrombolysis of peripheral arterial and graft occlusions: Improved results using high-dose urokinase. AJR 144:769–775, 1985.

Miller GAH, Hall RJC, Paneth M: Pulmonary embolectomy, heparin, and strepotokinase: Their place in the treatment of acute massive pulmonary embolism. Am Heart J 93(5):568–574, 1977.

Nenci GG, Gresele P, Taramelli M, et al: Thrombolytic therapy for thromboembolism of vertebrobasilar artery. Angiology 34(9):561–571, 1983.

Rowe JR, Rasmussen RL, Mader SL, et al: Successful thrombolytic therapy in two patients with renal vein thrombosis. Am J Med 77:1111–1114, 1984.

Sloan MA: Thrombolysis and stroke. Arch Neurol 44:748–766, 1987.

Tibbut DA, Davies JA, Anderson JA, et al: Comparison by controlled clinical trial of streptokinase and heparin in treatment of life-threatening pulmonary embolism. Br Med J 1:343–347, 1974.

Whitehouse G: Radiological diagnosis of deep vein thrombosis. Br Med J 295:801–802, 1987.

Wilcox RG, Olsson CG, Skene AM, et al: Trial of tissue plasminogen activator for mortality reduction in acute myocardial infarction Anglo-Scandinavian Study of Early Thrombolysis. Lancet 2:525–530, 1988.

Pulmonary Emboli

Delclos GL, Davila F: Thrombolytic therapy for pulmonary embolism in pregnancy: A case report. Am J Obstet Gynecol 155(2):375–376, 1986.

Hull RD, Raskob GE, Carter CJ, et al: Pulmonary embolism in outpatients with pleuritic chest pain. Arch Intern Med 148:838–844, 1988.

Overton DT, Bocks JJ: The alveolar arterial oxygen gradient in patients with documented pulmonary embolism. Arch Intern Med 146:1617–1619, 1988.

Parker JA, Markis JE, Palla A, et al: Pulmonary perfusion after rt-PA therapy for acute embolism: Early improvement assessed with segmental perfusion scanning. Radiology 166(2):441–445, 1988.

Raskob GE, Carter CJ, Hull RD: Heparin therapy for venous thrombosis and pulmonary embolism. Blood Reviews 2:251–258, 1988.

Sasahara AA, Sharma GVRK, McIntyre KM, Cella G: Does thrombolytic therapy alter the prognosis of pulmonary embolism. Hemostasis 16(Suppl 3):51–57, 1986.

Sharma GVRK, Burleson VA, Sasahara AA: Effect of thrombolytic therapy on pulmonary capillary blood volume in patients with pulmonary embolism. N Engl J Med 303(15):842–845, 1980.

Urokinase Pulmonary Embolism Trial Study Group: Urokinase-streptokinase embolism trial (phase 2 results): A cooperative study. JAMA 229(12):1606–1613, 1974.

Valenzuela TD: Pulmonary embolism. Ann Emerg Med 17(3):209–213, 1988.

Valenzuela TD: Pulmonary embolism. Emerg Clin North Am 6(2):253–266, 1988.

Wheeler AP, Jaquis EDB, Newman JH: Physician practices in the treatment of pulmonary embolism and deep venous thrombosis. Arch Intern Med 246:1321–1325, 1988.

Myocardial Infarction

Braunwald E: Myocardial reperfusion, limitation of infarct size, reduction of left ventricular dysfunction, and improved survival: Should the paradigm be expanded? Circulation 79(2):441–443, 1989.

O'Rourke M, et al (Sydney/Auckland Group for Study of Thrombolysis in Acute Coronary Occlusion [T.I.C.O]): Limitations of myocardial infarction by early infusion of recombinant tissue-type plasminogen activator. Circulation 77(6):1311–1315, 1988.

Van de Werf F, Arnold AER (for the European Cooperative Study Group for recombinant tissue type plasminogen activator): Intravenous tissue plasminogen activator and size of infarct, left ventricular function, and survival in acute myocardial infarction. Br Med J 279:1374–1379, 1988.

Arterial Occlusion

Sullivan KL, Minken SL, White RI: Treatment of a case of thromboembolism resulting from thoracic outlet syndrome with intra-arterial urokinase infusion. J Vasc Surg 7(4):568–571, 1988.

Ischemic Stroke

Duke RJ, Bloch RF, Turpie AGG, et al: Intravenous heparin for the prevention of stroke progression in acute partial stable stroke: A randomized controlled trial. Ann Intern Med 105:825–828, 1986.

Hakim AM, Furlan AJ, Hart RG, et al: Immediate anticoagulation of embolic stroke: A randomized trial. Stroke 4:668–676, 1983.

Miller VT, Hart RG: Heparin anticoagulation in acute brain ischemia. Stroke 19:403–406, 1988.

Putnam SF, Adams HP Jr: Usefulness of heparin in initial management of patients with recent transient ischemic attacks. Arch Neurol 42:960–962, 1985.

Ramirez-Lassepas M, Quinones MR, Nino HR: Treatment of acute ischemic stroke: Open trial with continuous intravenous heparinization. Arch Neurol 43:386–390, 1986.

Webster BB, Levin M: Anticoagulation in cerebral ischemia. Stroke 14:658–663, 1983.

CHAPTER 25

Muscle Relaxants

SCOTT A. SYVERUD, M.D.

INTRODUCTION

Neuromuscular blocking agents are divided into two broad categories: depolarizing agents (e.g., succinylcholine) and nondepolarizing agents (e.g., pancuronium bromide). Drugs in both categories block nerve transmission at the neuromuscular junction. When given in therapeutic doses by intravenous push, paralysis of the skeletal muscles and the muscles of respiration ensues within seconds to minutes. Neuromuscular blocking agents facilitate endotracheal intubation of patients with conditions such as head injury, drug overdose, and status epilepticus. They can also be used for suppression of patient movement during computed tomography (CT) scanning or other diagnostic studies, and to prevent sudden rises in intracranial pressure (ICP) associated with head trauma. When used correctly, these drugs can be efficacious and even lifesaving in these settings. When used incorrectly or in the wrong setting, airway obstruction and death can result. It is therefore critical that the clinician clearly understand the indications and proper use of these agents.

Physiology of Muscle Contraction

To understand the mechanism of action and side effects of muscle relaxants, one must understand the sequence of events occurring at the neuromuscular junction and inside the muscle cell. The neuromuscular junction is the point where the terminal axon meets the muscle cell membrane. The axonal membrane ("presynaptic membrane") and the muscle membrane ("postsynaptic membrane") are specialized at the synapse (or "motor end-plate") to allow neuromuscular conduction. A narrow synaptic cleft separates the axon from the muscle cell membrane at this end-plate.

Acetylcholine, the intrinsic neurotransmitter of the neuromuscular junction, is produced in the axonal cytoplasm from acetyl coenzyme A and choline and then stored in vesicles within the axon at the end-plate. When a nerve impulse (action potential) reaches the neuromuscular junction, the axonal presynaptic membrane depolarizes, causing an influx of calcium ions from the synaptic cleft into the axon. This influx results in the release of acetylcholine into the synaptic cleft. Acetylcholine then traverses the synaptic cleft and combines with receptors on the postsynaptic membrane. This in turn increases the postsynaptic membrane permeability and causes depolarization. With sufficient depolarization, a threshold is reached and an action potential is then generated, which causes depolarization of the entire muscle cell membrane.

Inside the muscle cell, depolarization of the cell membrane results in a massive release of calcium from the sarcoplasmic reticulum. This calcium initiates the chain of events that results in contraction of the sarcomere and muscle contraction.

After the muscle action potential has been generated, acetylcholine is rapidly hydrolyzed by the enzyme cholinesterase in the synaptic cleft, resulting in termination of contraction, a return to the resting state, and a supply of choline for the regeneration of acetylcholine inside the axon.

Muscle relaxants interfere with this sequence in several ways. The depolarizing neuromuscular blockers (e.g., succinylcholine) cause a depolarization of the postsynaptic muscle cell membrane similar to that produced by acetylcholine, except that depolarization persists. This results in transient contraction (fasciculation) followed by relaxation as the membrane remains depolarized and cannot respond to subsequent stimulation.

Nondepolarizing agents (e.g., pancuronium) work in a different manner. By competing directly with acetylcholine for receptor sites on the postsynaptic membrane, these agents block the depolarization caused by acetylcholine. No fasciculations occur. The action of these "competitive" neuromuscular blockers can be reversed by drugs (e.g., neostigmine) that increase the concentration of acetylcholine at the end-plate. Reversal agents inhibit the action of cholinesterase, thus slowing the breakdown of acetylcholine at the end-plate and allowing its concentration to increase to the point where it can effectively compete with the nondepolarizing agent for receptor sites and once again stimulate contraction.

In contrast to nondepolarizing agents, depolarizing agents cannot be reversed by drug therapy. Their duration of action is determined primarily by the rate of drug clearance and cannot be altered by further pharmacologic intervention.

A separate class of muscle relaxants (e.g., dantrolene) works by blocking calcium release from the sarcoplasmic reticulum within muscle cells. Agents in this class are active at the muscle cell level and do not block neural transmission at the end-plate. The agents discussed in this chapter are grouped by class in Table 25–1.

Although the preceding discussion focuses on the motor end-plate and skeletal muscle contraction, acetylcholine acts as a neurotransmitter at numerous sites in the body in addition to the neuromuscular junction. The

TABLE 25–1. Muscle Relaxants and Reversal Agents°

Neuromuscular Blocking Agents
Nondepolarizing
    pancuronium (Pavulon)
    vecuronium (Norcuron)
    atracurium (Tracrium)
    tubocurarine
    gallamine (Flaxedil)
    metocurine (Metubine Iodide)
Depolarizing
    succinylcholine (Anectine, others)
Sarcoplasmic Calcium Release Blocker
    dantrolene (Dantrium)
Reversal Agents (Anticholinesterases)
    neostigmine (Prostigmin)
    pyridostigmine (Mestinon)
    edrophonium (Tensilon)
    physostigmine (Antilirium)

°Common trade names are in parentheses.

side effects of neuromuscular blocking agents can partially be explained by the interaction of these agents with acetylcholine at other sites. Acetylcholine is a neurotransmitter within the central nervous system (CNS) and at parasympathetic ganglia (muscarinic) and sympathetic ganglia (nicotinic), as well as at skeletal muscle end-plates. Since neuromuscular blocking agents do not cross the blood–brain barrier, they do not interact with CNS acetylcholine receptors or cause CNS effects (a fact to remember when using these agents in awake patients). These agents do reach sympathetic and parasympathetic synapses, however. Depending on the drug

TABLE 25–2. Muscarinic and Nicotinic Actions of Acetylcholine

Site	Action
Muscarinic	
Sweat glands	Sweating
Pupils	Constriction
Lacrimal glands	Lacrimation
Salivary glands	Salivation
Bronchial tree	Constriction
Gastrointestinal tract	Increased motility
Heart	Bradycardia
Bladder	Contraction
Nicotinic	
Sympathetic ganglia	Tachycardia, hypertension
Skeletal muscle end-plate	Muscle contraction

°Note that, depending on drug and dosage, neuromuscular blocking agents may manifest toxicity by stimulating or inhibiting these effects of acetylcholine.

and the dose used, they may mimic or inhibit the action of acetylcholine at these sites. The common toxicities or side effects of these medications (as listed under each individual agent at the end of this chapter) are frequently due to their actions at receptors other than those at the skeletal muscle endplate. Muscarinic and nicotinic actions of acetylcholine are summarized in Table 25–2.

Emergency Uses of Muscle Relaxants

There are several emergent situations in which the clinician should consider pharmacologic muscle relaxation as an adjunct to airway or patient management (Table 25–3). The common characteristic of all these conditions is that muscle contraction causes increased morbidity or prevents needed therapeutic intervention. It should be clearly understood that neuromuscular blockers will abolish all respiratory effort, and mechanical ventilatory support will be necessary. Therefore, only individuals skilled in airway management and ventilatory support should use these agents.

Clearly, there are some patients with the conditions listed in Table 25–3 in whom the needed intervention can be accomplished without the use of muscle relaxants. For example, a gentle, blind nasotracheal intubation may avoid the need for neuromuscular blockade prior to intubation in a combative head-injured patient. Similarly, administration of an opiate or a sedative-hypnotic may make neuromuscular blockade unnecessary in suppressing movement during an emergent CT scan. These alternatives to neuromuscular blockade carry their own risks, however. Nasotracheal intubation is not always gentle or successful; sedation may not adequately suppress movement or may also depress respiratory function. A thorough understanding of the use of muscle relaxants for these indications should aid the clinician in choosing a proper approach to these difficult patient management problems.

In this context, muscle relaxants should be regarded as a valuable tool for airway management. They are an adjunct to the skills of a trained clinician and not a substitute for that skill or for experience. Optimal management of the difficult conditions that are discussed below requires skill and experience as well as the proper tools.

CONDITIONS

Acute Uses of Muscle Relaxants (Emergent Relaxation Required for Intubation)

When jaw clenching or muscular activity prevents intubation in a patient who urgently requires an endotracheal airway, muscle relaxants can be particularly useful. Common conditions that may present in this manner include head injury, status epilepticus, drug overdose, and hypoxia.

Diagnosis and Indications for Treatment
Head Injury

Recent studies have suggested that early endotracheal intubation improves outcome after severe closed head injury. Although evidence of head trauma may be obvious, the diagnosis of intracranial injuries requiring rapid intervention is more difficult. Physical signs of increased ICP clearly mandate aggressive intervention, including endotracheal intubation and hyperventilation. These signs include bradycardia, hypertension, unilateral pupillary dilation, and papille-

---

TABLE 25–3. Indications for the Use of Muscle Relaxants

Endotracheal Intubation
Head injury
    Obtunded patient requiring intubation for airway control and hyperventilation in the presence of combativeness or jaw clenching
Drug overdose
    Obtunded patient requiring gastric lavage in the presence of combativeness or jaw clenching
Status epilepticus/seizures
    Patients with prolonged seizure activity that compromises airway, ventilation, and oxygenation
Hypoxia/respiratory failure
Muscle Relaxation after Endotracheal Intubation
Suppression of patient movement during CT scanning or MRI scanning
Suppression of patient movement for ICP control
Control of agitation during helicopter transport
Facilitation of ventilation in hypoxic patient who fights the ventilator
Treatment of Pathologic Muscle Rigidity
Malignant hyperthermia
Neuroleptic malignant syndrome
Tetanus

DRUG TREATMENT: ENDOTRACHEAL INTUBATION USING MUSCLE RELAXANTS

First-Line Drug
Succinylcholine

Initial Dose	1.5 mg/kg IV push
Repeat Dose	1.5 mg/kg IV push 2–3 minutes after initial dose if adequate relaxation is not present
End-Point	Adequate relaxation to allow bag–mask ventilation and gentle orotracheal intubation
Caution	Atropine (0.01 mg/kg IV push) should be administered to children 1–3 minutes prior to succinylcholine.

Second-Line Drugs
Atracurium

Initial "Priming" Dose	0.1 mg/kg IV push
Repeat Dose	0.4 mg/kg IV push 2–3 minutes after initial dose. Used in this sequence, adequate relaxation for intubation will usually be present 1–2 minutes after the second dose.
End-Point	Adequate relaxation to allow bag–mask ventilation and gentle orotracheal intubation

OR

Vecuronium

Initial "Priming" Dose	0.02 mg/kg IV push
Repeat Dose	0.08 mg/kg IV push 2–3 minutes after initial dose. Used in this sequence, adequate relaxation for intubation will usually be present 1–2 minutes after the second dose.
End-Point	Adequate relaxation to allow bag–mask ventilation and gentle orotracheal intubation

dema. Unfortunately, these signs usually appear late in the progression of brain injury. Effective treatment should optimally be instituted before intracranial hypertension has progressed to this point.

For this reason, intubation and hyperventilation are often necessary before definitive evidence of intracranial hypertension is present. Because common causes of early morbidity and mortality in victims of closed head injury are unrecognized hypoxia, hypoventilation, and aspiration, some authorities recommend early intubation for any victim of closed head trauma whose Glasgow Coma Scale (GCS) is significantly depressed. Endotracheal intubation should be strongly

considered in any patient with altered mental status, declining level of consciousness, or decreased airway reflexes. Early airway intervention in all cases of closed head injury accompanied by a significantly depressed level of consciousness will ensure that patients with major intracranial pathology receive hyperventilation and oxygenation during the critical early stages of emergency care. After complete evaluation in a definitive care setting, including blood gas measurement, head CT scanning, and complete neurologic evaluation, an unneeded endotracheal airway can always be removed.

The optimal method of airway control in the combative patient with a significant head injury remains controversial. Endotracheal intubation carries inherent risks in such patients. Cervical spine injury may also be present and may be aggravated by neck motion during intubation. Prolonged intubation attempts may delay transport to definitive care and may worsen hypoxia. Bag–mask ventilation and blind nasotracheal intubation are alternatives to orotracheal intubation with the use of muscle relaxants in these patients. The best airway management technique in this setting is the subject of ongoing debate and study.

In many centers, orotracheal intubation after muscle relaxation is the preferred airway management technique in patients with closed head injury. Muscle relaxation allows rapid oral intubation and hyperventilation in combative, jaw-clenching patients with flailing extremities. It may also prevent cervical spinal injury due to neck movement in the patient who fights restraint and intubation. (See box.)

Seizures/Status Epilepticus

The diagnosis of seizures and status epilepticus is discussed in Chapter 10. Most seizures are of short duration and do not require invasive airway intervention. Indeed, in many instances more harm is done by unskilled attempts to secure the airway than would occur if the short seizure were allowed to run its course. Supplemental oxygenation and careful observation, along with anticonvulsant medication, are adequate treatment in these cases. In cases where seizure activity is prolonged or accompanied by airway obstruction or respiratory compromise, endotracheal intubation and ventilatory assistance are indicated.

Endotracheal intubation may be impossible during status epilepticus due to jaw clenching. Muscle relaxation will not stop seizure activity in the CNS, but it will allow endotracheal intubation, ventilation, oxygenation, and the termination of the motor activity that contributes to acidosis. Since neuromuscular blocking agents do not cross the blood–brain barrier, they have no activity against the seizure focus in the brain. Continued neuronal firing and CNS damage occur even though the outward evidence of seizure activity is abolished by paralysis. For this reason, neuromuscular blockers are always administered concomitantly with anticonvulsants and should never be used alone to treat status epilepticus. If a long-acting muscle relaxant is used in this setting, continuous electroencephalographic (EEG) monitoring should be established in order to assess continued CNS seizure activity during prolonged muscular paralysis.

Since muscle relaxants do stop the tonic–clonic activity of motor seizures, they also stop muscle lactate production, which is a major source of metabolic acidosis during status epilepticus. Controlled ventilation after endotracheal intubation corrects hypercarbia, hypoxia, and respiratory acidosis. Thus, although muscle relaxants do not treat the CNS focus of status epilepticus, they may be a useful adjunct in reversing the potentially lethal systemic derangements associated with this condition. (See box.)

Drug Overdose

Drug overdose patients, like patients with a simple grand mal seizure, usually do not require endotracheal intubation. When an obtunded or combative patient requires gastric emptying, muscle relaxants may be a useful adjunct to aid placement of an endotracheal tube for airway protection during gastric lavage. The indications for gastric lavage in overdose patients are controversial. Most authorities agree that patients who have recently (within 60 minutes) ingested a potentially fatal overdose should have some form of gastric emptying performed. Since the history is usually unreliable in such patients, other authorities recommend observation for signs of clinical intoxication prior to emptying. When a patient already is manifesting significant toxicity (i.e., hypotension, deteriorating mental status) after a recent ingestion, gastric lavage is clearly indicated. A common example of this scenario is the patient with a tricyclic antidepressant overdose who presents with obtundation and cardiac dysrhythmias.

Aspiration is a significant risk when gastric lavage is undertaken without an endotracheal airway. Gastric lavage without endotracheal intubation is best reserved for the cooperative patient with intact airway reflexes and may even then be complicated by aspiration. Since relatively few overdose patients requiring lavage are cooperative and have intact airway reflexes, muscle relaxants often prove useful in this setting. If poisoning with an organophosphate insecticide is suspected, a depolarizing agent (succinylcholine) should *not* be used. These insecticides inhibit the cholinesterases that normally metabolize succinylcholine. If succinylcholine is administered after organophosphate poisoning, apnea may persist for hours. (See box.)

Hypoxia/Respiratory Failure

Cyanosis, lethargy, and sudden slowing of the respiratory rate after a period of marked tachypnea all herald the onset of respiratory arrest in the patient with respiratory failure. When arterial blood gas results are available, a marked elevation of the pCO_2 with acute respiratory acidosis also signals the need for assisted ventilation. Patients with respiratory failure may actively resist attempts at endotracheal intubation, even when the clinical picture clearly mandates this procedure. Factors that contribute to combative behavior in such patients include hypoxia, hypercarbia, and increased dyspnea when the patients are forced to remain supine for standard oral intubation. Awake nasotracheal intubation in the sitting position should be attempted first in such patients.

Administration of a muscle relaxant should be approached with trepidation in such patients, since preexisting hypoxia and acidosis predispose to cardiac dysrhythmias or cardiac arrest after induction of apnea. Once respiratory drive has been abolished with muscle relaxation, the clinician may find such patients impossible to ventilate adequately with a bag–mask due to their underlying disease process. Whereas most patients are easier to ventilate after induction of muscle relaxation, patients with respiratory failure often have airway or pulmonary disease that makes ventilation difficult. If nasotracheal intubation is unsuccessful, orotracheal intubation without muscle relaxation should be attempted. Sedation with an opiate or a benzodiazepine may be useful in this instance. If intubation is still unsuccessful due to jaw clenching, muscle relaxation may be considered. Preoxygenation and ventilation should be optimized prior to administration of the relaxant to minimize the incidence of the complications discussed above. This is problematic, however, since oxygenation and ventilation unresponsive to other measures are the primary reasons endotracheal intubation is being attempted. When other techniques fail, muscle relaxation may be required as a last resort to aid intubation in this setting. (See box.)

Discussion

Succinylcholine is the first-line muscle relaxant for endotracheal intubation in the emergency setting. In the dosage range recommended for endotracheal intubation (1.5 mg/kg), succinylcholine has the most rapid onset of complete relaxation and the shortest duration of action of any muscle relaxant. This means that intubation can proceed sooner and paralysis will wear off sooner than with other agents. In the context of the head-injured patient, earlier onset is important since it will allow earlier hyperventilation and may speed transport to definitive care. Shorter duration is also important, since unsuccessful intubation attempts must be followed by bag–mask ventilation until paralysis resolves and spontaneous respirations return. In most cases spontaneous respirations return 5 to 10 minutes after an intubating dose of succinylcholine.

The search for newer, short-acting, nondepolarizing relaxants has continued largely because of the undesirable effects of succinylcholine. The initial depolarization caused by succinylcholine results in muscle fasciculations 30 to 60 seconds after an intubating dose. These transient fasciculations may increase intraocular pressure or displace unstable fractures, leading some clinicians to list penetrating globe injuries or long bone fractures as contraindications to the use of this agent.

It should be noted that the actual increase in intraocular pressure observed after succinylcholine administration is relatively small (<10 mmHg). Anesthesiologists at some eye hospitals use succinylcholine for crash induction of patients with globe injuries, believing the benefits of rapid onset outweigh the risk of intraocular content extrusion during induction. This theoretical complication has never actually occurred in large series of patients with penetrating eye injuries induced with succinylcholine. Displacement of fractures during fasciculations is also a theoretical risk that has rarely been reported. Fractures and eye injuries thus remain only *relative* contraindications to the use of succinylcholine.

Succinylcholine also causes a transient rise in ICP. In studies of patients undergoing neurosurgery for intracranial tumors, ICP increased an average of 5.0 mmHg after succinylcholine administration. The degree or clinical significance of this elevation in the setting of acute head injury remains unknown. ICP is also elevated in response to laryngoscopy. As is the case with eye injuries, most clinicians believe the benefits of rapid onset of induction with succinylcholine outweigh the risk of mild, transient elevation of ICP. Lidocaine, when administered in adequate doses prior to induction, has been shown to blunt the rise of ICP seen in response to succinylcholine and laryngoscopy.

Succinylcholine administration results in a transient elevation of serum potassium. In normal individuals, this elevation is usually small and not clinically important (<0.5 mEq/liter). In patients with certain disease states, however, it can be large and significant and can induce life-threatening dysrhythmias or cardiac arrest. These patients include those who may have preexisting high potassium levels (i.e., renal failure patients) and patients in whom damaged or abnormal cell membranes release large amounts of potassium in response to succinylcholine administration. Examples of the latter conditions include patients with major burns, muscle trauma, or upper motor neuron disease. The marked rise of serum potassium will only occur days to weeks after the initial insult and therefore need not be a concern in the initial treatment of trauma or burn patients.

In children, the effects of succinylcholine on the vagal ganglia are especially pronounced, as is vagal stimulation in response to laryngoscopy, leading to the common occurrence of bradycardia and, very rarely, asystole. For this reason, children should be pretreated with atropine (0.01 mg/kg) prior to succinylcholine administration. Bradycardia after succinylcholine administration should also be treated with atropine, along with simultaneous treatment of hypoxia, which may have occurred during intubation attempts.

If succinylcholine is contraindicated, a second-line agent should be used. These agents are nondepolarizing and therefore do not cause muscle fasciculations, with the attendant complications described above. When used for rapid-sequence induction and intubation, these agents are used with an initial priming dose. Use of the initial "priming" dose of the nondepolarizing relaxants will allow intubation almost as rapidly as with succinylcholine, but relaxation will persist for a much longer interval (approximately 20 to 40 minutes for atracurium and 25 to 50 minutes for vecuronium). This becomes a major disadvantage if intubation attempts are unsuccessful and bag–mask ventilations are required until spontaneous recovery of respiration occurs.

For most of the indications described above, prolonged paralysis may be undesirable. When seizures are present, the shorter duration of succinylcholine allows for earlier clinical assessment of continued seizure activity in order to assess the need for further anticonvulsant therapy. With head injury, the shorter duration of succinylcholine allows earlier reassessment of the neurologic examination in the absence of pharmacologic paralysis. Prolonged relaxation is rarely required for gastric lavage of overdose patients. Although some clinicians believe nondepolarizing agents are preferable to succinylcholine for "crash" intubations, most authorities believe succinylcholine remains the first-line drug due to its more rapid onset and shorter duration.

Since muscle relaxants do not affect the CNS, they are not a substitute for adequate sedation of a conscious patient. In such patients a sedative-hypnotic or an opiate should be administered prior to the muscle relaxant. When using nondepolarizing agents, care must be taken to maintain sedation throughout the period of neuromuscular blockade. Repetitive dosing of the sedative may be required. If the patient is paralyzed pharmacologically, outward signs that sedation is inadequate will be masked. It is a frightful experience indeed to be fully conscious *and* fully paralyzed. Empiric doses of sedatives/opiates will be required at regular intervals if prolonged muscle relaxation is induced.

Histamine release, with resultant flushing, tachycardia, and hypertension, has been a persistent problem with nondepolarizing agents. The newer nondepolarizing agents (atracurium, vecuronium) cause significant histamine release much less often than pancuronium. Vecuronium causes less histamine release than atracurium. Vecuronium is metabolized by the liver and will have a prolonged duration of action in patients with significant liver dysfunction. Atracurium is metabolized by two mechanisms (Hoffman degradation and serum cholinesterases) and is preferable to vecuronium in patients with hepatic dysfunction. General characteristics

TABLE 25–4. Characteristics of Neuromuscular Blocking Agents[*]

Drug	Metabolism	Excretion	Onset (min)	Peak Effect (min)	Duration (min)
Succinylcholine (Anectine)	Plasma pseudocholin-esterase	Renal	0.5	1.0	4–10
Pancuronium (Pavulon)	Hepatic	Renal/biliary	0.5	4.0	45–60
Atracurium (Tracrium)	Plasma esterases/ Hoffman degradation	Renal/biliary	1.5–2.0	3–5	20–60
Vecuronium (Norcuron)	Hepatic	Biliary/renal	2.5–3.0	3–5	25–65
Tubocurarine	Hepatic	Renal	1.0	2–5	25–90
Gallamine	None	Renal	1–2	3–5	15–30
Metocurine	None	Renal	1–4	3–5	60–90

[*]Times assume administration of a single dose sufficient to induce complete relaxation. Repeat dosing will prolong duration, especially if administered prior to partial recovery. Duration will be prolonged if metabolism is impaired or, in the case of nonmetabolized agents, if excretion is impaired.

of neuromuscular blocking agents are summarized in Table 25–4 and in the section on specific drugs at the end of this chapter.

Procedure for Endotracheal Intubation Using Muscle Relaxants

1. Assemble required equipment:
   Bag–valve–mask connected to functioning oxygen-delivery system
   Working suction at hand
   Endotracheal tube(s) with stylette and intact cuff
   Laryngoscope with blades and bright light
   Cricothyrotomy tray, #4 tracheostomy tube
   Atropine, 1.0 mg; muscle relaxant drawn up in labeled syringes
2. Check to be sure that a good, functioning, secure IV line is in place and running.
3. Connect patient to a cardiac monitor or pulse oximeter. One assistant assumes responsibility for administering IV premedication and muscle relaxant on the physician's order. After administration of the muscle relaxant, this assistant's main responsibility is to watch the cardiac monitor for ventricular dysrhythmia or bradycardia and a pulse oximeter for desaturation during subsequent endotracheal intubation. The physician and team member assisting with intubation should be notified immediately if dysrhythmia or a fall in O_2 saturation <90% occurs.
4. Allow the patient to breath 100% O_2 via the mask (gently assist ventilations if necessary).
5. Premedicate as appropriate:
   Diazepam, 3 to 5 mg IV push for sedation of awake patients *Alternatives:* other benzodiazepines or narcotics
   Atropine, 0.01 mg/kg IV push for children
   Lidocaine, 1.0 to 1.5 mg/kg IV push, for ICP control in head-injured patients, patients with CNS injury (hypertensive crisis, bleed), or for dysrhythmia control in patients at risk for ventricular arrhythmias
   Pancuronium, 1 mg IV push, prior to succinylcholine to prevent fasciculations
6. The third team member (a second physician or nurse) now applies cricoid pressure to occlude the esophagus until intubation is successfully completed and the endotracheal tube cuff is inflated.
7. Administer muscle relaxant.
8. After muscle fasciculations stop or after 60 to 90 seconds, demonstrate adequate relaxation by ventilating the patient 4 or 5 times with the bag–mask. Jaw relaxation and decreased resistance to bag–mask ventilation indicate that it is time to proceed with intubation.
9. Perform endotracheal intubation. If unable to intubate during the first 30-second attempt, stop and ventilate the patient with the bag–mask for 30 to 60 seconds. If inadequate relaxation is present or if laryngospasm persists and succinylcholine was the drug used, give a repeat dose of succinylcholine. If re-

peated intubation attempts fail, ventilate the patient with the bag–mask until spontaneous ventilations return (usually 6 to 10 minutes after succinylcholine administration). If endotracheal intubation fails and you are unable to adequately ventilate the patient with the bag–mask, perform cricothyrotomy.

10. Treat bradycardia occurring during intubation with atropine, 0.01 mg/kg IV push, and by temporarily halting intubation attempts and hyperventilating the patient with the bag–mask and 100% O_2.

11. Once intubation is completed, inflate the cuff and confirm endotracheal tube placement by auscultating for bilateral breath sounds.

12. Release cricoid pressure; secure the endotracheal tube.

Careful patient selection is key to the proper use of muscle relaxants in this setting. Administration of these agents commits the physician to manually ventilating the patient once paralysis has occurred. Endotracheal intubation should follow shortly thereafter. In the unlikely event that endotracheal intubation is not possible and bag–mask ventilations do not adequately ventilate the patient after paralysis, the airway must be secured by cricothyrotomy. This procedure is rarely necessary, but the required equipment for cricothyrotomy should always be at hand whenever neuromuscular blocking agents are used. These agents should be used with trepidation in cases where a cricothyrotomy would be difficult or impossible (i.e., children <2 years of age, massive neck swelling) or in cases where ventilation and intubation will be difficult after paralysis (upper airway obstruction).

Use of these agents requires the presence of a clinician who has competence in endotracheal intubation and cricothyrotomy, as well as familiarity with the contraindications and pharmacologic effects of the drug. It also requires the presence of at least two other competent assistants. When time allows, a neurologic examination should be performed prior to paralysis.

Any patient requiring emergent endotracheal intubation is assumed to have a full stomach. Fasciculations of the abdominal wall muscles may increase intragastric pressure and induce vomiting. To prevent passive aspiration of gastric contents, all intubations should be done in a "crash sequence" with continuous cricoid pressure until endotracheal tube position is confirmed and the cuff inflated. Active vomiting will not be prevented by cricoid pressure but rather requires thorough suctioning. Suctioning equipment should always be at hand and functioning prior to administration of a muscle relaxant.

Longer-Term Usages of Muscle Relaxants (Muscle Relaxation after Endotracheal Intubation)

After an endotracheal airway is secured, muscle relaxants may be indicated to prevent patient movement during critical procedures (e.g., CT scanning), to blunt rises in ICP associated with patient movement, or to allow controlled ventilation in a patient with respiratory failure who struggles against a ventilator.

It bears repeating that since these agents do not cross the blood–brain barrier, they are not a substitute for the adequate sedation of a conscious patient. When treating an awake individual, a sedative-hypnotic or an opiate should be administered prior to the muscle relaxant. When using longer-acting nondepolarizing agents, care must be taken to maintain sedation throughout the period of neuromuscular blockade. Since outward signs that sedation is inadequate will be masked by paralysis, empiric doses of sedatives/opiates will be required at regular intervals if prolonged muscle relaxation is induced.

Just as muscle relaxants abolish clinical signs of the need for sedation, they also abolish neurologic signs of significant disease. Eye opening, verbal response, motor response, and muscular reflexes are all eliminated. If the duration of paralysis is short, as with succinylcholine for endotracheal intubation, this problem is less worrisome. Normal muscular activity begins to return within minutes of intubation, often as the tube is being secured, and neurologic evaluation can then continue. When nondepolarizing agents are used for muscle relaxation, duration will be more prolonged, potentially hindering the normal neurologic evaluation of the patient.

Especially when neurologic disease is present, it becomes critical to perform an adequate neurologic examination prior to inducing muscle relaxation for prolonged intervals. In patients with head injury or focal neurologic signs prior to relaxation, progression of the deficit will be masked by paralysis. In such patients, CT scanning of the head should be performed as soon as possible in order to identify lesions requiring urgent intervention. The clinician should continue treatment for possible CNS injury (including efforts to reduce ICP) until CT results are available to guide further intervention.

Diagnosis and Indications for Treatment

Intracranial Pressure Control

Physical signs of increased ICP include bradycardia, hypertension, unilateral pupillary dilation, and papilledema. When these signs are present in the setting of acute brain injury, aggressive efforts to lower ICP are indicated. Unfortunately, these signs usually appear late in the progression of brain injury. Effective treatment should optimally be

---

DRUG TREATMENT: MUSCLE RELAXATION AFTER ENDOTRACHEAL INTUBATION

First-Line Drug
Vecuronium

Initial Dose	0.1 mg/kg IV push
Repeat Dose	0.02 mg/kg IV push
End-Point	Adequate muscle relaxation to produce immobility and allow controlled ventilation for 25 to 45 minutes

Second-Line Drugs
Succinylcholine

Initial Dose	1.5 mg/kg IV push
Repeat Dose	0.5 mg/kg IV push 2–3 minutes after initial dose if adequate relaxation is not present
End-Point	Adequate relaxation to produce immobility and allow controlled ventilation for 5–10 minutes
Caution	Pretreat children with atropine (0.01 mg/kg).

OR

Atracurium

Initial Dose	0.5 mg/kg IV push
Repeat Dose	0.1 mg/kg IV push
End-Point	Adequate relaxation to produce immobility and allow controlled ventilation for 20–40 minutes

OR

Pancuronium

Initial Dose	0.1 mg/kg IV push
Repeat Dose	0.025 mg/kg IV push
End-Point	Adequate relaxation to produce immobility and allow controlled ventilation for 45–90 minutes

instituted before intracranial hypertension has progressed to this point. In addition to elevation of the head, hyperventilation, and osmotic agents, muscle relaxants are useful in the control of intracranial hypertension.

Acute ICP elevations have been associated with endotracheal suctioning, agitation, coughing, and patient movement. Muscle relaxation prevents this elevation in ICP much more effectively than barbiturates, narcotics, or lidocaine. Paradoxically, succinylcholine administration causes a transient rise in ICP on the order of 5 mmHg. This rise is independent of muscle fasciculations and may not be clinically significant. In studies of patients with traumatic brain injuries, ICP rose an average of 22 mmHg in response to endotracheal suctioning. Pretreatment with fentanyl, thiopental, or lidocaine decreased this rise to 10 to 15 mmHg. Pretreatment with succinylcholine decreased this rise to 3 mmHg.

When intracranial hypertension is suspected, muscle relaxants are indicated if excessive patient movement must be controlled or if airway procedures (endotracheal suctioning, laryngoscopy) are required. For example, an intubated patient with a significant closed head injury who flails about during evaluation and treatment should receive muscle relaxation. Similarly, an intubated patient with a large intracranial bleed or with a large stroke accompanied by cerebral edema should receive a muscle relaxant prior to endotracheal suctioning if this procedure is required frequently and is accompanied by marked bucking and gagging. Muscle relaxation is also indicated in these patients if muscle activity prevents controlled hyperventilation. (See box.)

Controlling Patient Agitation

The administration of a neuromuscular blocking agent will certainly eliminate the outward signs of agitation. It will not eliminate the cause of the agitation and may indeed (by masking agitation as a symptom) delay diagnosis and treatment of life-threatening conditions. When the diagnosis is not in doubt, however, or when agitation prevents expeditious treatment for the underlying disorder, muscle relaxation may be indicated. The combative head-injured patient whose agitation causes rises in ICP and prevents diagnostic studies is an example of the latter scenario. Such patients are commonly

transported by helicopter; muscle relaxation may make transport safer in these instances.

Some centers have used muscle relaxants to facilitate the initial evaluation and resuscitation of agitated or uncooperative multiple trauma patients with life-threatening injuries, even in the absence of closed head injury. The use of muscle relaxants in this setting remains controversial. Alternatives to muscle relaxation include physical restraint and/or pharmacologic sedation using opiates, antipsychotics, or sedative-hypnotics. When immediate intervention is required, muscle relaxants may be preferable in such cases.

It should always be remembered that the underlying cause of patient agitation remains after relaxation and must be sought out, diagnosed, and simultaneously treated. It is a common error to forget to treat disorders such as hypoglycemia or hypoxia after the outward signs of agitation are eliminated by neuromuscular blockade. (See box.)

Controlled Ventilation

Critically ill patients frequently require mechanical ventilation. The interfacing of the mechanical ventilator and the patient can become quite difficult because of hypoxia, hypercarbia, acidemia, pain, apprehension, cerebral dysfunction, increased airway resistance, and decreased lung or chest wall compliance. Even as blood gases are returned toward normal, some patients continue to fight the ventilator; this incoordination of man and machine can seriously hinder oxygenation and ventilation as well as cause disturbances in hemodynamics (usually tachycardia and hypertension). Fortunately, sedative-hypnotics, analgesics, hyperventilation, intermittent mandatory ventilation (IMV), and/or tracheostomy usually can produce a successful man-machine interaction.[*]

There are conditions where other methods fail or where muscle relaxants may be preferable to other methods to allow controlled ventilation. Such instances may include severe status asthmaticus, tetanus, severe bronchiolitis, and adult respiratory distress syndrome. Muscle relaxation may increase chest wall compliance and decrease the incidence of complications associated with high peak airway pressures (i.e., pneumothorax). Muscle relaxation is indicated when

[*]Kravitz M, Pace NL: Management of the mechanically ventilated patient receiving pancuronium bromide. Heart Lung, 8:81–86, 1979.

muscle activity consistently decreases the effectiveness of controlled ventilation. (See box.)

Relaxation During Procedures

Patient immobility is sometimes critical to the successful completion of urgent diagnostic or therapeutic procedures. This is a major reason for the use of muscle relaxants in the operating room, and it is applicable to emergent and critical care settings as well. Head CT scanning of the disoriented or combative patient is a common situation where immobility is essential.

Immobility of the cervical spine before and during radiographic imaging can be improved by administration of muscle relaxants. Muscle relaxation may also aid visualization of the seven cervical vertebrae with standard cross-table lateral radiographs. Ventilatory assistance must be available and maintained throughout any procedure until relaxation wears off. In most cases this means that the agent with the shortest duration that will allow completion of the procedure should be used.

Sedative-hypnotics or opiates can also be used to accomplish this same purpose; however, immobility is less certain and delays in

TABLE 25–5. Factors That May Vary the Response to Neuromuscular Blockade

Factor	Effect	Agents Affected
Other Drugs		
Aminoglycosides	Prolonged duration of relaxation	All
Lidocaine (>5 mg/kg)	Prolonged duration of relaxation	All
Local anesthetics	Prolonged duration of relaxation	All
Trimethaphan	Prolonged duration of relaxation	All
Narcotics	Prolonged respiratory depression	All
Inhaled anesthetic agents	Prolonged duration of relaxation	All
Antimyasthenics (edrophonium)	Antagonize relaxation	Nondepolarizing agents
Calcium salts	Antagonize relaxation	Nondepolarizing agents
Beta-blockers	Prolong relaxation	Pancuronium Tubocurarine
Insecticides	Inhibit pseudocholinesterase	Succinylcholine
Cyclophosphamide	Prolong relaxation	Succinylcholine
Thiopental	Prolong relaxation	Succinylcholine
Digoxin	Increased cardiac effects	Succinylcholine
	Cardiac dysrhythmias	Pancuronium
Lithium	Prolonged relaxation	Succinylcholine Atracurium
Magnesium-procainamide, quinidine	Prolonged relaxation	All
Potassium-depleting medications	Prolonged relaxation	Nondepolarizing agents
Medical Conditions		
Burns (severe)	Hyperkalemia, cardiac dysrhythmias	Succinylcholine
Digoxin toxicity		
Neuromuscular disease	Hyperkalemia, cardiac dysrhythmias	Succinylcholine
Paraplegia	Hyperkalemia, cardiac dysrhythmias	Succinylcholine
Trauma (severe)	Hyperkalemia, cardiac dysrhythmias	Succinylcholine
(All > one week after onset)	Hyperkalemia, cardiac dysrhythmias	Succinylcholine
Bronchogenic carcinoma	Prolonged relaxation	All
Pseudocholinesterase deficiency (hereditary, pregnancy, dehydration, anemia, etc.)	Prolonged relaxation	Succinylcholine
Eye injury, glaucoma	Increased intraocular pressure	Succinylcholine
Unstable fractures	Fasciculations–fracture displacement	Succinylcholine
Liver disease	Decreased pseudocholinesterase, prolonged action	Succinylcholine
	Decreased metabolism, prolonged action	Vecuronium
Hyperthermia	Decreased activity	Succinylcholine
	Increased activity	Nondepolarizing agents
Hypothermia	Increased activity	Succinylcholine
	Decreased activity	Nondepolarizing agents
Myasthenia gravis	Prolonged duration	All
Renal dysfunction	Prolonged duration	Succinylcholine Pancuronium Gallamine

completing a critical procedure may be encountered while slowly titrating these alternative agents to effect. If an endotracheal airway is already in place, muscle relaxants may be the preferred method for inducing immobility during procedures. (See box.)

Discussion

By tailoring the drug and dosage of the drug to the duration of desired muscle relaxation, the clinician can minimize the problems associated with symptoms being masked by prolonged paralysis (i.e., seizures, progressing neurologic deficits, inadequate sedation) (see Table 25–4). Succinylcholine has the shortest onset and duration of action. For decades, these characteristics have secured its place as the primary muscle relaxant for intubation, despite the toxic side effects associated with muscle fasciculations, potassium release, and malignant hyperthermia. When the airway is already secured, rapid onset of action is less important. The increased safety of nondepolarizing agents (no muscle fasciculations, no potassium release) usually makes them preferable to succinylcholine for this indication, unless very short duration is clinically necessary. Children should be pretreated with *atropine (0.01 mg/kg IV push)* prior to succinylcholine use to prevent significant bradycardia, which commonly occurs in this age group.

The duration of muscle relaxation is dependent on the drug and dose given and on a variety of patient characteristics listed in Table 25–5. Organ failure, medications, disease states, and exogenous toxins may all prolong duration of action. In general, succinylcholine has the shortest duration of action, followed by atracurium, vecuronium, and pancuronium, respectively. In the dosage range recommended, relaxation after the initial dose usually lasts less than 10 minutes with succinylcholine, 20 to 40 minutes with atracurium, 25 to 45 minutes with vecuronium, and 45 to 90 minutes with pancuronium. Since pancuronium is excreted by the kidneys, its duration will be prolonged in renal failure. Vecuronium is metabolized by the liver and secreted in the bile. Duration will be prolonged in the setting of hepatic failure or biliary tract obstruction. Atracurium is metabolized by two independent pathways, and duration is usually not affected by renal or hepatic dysfunction. The relaxant effects of pancuronium are cumulative; duration is much greater with additional doses than with the initial dose. For this reason, dosage should be decreased significantly when giving additional doses of pancuronium.

Nondepolarizing agents (pancuronium, vecuronium, atracurium) control transient elevations in ICP without causing the initial transient ICP rise seen with succinylcholine. Nondepolarizing agents are therefore used more commonly than succinylcholine for this indication, although the clinical significance of the mild, transient ICP elevation seen with succinylcholine administration (5 mmHg) may be minimal.

Procedure for Muscle Relaxation After Endotracheal Intubation

1. Ensure that the endotracheal tube is in working order and in the proper position above the carina. Be sure the patient is receiving supplemental oxygen.
2. Assemble required equipment:
   Bag–valve–mask connected to functioning oxygen-delivery system (A ventilator should be used if prolonged relaxation is planned.)
   Working suction with suction tip attached
   Labeled syringe drawn up with muscle relaxant
3. The following equipment should be readily available for possible use in the event of inadvertent extubation after paralysis:
   Endotracheal tube(s) with stylette and intact cuff
   Laryngoscope with blades and bright light
   Cricothyrotomy tray and #4 tracheostomy tube
4. Check to be sure that a functioning, secure IV line is in place and running.
5. Connect patient to a cardiac monitor or pulse oximeter. One assistant assumes responsibility for administering IV premedication and the neuromuscular blocking agent on the physician's order. After administration of the drug, this assistant's main responsibility is to watch the cardiac monitor for dysrhythmias or bradycardia or the pulse oximeter for a fall in O_2 saturation.
6. In awake/oriented patients, use sedation (e.g., *diazepam*, 3 to 5 mg IV push).
7. Administer muscle relaxant.

8. If assisted ventilation is not already in progress, begin ventilating the patient as paralysis takes effect (usually 2 to 3 minutes after administration).

9. Repeat doses can be given if muscular activity begins to return sooner than desired.

10. Repeat sedation should be considered every 30 to 60 minutes in conscious patients who require continued paralysis.

11. In some cases where prolonged paralysis causes a problem in diagnosis or patient management, it may be appropriate to use pharmacologic reversal (see next section).

Use of these agents requires an endotracheal airway. Sedation, using an agent such as diazepam or lorazepam, should be administered prior to paralyzing any conscious patient. All members of the medical team should be aware that paralyzed patients, although appearing unconscious, are fully awake and aware of their surroundings unless adequate sedation is given. When time allows, a neurologic examination should be performed prior to relaxation. The presence of a mechanical ventilator does not obviate the need for constant supervision when neuromuscular blocking agents are used for this indication. Inadvertent ventilator disconnection will cause death if not detected and corrected promptly. All ventilator alarms must be functional and "on," and the patient must be constantly supervised to prevent this potential disaster.

Reversal of Neuromuscular Blockade

Diagnosis

Occasionally, prolonged paralysis after the administration of neuromuscular blocking agents presents a problem in patient evaluation or management. Pharmacologic reversal of drug-induced muscle relaxation may be useful in these cases. This technique is commonly used in the operating room to eliminate residual effects of the relaxants as an aid to extubation at the end of surgery. In emergency and critical care settings, the need for reversal is less frequently encountered. In most cases it is safer and simpler to allow normal drug metabolism and excretion to clear the neuromuscular agent while continuing treatment for the patient's underlying disorder. Selection of the proper agent (see

Table 25–4) should ensure that relaxation will resolve after the desired interval.

Pharmacologic reversal is useful primarily when nondepolarizing agents have been used. Even with nondepolarizing agents, reversal is not immediate, especially if only a short interval has passed since the muscle relaxant was administered. Sufficient acetylcholine must accumulate at the end-plate to successfully compete with the muscle relaxant. A peripheral nerve stimulator can be used to evaluate train-of-four response or response to tetanic stimulation. When the train-of-four response is returning to normal, relaxant concentrations at the end-point are decreasing to the point where reversal can be relied on to restore normal neuromuscular transmission.

Indications for Treatment

If drug metabolism is abnormally prolonged, muscle relaxation may linger even after the underlying condition has resolved. Certain drugs and conditions can lengthen the duration of neuromuscular blockade beyond a period that is clinically useful (see Table 25–5). It may also become necessary to reverse neuromuscular blockade in order to obtain a reliable neurologic examination and to discover if a neurologic deficit is progressing. In patients with head injury, this necessity may arise when CT scanning is not available or is unexpectedly delayed.

Neuromuscular blocking agents can be antagonized by increasing the concentration of acetylcholine at the motor end-plate. This will favor acetylcholine–receptor interactions over relaxant–receptor interactions and ultimately lead to a return of normal neuromuscular conduction. This process will only work if the relaxant is competitive; that is, if the relaxant competes with acetylcholine for receptors. Depolarizing agents (succinylcholine) are noncompetitive and therefore cannot be reversed pharmacologically in most circumstances. (See box.)

Discussion

These agents should be administered by slow intravenous push. The patient should be on a cardiac monitor. Reversal will only be effective when a nondepolarizing block has already begun to resolve. It will not be effective immediately after administration of a nondepolarizing agent, nor will it work for depolarizing agents (succinylcholine). Glycopyrrolate (0.2 mg for every 1.0 mg of neo-

DRUG TREATMENT: REVERSAL OF NEUROMUSCULAR BLOCKADE

First-Line Drug Combination

Neostigmine and *Atropine*

Initial Dose	Neostigmine, 0.05 mg/kg, and atropine, 15 μg/kg (normal adult dose: 2 mg neostigmine/1.0 mg atropine) Total initial dose not to exceed 5.0 mg
Repeat Dose	Not recommended (see Discussion)
End-Point	Return of normal train-of-four response to peripheral nerve stimulator and return of muscular tone/spontaneous respirations

Second-Line Drug Combination

Pyridostigmine and *Atropine*

Initial Dose	Pyridostigmine, 0.2 mg/kg, and atropine, 15 μg/kg (normal adult dose: 15 mg pyridostigmine/1.0 mg atropine)
Repeat Dose	Not recommended (see Discussion)
End-Point	Return of normal train-of-four response to peripheral nerve stimulator and return of muscular tone/spontaneous respirations

OR

Edrophonium and *Atropine*

Initial Dose	Edrophonium, 0.5 mg/kg, and atropine, 7 μg/kg (normal adult dose: 35 mg edrophonium/0.5 mg atropine), mixed thoroughly in same syringe
Repeat Dose	0.5 mg/kg 10 minutes after initial dose
End-Point	Return of normal train-of-four response to peripheral nerve stimulator and return of muscular tone/spontaneous respirations or maximum dose of 40 mg reached

stigmine or every 5 mg of pyridostigmine) can be used instead of atropine but should be administered several minutes before the anticholinesterase owing to its more delayed onset of action. Tachycardia from the atropine will usually occur 30 to 60 seconds after administration and will resolve in 5 to 10 minutes as the anticholinesterase begins to work. If atropine is not given, significant bradycardia may occur. Edrophonium should be used only after single doses of shorter-acting relaxants (atracurium, vecuronium) since its duration of action may be shorter than that of long-acting muscle relaxants, resulting in the possibility of a return of paralysis after the edrophonium wears off. Edrophonium's onset of action is faster (1 to 2 minutes) than that of neostigmine or pyridostigmine (3 to 5 minutes). As shorter-acting nondepolarizing agents (vecuronium, atracurium) become more popular, edrophonium may become more widely used as a reversal agent.

At large doses, physostigmine will reverse neuromuscular blockade. This drug crosses the blood–brain barrier, however, and produces CNS excitatory effects at the dosage required for reversal (4 to 8 mg). This untoward effect, in addition to a relatively slow onset of action, limits the usefulness of physostigmine for reversal.

Pyridostigmine and neostigmine are the most common agents used for neuromuscular reversal. Neostigmine has a slightly faster time of onset and time to peak activity than pyridostigmine. Neostigmine effects peak at 7 to 10 minutes, compared to 12 to 16 minutes for pyridostigmine. Onset time is usually 3 to 5 minutes but will vary depending on relaxant concentration at the motor endplate at the time of administration. In assessing onset and effect, the clinician should look at the patient rather than at the clock. The return of a normal response to peripheral nerve stimulation and the return of normal sustained muscle activity are indicators of successful reversal.

It should be remembered that in most cases it is safer to allow normal drug metabolism and excretion to clear the neuromuscular agent. Once a reversal agent has been administered, it will be difficult to reinduce muscle relaxation for a prolonged interval—a factor to keep in mind if the therapeutic effects of relaxation may still be required for patient management. The doses outlined above are sufficient to reverse neuromuscular blockade in the vast majority of individuals. Failure to respond to the initial dose should suggest that the patient was not ready for reversal (i.e., nondepolarizing block has not yet begun to resolve or the reversal agent was administered too soon after the nondepolarizing relaxant). Repeat dosing is not recommended in this situation because it will increase the toxic effects of the reversal agents without affecting neuromuscular blockade. Repeat doses of edrophonium may be required if relaxation recurs after initial reversal with this agent.

Malignant Hyperthermia

Diagnosis

Malignant hyperthermia is an inherited abnormality of the skeletal muscle membrane. In response to certain stresses or drugs (Table 25–6), patients with this disorder sus-

TABLE 25–6. Triggers for Malignant
Hyperthermia

Drugs
Halothane
Methoxyflurane
Enflurane
Diethyl ether
Cyclopropane
Succinylcholine
Tubocurarine
Lidocaine
Mepivacaine
(?) Nitrous oxide
(?) Isoflurane
(?) Gallamine
Conditions
Heat stress
Vigorous exercise
(?) Emotional stress

tain a massive efflux of calcium from skeletal muscle sarcoplasmic reticulum, resulting in contraction of the sarcomeres, skeletal muscle rigidity, increased skeletal muscle metabolism and heat production, and finally systemic hyperthermia. Hyperthermia is a late development, occurring after rigidity has been present for some time and the body's normal heat dissipation mechanisms have been overwhelmed. The earliest signs of malignant hyperthermia are increased carbon dioxide production, muscle rigidity, and tachycardia with increasing cardiac output and cutaneous blood flow to increase heat loss. The diagnosis of malignant hyperthermia can be confirmed by muscle biopsy and subsequent testing of muscle cells for calcium release in response to various agents. This test is useful in the preoperative testing of the relatives of persons with a history of malignant hyperthermia.

Malignant hyperthermia is diagnosed based on the clinical triad of (1) exposure to an agent or stress known to trigger the condition (see Table 25–6), (2) skeletal muscle rigidity, and (3) hyperthermia. High levels of expired carbon dioxide (from high skeletal muscle metabolism) may also indicate this diagnosis. Rapid resolution after treatment with dantrolene sodium is strongly suggestive. The diagnosis can be confirmed by muscle biopsy after the syndrome has resolved.

Malignant hyperthermia is usually encountered in the operating room while patients are undergoing general anesthesia. Cases of malignant hyperthermia may be encountered anywhere that general anesthetics or neuromuscular blocking agents are used. Patients with malignant hyperthermia triggered by environmental or emotional stress may present to the emergency department. Complications of malignant hyperthermia include circulatory collapse, acidosis, coagulopathy, myoglobinuria with acute tubular necrosis, and hyperthermic organ damage.

Indications for Treatment

Successful treatment of malignant hyperthermia requires early diagnosis and prompt drug therapy. The clinical suspicion of this diagnosis may be enough to justify a trial of dantrolene therapy. Patients who present with the clinical triad of muscle rigidity, hyperthermia, and exposure to a triggering agent (see Table 25–6) should receive dantrolene. Since a prompt response to this drug helps make the diagnosis, a trial of dantro-

DRUG TREATMENT: MALIGNANT HYPERTHERMIA

First-Line Drug

Dantrolene Sodium

Initial Dose	1.0 mg/kg IV push
Repeat Doses	1.0 mg/kg IV push every 1–3 minutes
End-Point	Muscle relaxation (no detectable rigidity) or total dose of 10 mg/kg

lene may be indicated before the diagnosis is confirmed.

The history of exposure to a triggering agent may not be available. Many conditions other than malignant hyperthermia may present with hyperthermia and muscle rigidity (i.e., cocaine overdose, status epilepticus). In cases of muscle rigidity and hyperthermia of unknown etiology, dantrolene should be administered if standard measures fail to induce relaxation and lower body temperature. (See box.)

Discussion

Once the diagnosis of malignant hyperthermia is suspected, the precipitating drug or stimulus should be discontinued immediately. This means stopping all surgical procedures and discontinuing all anesthetic or neuroleptic agent(s) that may be in use. The patient should be placed on 100% oxygen. If the patient is not intubated, the airway should be assessed and endotracheal intubation and controlled ventilation should be considered. Cooling measures should be instituted as the dantrolene is being prepared. Other drugs may be indicated for supportive care (mannitol to maintain brisk urine output if myoglobinuria occurs, bicarbonate to correct metabolic acidosis, pressors to maintain blood pressure and cardiac output).

Dantrolene is poorly soluble in water. To promote solubility for parenteral administration, each 20 mg of dantrolene is supplied in a vial that also contains 3.0 g of mannitol and sufficient sodium hydroxide to yield a solution pH of 9.5 when reconstituted with 60 ml of sterile water. Several minutes of agitation may be required to get the drug into solution. If extravasated, dantrolene solution may cause tissue necrosis because of its alkaline pH. Dantrolene availability may be a problem. Malignant hyperthermia occurs in-

frequently in the operating room and even less often in other critical care settings. Dantrolene is rarely stocked with emergency drug supplies in critical care or emergency units. Although rapid administration of this agent is key to proper treatment, the clinician may have to wait a prolonged interval while the drug is obtained and reconstituted. For this reason, the clinician should begin efforts to obtain and reconstitute the drug as soon as the diagnosis of malignant hyperthermia is suspected.

Treatment of malignant hyperthermia requires elimination of the triggering factor as well as administration of an agent (dantrolene sodium) that blocks calcium release at the level of the sarcoplasmic reticulum. Since the genetic disorder of malignant hyperthermia involves skeletal muscle membranes (below the level of the neuromuscular junction), neuromuscular blocking agents will not reverse muscle rigidity in malignant hyperthermia. In fact, succinylcholine is one of the most common pharmacologic triggers implicated in malignant hyperthermia. Standard cooling and supportive measures must be instituted simultaneously with dantrolene administration.

Neuroleptic Malignant Syndrome

Diagnosis

Neuroleptic malignant syndrome (NMS) was first described in the late 1960s and is characterized by fever, muscle rigidity, altered level of consciousness, and autonomic instability. This uncommon disorder follows the therapeutic use of neuroleptic drugs, including phenothiazines, butyrophenones, thioxanthenes, lithium, and tricyclic antidepressants. Muscle rigidity can manifest as oculogyric crisis, dyskinesia, akinesia, dysphagia, dysarthria, or opisthotonos. Temperatures can reach 107°F (42°C) or higher. Initial agitation often progresses to stupor and coma. Catatonia and mutism may also be present. Autonomic instability is manifested as tachycardia, hypotension or hypertension, sweating, and incontinence. Ventilations may be impaired by chest wall rigidity.

This syndrome is more likely to occur at the initiation or after an increase in neuroleptic dosage. It may occur if antiparkinsonian drugs are suddenly discontinued. NMS resembles malignant hyperthermia but usually takes considerably longer to develop (2 to 3 days) and lasts longer (5 to 10 days) after the inciting drug is discontinued. Mortality is high (30%) and is usually caused by respiratory failure, renal failure, cardiovascular collapse, or thromboembolic disease. Unlike malignant hyperthermia, NMS is thought to be caused by a central disorder of thermoregulation. Neuromuscular function is normal; either neuromuscular blocking agents or dantrolene will reverse the muscle rigidity associated with this condition.

Indications for Treatment

The presence of muscle rigidity alone in a patient on neuroleptic agents may justify a trial of oral dantrolene therapy. When muscle rigidity is accompanied by fever, altered mental status, and autonomic instability, parenteral dantrolene administration is indicated. For example, a patient who presents from a psychiatric institution with fever, coma, and muscle rigidity should receive dantrolene as both a diagnostic and therapeutic aid. A patient with Parkinson's disease who recently stopped taking his medications and now presents with stupor, hyperpyrexia, hypotension, and muscle rigidity should also receive intravenous dantrolene. The response to drug treatment may help confirm the diagnosis. (See box.)

Discussion

Fewer than 100 cases of NMS have been reported since the original description of this disorder in 1968. The recommended treatment is therefore based on limited clinical experience. Dantrolene and bromocriptine have been used successfully (alone or in combination) to treat reported cases. Neuromuscular blocking agents combined with benzodiazepines have been used with less success.

Treatment of severe NMS (i.e., hypotension, hyperthermia, marked rigidity) closely follows that of malignant hyperthermia, with the noted difference that therapy must be maintained for several days until symptoms resolve. Discontinuation of the triggering neuroleptic, cooling, and supportive treatment for ensuing organ failure remain cornerstones of therapy. Bromocriptine is only available in oral form, limiting its usefulness to less severe cases or to use concomitantly with dantrolene. Oral dantrolene and bromocriptine can be administered after reso-

---

DRUG TREATMENT: NEUROLEPTIC MALIGNANT SYNDROME

First-Line Drug
Dantrolene Sodium

Initial Dose	1.0 mg/kg IV push
Repeat Doses	1.0 mg/kg IV push every 1–3 minutes
End-Point	Muscle relaxation (no detectable rigidity) or total dose of 10 mg/kg

Second-Line Drug
Bromocriptine Mesylate

Initial Dose	5.0-mg tablet PO
Repeat Doses	2.5 mg PO every 8 hours
End-Point	Muscle relaxation (no detectable rigidity)

lution of the acute symptoms to maintain relaxation over the days to weeks it takes for this syndrome to resolve. Osmotic diuretics, pressors, ventilatory support, and anticoagulation are frequently required adjunctive treatments.

As mentioned previously, dantrolene is poorly soluble in water. Several minutes of agitation may be required to get the drug into solution. If extravasated, dantrolene solution may cause tissue necrosis owing to its alkaline pH. Dantrolene availability may be a problem. NMS is a rare condition that is infrequently diagnosed in critical care settings. Dantrolene is rarely stocked with emergency drug supplies in critical care or emergency units. Treatment of NMS also requires elimination of the triggering factor. Neuroleptic agents should be discontinued as soon as the diagnosis is suspected.

SPECIFIC AGENTS

Atracurium Besylate (Tracrium)

Pharmacology

Atracurium is an intermediate-duration, nondepolarizing skeletal muscle relaxant. Atracurium loses potency slowly when refrigerated and more rapidly at room temperature. The drug should be used within 14 days of removal from refrigeration.

Distribution

Atracurium administered by bolus injection is rapidly distributed to the intravascular and extracellular compartments. The drug does not cross the blood–brain barrier. Small amounts do cross the placenta. The exact volume of distribution has not been identified.

Elimination

Atracurium is metabolized in the plasma by two mechanisms: ester hydrolysis, catalyzed by nonspecific esterases, and Hoffman degradation. The metabolites are inactive and are later excreted in the bile and urine. Neither renal nor kidney function is required for drug inactivation and elimination.

Actions

Atracurium competes with acetylcholine for cholinergic receptors at the motor endplate. The resultant neuromuscular blockade is nondepolarizing; fasciculations do not occur.

Indications

Atracurium is indicated for intermediate-duration muscle relaxation in clinical settings where muscle contraction or voluntary movement may impede therapeutic interventions. This includes use for intracranial pressure control, for agitation control, and as an aid to controlled ventilation, and to suppress patient movement during critical procedures.

This drug is also indicated as an adjunct for endotracheal intubation, including use for patients in whom succinylcholine is contraindicated. Onset of action is not as fast as with succinylcholine; duration of action is longer than with succinylcholine but shorter than with vecuronium.

Cautions

RENAL FAILURE. No modification of dosage is needed.

HEPATIC FAILURE. No modification of dosage is needed.

CARDIAC FAILURE. A 20 to 40% decrease in the initial dose and incremental administration over 1 minute are recommended in any patient with significant cardiovascular disease or with a history (asthma, anaphylactic reactions) suggesting a greater risk of histamine release.

USE IN PREGNANCY. Category C. Atracurium is potentially teratogenic in rabbit studies; no human studies in early pregnancy exist to date. Atracurium has been used during labor and delivery without adverse effect on the newborn. Small amounts of the drug are recovered in cord blood. Repeated dosing for a prolonged period prior to delivery may cause flaccid paralysis in the newborn.

USE IN PEDIATRIC PATIENTS. Safety and effectiveness in children below the age of 1 month have not been established.

OTHER. A few cases have been reported where malignant hyperthermia occurred after administration of atracurium in addition to other agents known to trigger this disorder. Atracurium is probably not a triggering agent for malignant hyperthermia, although more extensive experience may be required to prove this.

Onset and Duration of Action

Dosage

Adults and children older than 2 years: 0.5 mg/kg IV push

Children 1 month to 2 years: 0.3 to 0.4 mg/kg IV push

Atracurium is compatible with all intravenous solutions except lactated Ringer's. Spontaneous degradation of the drug occurs more rapidly in lactated Ringer's; this fluid should not be used as a diluent.

Limits

Onset of action after an initial bolus is 1.5 to 2 minutes, with peak relaxation after 3 to 5 minutes. Time to peak relaxation can be decreased by using a priming dose (20% of the initial dose 2 to 3 minutes before the initial dose is administered). Duration of relaxation with 0.5 mg/kg is 20 to 60 minutes. Additional doses should be administered based on the need for continued relaxation in the face of resolving blockade. Since atracurium lacks cumulative effects, total dosage is limited only by clinical evidence of prolonged relaxation in individual patients.

Repeat Dosing

Repeat doses of 0.1 mg/kg may be administered 20 to 60 minutes after the initial dose and should be based on the response to peripheral nerve stimulation or the return of spontaneous muscle activity.

Toxicity

Drug Interactions (See Table 25–5)

Prior use of succinylcholine does not prolong the effect of atracurium but will speed onset and increase depth of relaxation induced with atracurium. Volatile anesthetics (enflurane, halothane, isoflurane), antibiotics (aminoglycosides, tetracyclines), lithium, magnesium salts, procainamide, and quinidine may prolong the duration of relaxation with atracurium.

Adverse Effects

Less than 1% of patients have reactions attributable to histamine release after atracurium administration. These reactions include skin flushing, itching, wheezing, hives, and hypotension. Histamine release is more common in patients with underlying cardiovascular or allergic (e.g., asthma) disorders.

Prolonged relaxation is rarely a problem with this intermediate-acting muscle relaxant.

Since atracurium does not cross into the brain, it has no CNS effects. Adequate anesthesia or sedation should always be administered concomitantly with this agent.

Treatment of Toxicity

Most histamine reactions are self-limited and require no specific treatment. Severe reactions respond to antihistamines (diphenhydramine, 25 to 50 mg IV bolus) and bronchodilators.

Prolonged relaxation can be reversed with anticholinesterases (see Reversal of Neuromuscular Blockage, earlier in this chapter).

Dantrolene Sodium (Dantrium)

Pharmacology

Dantrolene is a direct-acting skeletal muscle relaxant. The intravenous preparation is supplied in 70-ml vials containing 20 mg of dantrolene, 3 g of mannitol, and sodium hydroxide to yield a solution of pH 9.5 when reconstituted with sterile water.

Distribution

Significant amounts of dantrolene are reversibly bound to plasma proteins and red blood cells after intravenous administration. Serum half-life is 5 hours. Volume of distribution and the ability of this drug to cross the blood–brain barrier have not been determined. Dantrolene readily crosses the placenta.

Elimination

Dantrolene is metabolized in the liver (probably by microsomal enzymes) to 5-hydroxydantrolene and other metabolites. Most of an administered dose is excreted in the urine as metabolites. A small amount of unchanged dantrolene is excreted in the urine.

Actions

Dantrolene interferes with the release of calcium from the sarcoplasmic reticulum of skeletal muscle. This action, in turn, blocks excitation-contraction coupling and induces skeletal muscle relaxation. The site of action is beyond the level of the myoneural junction; this drug's action is not dependent on acetylcholine-mediated neural transmission.

Indications

Dantrolene is indicated for treatment of skeletal muscle rigidity resulting from malignant hyperthermia and neuroleptic malignant syndrome.

Cautions

RENAL FAILURE. No modification of dosage is needed.

HEPATIC FAILURE. No modification of dosage is needed. Long-term oral use of this agent is associated with hepatotoxicity. Toxicity has not been a problem with short-term intravenous use for hyperthermic crisis.

CARDIAC FAILURE. No modification of dosage is needed. There is no effect on cardiac or smooth muscle at recommended dosage. Long-term oral use is associated with pleural effusion and pericarditis.

USE IN PPREGNANCY. Category C. Animal studies show an adverse effect of dantrolene on embryo survival in rats and rabbits. The drug readily crosses the placenta. Low oral doses administered to women prior to delivery did not result in newborn cardiac or respiratory depression.

USE IN PEDIATRIC PATIENTS. No modification of dosage is needed.

PULMONARY FAILURE (COPD). No modification of dosage is needed. Chronic oral use of dantrolene in patients with obstructive pulmonary disease is associated with respiratory depression and pleural effusion.

Onset and Duration of Action

Dosage

Adult and children: 1 mg/kg rapid IV push

Limits

10 mg/kg total dose

Repeat Dosing

In the setting of malignant hyperthermia the drug should be administered continuously in 1 mg/kg increments every 1 to 3 minutes until symptoms (muscle rigidity) have subsided or the maximum dose (10 mg/kg) is reached. Duration of action of the intravenous preparation is 4 to 8 hours. After resolution of a hyperthermic crisis, oral dantrolene should be administered for 1 to 3 days (5 mg/kg/day divided every 6 hours) beginning within 6 hours of the initial intravenous dose.

Toxicity

Drug Interactions

Alcohol, CNS depressants, and magnesium salts may cause increased CNS depression when used concurrently with dantrolene. Combined use of dantrolene and verapamil has resulted in hyperkalemia and ventricular fibrillation in swine. Calcium channel blockers should not be administered with dantrolene in the clinical setting of malignant hyperthermia.

Adverse Effects

The most significant adverse effects of dantrolene are seen with chronic oral administration (hepatotoxicity, pericarditis, seizures). These effects are not seen with short-term (up to 3 days) use.

Common adverse effects with short-term use include diarrhea, dizziness, drowsiness, malaise, muscle weakness, nausea, and abdominal cramps.

Extravasation of the drug can cause soft tissue necrosis and sloughing due to the alkaline pH of the solution.

Rare adverse effects that have been reported after intravenous administration of dantrolene for malignant hyperthermia include pulmonary edema, thrombophlebitis, urticaria, and cutaneous flushing. Causation by dantrolene has not been established in these cases.

Treatment of Toxicity

Common adverse effects of intravenous dantrolene are self-limited. Rare severe effects require symptomatic and supportive care. There is no antidote.

Edrophonium Chloride (Tensilon)

Pharmacology

Edrophonium is a short-acting cholinesterase inhibitor that is structurally related to neostigmine. It is supplied in solution that is pH corrected to 5.4.

Distribution

After intravenous administration, 15 to 25% of the administered dose is bound to serum albumin. Plasma half-life is 47 to 60 minutes. This drug does not cross the blood–brain barrier in appreciable quantities. It is not known whether edrophonium crosses the placenta or is excreted in breast milk.

Elimination

Edrophonium is hydrolyzed by plasma cholinesterase and is also metabolized by hepatic microsomal enzymes. Fifty percent of an administered dose is excreted unchanged in the urine. Another 30% is excreted in the urine as metabolites.

Actions

Edrophonium inhibits destruction of acetylcholine by acetylcholinesterase. Increased concentration of acetylcholine improves transmission of nerve impulses across the myoneural junction.

The drug also mimics acetylcholine and has a direct effect on skeletal muscle and, to a lesser degree, on autonomic ganglia.

Edrophonium has a more rapid onset and a shorter duration of action than neostigmine.

Indications

Edrophonium is indicated for reversal of nondepolarizing neuromuscular blocking agents. Prolonged muscle relaxation with these agents can be reversed by increasing the concentration of acetylcholine at the motor end-plate.

Edrophonium is also indicated for treatment and diagnosis of myasthenia gravis.

Cautions

RENAL FAILURE. No modification of dosage is needed.

HEPATIC FAILURE. No modification of dosage is needed.

CARDIAC FAILURE. In severe cardiac failure, the dose can be slowly titrated to effect using a peripheral nerve stimulator. If bradycardia is present, heart rate should be increased to 80 or greater using atropine prior to edrophonium administration.

USE IN PREGNANCY. Category C. Anticholinergics may cause uterine irritability and preterm labor when administered near term.

USE IN PEDIATRIC PATIENTS. No modification of dosage is needed.

OTHER. The drug should be used with caution in patients with epilepsy, asthma, bradycardia, or hyperthyroidism. In such patients, the smallest dose needed to produce the desired effect should be used. Dosage can be slowly titrated upward using a peripheral nerve stimulator.

Onset and Duration of Action

Dosage

For reversal of nondepolarizing muscle relaxants, 0.5 mg/kg is administered by intra-venous push concurrently with atropine, 7 µg/kg. *Constant cardiac monitoring should be used when this agent is administered.*

Limits

A maximum dose of 40 mg should not be exceeded. Onset of action is 30 to 60 seconds, and duration of action is 10 minutes.

Repeat Dosing

Repeat doses (same as initial dose) can be administered every 10 minutes up to the maximum dose if symptoms of neuromuscular relaxation (respiratory depression) recur. Because the duration of this agent is considerably shorter than the duration of relaxation induced by some nondepolarizing neuromuscular blocking agents, its use should be reserved for reversal of single doses of short- or intermediate-acting muscle relaxants. Use of this agent after repeated doses of muscle relaxants or after single doses of long-acting relaxants may result in transient reversal (return of respirations). Neuromuscular blockade could return after edrophonium effects have cleared, and unnoticed respiratory arrest could result.

Toxicity

Drug Interactions

The following drugs may have weak neuromuscular blocking properties, which antagonize the effects of edrophonium: aminoglycosides, inhalation anesthetics, lidocaine, procainamide, and quinidine.

Ganglionic blocking agents (guanadrel, guanethidine, mecamylamine, trimethaphan) antagonize the effects of edrophonium. Reversal may be incomplete or myasthenic symptoms may become more severe in patients taking these medications. Administration of edrophonium to a patient taking a ganglionic blocker for hypertension control may result in elevated blood pressure.

Adverse Effects

Overdosage with edrophonium may be difficult to distinguish from myasthenic crisis. Both present with severe muscle weakness. Continued failure to respond to edrophonium in a myasthenic patient should suggest the diagnosis of cholinergic crisis.

Most of the adverse effects of edrophonium result from ganglionic or muscarinic stimulation. Increased respiratory tract secretions and bronchospasm are common.

Rash, urticaria, and anaphylaxis may occur, as may dizziness, headache, drowsiness, and seizures. Nausea, flatulence, increased peristalsis, urinary frequency, and muscle cramps are common.

Cardiac dysrhythmias, particularly conduction blocks and bradycardia, occur after administration of intravenous edrophonium. These dysrhythmias are much more common in patients who have not been treated with atropine.

Treatment of Toxicity

Due to the short duration of action of edrophonium, most adverse effects clear rapidly and do not require specific therapy. Bradycardia is treated with atropine, 0.01 mg/kg IV push. Atropine should be readily available whenever this agent is used. When this drug is used for reversal of neuromuscular blockade, continued close monitoring is necessary to ensure that muscle relaxation does not recur as the effect of edrophonium wears off.

Neostigmine Methylsulfate (Prostigmin)

Pharmacology

Neostigmine is a quaternary ammonium salt of a phenol methylcarbamate. It is a reversible acetylcholinesterase inhibitor structurally related to edrophonium, physostigmine, and pyridostigmine. The parenteral form of this drug is the methyl sulfate salt supplied in various dilutions that are pH adjusted to 5.9.

Distribution

After intravenous administration, 15 to 25% of the administered dose is bound to serum albumin. Plasma half-life is 47 to 60 minutes. This drug does not cross the blood–brain barrier in appreciable quantities. It is not known whether neostigmine crosses the placenta or is excreted in breast milk.

Elimination

Neostigmine is hydrolyzed by plasma cholinesterase and is also metabolized by hepatic microsomal enzymes. Fifty percent of an administered dose is excreted unchanged in the urine. Another 30% is excreted in the urine as metabolites.

Actions

Neostigmine inhibits destruction of acetylcholine by acetylcholinesterase. Increased concentrations of acetylcholine improve transmission of nerve impulses across the myoneural junction.

The drug also mimics acetylcholine and has a direct effect on skeletal muscle and, to a lesser degree, on autonomic ganglia.

Indications

REVERSAL OF NONDEPOLARIZING NEUROMUSCULAR BLOCKING AGENTS. Prolonged muscle relaxation with these agents can be reversed by increasing the concentration of acetylcholine at the motor end-plate.

MYASTHENIA GRAVIS. Muscle strength can be increased by administration of neostigmine. The drug is useful in the acute treatment of myasthenic crisis or as a diagnostic aid in patients with muscle weakness and suspected myasthenia.

Cautions

RENAL FAILURE. No modification of dosage is needed.

HEPATIC FAILURE. No modification of dosage is needed.

CARDIAC FAILURE. In severe cardiac failure, dose can be slowly titrated to effect using a peripheral nerve stimulator. If bradycardia is present, heart rate should be increased to 80 or greater using atropine prior to neostigmine administration.

USE IN PREGNANCY. Category C. Anticholinergics may cause uterine irritability and preterm labor when administered near term.

USE IN PEDIATRIC PATIENTS. No modification of dosage is needed.

OTHER. The drug should be used with caution in patients with epilepsy, asthma, bradycardia, or hyperthyroidism. In such patients, the smallest dose needed to produce the desired effect should be used. Dosage can be slowly titrated upward using a peripheral nerve stimulator.

Onset and Duration of Action

Dosage

For reversal of neuromuscular blockade, 0.05 mg/kg, up to 2.0 mg, is administered by slow intravenous injection. Atropine (15 μg/kg) should be administered concurrently to block muscarinic side effects of neostigmine.

Constant cardiac monitoring should be used during administration of this agent.

Limits

Onset of action with intravenous neostigmine is 4 to 8 minutes. Peak effect occurs in 20 to 30 minutes. Duration of action of a single intravenous dose is 2 to 4 hours. Total dosage should not exceed 5 mg.

Repeat Dosage

Although a second dose can be administered 30 minutes after the initial dose, the failure of an initial dose to reverse neuromuscular blockade is usually due to continued high concentrations of the nondepolarizing neuromuscular blocking agent at the motor end-plate. Time to clear the nondepolarizing agent, rather than additional doses of neostigmine, is required for reversal in this setting. The response to a peripheral nerve stimulator (partial return of train-of-four response) can be used to ascertain when neostigmine will successfully reverse a nondepolarizing blockade.

Toxicity

Drug Interactions

The following drugs may have weak neuromuscular blocking properties, which antagonize the effects of neostigmine: aminoglycosides, inhalation anesthetics, lidocaine, procainamide, and quinidine.

Ganglionic blocking agents (guanadrel, guanethidine, mecamylamine, trimethaphan) antagonize the effects of neostigmine. Reversal may be incomplete or myasthenic symptoms may become more severe in patients taking these medications. Administration of neostigmine to a patient taking a ganglionic blocker for hypertension control may result in elevated blood pressure.

Adverse Effects

Overdosage with neostigmine may be difficult to distinguish from myasthenic crisis. Both present with severe muscle weakness. Continued failure to respond to neostigmine in a myasthenic patient should suggest the diagnosis of cholinergic crisis.

Most of the adverse effects of neostigmine result from ganglionic or muscarinic stimulation. Increased respiratory tract secretions and bronchospasm are common. Rash, urticaria, and anaphylaxis may occur, as well as dizziness, headache, drowsiness, and seizures. Nausea, flatulence, increased peristalsis, urinary frequency, and muscle cramps are common.

Cardiac dysrhythmias, particularly conduction blocks and bradycardia, may occur after administration of intravenous neostigmine. These dysrhythmias are much more common in patients who have not been treated with atropine.

Treatment of Toxicity

Bradycardia is treated with atropine, 0.01 mg/kg IV push. Atropine will also reverse other muscarinic side effects of neostigmine.

Cholinergic crisis (overdosage with neostigmine) is treated by discontinuation of the drug and all other cholinesterase inhibitors as well as administration of intravenous atropine.

Pancuronium Bromide (Pavulon)

Pharmacology

Pancuronium is a long-acting, nondepolarizing neuromuscular blocking agent. It is an aminosteroid. Pancuronium is supplied in water, with sodium acetate and benzyl alcohol as preservatives. Sodium chloride is added to maintain isotonicity; the pH of the drug solution is adjusted to 4.0.

Distribution

After a single intravenous dose, pancuronium is rapidly distributed to the intravascular and extracellular compartments. This drug does not cross the blood–brain barrier in appreciable amounts. The volume of distribution ranges from 240 to 280 ml/kg. From 85 to 90% of an administered dose is protein bound.

Elimination

Pancuronium is eliminated unchanged in the bile (10% of administered dose) and urine (40% of administered dose). In addition, it is metabolized in the liver to 3-hydroxy-pancuronium, which has approximately half the muscle relaxant potency of pancuronium. The elimination half-life is 90 to 160 minutes and is significantly prolonged by hepatic or renal failure.

Actions

Pancuronium competes for cholinergic receptors at the motor end-plate. This action blocks acetylcholine and prevents neuromuscular transmission. Prolonged relaxation of skeletal muscle and the muscles of respiration results. The block is nondepolarizing;

that is, no muscle stimulation/fasciculations precede relaxation.

Indications

Pancuronium is indicated for prolonged muscle relaxation in clinical settings where muscle contraction or voluntary movement may impede therapeutic interventions. This includes use for suppression of patient movement during critical procedures, for intracranial pressure control, and as an aid to controlled ventilation.

This drug is also indicated as an adjunct to endotracheal intubation, although slow onset and prolonged duration make it less desirable than other relaxants for this indication.

Cautions

RENAL FAILURE. The elimination half-life is approximately doubled in renal failure. Duration of muscle relaxation is much longer in these patients, and half or less of the normal dose is indicated for them. A different non-depolarizing agent that is not as dependent on renal excretion (atracurium, vecuronium) may be preferred in this setting.

HEPATIC FAILURE. Elimination half-life is doubled and plasma clearance is reduced in patients with hepatic disease or biliary tract obstruction. Muscle relaxation will be prolonged in patients with these conditions. A lower initial dose or an alternative agent (atracurium) should be considered in patients with hepatic failure.

CARDIAC FAILURE. Edematous states increase the volume of distribution. Slow circulation times (as seen in cardiac failure) may delay onset of relaxation. The normal dose should be used, but it will require a longer period to induce paralysis.

USE IN PREGNANCY. Category C. Animal reproductive studies have not been performed. Pancuronium does cross the placenta, although slowly. Prolonged administration prior to delivery may cause flaccid paralysis in the newborn. Magnesium salts prolong neuromuscular blockade. Women receiving magnesium for treatment of toxemia should receive a lower dose of pancuronium.

USE IN PEDIATRIC PATIENTS. Neonates are especially sensitive to nondepolarizing muscle relaxants during the first month of life. In this group, a test dose (0.02 mg/kg) should be given initially to gauge response. After the age of 1 month, pediatric dosage requirements are the same as for adults.

OTHER. Paralysis will be markedly prolonged in patients with myasthenia gravis. Dosage should be reduced; a small test dose (0.02 mg/kg) should be administered first to gauge response.

Onset and Duration of Action

Dosage

For prolonged muscle relaxation, pancuronium is usually administered as an intravenous bolus of 0.1 mg/kg. Onset of action at this initial dose is approximately 1 minute, with complete relaxation in 3 to 5 minutes. Duration of paralysis is 45 to 60 minutes.

Limits

After initial dosing, further pancuronium administration should be based on return of muscular activity or response to peripheral nerve stimulation. Small repeat doses will greatly prolong the duration of relaxation.

Repeat Dosing

If muscle activity returns, or if peripheral nerve stimulation reveals that relaxation is spontaneously resolving, additional doses of 0.025 mg/kg can be administered.

Toxicity

Drug Interactions (See Table 25–5)

Prior use of succinylcholine or concomitant use of inhaled anesthetics (isoflurane, enflurane, halothane) will prolong the duration of relaxation with pancuronium. The action of pancuronium is prolonged by certain antibiotics, including aminoglycosides, tetracyclines, bacitracin, and polymixins.

Adverse Effects

Prolonged duration of action requiring prolonged ventilation or pharmacologic reversal is the most common adverse effect of this agent.

Administration of pancuronium causes a moderate rise in heart rate, blood pressure, and cardiac output. It can also cause histamine release and hypersensitivity reactions, including bronchospasm, cutaneous flushing, hypotension, and tachycardia.

Pancuronium has no anesthetic effect and should always be administered concomitantly with an anesthetic or a sedative hypnotic agent in awake patients.

Treatment of Toxicity

The muscle relaxation induced by pancuronium can be pharmacologically reversed (see Reversal of Neuromuscular Blockade, earlier in this chapter), but only after substantial spontaneous recovery has occurred. Prolonged relaxation requires continued ventilation until spontaneous ventilations resume or until reversal is effective.

Cardiovascular changes induced by pancuronium can be blunted by pretreatment with atropine or narcotics. Histamine reactions usually respond to intravenous diphenhydramine. The reactions are usually of short duration and resolve spontaneously without drug treatment. More severe or prolonged reactions require antihistamine administration.

Pyridostigmine Bromide (Mestinon)

Pharmacology

Pyridostigmine is structurally related to neostigmine and other cholinesterase inhibitors. Like other agents in this class, it is the methylcarbamate of a substituted phenol. As supplied for intravenous use, each milliliter of solution contains 5 mg of the drug and is pH adjusted to 5.0.

Distribution

After intravenous administration, 15 to 25% of the administered dose is bound to serum albumin. Plasma half-life is 47 to 60 minutes. This drug does not cross the blood–brain barrier in appreciable quantities. It is not known whether pyridostigmine crosses the placenta or is excreted in breast milk.

The serum half-life of pyridostigmine is approximately 90 minutes.

Elimination

Pyridostigmine is metabolized by plasma cholinesterase and by hepatic microsomal enzymes. Both metabolites and unchanged drug are excreted in the urine.

Actions

Pyridostigmine inhibits destruction of acetylcholine by acetylcholinesterase. Increased concentration of acetylcholine improves transmission of nerve impulses across the myoneural junction.

The drug also mimics acetylcholine and has a direct effect on skeletal muscle and, to a lesser degree, on autonomic ganglia.

Pyridostigmine has a longer duration of action and fewer gastrointestinal side effects than neostigmine.

Indications

Pyridostigmine is indicated for reversal of nondepolarizing muscle relaxants. Prolonged muscle relaxation with these agents can be reversed by increasing the concentration of acetylcholine at the motor end-plate.

Pyridostigmine is also indicated for treatment of myasthenic crisis.

Cautions

RENAL FAILURE. No modification of dosage is needed.

HEPATIC FAILURE. No modification of dosage is needed.

CARDIAC FAILURE. In severe cardiac failure, the dose can be slowly titrated to effect using a peripheral nerve stimulator. If bradycardia is present, heart rate should be increased to 80 or greater using atropine prior to pyridostigmine administration.

USE IN PREGNANCY. Category C. Anticholinergics may cause uterine irritability and preterm labor when administered near term.

USE IN PEDIATRIC PATIENTS. No modification of dosage is needed.

OTHER. The drug should be used with caution in patients with epilepsy, asthma, bradycardia, or hyperthyroidism. In such patients, the smallest dose needed to produce the desired effect should be used. Dosage can be slowly titrated upward using a peripheral nerve stimulator.

Pyridostigmine will increase peristalsis and bladder muscle tone. Its use is contraindicated in the presence of mechanical bowel or bladder obstruction.

Onset and Duration of Action

The dosage for reversal of nondepolarizing muscle relaxants in adults and children is 0.2 mg/kg slow IV push. Atropine, 15 μg/kg, should be administered concurrently with pyridostigmine. A normal adult dose for reversal would be 15 mg pyridostigmine/1.0 mg atropine.

For the dosage for myasthenic crisis, see Chapter 21.

Constant cardiac monitoring should be used during the administration of this agent.

Limits and Repeat Dosing

Because of the longer duration of action of this agent, repeat dosing is not indicated.

Onset of action of pyridostigmine is 2 to 5 minutes, and duration of action is 2 to 4 hours. Failure to respond to an initial dose of this agent usually requires prolonged ventilation until spontaneous respirations return. Additional doses will not reverse neuromuscular blockade in the presence of continued high concentrations of the muscle relaxant at the motor end-plate.

Toxicity

Drug Interactions

The following drugs may have weak neuromuscular blocking properties, which antagonize the effects of pyridostigmine: aminoglycosides, inhalation anesthetics, lidocaine, procainamide, and quinidine.

Ganglionic blocking agents (guanadrel, guanethidine, mecamylamine, trimethaphan) antagonize the effects of pyridostigmine. Reversal may be incomplete or myasthenic symptoms may become more severe in patients taking these medications. Administration of pyridostigmine to a patient taking a ganglionic blocker for hypertension control may result in elevated blood pressure.

Adverse Effects

Overdosage with pyridostigmine may be difficult to distinguish from myasthenic crisis. Both present with severe muscle weakness. Continued failure to respond to pyridostigmine in a myasthenic patient should suggest the diagnosis of cholinergic crisis.

Most of the adverse effects of pyridostigmine result from ganglionic or muscarinic stimulation. Increased respiratory tract secretions and bronchospasm are common. Rash, urticaria, and anaphylaxis may occur, as may dizziness, headache, drowsiness, and seizures. Nausea, flatulence, increased peristalsis, urinary frequency, and muscle cramps are common.

Cardiac dysrhythmias, particularly conduction blocks and bradycardia, occur after administration of intravenous pyridostigmine. These dysrhythmias are much more common in patients who have not been treated with atropine.

Pyridostigmine causes less bradycardia and fewer gastrointestinal side effects than neostigmine.

Treatment of Toxicity

Bradycardia is treated with atropine, 0.01 mg/kg IV push. Atropine will also reverse other muscarinic side effects of pyridostigmine, as outlined above.

Cholinergic crisis (overdosage with pyridostigmine) is treated by discontinuation of the drug and all other cholinesterase inhibitors, and by administration of intravenous atropine.

Succinylcholine Chloride (Anectine)

Pharmacology

Succinylcholine is a short-acting, depolarizing, skeletal muscle relaxant for intravenous administration. The drug is unstable in alkaline solutions and should be refrigerated while in solution to maintain potency.

Distribution

After intravenous administration, succinylcholine is rapidly distributed to the intravascular and interstitial spaces. It is poorly lipid soluble and does not cross the blood–brain barrier. Because this agent is so rapidly metabolized (see Elimination, below), volume of distribution has not been accurately determined.

Elimination

Succinylcholine is rapidly hydrolyzed by plasma and liver cholinesterases to succinylmonocholine. Succinylmonocholine has weak nondepolarizing muscle relaxant properties and is, in turn, metabolized to succinic acid and choline. About 10% of an administered dose is excreted unchanged in the urine.

Actions

Succinylcholine combines with cholinergic receptors at the motor end-plate to produce depolarization. This depolarization causes initial muscle contraction (fasciculations). Subsequent muscle contraction is blocked as long as a sufficient concentration of the drug remains at the end-plate.

Indications

Succinylcholine is indicated for endotracheal intubation in critical care situations where jaw clenching or muscle tone make direct laryngoscopy difficult or impossible. It is also used for muscle relaxation of very short duration (5 to 10 minutes) to facilitate procedures in patients who are already endotracheally intubated.

Cautions

RENAL FAILURE. Succinylcholine causes an acute elevation in serum potassium concentration. Because patients with renal failure are more likely to have a baseline elevation of their serum potassium, succinylcholine administration to these patients may cause clinically significant hyperkalemia manifested by cardiac arrhythmias.

CARDIAC FAILURE. Patients taking quinidine or digoxin and patients who have recently been digitalized or who are suffering from digoxin toxicity are more likely to have cardiac arrhythmias after succinylcholine administration.

HEPATIC FAILURE. Severe hepatic failure may result in decreased levels of plasma cholinesterase. Duration of muscle relaxation will therefore be prolonged. The clinician should anticipate the possibility of prolonged paralysis (more than 10 minutes) in such patients.

USE IN PREGNANCY. Category D. This drug may cause congenital fetal contractures if large and repeated doses are administered during the first trimester of pregnancy. Muscle weakness of the newborn may occur if large, repeated doses are administered near delivery. Pregnancy may cause lower plasma cholinesterase levels, leading to an increased duration of muscle relaxation.

USE IN PEDIATRIC PATIENTS. Intravenous bolus administration of succinylcholine to infants and children may result in profound bradycardia or asystole. This effect results from vagal stimulation. *Prior treatment with atropine (0.01 mg/kg IV) prevents this response.*

HYPERKALEMIA. Patients with preexisting hyperkalemia, patients who are more than 1 week status post severe trauma or burns, patients who are paraplegic, and patients who have suffered extensive denervation of skeletal muscle (CNS disease or injury, neuromuscular disorders) tend to become severely hyperkalemic after administration of succinylcholine. Cardiac dysrhythmias frequently result. Caution should be used when administering succinylcholine to such patients; a different muscle relaxant (nondepolarizing) is often preferable to succinylcholine.

LOW LEVELS OF PSEUDOCHOLINESTERASE. Certain conditions may lower plasma cholinesterase levels. These conditions include pregnancy, burns, severe liver disease, cancer, severe anemia, malnutrition, severe dehydration, collagen diseases, hypothyroidism, hypothermia, and hyperthermia. The duration of muscle relaxation after succinylcholine administration may be prolonged in patients with these conditions. In patients who have been exposed to organophosphate insecticides, or in the rare patients who have hereditary pseudocholinesterase deficiency, the paralysis caused by succinylcholine will be markedly prolonged (hours to days).

If low pseudocholinesterase levels are suspected, a test dose (0.1 mg/kg) of succinylcholine should be administered. Relaxation or muscle fasciculations after the test dose are indications for a reduction or elimination of subsequent dosage.

MALIGNANT HYPERTHERMIA. Succinylcholine use is contraindicated by a history of malignant hyperthermia. The physician should also select a different relaxant if the patient has a positive family history for this disorder, since the patient may carry the genetic predisposition to malignant hyperthermia.

Onset and Duration of Action

Dosage

For adults and children, the dosage is 1.0 to 1.5 mg/kg by rapid IV push. The drug should not be administered concomitantly with alkaline intravenous medications. It is rapidly hydrolyzed in such solutions and loses potency.

Limits

The initial dose should not exceed 2 mg/kg in children or 150 mg in adults.

Repeat Dosing

A second dose of 1.0 to 1.5 mg/kg can be administered if there is inadequate relaxation after the first dose. Adverse effects (arrhythmias, hyperkalemia) are much more common after repeat doses. For this reason, the initial dose should be at the upper end of the suggested dosage range in order to ensure adequate relaxation after the first dose.

Toxicity

Drug Interactions

See Table 25–5.

Adverse Effects

Bradycardia and, rarely, asystole may occur secondary to vagal stimulation. This adverse effect is much more common in infants and children and can be avoided by pretreatment with atropine.

Hyperkalemia can occur after succinylcholine administration to patients with the conditions listed under Cautions, above. It occurs primarily because of potassium release from chronically denervated muscle and is not important in the setting of acute burns, trauma, or CNS injury (less than 1 week since injury).

Fasciculations can cause aching and deep muscle pain after recovery. Fasciculations may be responsible for the mild, transient elevation in intraocular pressure that occurs with succinylcholine use. Fasciculations may also be responsible for elevation of intragastric pressure, which can cause forceful vomiting and aspiration, particularly in patients with full stomachs.

Myoglobinemia and myoglobinuria may occur after succinylcholine use, particularly in children. This adverse effect is probably the result of fasciculations and can also be blocked by premedication with a small dose of a nondepolarizing relaxant.

Malignant hyperthermia may be triggered by succinylcholine (see earlier in this chapter).

Prolonged intravenous administration of succinylcholine may result in tachyphylaxis and a "Phase II" nondepolarizing-type muscle relaxation. The time before spontaneous recovery of muscle tone is prolonged; pharmacologic reversal of muscle relaxation may be required.

Treatment of Toxicity

Bradycardia and asystole are treated with immediate intravenous atropine, 0.01 mg/kg, as well as hyperventilation with 100% oxygen. Attempts at intubation should be discontinued immediately if bradyarrhythmias occur. Most patients respond rapidly with increased heart rate; intubation can then proceed. Failure to respond to atropine and 100% oxygen may require the initiation of cardiopulmonary resuscitation.

Malignant hyperthermia is treated with dantrolene sodium (outlined elsewhere in this chapter). Ventricular dysrhythmias (premature ventricular contractions, ventricular tachycardia) are treated with the standard agents outlined elsewhere in this text. If dysrhythmias are caused by hyperkalemia, they may resolve with bicarbonate or calcium therapy.

Vecuronium Bromide (Norcuron)

Pharmacology

Vecuronium is an intermediate-duration nondepolarizing muscle relaxant.

Distribution

The distribution half-life of a single intravenous dose of vecuronium is approximately 4 minutes. From 60 to 80% of the drug is protein bound. The volume of distribution is 300 to 400 ml/kg. This drug does not cross the blood–brain barrier in appreciable quantities.

Elimination

The elimination half-life is approximately 70 minutes. From 3 to 35% of an administered dose is excreted in the urine, and from 25 to 50% is excreted in the bile. The metabolite 3-deacetyl-vecuronium is also excreted in the bile (25%) and urine (10%). This metabolite has about half the relaxant potency of vecuronium.

Actions

Vecuronium competes with acetylcholine for cholinergic receptors at the motor endplate. The resulting muscle relaxation is nondepolarizing; initial muscle stimulation/fasciculations do not occur. Muscle relaxation produced by vecuronium is of intermediate duration when compared to that produced by other nondepolarizing agents.

Indications

Vecuronium is indicated for intermediate-duration muscle relaxation in clinical settings where muscle contraction or voluntary movement may impede therapeutic interventions. This includes use for suppression of patient movement during critical procedures, for intracranial pressure control, and as an aid to controlled ventilation.

This drug is also indicated as an adjunct for endotracheal intubation, including use in patients for whom succinylcholine is contraindicated. Onset of action is not as fast as for succinylcholine; duration is longer than with succinylcholine.

Cautions

RENAL FAILURE. In patients who have been recently and adequately dialyzed, duration of paralysis is not prolonged compared to patients with normal renal function. Standard dosage can be used. Under emergency conditions, some prolongation of relaxation may be observed in renal failure patients. A lower dose should be used in this setting.

HEPATIC FAILURE. Duration of action will be prolonged in patients with hepatic dysfunction or biliary tract obstruction. A lower dose or an agent that is not dependent on hepatic clearance (atracurium) should be used in patients with these conditions.

CARDIAC FAILURE. No modification in dosage is required. Vecuronium has no clinically significant cardiovascular effects.

USE IN PREGNANCY. Category C. Animal reproduction studies have not been performed. In late pregnancy, the elimination half-life may be shortened to 35 to 45 minutes (duration may be shortened as well).

USE IN PEDIATRIC PATIENTS. Infants 7 weeks to 1 year of age are slightly more sensitive to vecuronium than are older children and adults. Duration of relaxation will be one and one-half times longer in this age group at the same mg/kg dose. Use in neonates less than 7 weeks of age has been limited.

Onset and Duration of Action

Dosage

Adults and children: 0.1 mg/kg IV push
Neonates (age <8 weeks): not recommended

Vecuronium is compatible with all intravenous solutions. The drug should be administered within 24 hours of mixing with intravenous solutions.

Limits

Unlike pancuronium, vecuronium has little cumulative effect. Onset of action is 2 to 3 minutes, with peak relaxation in 3 to 5 minutes. Use of a priming dose (see Drug Treatment: Endotracheal Intubation Using Muscle Relaxants) decreases the time to peak relaxation to 1 to 2 minutes. Total dosage administered is limited by the patient's response. If repeated doses are required, the monitoring of muscle twitch response to peripheral nerve stimulation is advised. Initial doses up to 0.28 mg/kg and total doses in excess of 0.6 mg/kg have been administered without ill effects to the cardiovascular system as long as adequate ventilation is maintained.

Repeat Dosage

Duration of action of an initial dose is 45 to 65 minutes. After 25 to 45 minutes, 25% of normal muscle contraction has returned. Repeat doses of 0.02 to 0.08 mg/kg may be administered. Repeat dosing is usually required 25 to 45 minutes after the initial dose and should be guided by response to nerve stimulation or by the return of muscle activity.

Toxicity

Drug Interactions (See Table 25–5)

Prior use of succinylcholine may prolong the effect of vecuronium. Volatile anesthetics (enflurane, isoflurane, halothane) may enhance and prolong the neuromuscular blockade induced with vecuronium. This is also true of certain antibiotics (aminoglycosides, tetracyclines, bacitracin, polymixins).

Adverse Effects

The most common adverse reaction observed with nondepolarizing agents is prolonged relaxation beyond the time required. Adequate ventilation is mandatory as long as relaxation persists.

Histamine release, accompanied by bronchospasm, flushing, tachycardia, and hypotension, has rarely been reported with this drug.

Since vecuronium does not cross the blood–brain barrier, it has no CNS effects. Adequate anesthesia or sedation should always be administered when this agent is used.

Treatment of Toxicity

Prolonged relaxation can be pharmacologically reversed using anticholinesterases.

Severe histamine reactions are treated with intravenous antihistamines (diphenhydramine, 25 to 50 mg IV). Most reactions are self-limited.

REFERENCES

Aldrete JA, Hendricks PL: Cost of muscle relaxant drugs (letter). Anesth Analg 64:941–944, 1985.

Bourke DL, Rosenberg M: Changes in total serum Ca^{++}, Na^{++}, and K^+ with administration of succinylcholine. Anesthesiology 49:361–363, 1978.

Breen PJ, Doherty WG, Donati F, Bevan DR: The potencies of edrophonium and neostigmine as antagonists of pancuronium. Anaesthesia 40:844–847, 1985.

Cordell WH, Nugent SK, Ehrenwerth J: Using neuromuscular blocking agents to facilitate tracheal intubation. Emergency Medicine Reports 5(19):141–145, 1984.

Dronen SC, Merigian KS, Hedges JR, et al: A comparison of blind nasotracheal and succinylcholine-assisted intubation in the poisoned patient. Ann Emerg Med 16(6):650–652, 1987.

Foldes FF: The rational use of neuromuscular blocking agents: The role of pancuronium (editorial). Drugs 4:153–162, 1972.

Gronert GA, Theye RA: Pathophysiology of hyperkalemia induced by succinylcholine. Anesthesiology 43(1):89–99, 1975.

Katz RL (ed): Muscle Relaxants: Basic and Clinical Aspects. Orlando, FL, Grune & Stratton, 1985.

Kunjappan VE, Brown EM, Alexander GD: Rapid sequence induction using vecuronium. Anesth Analg 65:503–506, 1986.

Lebrault C, Berger JL, D'Hollander AA, et al: Pharmacokinetics and pharmacodynamics of vecuronium (ORG NC 45) in patients with cirrhosis. Anesthesiology 62:601–605, 1985.

Leigh MD, McCoy DD, Belton MK, Lewis GB: Bradycardia following intravenous administration of succinylcholine chloride to infants and children. Anesthesiology 18(5):698–702, 1957.

Libonati MM, Leahy JJ, Ellison N: The use of succinylcholine in open eye surgery. Anesthesiology 62:637–640, 1985.

Martin ML, Lucid EJ, Walker RW: Neuroleptic malignant syndrome. Ann Emerg Med 14(4):354–358, 1985.

Meistelman C, Agoston S, Kersten UW, et al: Pharmacokinetics and pharmacodynamics of vecuronium and pancuronium in anesthetized children. Anesth Analg 65:1319–1323, 1986.

Miller RD: Antagonism of neuromuscular blockade. Anesthesiology 44(4):318–329, 1976.

Millis RM, Wood DH, Trouth CO: Amelioration of hypoxemia by neuromuscular blockade following brain injury. Life Sciences 37:739–747, 1985.

Mirakhur RK, Lavery GG, Gibson FM, McAteer E: Atracurium in clinical anaesthesia: Effect of dosage on onset, duration and conditions for tracheal intubation. Anaesthesia 40:801–805, 1985.

Nelson TC, Burritt MF: Pesticide poisoning, succinylcholine-induced apnea, and pseudocholinesterase. Mayo Clin Proc 61:750–755, 1986.

Nugent SK, Laravuso R, Rogers MC: Pharmacology and use of muscle relaxants in infants and children. J Pediatr 94(3):481–487, 1979.

Pansard J-L, Chauvin M, Lebrault C, et al: Effect of an intubating dose of succinylcholine and atracurium on the diaphragm and the adductor pollicis muscle in humans. Anesthesiology 67:326–330, 1987.

Physicians' Desk Reference, 44th ed. Oradell, NJ, Medical Economics, 1990.

Roizen MF, Feeley TW: Pancuronium bromide. Ann Intern Med 88(1):64–68, 1978.

Rupp SM, McChristian JW, Miller RD, et al: Neostigmine and edrophonium antagonism of varying intensity neuromuscular blockade induced by atracurium, pancuronium, or vecuronium. Anesthesiology 64:711–717, 1986.

Selden BS, Curry SC: Prolonged succinylcholine-induced paralysis in organophosphate insecticide poisoning. Ann Emerg Med 16(2):215–217, 1987.

Sohn YJ, Bencini AF, Scaf AHJ, et al: Comparative pharmacokinetics and dynamics of vecuronium and pancuronium in anesthetized patients. Anesth Analg 65:233–239, 1986.

Symposium on malignant hyperthermia. Br J Anaesth 60:251–319, 1988.

Syverud SA, Borron SW, Storer DL, et al: Prehospital use of neuromuscular blocking agents in a helicopter ambulance program. Ann Emerg Med 17(3):236–242, 1988.

Talucci RC, Shaikh KA, Schwab CW: Rapid sequence induction with oral endotracheal intubation in the multiply injured patient. Am Surg 54(4):185–187, 1988.

Thompson JD, Fish S, Ruiz E: Succinylcholine for endotracheal intubation. Ann Emerg Med 11:526–529, 1982.

Tilson HH, Weakly JN, Lineberry CG, et al: Postmarketing surveillance of tracrium, 1983–1986. J Clin Res Drug Dev 2:89–99, 1988.

USP DI Drug Information for the Health Care Provider. Rockville, MD, The United States Pharmacopeial Convention, Inc., 1985, pp 1058–1070.

White PF, Schlobohm RM, Pitts LH, Lindauer JM: A randomized study of drugs for preventing increases in intracranial pressure during endotracheal suctioning. Anesthesiology 57:242–244, 1982.

CHAPTER 26

THERAPEUTIC GASES

DANIEL L. SAVITT, M.D.

INTRODUCTION

Therapeutic gases are a class of drugs administered and assimilated through the lungs. These gases owe their therapeutic effect to pharmacologic as well as physical properties. In each case, however, the gases should be viewed as drugs with therapeutic dose ranges as well as toxic side effects. Gases, particularly oxygen, are one of the most widely prescribed groups of drugs in modern medicine. Newer uses are evolving with continued research and clinical experience. It is the intent of this chapter to familiarize the reader with the uses of hyperbaric oxygen, helium–oxygen, carbon dioxide, and nitrous oxide in clinical medicine and to provide guidelines for their use in specific conditions.

The conditions discussed in this chapter include decompression sickness, gas embolism, carbon monoxide poisoning, acute management of painful conditions, upper airway obstruction, and gas gangrene. None of the conditions is common, but many will be encountered in a routine practice of medicine. Thus, an understanding of the conditions and their specific treatments can be of great benefit to both the physician and the patient.

The actions of various gases discussed in this chapter are due to a combination of biologic and physical properties. Oxygen, nitrous oxide, and carbon dioxide are drugs in the true sense of the word and cause specific biochemical reactions and interactions within the body. Helium is totally inert and owes its therapeutic effect soley to physical properties that may be predicted from a knowledge of physics. Hyperbaric oxygen results in both biochemical and physical effects that combined are more effective than either pressure or normobaric oxygen used individually. Because of the variety of pathophysiologic actions caused by the class of therapeutic gases, each is discussed individually. Guidelines are provided for their use under urgent conditions.

CONDITIONS

Decompression Sickness

Decompression sickness is a condition that was first recognized in the 1800s when the entity was discovered in workers building tunnels in a compressed-air environment. Today decompression sickness is more frequently associated with diving, whether it be commercial or sport SCUBA. Decompression sickness is the result of a pressure change, and its occurrence can be predicted from knowledge of the physical properties of gases and the laws that govern their behavior. As one goes underwater the ambient pressure increases at a rate of 1 atmosphere for each 33 feet one descends. Diving equipment allows one to breathe by delivering the breathing mix at this increased pressure. For most applications, conventional air is the breathing mix.

Nitrogen is the gas responsible for decompression sickness, with air as the breathing mix. Other gases are present in inconsequential amounts or are metabolized (oxygen). Nitrogen moves from the air to plasma to tissues at variable rates as a result of its solubility in that tissue and blood flow. As long as the nitrogen remains dissolved it is of little consequence. Once ascent occurs, however, the nitrogen becomes less soluble and will come out of solution. A certain amount of this nitrogen comes out and will be cleared by the lungs, causing no ill effect. Any excess above this amount caused by too rapid an ascent after too long a period at depth will cause the formation of nitrogen bubbles. The bubbles accumulate in tissues such as tendons, causing pain in joints (the bends) or acting as emboli to blood vessels and thus producing ischemia distal to the occlusion. Once bubble formation occurs, the clotting cascade is activated and platelets aggregate around the bubble, making the situation less reversible.

Diagnosis

Classically, decompression sickness has been divided into two categories: Type I, which is pain in extremities only, and Type II, or neurologic decompression sickness, which includes all other symptoms. This rather simplistic approach has several shortcomings. Frequently patients have symptoms in both categories. Patients may also have symptoms or signs that may be due to arterial gas embolism, further confusing the picture. If patients have symptoms of only Type I decompression sickness, their treatment may be simplified and their outcome is predictably good.

Typically, symptoms will begin to appear anywhere from 10 minutes to 36 hours after the completion of a dive. The majority of patients become symptomatic within the first 12 hours. Any symptoms, particularly those of a neurologic nature, that occur *immediately* following a dive are usually the result of pulmonary overpressure and arterial gas embolism.

Type I symptoms are pains that occur in a joint or extremity. This is frequently described as a deep pain like a "toothache" that is unaffected by movement but is relieved by pressure. It may be quite difficult to distinguish from the pain resulting from a strained muscle. Pain should be differentiated from paresthesias, which are considered a Type II symptom. Type I symptoms respond rapidly to pressurization in a hyperbaric chamber. This can be used as a diagnostic maneuver if there is doubt as to diagnosis. (See box, Drug Treatment: Decompression Sickness, Type I: Pain Only.)

DRUG TREATMENT: DECOMPRESSION SICKNESS, TYPE I: PAIN ONLY

First-Line Drug

Surface Oxygen

Initial Dose	100% by tight-fitting non-rebreathing mask
Repeat Dosing	Continuous administration
End-Point	Discontinue when hyperbaric oxygen therapy initiated.

Second-Line Drug

Hyperbaric Oxygen

Initial Dose	Treat according to United States Navy Treatment Table 5.* Immediate compression to 60 feet sea water (fsw) over 24 minutes breathing 100% oxygen Oxygen breathing for two periods of 20 minutes spaced by 5-minute air break Ascent to 30 fsw over 30 minutes breathing oxygen

Chart continued on following page

DRUG TREATMENT: DECOMPRESSION SICKNESS, TYPE I:
PAIN ONLY *Continued*

	5-minute air break followed by 20-minute period of oxygen breathing followed by 5-minute air break Ascent to surface over 30 minutes breathing oxygen Total treatment time 2 hours and 15 minutes
Repeat Dosing	No standard guideline United States Navy Treatment Table 5 or a monoplace protocol or Treatment Table 6 could be used after appropriate surface interval if clinically indicated.
End-Points	Completion of treatment outlined in table Signs of oxygen toxicity Patient deterioration Clinical resolution of symptoms at completion of treatment outlined in table

---

*The United States Navy Manual should be consulted in detail before utilizing any recompression treatment table, and treatment should be conducted by only those trained in hyperbaric and diving medicine.

Type II symptoms are classically thought of as neurologic, although they also include painful areas in the head or trunk. Typically patients have accumulation of bubbles that cause symptoms referable to the spinal cord, such as urinary retention or lower limb paralysis. Frequently patients present with complaints that are much less straightforward, such as extreme lethargy, a feeling of detachment, or a change in personality. Although to the uninitiated these symptoms would not seem to be due to decompression sickness, they will respond to treatment and are well recognized as part of the symptom complex. It is important to consider decompression sickness with any complaint in a patient who has been diving within the previous 24 hours. Consultation with a diving physician is available 24 hours a day through the Divers' Alert Network (DAN) at Duke University.° This facility can also advise you of the nearest hyperbaric chamber and can coordinate treatment if necessary. (See box, Drug Treatment: Decompression Sickness, Type II: Neurologic.)

°Telephone (919) 684-8111.

DRUG TREATMENT: DECOMPRESSION SICKNESS, TYPE II:
NEUROLOGIC

First-Line Drug

Surface Oxygen

Initial Dose	100% by tight-fitting non-rebreathing mask or endotracheal tube
Repeat Dosing	Continuous administration
End-Point	Initiation of hyperbaric oxygen therapy

Second-Line Drug

Hyperbaric Oxygen

Initial Dose	Treat according to United States Navy Treatment Table 6.* Immediate compression to 60 fsw over 24 minutes breathing 100% oxygen 5-minute air breaks alternating with three periods of 20 minutes of oxygen breathing for 75 minutes Ascent to 30 fsw breathing oxygen over 30 minutes

DRUG TREATMENT: DECOMPRESSION SICKNESS, TYPE II: NEUROLOGIC *Continued*

	Air break of 15 minutes alternating with 60 minutes of oxygen breathing for 90 minutes Ascent to surface breathing oxygen over 30 minutes Total treatment time 4 hours and 45 minutes
Repeat Dosing	Treatment time can be extended for 25 minutes at 60 fsw and/or 75 minutes at 30 fsw if clinically indicated. Saturation treatment can be entertained. Repeat treatment of residua after initial treatment using a monoplace regimen may be conducted daily for as long as clinical improvement continues. No standard guideline; clinical judgment paramount
End-Points	Completion of treatment outlined in table Clinical resolution of symptoms at completion of treatment outlined in table Patient deterioration Signs of oxygen toxicity

Third-Line Drugs

Crystalloid Infusion

Initial Dose	Infusion of Ringer's lactate or normal saline to maintain hydration and urine output
Repeat Dosing	Constant infusion during treatment
End-Point	Completion of treatment

Aspirin

Initial Dose	Standard dose for age or 650 mg for adult
Repeat Dosing	No standard guidelines May repeat in 24 hours
End-Point	No clinical end-point

Dexamethasone

Initial Dose	6–10 mg IM or IV
Repeat Dosing	No standard guidelines May be repeated in 6 hours
End-Point	No clinical end-point

*The United States Navy Manual should be consulted in detail before using any recompression treatment table, and treatment should be conducted by only those trained in hyperbaric and diving medicine.

Indications for Treatment

Hyperbaric oxygen therapy should be instituted once the diagnosis of decompression sickness is considered. Delay in obtaining additional tests will only serve to complicate treatment in those patients. Cases of pain-only decompression sickness should respond quickly to a test of pressure, confirming the diagnosis. Most cases that are rapidly treated will demonstrate significant improvement soon after treatment is initiated. If there is a question of air embolism, the patient should receive immediate recompression as well; however, many authorities recommend the use of greater pressures to treat this condition. Simple pneumothorax or subcutaneous air caused by pulmonary overpressure, *without any other complaints or findings,* can be observed.

Discussion

Once the decision to treat has been made, many experts will advise that the patient be hydrated with a crystalloid solution such as Ringer's lactate to improve blood rheology as much as possible. Some authorities use steroids such as dexamethasone and platelet inhibitors such as aspirin in their treatment of decompression sickness as well. No medical management replaces hyperbaric oxygen therapy, however.

Hyperbaric oxygen is the primary treatment modality for several serious conditions and adjunctive therapy for numerous others. Research into potential uses is active. Hyperbaric oxygen therapy is technically defined as the intermittent administration of oxygen under pressure for therapeutic benefit. In practice this is accomplished through the use of a hyperbaric chamber. Hyperbaric chambers are divided into either monoplace or multiplace types depending on their structure. A monoplace chamber accommodates only one patient at a time. Treatment time is limited by oxygen toxicity since the patient usually breathes 100% oxygen for the entire treatment. At the maximum pressure, this is roughly 90 minutes for routine cases.

Multiplace chambers are much larger units and can accommodate more than one patient as well as medical personnel. Since these chambers are much larger, it is neither safe nor cost-effective to pressurize the entire unit with oxygen. Instead, the chamber is pressurized with air and the patient breathes 100% oxygen at pressure, using a tight-fitting mask or hood. Multiplace chambers may utilize pressures of up to 6 atmospheres. For practical purposes, treatment time is indefinite since the patient can breathe air or other therapeutic gases intermittently to limit oxygen toxicity.

Proponents of each type of chamber exist, as there clearly are differences between them. Critically ill patients can be treated in monoplace chambers by skilled operators. The wide availability of these units makes them appropriate for general treatment of carbon monoxide poisoning. Many experienced physicians in the field of diving medicine prefer to treat decompression sickness and air embolism in multiplace chambers initially because treatment schedules can be varied extensively depending on clinical condition. The appropriate chamber choice for a particular patient is best determined in consultation with a hyperbaric specialist.

Diving accidents are best treated by physicians trained in diving and hyperbaric medicine. Most authorities prefer to treat decompression sickness in multiplace chambers and

use a variety of treatment regimens, which include those developed by the United States, French, and British navies, as well as commercial treatment tables. The extent of treatment, use of variable mixtures of gases, and potential for causing decompression sickness in medical attendants are some of the considerations involved and are best dealt with by experts. The availability of multiplace chambers, however, is limited. Time to treatment is directly related to outcome in acute cases of decompression sickness. Under emergency circumstances it is possible to carry out an initial treatment in a monoplace chamber using modified treatment tables. Furthermore, monoplace chambers can be modified to allow the patient to breathe air intermittently via a mask, allowing for complete use of United States Navy treatment tables without risking oxygen toxicity. If presented with an acute case of decompression sickness when the only chamber available within a reasonably short period of time is a monoplace chamber, emergency treatment should probably be carried out in this chamber while arrangements are made for more definitive treatment. Once again the Divers' Alert Network is a resource in these circumstances.

Standard treatment for decompression sickness in the United States is United States Navy Treatment Table 6. Table 5 is occasionally used for cases of pain-only decompression sickness (Type I). There are, however, many more tables and treatment options available to the treating physician. The specific treatment of decompression sickness can be quite complex in certain cases and is beyond the scope of this discussion. The approach to treatment of decompression sickness is summarized in Figure 26–1.

Carbon Monoxide Poisoning

Poisoning by carbon monoxide is a serious public health problem in the United States. One-half of all fatal poisonings each year are caused by carbon monoxide (CO). Annually this results in 3800 deaths, the majority of which are suicides. Overall, approximately 10,000 people yearly seek medical attention for the toxic effects of CO.

CO is a colorless, tasteless, odorless gas that is lighter than oxygen. The major source of CO is incomplete combustion of organic fuels. Without combustion, these fuels do not produce CO. Motor vehicles can pro-

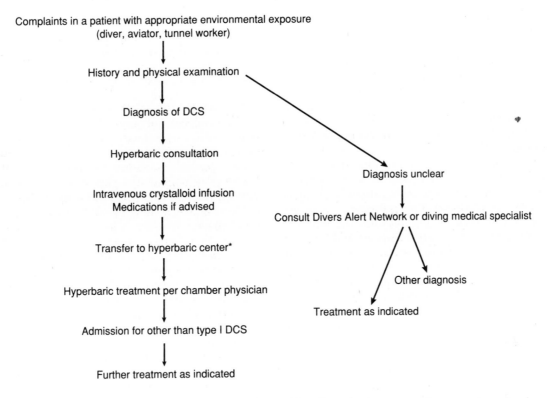

FIGURE 26-1. Treatment algorithm: decompression sickness. (*See discussion in text regarding monoplace chambers for emergency treatment.)

duce up to 7% CO in exhaust fumes, although this is severely curtailed with efficient catalytic conversion devices. Cigarette smoke contains up to 4% CO, accounting for low levels of carboxyhemoglobin in smokers. An unusual source of CO is methylene chloride, which is contained in paint strippers. This compound is metabolized within the body to carbon monoxide in significant quantities.

Hemoglobin that binds CO does not carry oxygen. Thus, a patient with a hematocrit of 50% and a carboxyhemoglobin level of 50% has an effective oxygen-carrying hematocrit of 25%. Additionally, the presence of CO on hemoglobin molecules causes a leftward shift of the hemoglobin–oxygen dissociation curve, called the Haldane effect. The Haldane effect makes the oxygen carried less available to tissues. Carbon monoxide also binds to other heme-containing proteins in the body, such as myoglobin, but the clinical significance of this is not known. There is a further aspect to CO poisoning that goes beyond a decrease in oxygen-carrying capacity. Accumulating evidence indicates that a serious consequence of CO poisoning is inhibi-

tion of cellular respiration, which may occur at the level of the cytochrome system. Thus, the result of CO poisoning is a nonischemic hypoxia coupled with an inhibition of cellular respiration. Clinically the heart and brain are the organs most commonly affected. Signs and symptoms are most frequently hemodynamic or neuropsychiatric.

Diagnosis

CO poisoning is a protean illness that is well known as an imitator of other conditions. The literature abounds with studies pointing out the difficulties associated with making the diagnosis, particularly in cases of low-level poisoning. Signs and symptoms follow a general trend that can be correlated with levels of carboxyhemoglobin. However, it should be cautioned that levels only serve to confirm the diagnosis and should not be used to guide therapy since they do not reflect the degree of cellular poisoning or the duration of exposure.

At levels of up to 20%, symptoms are easily ascribed to a viral syndrome. The patient complains of nausea, headache, or malaise. Patients with coronary artery disease are stressed by decreases in oxygen available to an already ischemic myocardium and may demonstrate an accelerated pattern of angina. Levels of 20 to 40% will produce severe headache, vomiting, difficulties with mentation, and visual disturbances. Above 40%, syncopal episodes may occur and frank confusion may be present. Seizures, coma, and death complete the continuum as levels approach 70%.

In recent years a second component of CO poisoning, termed the *delayed syndrome*, has been recognized. Following successful treatment of significant CO poisoning, patients will present with rapid deterioration of their neuropsychiatric status after a lucid interval of 2 to 3 weeks from the initial insult. About two-thirds of these patients will significantly improve with hyperbaric oxygen therapy at this point. Several studies in the literature indicate that this delayed syndrome may be prevented with hyperbaric oxygen therapy at the time of initial insult.

The laboratory serves to confirm the diagnosis of CO poisoning. Carboxyhemoglobin levels can be dramatically altered by oxygen administered prior to determination, and thus laboratory results do not reflect the cellular aspect of poisoning. Clinical status of the patient is much more relevant in determining a therapeutic plan. Arterial blood gases will show a normal pO_2 since this number reflects dissolved oxygen. If PaO_2 is decreased, one should seek other causes such as significant smoke inhalation or pulmonary pathology. An acidosis will be present in serious cases of poisoning. This acidosis tends to shift the hemoglobin–oxygen curve to the right, normalizing it and offering the patient an advantage with regard to tissue oxygen delivery. Acidosis should be tolerated whenever possible and treated with caution. Lactate is responsible for much of the acidosis, and lactate levels can be measured. The measurement of creatine phosphokinase levels and checking the urine for the presence of myoglobin will allow for prediction and prevention of renal failure. All patients at risk for myocardial ischemia should have an electrocardiogram. Monitoring is also advisable in these patients since cardiac arrhythmias account for significant mortality and morbidity. The chest radiograph is usually normal but may reflect smoke inhalation or noncardiogenic pulmonary edema. Availability of toxic screen or blood alcohol determinations will aid the clinician since other compounds frequently complicate both intentional and accidental exposures. Increased experience with computed tomography and magnetic resonance imaging has shown characteristic lesions in the globus pallidus, which are associated with a poor prognosis.

Indications for Treatment

The treatment of carbon monoxide poisoning centers on administering oxygen. The administration of 100% oxygen at 1 atmosphere (ambient) pressure shortens the half-life of the carboxyhemoglobin complex from 320 minutes to about 80 minutes. Administration of 100% oxygen at 3 atmospheres (hyperbaric) pressure diminishes the half-life to 23 minutes. Increasing clinical evidence indicates that more aggressive use of hyperbaric oxygen may act to ameliorate the cellular aspect of poisoning and prevent occurrence of the delayed syndrome. Despite an increasing body of clinical evidence favoring the use of hyperbaric oxygen, its use is still controversial.

Currently accepted guidelines for treatment with hyperbaric oxygen will identify patients who should be treated even if this necessitates transfer to another facility (Table 26–1). Advocates of hyperbaric therapy frequently treat patients who are not seriously ill, pointing out that careful neuropsychiatric testing of these patients often shows abnormalities.

When assessing a patient who has relatively mild symptoms, such as headache, nausea, and vomiting, the physician should pay careful attention to a neuropsychiatric assessment. The Maryland Institute for Emergency Medical Services has assembled a collection of tests that have been found

TABLE 26–1. Indications for Hyperbaric Oxygen in Carbon Monoxide Poisoning

Comatose patient
History of loss of consciousness
Pregnancy°
Acidosis
Abnormal neurologic examination
Evidence of myocardial ischemia
Carboxyhemoglobin level >40% regardless of symptoms
Abnormal neuropsychiatric testing
Persistent symptoms after 3 hours of treatment with 100% O_2 at 1 atmosphere absolute

°Physiologically the fetus is at greater risk than the mother. Several cases of poor fetal outcome with standard treatment in cases of CO poisoning exist. Clinical experience with treating pregnant patients is limited, and each case should be considered individually.

DRUG TREATMENT: CARBON MONOXIDE POISONING

First-Line Drug

Surface Oxygen

Initial Dose	100% via non-rebreathing mask or endotracheal tube
Repeat Dosing	Continuous administration for approximately 3 hours If further treatment deemed necessary, consider hyperbaric oxygen
End-Points	Resolution of symptoms Initiation of hyperbaric therapy

Second-Line Drug

Hyperbaric Oxygen

Initial Dose	2.8 atmospheres of pressure for 90 minutes (standard monoplace protocol)*
Repeat Dosing	No standard guidelines Suggest repeating initial dose after surface air break of 5–6 hours or daily as long as clinical improvement continues
End-Points	Resolution of clinical symptoms Completion of treatment protocol

*Most authorities feel treatment in monoplace chambers is adequate. Those facilities that have multiplace chambers may utilize United States Navy Treatment Table 5 or 6 or their own protocol.

useful in predicting significant intoxication in borderline patients as well as in documenting abnormalities in others. A tool such as this should be employed in making the decision to treat patients who otherwise appear well enough to be treated with surface oxygen.

When treating CO poisoning, early consultation with a hyperbaric specialist is useful. The hyperbaric specialist can lend judgment in regard to questionable cases and expedite therapy in clear-cut cases. (See box.)

Discussion

Treatment of patients with suspected CO poisoning should start with stabilization measures. If there is any doubt about the patient's airway, especially in the face of inhalation injury, early intubation is warranted. Once CO poisoning is suspected, administration of 100% oxygen should begin. Thereafter a carboxyhemoglobin level will serve to confirm the diagnosis. The absolute level frequently does not correlate with symptoms and should not be used to guide therapy unless it is very high. Further laboratory studies should be obtained as previously discussed. Stabilization should include treatment of hypotension, using pressors only if fluids are inadequate. In the face of ventricular ectopy and potential myocardial ischemia, lidocaine should be administered. Mild acidosis should be tolerated since it affords the patient some protection against tissue hypoxia.

If patients have only mild symptoms such as nausea and headache and a carboxyhemoglobin level under 25 to 35%, a trial of 100% surface oxygen is warranted. Standard plastic non-rebreathing masks deliver only about 60 to 70% oxygen. Tight-fitting masks such as aviator's masks are preferable. Once therapy has been initiated, a careful neuropsychiatric assessment should be performed. Any patient with other than mild abnormalities should be referred for hyperbaric oxygen therapy. If the patient's symptoms or signs do not resolve with 3 hours of treatment with surface oxygen, he or she should be referred for hyperbaric oxygen therapy. The approach to treatment of carbon monoxide poisoning is summarized in Figure 26–2.

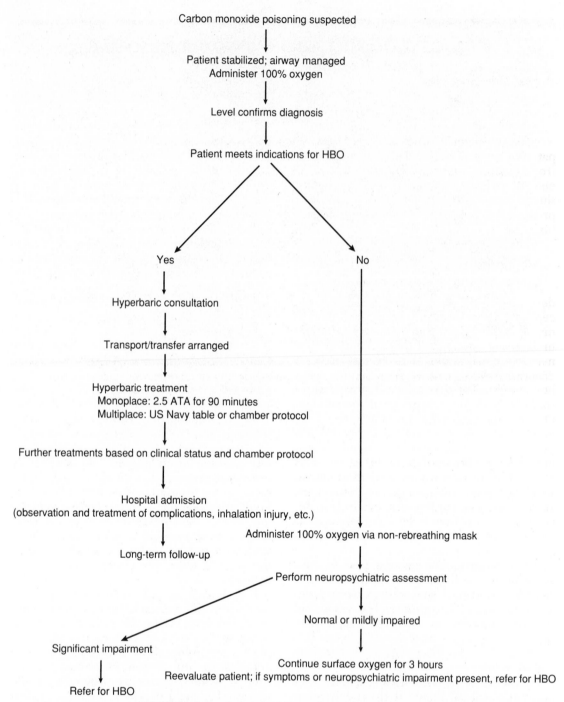

FIGURE 26–2. Treatment algorithm: carbon monoxide poisoning.

Standard treatment protocols using hyperbaric oxygen depend on the type of chamber being utilized. Monoplace chambers accommodate only the patient in an environment of 100% oxygen. Patients may be on ventilators and have intravenous lines in place. Treatment time is limited by central nervous system oxygen toxicity to about 90 minutes at 2.5 atmospheres. Multiplace chambers are pressurized with air, and the patient breathes oxygen at pressure through a tight-fitting mask or hood. These chambers are larger, and usually a technician or nurse will accompany the patient. If the patient intermittently breathes air, the total duration of oxygen treatment can be increased without risking oxygen toxicity. Multiplace chambers utilize protocols such as those published by the United States Navy.

Repetitive treatments may be administered after a hiatus of 5 to 6 hours. Continued improvement is an indication for repeat treatments. Some facilities routinely treat all patients several times. There are no controlled data to support this practice at present. All patients who have had CO poisoning should have follow-up within one month of presentation to assess neuropsychiatric status.

Air Embolism

Air embolism as a medical entity was first described in the early 1800s. Until very recently, it has been mostly a disease limited to divers and is manifested primarily in sailors undergoing emergency ascents during submarine escape training. However, in the past 25 years there have been an increasing number of reports of iatrogenic air embolism associated with invasive medical technology. One author estimates the incidence of air embolisms in the United States to be 20,000 per year, although most of these are unrecognized and untreated.

Gas introduced into the venous circulation may also result in an arterial embolus if the patient has a patent foramen ovale. The cardiac defect responsible for this "paradoxical embolus" is present in up to one-third of the population according to some autopsy series. Thus, a central venous line that becomes disconnected can result in a cerebral air embolus. Neurosurgical procedures carried out with the patient in a sitting position are high-risk situations for venous (and thus paradoxical) emboli, which may occur in up to 40% of these patients. There are reported cases where venous gas has resulted in arterial emboli without a patent foramen ovale. These are thought to be the result of an overloading of the capacity of the lung to filter bubbles with a massive injection of gas.

Once gas enters the arterial circulation it can embolize anywhere; however, the cerebral circulation appears to be at highest risk due to the normal upright position of humans. Coronary arteries can also be affected, producing infarction. With central nervous system embolization, cortical deficits predominate.

Diagnosis

The diagnosis of air embolism should be suspected in any patient in the appropriate setting who develops symptoms referable to the cerebrum. With diving accidents, as with all other causes, signs and symptoms occur immediately following the embolus. Thus, the diver who surfaces and becomes unconscious within minutes is suffering from an air embolism and not decompression sickness, which usually presents in a more delayed fashion. The same reasoning applies for a patient undergoing an invasive procedure.

A change in mental status is the most frequent symptom. Other signs and symptoms include difficulty with mentation, difficulty with balance, hemianopsia, and apraxias, depending on the location of the embolus. Usually the location of a single embolus can be surmised; however, emboli may be numerous, producing diffuse defects that are not easy to sort out. Emboli may produce syndromes that can be missed by simple neurologic examination, so a careful examination of the patient is mandatory. The temporal relationship of symptom onset to the causative event is the most important historical factor.

Embolization to the coronary arteries may result in infarction or arrhythmia. Additionally, an embolus to the brain stem may produce cardiac instability.

The diagnosis of air embolism should be a clinical one. Time to treatment is directly related to outcome in most series. One should not delay treatment in order to confirm the diagnosis unless there is serious doubt. Once the clotting cascade is activated and edema formation begins, the result of recompression is less likely to be beneficial. If doubt exists, a cranial computed tomography scan will frequently demonstrate air if the bubbles are within the limits of resolution of the machine.

Indications for Treatment

Hyperbaric treatment should be instituted whenever there is a reasonable suspicion of the diagnosis of air embolism. Appropriate diagnosis and treatment result in a good outcome. Delays in diagnosis or other forms of treatment are associated with poor outcomes. (See box.)

Discussion

Once the diagnosis of air embolism is considered likely, the patient should be imme-

DRUG TREATMENT: AIR EMBOLISM

First-Line Drug

Surface 100% Oxygen

Initial Dose	Apply via tight-fitting non-rebreathing mask or endotracheal tube.
Repeat Dosing	Continuous administration Continue until hyperbaric oxygen is available.
End-Point	Initiation of hyperbaric oxygen

Hyperbaric Oxygen

Initial Dose	Utilize United States Navy Treatment Table 6A if a multiplace facility is available.* Immediate compression to 165 fsw as rapidly as possible Total time at 165 fsw equals 30 minutes. Ascent to 60 fsw over 4 minutes and initiation of 100% oxygen breathing Periods of 20 minutes breathing oxygen alternating with 5 minutes breathing air Ascent to 30 fsw over 30 minutes breathing 100% oxygen after 75 minutes at 60 fsw Periods of 60 minutes breathing oxygen alternating with 15 minutes breathing air Ascent to surface over 30 minutes breathing 100% oxygen after 150 minutes at 30 fsw Total treatment time 5 hours 19 minutes
Repeat Dosing	No standard protocol May use 100% oxygen at 2.4 to 3.0 atmospheres for 90 to 120 minutes if residua exist after surface interval
End-Points	Clinical resolution of signs and symptoms Completion of United States Navy Treatment Table 6A Patient decompensation during treatment Signs of oxygen toxicity

*The United States Navy Diving Manual should be consulted in detail before utilizing this or other treatment tables. Under emergency circumstances some authors recommend utilization of monoplace chambers if a multiplace chamber is unavailable (see discussion in text).

diately removed from further risk of cerebral embolization by being placed in the head-down position. If the air has entered through a vein, placement of the patient with the right side up is indicated. In this way, large quantities of venous air may collect in the right ventricle and can be aspirated by catheter. If there is no further risk of embolization (i.e., procedure is terminated), a supine position is adequate and will not exacerbate edema formation. Administration of 100% oxygen initiates treatment by minimizing hypoxia and decreasing some of the nitrogen within the bubble embolus. At this point, any other measures required to stabilize the patient may be completed and plans for hyperbaric therapy should begin.

In the majority of cases, treatment of gas embolism employs United States Navy Treatment Table 6A. This treatment table contains an initial recompression to 6 atmospheres absolute on air to maximize the effects of Boyle's law in reducing the size of the bubble. Some authorities utilize mixtures of nitrogen and oxygen with higher concentrations of oxygen than air at this depth; however, the risk of oxygen toxicity precludes the use of pure oxygen. After a short period at this great depth the patient ascends to 60 feet for several periods of pure oxygen breathing broken by periods of air breathing. The last portion of the treatment table is similar but is carried out at a depth of 30 feet. The entire treatment table takes over 5 hours to complete. Because of the extreme depth and requirement for air breaks, the

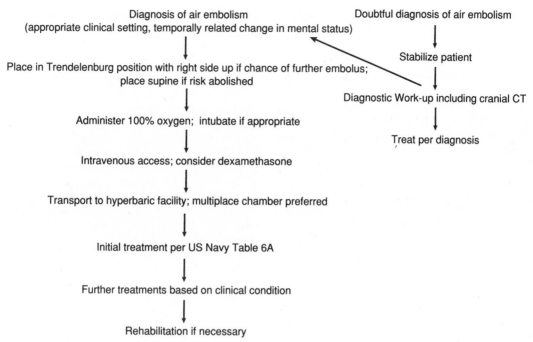

FIGURE 26–3. Treatment algorithm: air embolism.

treatment using this table cannot be performed in a monoplace chamber.

There is some controversy regarding the necessity of treating patients in multiplace chambers. Evidence from animal experiments indicates that outcome is no better when using United States Navy Treatment Table 6A than when using Table 6, which does not include the 6-atmosphere segment. No clinical studies have been performed comparing monoplace versus multiplace treatment of air embolism. Clearly most authorities recommend the use of Treatment Table 6A and multiplace chambers if at all available. The Divers' Alert Network can act as consultant and facilitate transfer for treatment if necessary.

Rapidly instituted therapy often has dramatic results. Residua are often treated with wash-out hyperbaric treatments that vary according to clinical condition and chamber protocol. The approach to treatment of gas embolism is summarized in Figure 26–3. Permanent or long-standing disability may occur and require rehabilitation.

Gas Gangrene

Gas gangrene caused by *Clostridium perfringens* is a dreaded complication of trauma. Despite many advances in the treatment of this disease, mortality in the best of series is approximately 20%, with morbidity approaching 100% in the form of amputation or other disfiguring surgery. A multidisciplinary approach combining surgery, antibiotic therapy, supportive medical care, and hyperbaric oxygen therapy has provided the best results, but no one therapy alone yields an adequate response.

Diagnosis

The diagnosis of gas gangrene is clinical. If the diagnosis is suspected, the patient should be treated presumptively since the infection progresses rapidly and can result in death within 12 hours from the time of diagnosis. Furthermore, the causative agent is difficult to isolate in the laboratory, and up to 20% of cases may never have laboratory confirmation of the diagnosis. Traditionally the disease has followed major trauma such as open fractures or war wounds. Recent experience indicates that there is an equally large group of patients in whom the etiology is nontraumatic or related to minor trauma. In some cases the infection arises spontaneously. Diabetes, malignancy, and peripheral vascular disease are all risk factors.

Clinical manifestations follow a continuum. Classically the wound is edematous with a bronze or purple discoloration. Margins of infection may be red and can progress proximally up a limb within an hour. Drainage from the wound is watery, malodorous, and brown and may contain bubbles of gas. A Gram stain of the fluid should be made rapidly as it is the quickest means of confirming the diagnosis. *Clostridium* is a gram-positive bacillus whose appearance is said to resemble boxcars. Patients frequently complain of severe pain, although the area can often be examined without significant discomfort. Fever is often low grade, but a prominent tachycardia is usually observed. Later cases will demonstrate signs of septicemia, shock, and organ failure.

The presence of gas in the tissue by palpation or radiograph is neither pathognomonic nor regularly observed. Gas is often a late finding and typically has the appearance of dissecting along fascial planes rather than being localized. Other bacteria including *Escherichia coli* and *Streptococcus* can result in gas formation. Laboratory values are nonspecific.

Indications for Treatment

Since the disease is rapidly progressive and the diagnosis is clinical, any patient suspected of having gas gangrene should be aggressively treated until the infection is ruled out. As indicated previously, the approach to this infection requires a rapid coordination of multiple techniques to arrest the infection and limit damage. No single approach is effective in the absence of others.

Hyperbaric oxygen therapy acts directly on the bacteria to prevent further production of alpha toxin, which is the primary lethal exotoxin of *Clostridium perfringens*. Tissue oxygen tensions of greater than 80 mmHg are required to stop the production of alpha toxin. Usual conditions in the edematous wounds of gangrene are quite hypoxic. At 2 atmospheres of pressure in a hyperbaric chamber, the measured tissue oxygen tension approaches 250 mmHg. Under experimental conditions, hyperbaric oxygen has proven to be bactericidal as well as bacteriostatic to clostridia. In addition to direct effects on the bacteria, improved oxygenation of infected tissue results in improved white cell function and production of peroxides that are destructive to anaerobic bacteria. (See box.)

Discussion

Once a clinical diagnosis of gas gangrene is made, no time should be wasted in initiating therapy. Immediate fluid resuscitation should be started along with obtaining base-

---

DRUG TREATMENT: GAS GANGRENE

First-Line Drug

Penicillin

Initial Dose	2–4 million units IV
Repeat Dosing	Same Repeated every 4 hours
End-Points	No clinical end-points Continue as long as infection persists or for 7–10 days.

Other Antibiotics

Tetracycline for penicillin-allergic patients
Consider gram-negative coverage and broader anaerobic coverage.

Second-Line Drug

Hyperbaric Oxygen

Initial Dose	2.4–3.0 atmospheres absolute for 90–120 minutes
Repeat Dosing	Same No standard protocol Suggest repeating 3 times daily for first 48 hours
End-Point	Clinical resolution of active infection or toxicity

line data from laboratory studies. Frequently, tissue destruction results in hyperkalemia and eventual renal failure.

Antibiotics should be rapidly administered. Penicillin is the drug of choice and should be administered in high doses since diffusion may be the main route of delivery to infected tissues. Experts recommend doses of 10 to 24 million units of penicillin per day and favor the sodium salt over the potassium salt due to existing hyperkalemia in many cases. Many authorities will also cover the patient for gram-negative organisms with an aminoglycoside such as gentamicin and for gram-positive anaerobic organisms with metronidazole or clindamycin. Penicillin-allergic individuals should be treated with tetracycline.

Surgical consultation should be concomitant with the initiation of medical therapy because surgery is the mainstay of therapy and virtually all patients require some form of debridement. Routinely the surgeon coordinates and directs care of these patients. Hyperbaric therapy is best administered by a specialist in close association with surgical therapy. Frequently the initial treatment can be given while the operating room is being readied and will not delay debridement. Surgical margins may be easier to define following hyperbaric therapy. The approach to treatment of gas gangrene is summarized in Figure 26–4.

Hyperbaric treatments can be repeated in the immediate postoperative period. Many authorities treat three times a day at 2 to 2.5 atmospheres for the initial 48 hours and then less frequently depending on clinical condition. Patients frequently require repeat surgery and should be regularly assessed in this regard. There is no clear advantage of multiplace chambers over monoplace chambers

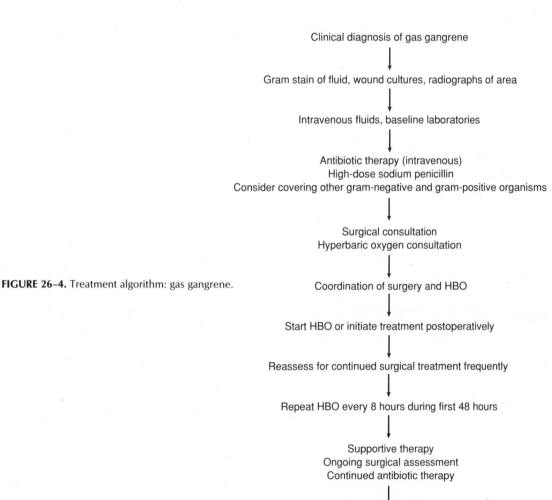

FIGURE 26–4. Treatment algorithm: gas gangrene.

Clinical diagnosis of gas gangrene

↓

Gram stain of fluid, wound cultures, radiographs of area

↓

Intravenous fluids, baseline laboratories

↓

Antibiotic therapy (intravenous)
High-dose sodium penicillin
Consider covering other gram-negative and gram-positive organisms

↓

Surgical consultation
Hyperbaric oxygen consultation

↓

Coordination of surgery and HBO

↓

Start HBO or initiate treatment postoperatively

↓

Reassess for continued surgical treatment frequently

↓

Repeat HBO every 8 hours during first 48 hours

↓

Supportive therapy
Ongoing surgical assessment
Continued antibiotic therapy

↓

Eventual wound closure (infection eradicated)
Rehabilitation

in this illness. Since the patients are frequently seriously ill, it is recommended that invasive hemodynamic monitoring be utilized to guide resuscitation.

Painful Procedures and Conditions

Physicians practicing emergency medicine and prehospital care personnel frequently treat patients experiencing pain. Treatment may require utilizing a procedure that itself is painful. The practitioner must be adept at limiting the pain that a patient experiences in order to facilitate treatment as well as provide comfort.

Analgesia is defined as loss of painful sensation without alteration of consciousness, whereas *anesthesia* is reduction of pain with or without loss of consciousness. The term *conscious sedation* is applied to application of agents that produce anesthesia/analgesia with sedative effects but no loss of consciousness or respiratory drive. Nitrous oxide analgesia is a technique that has wide application in dental surgery and has more recently gained acceptance in emergency medicine and prehospital care.

Indications for Treatment

The conditions that respond favorably to application of nitrous oxide (N_2O) are varied. Its use as an analgesic is limited to minor surgical procedures as well as a variety of painful nonsurgical conditions. Table 26–2 provides a summary of common applications. Recent experience shows that N_2O may be used in prehospital settings for almost any painful procedure or condition, including ex-

TABLE 26–2. Indications for Application of Nitrous Oxide Analgesia

Conditions Suitable for Nitrous Oxide Analgesia
Burns
Fractures
Soft tissue trauma
Labor and delivery
Myocardial ischemia
Drug withdrawal
Renal colic
Pain associated with malignancy

Procedures Appropriate for Nitrous Oxide Analgesia
Dental extraction
Incision and drainage of abscesses and thrombosed hemorrhoids
Reduction of joints, fractures
Culdocentesis
Debridement of burns; dressing changes
Dilatation and curettage

trications and ischemic cardiac pain, because of its ease of application, short duration of action, and lack of significant side effects.

Since indications for treatment encompass the scope of modern medicine, the physician is best guided by knowledge of conditions in which the application of N_2O is contraindicated. Conditions in which constant observation of mental status is important, such as head trauma, are considered to be contraindications. N_2O will also exacerbate decompression sickness and air embolism and should be avoided in the treatment of diving accidents.

The most common formulation of N_2O involves the use of an increased FiO_2 and could lead to respiratory depression if administered to a patient with chronic obstructive lung disease. Patients who are not capable of performing the procedure (self-application)

DRUG TREATMENT: NITROUS OXIDE ANALGESIA

First-Line Drug

Nitrous Oxide

Initial Dose	Patient applies 50% N_2O/50% O_2 via demand valve mask or mouthpiece with tight seal.
Repeat Dosing	Administration is continuous. May be reapplied by patient if pain persists or recurs after initial administration in same dose
End-Points	Clinical relief of pain and onset of sedation are rapid. Administration is discontinued by patient when level of sedation is too great. May be discontinued by patient for any reason at any time

should be considered a relative contraindication, and each case should be considered individually. (See box.)

Discussion

Once an appropriate patient has been identified, application of N_2O analgesia is a relatively simple procedure. A commercially available apparatus for delivering 50% N_2O/ 50% O_2 (Nitronox) is based on patient self-administration. The patient places the mask over the face or the mouthpiece into the mouth and breathes at a normal rate. As long as the patient requires analgesia, self-administration continues. Oversedation is prevented by the patient's inability to maintain an adequate seal. Without a seal the necessary negative pressure to trigger the demand valve is lost and the mouthpiece or mask simply falls off the face, exposing the patient to room air.

During N_2O administration, the patient should have frequent monitoring of vital signs, although this form of sedation rarely produces significant changes. If side effects occur, the mask should be removed. Once administration is complete, usual practice is to have the patient breathe high-flow oxygen for several minutes to counteract any backflow of N_2O from the blood into the alveoli that might displace inspired oxygen. This is termed *diffusion hypoxia* and may not be a clinically relevant phenomenon with the N_2O concentrations used for sedation.

Exposure of health care workers to high levels of N_2O in the workplace should be minimized. Scavenging devices should be used if available. General guidelines for exposure in the operating room allow for 25 parts per million (ppm), but levels measured transiently in the emergency department have approached 1200 ppm and levels in unventilated ambulances have reached 9000 ppm. Thus, short periods of use, ventilated rooms, and use of scavenging devices are of great importance.

Upper Airway Obstruction

Obstruction of the upper airway may result from a variety of causes. These conditions produce a mechanical reduction in the cross-sectional area of the airway, which reduces air flow to the lungs and increases work effort on the part of the patient to get oxygen to the lungs. The causes of upper airway obstruction, though resulting in the same narrowing of the airway, have not all been studied with respect to the therapeutic gas helium–oxygen and thus all causes of obstruction may not represent indications for treatment.

Tumor can cause intrinsic or extrinsic mechanical compression of the trachea. Additionally, edema related to radiation treatment of tumor masses can result in obstruction. Further causes of edema of the airway may be related to the presence of an endotracheal tube, and symptoms may occur after extubation. Viral laryngotracheobronchitis or "croup" may produce a degree of upper airway obstruction due to edema. Clinical experience with these causes of upper airway obstruction has been positive with regard to the use of helium–oxygen as a therapeutic maneuver.

No data exist, however, about its use in other conditions such as foreign body obstruction of the airway or epiglottitis. Theoretically, the use of helium–oxygen in these situations could provide temporary relief prior to definitive airway control. Until this method of treatment has been studied, however, it cannot be recommended.

Diagnosis

Signs and symptoms of upper airway obstruction are not subtle. Patients present in respiratory distress exhibiting air hunger. Stridor is frequently audible. Use of the accessory muscles of respiration is common, and retractions above the clavicle may be evident. Further signs of distress will be evidenced by tachypnea, tachycardia, and diaphoresis. Many of these clinical signs respond rapidly and dramatically to the use of helium–oxygen in appropriate patients.

Further evaluation is required in the patient with respiratory distress of unclear etiology. Primary pulmonary pathology such as shunting, infectious processes, and atelectasis do not respond to helium–oxygen therapy, and patients will probably deteriorate if more appropriate therapy is not instituted. Bronchospastic diseases such as asthma and chronic obstructive pulmonary disease show a limited response in clinical studies, and helium–oxygen can only be considered an adjunctive therapy.

Indications for Treatment

Much of the recent experience with helium–oxygen in upper airway obstruction utilizes it as a temporary solution to the problem. Application of this therapeutic gas allows the patient to breathe with an obstruction until the obstruction resolves with therapy or can be treated with other modalities. Thus, the gas should be viewed as an adjunctive measure only.

In cases where edema is responsible for the obstruction, use of the gas potentially allows time for standard therapies such as neb-ulized racemic epinephrine or systemic steroids to work and may preclude the need for intubation. In cases of mechanical obstruction by tumor, it allows radiation treatment to proceed. Emergency tracheostomy may be averted, allowing the patient to have the tracheostomy done under urgent but more

---

DRUG TREATMENT: UPPER AIRWAY OBSTRUCTION

First-Line Drug

Racemic Epinephrine

Initial Dose	Racemic epinephrine (0.5 ml in 2 ml saline) aerosol inhalation via nebulizer
Repeat Dosing	Same May be repeated in 20–30 minutes Not to exceed 3 doses in 60 minutes
End-Point	Improvement in symptoms

Second-Line Drug

Helium–Oxygen

Initial Dose	Apply 80%/20% mixture via tight-fitting mask.
Repeat Dosing	Administration is continuous and may be continued for several days if necessary.
End-Point	Clinical response is rapid; continue until underlying obstruction is resolved.

Third-Line Drug

Diphenhydramine

Initial Dose	1 mg/kg, up to 50 mg IV or IM
Repeat Dosing	Same May repeat every 6 hours
End-Points	No clinical end-points Continue for 24–72 hours.

Fourth-Line Drugs

Methylprednisolone

Initial Dose	1–2 mg/kg IV
Repeat Dosing	No standard guidelines Suggest repeat of initial dose every 6–8 hours
End-Point	No clinical end-point

OR

Dexamethasone

Initial Dose	1.0–1.5 mg/kg, up to 20 mg IV or IM
Repeat Dosing	See Methylprednisolone, above.
End-Point	See Methylprednisolone, above.

controlled circumstances in the operating room. Laser excision of tumor masses may be a feasible alternative in patients with otherwise inoperable lesions below the level where tracheostomy is technically possible. Availability of helium–oxygen mixtures may provide the modality for temporary stabilization of these difficult patients and allow appropriate plans to be made for more definitive therapies. (See box.)

Discussion

Once a patient presents with upper airway obstruction that may be amenable to helium–oxygen treatment, use of this therapeutic gas can be considered. Many patients respond to standard therapy such as steroid administration and application of supplemental oxygen. If a patient stabilizes with this therapy, there is no need to proceed to using helium–oxygen, and the patient can be managed in a standard fashion.

Patients who do not show adequate response to standard measures can be considered for a trial of helium–oxygen. For this therapy to be valuable, it should be readily available within the emergency department or other critical care environment in which the patient is being treated. If helium–oxygen is not immediately available, the patient should be intubated or a tracheostomy or cricothyrotomy should be performed. The approach to patients with upper airway obstruction is summarized in Figure 26–5.

Helium–oxygen is available premixed in concentrations of 80% helium/20% oxygen, which approximates the FiO_2 in air. Although other mixtures may be available, this percentage maximizes the desired effect of helium. The simplest method of increasing the amount of inspired oxygen is to supplement it at the level of the patient with a nasal cannula or a Venturi system that will add oxygen to the mask. An oxygen meter at the level of the mask will then guide adjustments. Arterial blood gases as well as clinical response should be monitored to guide therapy. Masks used to administer the gas should be of the tight-fitting variety such as those designed for anesthesia use or continuous positive airway pressure devices.

It is hoped the patient will respond to this therapy for a sufficient length of time to allow medication to work or alternative therapies to be arranged. It should be noted that pharmacologic agents should continue to be administered (e.g., racemic epinephrine) even though the patient is breathing helium–oxygen. The response to helium–oxygen is usually rapid and can be seen within

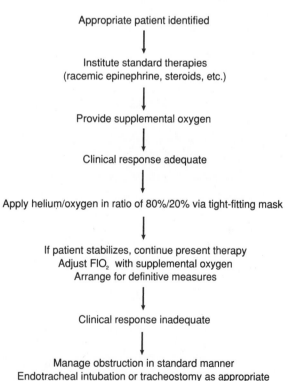

FIGURE 26–5. Treatment algorithm: upper airway obstruction.

Appropriate patient identified

↓

Institute standard therapies
(racemic epinephrine, steroids, etc.)

↓

Provide supplemental oxygen

↓

Clinical response adequate

↓

Apply helium/oxygen in ratio of 80%/20% via tight-fitting mask

↓

If patient stabilizes, continue present therapy
Adjust FIO_2 with supplemental oxygen
Arrange for definitive measures

↓

Clinical response inadequate

↓

Manage obstruction in standard manner
Endotracheal intubation or tracheostomy as appropriate

minutes of administration. Patients who do not respond within this time frame should immediately be considered for other forms of therapy such as airway control via endotracheal intubation. Patients have been maintained successfully on this gas mixture for several days while radiation and other measures are instituted.

Central Retinal Artery Occlusion

Perhaps the most common use of carbogen (carbon dioxide 5%, oxygen 95%) under emergency conditions is in the treatment of acute central retinal artery occlusion. This condition results in an acute loss of vision in one eye and is most commonly due to thrombosis of an atherosclerotic vessel but may be caused by an embolus or primary vasospasm. Most authorities believe that rapid treatment is required for good outcome. Emergency measures include massage of the globe to dislodge an embolus, retrobulbar block to produce local sympathectomy, anterior chamber paracentesis, and the administration of carbogen.

Diagnosis

This condition is characterized by the sudden painless loss of vision in one eye. Physical examination is remarkable for a marked decrease in visual acuity. Examination of the fundus will demonstrate a pale disc and distinctive cherry-red macular spot.

Indications for Treatment

Most authorities believe that rapid treatment is required for good outcome. Carbogen is often used in conjunction with other interventions. It is administered intermittently for short periods (e.g., 10 minutes every hour) depending on the response.

Numerous chemoreceptors within the body are sensitive to carbon dioxide. Two primary effects will occur. First, the increase in levels of carbon dioxide stimulates the respiratory drive through direct action as well as that produced by the associated acidosis. Second, the gas, which is highly soluble, acts as a vasodilator of many vessels. It should be noted that carbogen is a combination of oxygen and carbon dioxide and that oxygen is a potent vasoconstrictor of cerebral vessels, directly opposing the effect of carbon dioxide.

In clinical studies of normal volunteers, oxygen is a potent vasoconstrictor of the retinal vessels, and this effect is not countered by the addition of 5% carbon dioxide. Other studies using 10% carbon dioxide demonstrated an increased diameter of retinal vessels; however, this is not the concentration employed clinically. Theoretically the dilation of retinal vasculature in concert with the administration of oxygen could reduce the

---

DRUG TREATMENT: CENTRAL RETINAL ARTERY OCCLUSION

First-Line Drugs

Acetazolamide

Initial Dose	500 mg IV
Repeat Dosing	250 mg PO/IV in 6–8 hours
End-Points	Dehydration Clinical improvement

AND

Carbon Dioxide 5%/Oxygen 95% (Carbogen)

Initial Dose	Inhalation at 3 liters/min for 10 minutes
Repeat Dosing	No standard guidelines Same as initial dose May be repeated every hour for up to 48 hours
End-Points	Clinical improvement Evidence of toxicity

ischemic insult of arterial occlusion and limit visual loss. Treatment of this condition is largely empiric and should only be carried out in close consultation with an ophthalmologist. (See box.)

SPECIFIC AGENTS

Carbon Dioxide (Carbogen)

Pharmacology

Chemical Structure

Carbon dioxide as a gas has the formula CO_2. Carbogen gas is a mixture of 5% carbon dioxide and 95% oxygen.

Distribution

Carbon dioxide is distributed into all body compartments. Once in solution it is in equilibrium with bicarbonate and is a dynamic component of acid–base equilibrium.

Elimination

Elimination occurs primarily through exhalation via the lungs although minor renal mechanisms of elimination exist. Elimination is tied to concentration gradients as well as to minute volume.

Actions

The effects produced by altering the pH and pCO_2 are seen throughout the body. Increased levels of carbon dioxide act to stimulate respiratory drive both through central mechanisms and peripheral chemoreceptors. Carbon dioxide acts as a peripheral vasodilator although central vasoconstriction can be stimulated through sympathetic mechanisms. Low doses provide a general central nervous system depressant effect, whereas high doses can result in excitability displayed as seizure activity.

Indications

Central retinal artery occlusion
Acute deafness
Panic disorder/anxiety
Anesthesia

Cautions

Respiratory disease/failure—use with caution if at all.
Cardiac disease—may promote arrhythmias
Hepatic failure—no known guidelines

Renal failure—no known guidelines; use with caution in presence of acidosis.
Use in pregnancy—Category C; no known guidelines
Use in childhood—no known guidelines

Onset and Duration of Action

Dosage

Inhalation of 5% mixture for 10 minutes every hour

Limits

Will be based on clinical evidence of improvement or toxicity

Repeat Dosing

May be repeated every hour for up to 48 hours depending on clinical response (for central retinal artery occlusion)

Toxicity

Drug Interactions

None specifically reported
May potentiate antihypertensive medications.

Adverse Effects

Adverse effects are usually found only when concentrations greater than 5% are used. Most frequent are acidic taste, headache, dizziness, dyspnea, diaphoresis, paresthesias, and apprehension. High concentrations may produce seizures, arrhythmias, and coma.

Treatment of Toxicity

Withdrawal of the gas from the patient will result in rapid reversal of symptoms.

Helium–Oxygen (Heliox)

Pharmacology

Chemical Structure

Heliox is a mixture of oxygen (O_2) and helium (He). It is available commercially in mixtures ranging from 60 to 90% helium with the remainder being oxygen. For use at 1 atmosphere (surface conditions), concentrations of oxygen less than 20% are not useful. However, the maximization of the concentration of helium gives the greatest therapeutic effect since the physical properties of the gas are responsible for its benefit.

For these reasons a relative mixture of 80% helium and 20% oxygen is used most commonly for medical applications.

Distribution

Helium is inert and only slightly soluble. For all intents and purposes it is not distributed within the body and remains within the respiratory tree.

Elimination

Helium is eliminated from the respiratory tree via respiration.

Actions

The physical properties of helium are responsible for its benefit when used as a breathing medium. Helium has the second lowest specific gravity of all gases after hydrogen. In contrast to hydrogen it is inert rather than explosive. Within the body it is metabolically inactive. Because it is less dense than nitrogen, heliox has a density of about one-third that of air. Graham's law states that gas flow through a given cross-sectional area is inversely proportional to the square root of its density. Thus, as cross-sectional area of the airway is reduced by obstruction, flow of a gas through that obstruction may be increased by decreasing the density of the gas.

The therapeutic effect of helium–oxygen is attributed to this direct increase in flow as predicted by Graham's law as well as to a reduction in turbulent flow in the poststenotic portion of the airway. Additionally, it is believed that distal segments of the airway will be less likely to collapse if flow is increased.

Indications

Upper airway obstruction
   Asthma and croup (investigational)
   Commercial diving

Cautions

Renal failure—no dosage adjustment necessary
Cardiac failure—no dosage adjustment necessary
Hepatic failure—no dosage adjustment necessary
Use in pregnancy—toxicity in this setting is unknown. Theoretically the risk should be small or absent.
Childhood—may be used

Onset and Duration of Action

Dosage

Administer 20% oxygen/ 80% helium via tight-fitting mask.

Repeat Dosing

Oxygen/helium is given by continuous administration; it may be continued for several days if necessary.

Limits

Limits will be determined by clinical response and response to other forms of therapy.

Toxicity

Drug Interactions

None known

Specific Adverse Effects

Use will alter speech, producing a "Donald Duck" phonation. Prolonged use may result in increased heat loss via the respiratory tree.

Treatment of Toxicity

Discontinue heliox.

Hyperbaric Oxygen (HBO)

Pharmacology

Chemical Structure

Hyperbaric oxygen is structurally the same as atmospheric oxygen and has the formula O_2.

Distribution

Inspired oxygen is carried by hemoglobin throughout the body. Under normobaric circumstances a small amount is also carried in solution. Hyperbaric administration greatly increases the dissolved fraction. In the body a small amount is bound by myoglobin within muscle tissue.

Elimination

Oxygen is metabolized rather than eliminated. The products of aerobic respiration are carbon dioxide and water, which are eliminated through pulmonary and renal mechanisms.

Actions

Normally oxygen is the primary component of aerobic metabolism. When administered under hyperbaric conditions, sufficient oxygen is dissolved in the plasma to support life in the absence of hemoglobin. The paO_2 is greater than 2000 mmHg at 3 ATA. This elevated level of oxygen allows diffusion into hypoxic areas as well as into nitrogen bubbles, where it is eventually metabolized. High levels of oxygen favor dissolution of the carboxyhemoglobin complex and account for shortening the half-life in cases of poisoning. Hyperbaric oxygen augments wound healing via diffusion into hypoxic segments of the wound and by improving white cell function. Oxygen is a vasoconstrictor and will act to reduce edema and intracranial pressure. High concentrations of oxygen directly inhibit anaerobic bacteria.

Indications

Indications for hyperbaric oxygen therapy have varied throughout the history of its use, and many applications are clearly controversial in this regard. The indications listed below are those currently accepted by the Undersea and Hyperbaric Medical Society.

Decompression sickness°
Gas embolism°
Carbon monoxide poisoning°
Gas gangrene†
Compromised skin grafts/reconstructive surgery†
Crush injuries†
Chronic skin ulcers/problem wounds†
Osteomyelitis†
Osteoradionecrosis†
Thermal injury†
Necrotizing fasciitis†
Cyanide poisoning†
Exceptional blood loss anemia†
Actinomycosis†

Cautions

Renal failure—none
Cardiac failure—none
Hepatic failure—none
Use in pregnancy—effects are unknown although toxicity has not been demonstrated. Its use is recommended by authorities in cases of carbon monoxide poisoning where fetal damage is likely.
Respiratory failure/CO_2 retention—although theoretically patients with chronic obstructive pulmonary disease

°Primary modality of treatment.
†Adjunctive modality.

might be thought to lose respiratory drive, this is generally not a problem in clinical practice. It may be more of a concern if the patient is treated during an exacerbation, and all such patients should be monitored closely.
Seizure disorder—seizures may be precipitated by oxygen toxicity. Elective treatments should only be undertaken with therapeutic anticonvulsant levels and careful patient monitoring.
Air-trapping—patients with severe bronchospasm may develop pneumothorax or air embolism with rapid decompression. Small bowel obstruction and untreated pneumothorax are relative contraindications to treatment.
Children—may be used

Onset and Duration of Action

Dosage

Oxygen is administered in a concentration of 100% at pressures from 2.0 to 6.0 atmospheres for varying periods of time depending on the condition being treated. Standard protocol for any condition in a monoplace chamber is 2.0 to 2.8 atmospheres for 90 minutes.

Limits

Oxygen may be administered under pressure for only a limited period of time before acute oxygen toxicity is manifested. Intermittent breathing of air will allow protracted administration.

Repeat Dosing

Treatments may be repeated after surface intervals of at least 4 hours depending on the treatment table being utilized. It is not uncommon to repeat monoplace protocols on a daily basis for some conditions.

Toxicity

Drug Interactions

Generally not clinically relevant

Adverse Effects

The adverse effects of oxygen may be divided into two components. Acute toxicity is most relevant to hyperbaric oxygen and is also termed *central nervous system toxicity.* The primary component is increased irritability resulting in seizures. This type of toxicity is exacerbated by increased body temperature, increased level of activity, acidosis, pressure, and time. The second or more chronic form of oxygen toxicity is termed *pulmonary toxicity.* Prolonged exposure to high concentrations of oxygen results in subjective respiratory distress displayed as burning, painful breathing during therapy utilizing longer treatment tables. Patients with pulmonary oxygen toxicity will have a measurable and predictable decrease in vital capacity. The mechanism of oxygen poisoning is not well understood. Other minor effects occur with prolonged exposure.

Treatment of Toxicity

Both acute and chronic oxygen toxicity may be treated by discontinuation of hyperbaric therapy. Seizures may be treated with intravenous benzodiazepines acutely if necessary. Treatment may be resumed if necessary after a break of breathing air.

Nitrous Oxide (Nitronox)

Pharmacology

Chemical Structure

Nitrous oxide has the formula N_2O. It is available commercially as a mixture of 50% oxygen/50% nitrous oxide.

Distribution

Inhaled nitrous oxide is taken up rapidly via dissolution in the plasma. It may exchange with pure nitrogen in gas form in the body and thus lead to expansion of pockets of gas such as an existing pneumothorax. It does not react chemically within tissues.

Elimination

Nitrous oxide is eliminated unchanged via the pulmonary tree. It is unknown whether any degree of metabolism occurs.

Actions

At low concentrations its actions are primarily sedative; higher concentrations produce analgesia and anesthesia. A vasodilatory effect within the body has been shown to slightly decrease blood pressure and myocardial function to a mild degree.

Indications

The use of nitrous oxide as an analgesic is indicated for almost any painful condition or procedure in which the period of administration is brief and contraindications do not exist. See earlier in this chapter for a more complete discussion.

Cautions

Renal failure—no dosage adjustment necessary

Cardiac failure—may decrease blood pressure and cardiac output; use with caution.

Hepatic failure—no dosage adjustment necessary

Use in pregnancy—believed to be a teratogen; use *not* recommended

Respiratory failure—may exacerbate hypoxia through decreasing respiratory drive; use *not* recommended

Sickle cell disease—may precipitate crisis; use *not* recommended

Closed gas pocket—may increase size; use *not* recommended

Children—may be used

Onset and Duration of Action

Dosage

The mixture is self-administered by the patient as necessary via hand-held mask or mouthpiece.

Onset of Effect

Minutes

Limits

No clinically applicable limits for short-term use

Removal of administration if side effects appear

Repeat Dosing

The patient may reapply the mask if pain recurs.

Toxicity

Drug Interactions

Central nervous system depressants potentiate sedation.

Adverse Effects

Adverse effects with short-term administration are mild. Patients may complain of nausea and vomiting most commonly. Long-term exposure, primarily of health care workers, is thought to result in a high incidence of neurologic complaints, spontaneous abortions, and possibly liver and kidney disease. Long-term therapeutic use has resulted in bone marrow depression through interference with B_{12} metabolism.

Treatment of Toxicity

Minor side effects can be treated by removal of the mask and discontinuation of administration. Prevention of chronic toxicity is best effected through the prudent use of scavenging devices, adequate ventilation, and short-term administration.

REFERENCES

Arthur DC, Margulies RA: A short course in diving medicine. Ann Emerg Med 16:689–701, 1987.

Bakker DJ: Necrotizing soft tissue infections. J Hyperbaric Med 2:161–168, 1987.

Barach AL: The therapeutic use of helium. JAMA 107:1273–1280, 1936.

Barnett TB: Effects of helium and oxygen mixtures on pulmonary mechanics during airway constriction. J Appl Physiol 22:707–713, 1967.

Bayne CG: Acute decompression sickness. J Am Coll Emerg Physicians 7:351–354, 1978.

Bennett PB, Elliot DH (eds): The Physiology and Medicine of Diving. San Pedro, CA, Best Publishing, 1982.

Bergofsky EH, Wang MC, Yamaki T, et al: Tissue oxygen and carbon dioxide tensions during hyperbaric oxygenation. JAMA 189:841–844, 1964.

Boerema I, Meyne NG, Brummelkamp WK, et al: Life without blood. J Cardiovasc Surg 1:133–146, 1960.

Boettger ML: Scuba diving emergencies: Pulmonary overpressure accidents and decompression sickness. Ann Emerg Med 12:563–567, 1983.

Bowersox JC, Strauss MB, Hart GB: Clinical experience with hyperbaric oxygen therapy in the salvage of ischemic skin flaps and grafts. J Hyperbaric Med 1:141–149, 1986.

Bretzke ML, Bubrick MP, Hitchcock CR: Diffuse spreading Clostridium septicum infection, malignant disease and immune suppression. Surg Gynecol Obstet 166:197–199, 1988.

Brodsky JB, Cohen EN, Brown BW, et al: Exposure to nitrous oxide and neurologic disease among dental professionals. Anesth Analg 60:297–301, 1981.

Butler FK, Pinto CV: Progressive ulnar palsy as a late complication of decompression sickness. Ann Emerg Med 15:738–741, 1986.

Clark JM: Oxygen toxicity. In Bennett PB, Elliot DH (eds): The Physiology and Medicine of Diving. San Pedro, CA, Best Publishing, 1982, pp 200–238.

Cohen EN, Gift HC, Brown BW: Occupational disease in dentistry and chronic exposure to trace anesthetic gases. J Am Dent Assoc 101:21–31, 1980.

Coppa GF, Gouge TH, Hofstetter SR: Air embolism: A lethal but preventable complication of subclavian vein catheterization. J Parenter Enter Nutr 5:166–168, 1981.

Crocker PJ, Walker JS: Pediatric carbon monoxide toxicity. J Emerg Med 3:443–448, 1985.

Curtis JL, Mahlmeister M, Fink JB, et al: Helium-oxygen gas therapy: Use and availability for the emergency treatment of inoperable airway obstruction. Chest 90:455–457, 1986.

Davis JC: Hyperbaric Oxygen Therapy: A Committee Report. Bethesda, MD, Undersea Medical Society, 1983.

Davis JC, Hart GK (eds): Hyperbaric Oxygen Therapy. Bethesda, MD, Undersea Medical Society, 1978.

Davis JC, Heckman JD, DeLee JC, et al: Chronic nonhematogenous osteomyelitis treated with adjuvant hyperbaric oxygen. J Bone Joint Surg 68A:1210–1217, 1986.

Deacon R, Lumb M, Perry J: Selective inactivation of vitamin B_{12} in rats by nitrous oxide. Lancet 2:1023–1090, 1978.

Deitsch TA, Read JS, Ernest JT, et al: Effects of oxygen and carbon dioxide on the retinal vasculature in humans. Arch Ophthalmol 101:1278–1280, 1983.

Demello FJ, Haglin JJ, Hitchcock CR: Comparative study of experimental Clostridium perfringens infection in dogs treated with antibiotics, surgery, and hyperbaric oxygen. Surgery 73:936–941, 1973.

Dolan MC, Haltom TL, Barrows GH, et al: Carboxyhemoglobin levels in patients with flu-like symptoms. Ann Emerg Med 16:782–786, 1987.

Dula DJ, Skiendzielewski JJ, Royco MM: Nitrous oxide levels in the emergency department. Ann Emerg Med 10:575–578, 1981.

Dula DJ, Skiendzielewski JJ, Snover SW: The scavenger device for nitrous oxide administration. Ann Emerg Med 12:759–761, 1983.

Duncan PG: Efficacy of helium-oxygen mixtures in the management of severe viral and post intubation croup. Can Anaesth Soc J 26:206–212, 1979.

Ellis ME, Mandal BK: Hyperbaric oxygen treatment: 10 years' experience of a regional infectious diseases unit. J Infect 6:17–28, 1983.

Fink BR: Diffusion anoxia. Anesthesiology 16:511–519, 1955.

Flomenbaum N, Gallagher EJ, Eagen K, et al: Self administered nitrous oxide: An adjunct analgesic. J Am Coll Emerg Physicians 8:95–97, 1979.

Fosberg MT, Crone RK: Nitrous oxide analgesia for refractory pain in the terminally ill. JAMA 250:511–513, 1983.

Frayser R, Hickam J: Retinal vascular response to breathing increased carbon dioxide and oxygen concentrations. Invest Ophthalmol Vis Sci 3:427–431, 1964.

Gibson A, Davis F: Hyperbaric oxygen therapy in the management of Clostridium perfringens infections. NZ Med J 99:617–620, 1986.

Gillman MA, Lichtigfeld FJ: Minimal sedation required with nitrous oxide-oxygen treatment of the alcohol withdrawal state. Br J Psychiatry 148:604–606, 1986.

Gillman MA, Lichtigfeld FJ: Analgesic nitrous oxide: Adjunct to clonidine for opioid withdrawal (letter). Am J Psychiatry 142:6, 1985.

Ginsberg MD: Carbon monoxide intoxication: Clinical features, neuropathology and mechanisms of injury. Clin Toxicol 23:281–288, 1985.

Glass M, Forman HJ, Rotman EI, et al: Bronchoalveolar polymorphonuclear leukocytes in pulmonary oxygen toxicity. J Hyperbaric Med 1:107–121, 1986.

Goldbaum LR, Orellano T, Dergal E: Mechanism of the toxic action of carbon monoxide. Ann Clin Lab Sci 6:372, 1976.

Goodman MW, Workman RD, Hedgepeth CG: Minimal recompression oxygen breathing approach to treatment of decompression sickness. BUSHIPS Res Report 5:65, 1965.

Gronert GA, Messick JM, Cucchiara RF, et al: Paradoxical air embolism from a patent foramen ovale. Anesthesiology 50:548–549, 1979.

Grossman RA, Grossman AJ: Update on hyperbaric oxygen treatment of burns. Hyperbaric Oxygen Review 3:52–59, 1983.

Haddad LM: Carbon monoxide poisoning: To transfer or not to transfer? Ann Emerg Med 15:1375, 1986.

Hart GB, Lamb RC, Strauss MB: Gas gangrene: I. A collective review. II. A 15 year experience with hyperbaric oxygen. J Trauma 23:991–1000, 1983.

Hart GB, Rowe MJ, Meyers LW, et al: A controlled study of hyperbaric oxygen treatment in multiple sclerosis. J Hyperbaric Med 2:1–5, 1987.

Heckerling PS, Leikin JB, Maturen A, et al: Predictors of occult carbon monoxide poisoning in patients with headache and dizziness. Ann Intern Med 107:174–176, 1987.

Horowitz AL, Kaplan R, Sarpel G: Carbon monoxide toxicity: MR imaging in the brain. Radiology 162:787–788, 1987.

Jacobsen WK, Briggs BA, Mason LJ: Paradoxical air embolism associated with a central total parenteral nutrition catheter. Crit Care Med 11:388–389, 1983.

Jacobsen JH, Morseh JC, Rendell-Baker L: The historical perspective of hyperbaric therapy. Ann NY Acad Sci 117:651–670, 1965.

Jastak TJ, Malamed SF: Nitrous oxide sedation and sexual phenomena. J Am Dent Assoc 101:38–40, 1980.

Kindwall EP: Hyperbaric treatment of carbon monoxide poisoning. Ann Emerg Med 14:1233–1234, 1985.

Kindwall EP, Goldmann RW, Thombs PA: Use of the monoplace vs multiplace chamber in the treatment of diving diseases. J Hyperbaric Med 3:5–10, 1988.

Kizer KW: Dysbaric cerebral air embolism in Hawaii. Ann Emerg Med 16:535–541, 1987.

Kizer KW: The management of dysbaric diving casualties. Emerg Med Clin North Am 1:659–670, 1983.

Kizer KW: Delayed treatment of dysbarism. JAMA 247:2555–2558, 1982.

Kripke BJ, Justice RE, Hechtman HB: Postoperative nitrous oxide analgesia and the functional residual capacity. Crit Care Med 11:105–109, 1983.

Lanphier EH, Camporesi EM: Respiration and exercise. In Bennet PB, Elliot DH (eds): The Physiology and Medicine of Diving. San Pedro, CA, Best Publishing, 1982, pp 99–156.

Lassen H, Henricksen E, Neukirch F, et al: Treatment of tetanus: Severe bone marrow depression after prolonged nitrous oxide anesthesia. Lancet 1:527–530, 1956.

Leitch DR, Greenbaum LJ, Hallenbeck JM: Cerebral air embolism I, II, III. Undersea Biomed Res 11:221–263, 1984.

Lunsford JM, Wynn MH, Kwan WH: Nitrous oxide induced myeloneuropathy. J Foot Surg 22:222–225, 1983.

Mader JT, Adams KR, Sutton TE: Infectious diseases: Pathophysiology and mechanisms of hyperbaric oxygen. J Hyperbaric Med 2:133–140, 1987.

Manson PN, Im MJ, Meyers RA, et al: Improved capillaries by hyperbaric oxygen skin flaps. Surg Forum 31:564–566, 1980.

Margulies JL: Acute carbon monoxide poisoning during pregnancy. Am J Emerg Med 4:516–519, 1986.

Marx RE, Johnson RP, Kline SN: Prevention of osteoradionecrosis: A randomized prospective clinical trial of hyperbaric oxygen versus penicillin. J Am Dent Assoc 111:49–54, 1985.

Mathieu D, Nolf M, Durocher A, et al: Acute carbon monoxide poisoning: Risk of late sequelae and treatment by hyperbaric oxygen. Clin Toxicol 23:315–324, 1985.

Messier LD, Meyers RA: The carbon monoxide screening battery manual of instructions. Baltimore, The Maryland Institute for Emergency Medical Services Systems, 1987.

Meyers RA, Bray P: Delayed treatment of serious decompression sickness. Ann Emerg Med 14:254–257, 1985.

Meyers RA, Snyder SK, Emhoff TA: Subacute sequelae of carbon monoxide poisoning. Ann Emerg Med 14:1163–1167, 1985.

Meyers RA, Snyder SK, Majerus TC: Cutaneous blisters and carbon monoxide poisoning. Ann Emerg Med 14:603–606, 1985.

Mink SN, Wood LH: How does $He-O_2$ increase maximum expiratory flow in human lungs? J Clin Invest 66:720–729, 1980.

Michel L, Poskanzer DC, McKusick KA, et al: Fatal paradoxical air embolism to the brain—complication of central venous catheterization. J Parenter Enter Nutr 6:68–70, 1982.

Mizrahi S, Yaari Y, Lugassy G, et al: Major airway obstruction relieved by helium-oxygen breathing. Crit Care Med 14:986–987, 1986.

Murphy BP, Harford FJ, Cramer FS: Cerebral air embolism resulting from invasive medical procedures. Ann Surg 201:242–245, 1985.

Nelson DS, McClellan R: Helium-oxygen mixtures as adjunctive support for refractory viral croup. Ohio State Med J 78:729–730, 1962.

Neuman TS, Hallenbeck JM: Barotraumatic cerebral air embolism and the mental status examination: A report of four cases. Ann Emerg Med 16:220–223, 1987.

Nielson NV: Treatment of acute occlusion of the retinal arteries. Acta Ophthalmol 57:1078–1082, 1979.

Norkool DM, Kirkpatrick JN: Treatment of acute carbon monoxide poisoning: A review of 115 cases. Ann Emerg Med 14:1168–1171, 1985.

Peters EJ, Boyars MC: Arterial air embolism after a percutaneous needle lung aspiration. J Hyperbaric Med 1:151–155, 1986.

Pierce EC: Treating acidemia in carbon monoxide poisoning may be dangerous. J Hyperbaric Med 1:87–97, 1986.

Pingleton SK, Bone RC, Ruth WC: Helium-oxygen mixtures during bronchoscopy. Crit Care Med 8:50–53, 1980.

Schweigel JF, Shim SS: A comparison of the treatment of gas gangrene with and without hyperbaric oxygen. Surg Gynecol Obstet 136:969–970, 1973.

Simmons K: Some sobering facts about laughing gas. JAMA 253:2334–2337, 1985.

Skrinskas GJ, Hyland RH, Hutcheon MA: Using helium-oxygen mixtures in the management of acute upper airway obstruction. Can Med Assoc J 128:555–558, 1983.

Stewart RD: Nitrous oxide sedation/analgesia in emergency medicine. Ann Emerg Med 14:139–148, 1985.

Stewart RD, Gorayeb MJ, Pelton GH: Arterial blood gases before, during and after nitrous oxide:oxygen administration. Ann Emerg Med 15:1177–1180, 1986.

Stewart RD, Paris PM, Stoy WA, et al: Patient-controlled inhalation analgesia in prehospital care: A study of side-effects and feasibility. Crit Care Med 11:851–855, 1983.

Stone R, Zink H, Klingele T, et al: Visual recovery after

central retinal artery occlusion: Two cases. Ann Ophthalmol 9:445–450, 1977.

Sturman K, Mofenson H, Caraccio T: Methylene chloride inhalation: An unusual form of drug abuse. Ann Emerg Med 14:903–905, 1985.

Sukoff HM: Central nervous system review and update: Cerebral edema and spinal cord injuries. Hyperbaric Oxygen Review 3:189–195, 1980.

Swidwa DM, Montenegro HD, Goldman MD, et al: Helium-oxygen breathing in severe chronic obstructive pulmonary disease. Chest 87:790–795, 1985.

TenEyck LG, Colgan FJ: Methods and guidelines for mechanical ventilation with helium-oxygen for severe upper airway obstruction. Respir Care 29:155–159, 1984.

Thal ER, Montgomery SJ, Atkins JM, et al: Self-administered analgesia with nitrous oxide: Adjunctive aid for emergency medical care systems. JAMA 242:2418–2419, 1979.

Thalman ED: Phenytoin sodium in oxygen toxicity induced seizures (letter). Ann Emerg Med 12:592–593, 1983.

Thomas AN, Stephens BG: Air embolism: A cause of morbidity and death after penetrating chest trauma. J Trauma 14:633–637, 1974.

Thompson PL, Lown B: Nitrous oxide as an analgesic in acute myocardial infarction. JAMA 235:924–927, 1976.

Thonton J, Fleming J, Goldberg A, et al: Cardiovascular effects of 50% nitrous oxide and 50% oxygen mixture. Anesthesia 28:484–489, 1973.

Torrey SA, Webb SC, Zwingelberg KM, et al: Comparative analysis of decompression sickness: Type and time of onset. J Hyperbaric Med 2:55–62, 1987.

United States Navy Diving Manual. NAVSEA 0994-001-9010. Washington, DC, Department of the Navy, US Government Printing Office, 1978.

Unsworth IP, Sharp PA: Gas gangrene: An 11 year review of 73 cases managed with hyperbaric oxygen. Med J Aust 140:256–259, 1984.

VanRynen JL, Taha AM, Erlich R, et al: Treatment of cerebral air embolism in the pediatric patient. J Hyperbaric Med 2:199–204, 1987.

Voorhies RM, Fraser RA: Cerebral air embolism occurring at angiography and diagnosed by computerized tomography. J Neurosurg 60:177–178, 1984.

Werner B, Back W, Akerblom H, et al: Two cases of acute carbon monoxide poisoning with delayed neurological sequelae after a "free" interval. Clin Toxicol 23:249–265, 1985.

Wolfson MR, Bhutani VK, Shaffer TH, et al: Mechanics and energetics of breathing helium in infants with bronchopulmonary dysplasia. J Pediatr 104:752–757, 1984.

Wynne J, Mann T, Alpert JS, et al: Hemodynamic effects of nitrous oxide administered during cardiac catheterization. JAMA 243:1440–1443, 1980.

Yee ES, Verrier ED, Thomas AN: Management of air embolism in blunt and penetrating thoracic trauma. J Thorac Cardiovasc Surg 85:661–668, 1983.

Zaltzman JI: Therapeutic nitrous oxide analgesia (letter). Crit Care Med 11:837–838, 1983.

Ziser V, Shupak A, Halpern P, et al: Delayed hyperbaric oxygen treatment for carbon monoxide poisoning. Br Med J 289:960, 1984.

Guidelines for Intravenous Dosing in Pediatric Patients*

The definitions needed to use the following table properly are:

Continuous infusion: Continuous administration of medication in intravenous fluids

D_5W: 5% dextrose in water

Intermittent infusion: Periodic administration of medication diluted in intravenous fluids, usually by minibags, minibottles, or a volume control set

IV push: A specific undiluted amount of medication given directly into the vein within 30 to 60 seconds

MD: Licensed physician

NI: No information available

NR: Not recommended

NS: Normal saline

pt: Patient

Rapid IV push: A specific undiluted amount of medication given directly into the vein in less than 30 seconds

RN: Registered nurse

Slow IV push: A specific undiluted amount of medication given directly into the vein within 3 to 5 minutes

TDD: Total daily dose

*From Ford DC, Leist ER, Algren JT, et al: Guidelines for the administration of intravenous medications to pediatric patients. American Society of Hospital Pharmacists, 1982.

Guidelines for Administration of Intravenous Medications in Pediatric Patients (17 Years and Under)

Generic Name	Initial Dilution	Maximum Dose	IV Push Administered by Critical Care RN		Intermittent or Continuous Infusion Recommended Rates/Further Dilution	Cautions and Comments
			IV Push Recommended Rate	Exceptions		
Aminophylline	250 mg/10 ml	6 mg/kg/dose as loading dose; 6 mg/kg/dose as loading dose in neonates	NR		Dilute with at least an equal volume of IV fluid; infuse dose over 15–30 min; continuous infusion rate 0.9–1.5 mg/kg/hour (do not use in neonates)	Observe for cardiac arrhythmias and hypotension. Adjust dosage based on serum levels.
Amobarbital sodium	100 mg/ml	10 mg/kg/dose, up to 500 mg	5–10 mg/kg over 1–2 min; not >60 mg/m²/min	Critical care RN may give only if pt on ventilator or MD present	Usual dose and rate 5 mg/kg/hour as 10% solution in saline (change solution every 4 hours) or dextrose (change every 2 hours)	Observe for hypotension and apnea. Titrate dose according to clinical response and EEG.
Ampicillin sodium	500 mg/5 ml	400 mg/kg/day, up to 14 g/day; 200 mg/kg/day in neonates	Not >100 mg/min		Minimum dilution 1 g/10 ml over 20–30 min (maximum 1 hour)	Observe for possible hypersensitivity reaction.
Atropine sulfate	0.1 mg/ml 0.4 mg/ml	0.01 mg/kg/dose, up to 0.5 mg; 0.03 mg/kg dose in neonates			NR	In multiple dosing, watch for tachycardia and ventricular fibrillation. May repeat dose two or three times.
Bretylium tosylate	500 mg/10 ml	5–10 mg/kg/ dose, up to 30 mg/kg/day	Rapidly if life threatening; slow IV push over >8 min	MD must be present	Dilute 1:4 in NS or D₅W; infuse over >8 min	Observe for hypotension.
Calcium chloride	1 g/10 ml (13.6 mEq Ca⁺⁺/10 ml)	300 mg/kg/day, up to 5 g/day (70 mEq Ca⁺⁺)	Slow IV push, not >0.5 ml/min		Give as constant infusion if possible; minimum dilution 200 mg/10 ml over at least 30 min	Observe for bradycardia. Do not use in neonates. Avoid extravasation.

Drug	Concentration	Dose	IV push		Dilution/infusion	Comments
Calcium gluconate	1 g/10 ml (4.8 mEq Ca^{++}/10 ml)	700 mg/kg/day, up to 15 g/day (70 mEq Ca^{++})	Slow IV push, not >2 ml/min		Give as constant infusion if possible; minimum dilution 200 mg/10 ml over at least 30 min	Observe for bradycardia. Avoid extravasation.
Chloramphenicol sodium succinate	1 g/10 ml	25 mg/kg/dose, up to 1 g	100 mg/ml over at least 1 min		Minimum dilution 1 g/50 ml over 30–60 min	Observe for potential vein irritation. Adjust dosage based on serum levels.
Cimetidine hydrochloride	300 mg/2 ml	10 mg/kg/dose, up to 600 mg	Dilute 300 mg/20 ml over at least 2 min (infusion preferred)		Minimum dilution 300 mg/50 ml in D$_5$W over 15–20 min	Cardiac arrest reported with bolus doses.
Clindamycin phosphate	300 mg/50 ml	10 mg/kg/dose, up to 1.2 g	NR		Minimum dilution 300 mg/50 ml over at least 10 min	Use with caution in infants and neonates.
Dexamethasone sodium phosphate	4 mg/ml	6 mg/kg/dose	Slow		Dilute in at least an equal volume; infuse over at least 10 min	
Dextrose	Varies	Usual dose 0.5 g/kg/dose	Slow; in neonates, dilute D$_{50}$W to D$_{25}$W		Run at convenient rate and volume; maximum concentration by peripheral vein 12%	Observe for potential vein irritation if hypertonic solution. No specific information available on maximum dose.
Diazepam	5 mg/ml	0.3 mg/kg/dose, up to 5 mg in infants and 15 mg in older children	Slow IV push over 3 min unless on ventilator	Critical care RN may give only if pt on ventilator or MD present	NR	Observe for hypotension and respiratory depression.
Diazoxide	300 mg/20 ml	10 mg/kg/dose, up to 300 mg/dose	Dose over 30 sec	Critical care RN may give only if MD present	NR	Observe for hypotension, arrhythmias, and hyperglycemia.
Digoxin	0.1 mg/ml 0.25 mg/ml	Maximum TDD 2–2.5 mg; maximum single digitalizing dose 1–1.25 mg; maximum maintenance dose 0.25 mg/day	1–5 min		NR	Monitor cardiac status. TDD and maintenance dose should be calculated on a per kilogram basis for infants and children. Recommendations may vary. Consult a cardiologist.

Table continued on following page

Generic Name	Initial Dilution	Maximum Dose	IV Push Administered by Critical Care RN		Intermittent or Continuous Infusion Recommended Rates/Further Dilution	Cautions and Comments
			IV Push Recommended Rate	*Exceptions*		
Diphenhydramine hydrochloride	50 mg/ml	100 mg/dose	1–2 mg/kg slowly		NI	No specific information available on maximum dose per kilogram.
Dobutamine hydrochloride	250 mg/10 ml	20 µg/kg/min	NR		Dilution can vary, 2.5–20 µg/kg/min; maximum concentration 5000 µg/ml	Observe for increased heart rate, blood pressure, and ventricular ectopic activity. Precipitate may occur if concentration >5000 µg/ml. No loss of potency with slight discoloration.
Dopamine hydrochloride	200 mg/5 ml	20 µg/kg/min	NR		Dilution can vary, 2–20 µg/kg/min	Observe for arrhythmias, tachycardia, and vasoconstriction. Infiltration may cause local ischemic tissue injury.
Epinephrine	1 mg/10 ml	0.01 mg/kg/dose, up to 0.5–1 mg; for infusion 1.5 µg/kg/min	0.01 mg/kg over 1–3 min	MD must be present	Dilution can vary; usual dose 0.02–1.0 µg/kg/min	Observe for hypertension and arrhythmias. Higher doses may cause excessive vasoconstriction. Do not use discolored solutions.
Erythromycin lactobionate	50 mg/ml	10 mg/kg/dose, up to 1 g	NR		Minimum dilution 50 mg/10 ml over at least 20 min	Observe for vein irritation and thrombophlebitis.
Furosemide	10 mg/ml	Usual maximum 2 mg/kg/dose, not to exceed 6 mg/kg/dose	1 mg/kg over at least 1 min; not >20 mg/min		Rate not >4 mg/min; dilute in at least an equal volume of IV fluid	In patients with impaired renal function, ototoxicity associated with dosage >4 mg/min.
Gentamicin sulfate	10 mg/ml 40 mg/ml	2.5 mg/kg/dose	NR		Concentration not >1 mg/ml over 30–120 min	Observe for respiratory depression. Adjust dosage based on serum levels.

Drug	Concentration	Dose	IV push	IV infusion	Comments
Heparin sodium	1000 units/ml	10,000 units/dose	NI	25 units/kg/hour; adjust according to prothrombin time (two to three times control)	Have protamine available to reverse anticoagulation. No specific information available on maximum dose. Titrate dose according to response.
Hydralazine hydrochloride	20 mg/ml	0.2–0.5 mg/kg/dose, up to 20 mg/dose	Slow	NR	Monitor blood pressure and heart rate for 30–60 min after dose. No specific information available on maximum dose.
Hydrocortisone sodium succinate	50 mg/ml	50 mg/kg/day	Slow	Concentration not >1 mg/ml over at least 30 min	
Insulin, regular U 100	100 units/ml	Usual dose 25 units/m² or 0.1–0.2 unit/kg, followed by infusion not to exceed 5 units/hour	Slow	Usual dose 0.1 unit/kg/hour; dilute with NS so rate is 6 ml/hour	Change infusion to 0.04 unit/kg/hour when blood sugar ≤200 and/or pH ≥7.2.
Isoproterenol hydrochloride	1 mg/5 ml	1.0 µg/kg/min	NR	5 ml (1 mg) diluted to 100 ml; infuse at 0.02–0.5 µg/kg/min (usual dose dilution can vary)	Observe for tachycardia and dysrhythmia.
Lidocaine hydrochloride	2%: 100 mg/5 ml 4%: 1 g/25 ml	1.5 mg/kg/dose; infusion up to 88 µg/kg/min	1 mg/kg over 2 min	20–50 µg/kg/min, 2 g/500 ml; dilution can vary	Observe for seizures, hypotension, and depression of cardiac conductivity.
Magnesium sulfate	1%: 10 mg/ml	100 mg/kg/dose	Slow	Dilute to 10 mg/ml; infuse over at least 15–30 min	Observe for respiratory depression. Monitor blood pressure.
Mannitol	20%: 1 g/5 ml 25%: 1 g/4 ml	2 g/kg/dose	Slow	1–2 g/kg over at least 30–60 min	Monitor serum osmolality. Use IV filters.
Meperidine hydrochloride	50 mg/ml	2 mg/kg/dose, up to 100 mg/dose	Dilute to 10 mg/ml; infuse slowly	Not usually recommended; dilute to 1 mg/ml; infuse over at least 15–30 min	Observe for respiratory depression. Use naloxone to reverse.
Methicillin sodium	500 mg/ml	50 mg/kg/dose, up to 4 g	500 mg/25 ml, 10 ml/min	Minimum dilution 1 g/50 ml; minimum infusion time 200 mg/min	Observe for vein irritation, thrombophlebitis, and possible hypersensitivity reaction.

Table continued on following page

Guidelines for Administration of Intravenous Medications in Pediatric Patients (17 Years and Under) *Continued*

Generic Name	Initial Dilution	Maximum Dose	IV Push Administered by Critical Care RN		Intermittent or Continuous Infusion Recommended Rates/Further Dilution	Cautions and Comments
			IV Push Recommended Rate	*Exceptions*		
Methohexital sodium	500 mg/50 ml	120 mg/dose	10 mg/ml/5 sec	Critical care RN may give only if pt on ventilator or MD present	Dilute to 2 mg/ml; infuse at 3 ml/min	Observe for respiratory depression, hypotension, convulsions, thrombophlebitis, and extravasation. No specific information available on recommended dose.
Methylprednisolone sodium succinate	40 mg/ml 62.5 mg/ml	30 mg/kg/dose	Slow		40 mg/50 ml over 20–30 min	Observe for hypotension and respiratory depression.
Morphine sulfate	10 mg/ml	0.2 mg/kg/dose, up to 15 mg	Slow		NI	
MVI concentrate	5 ml	NI	NR		Dilute to at least 1 ml/100 ml in continuous infusion	Observe for possible anaphylaxis.
Nafcillin sodium	250 mg/ml	37.5 mg/kg/dose, up to 2.5 g	Dilute in 15–30 ml over 5–10 min		Minimum dilution 1 g/30 ml; minimum infusion time 200 mg/min	Observe for thrombophlebitis and possible hypersensitivity reaction.
Naloxone hydrochloride	0.02 mg/ml 0.4 mg/ml	NI	0.005–0.01 mg/kg rapid IV push; usual adult dose 0.4 mg		NR	Use caution if pt may be narcotic dependent.
Pancuronium bromide	2 mg/ml	100 μg/kg/dose	NI	Critical care RN may give only if pt on ventilator	NR	
Penicillin G potassium	500,000 units/ml	50,000 units/kg/dose, up to 5 million units/dose and 30 million units/day	NR		Dilute 1–5 million units in 50–100 ml; infuse over 20–60 min	Observe for vein irritation, thrombophlebitis, and possible hypersensitivity reaction.

Drug	Concentration	Dose	Rate	Special considerations	Dilution	Nursing considerations
Pentobarbital sodium	50 mg/ml	3–5 mg/kg/dose	Usually 1–2 mg/kg slow IV push	Critical care RN may give only if pt on ventilator or MD present	NI	Observe for respiratory depression and hypotension. Dose may be divided and given over 10–20 min.
Phenobarbital sodium	65 mg/ml	10 mg/kg dose; may repeat up to 20 mg/kg or 400–600 mg	Not >1 mg/kg/min		Dilute with at least an equal volume of IV fluid; infuse at not >1 mg/kg/min	Observe for hypotension and respiratory depression. Adjust dosage based on serum levels.
Phenytoin sodium	50 mg/ml	18 mg/kg/dose	Not >1 mg/kg/min, up to maximum 50 mg/min; do not dilute; flush line		NR	Observe for hypotension, cardiotoxic effects, vein irritation, and thrombophlebitis. Use caution if pt on dopamine—may cause hypotension.
Physostigmine salicylate	1 mg/ml	2 mg (pediatric) 4 mg (adult)	1 mg/min or 0.5 mg slowly	Critical care RN may give only if MD present	NR	Observe for bradycardia, convulsions, and hypersalivation.
Phytonadione	1 mg/0.5 ml 10 mg/ml	25–50 mg (adult)	Not >1 mg/min		1 mg/25–50 ml at not >1 mg/min	Observe for hypotension, fever, chills, anaphylaxis, and dysrhythmias.
Potassium supplements	Varies	250 mEq/m²/day	NR		Usual concentration 40 mEq/liter; maximum rate 20 mEq/hour or 0.3 mEq/kg/hour	Avoid extravasation. Observe for dysrhythmias.
Promethazine hydrochloride	25 mg/ml	0.5 mg/kg/dose	Not >25 mg/min		Dilute with at least an equal volume of IV fluid; infuse at not >25 mg/min	Monitor blood pressure.
Propranolol hydrochloride	1 mg/ml	3 mg	0.01–0.15 mg/kg/dose *slow* push	Only MD may give	NR	Observe for hypotension, bradycardia, hypoglycemia, and bronchospasm. Monitor for 2–3 hours after dose.
Protamine sulfate	10 mg/ml	50 mg/dose	1 ml/min		1 mg for every 100 units heparin	Flush line.
Sodium bicarbonate	1 mEq/ml; 0.5 mEq/ml in neonates	100 mEq/dose	1–3 mEq/kg over 1–2 min		Dilute to at least 0.5 mEq/ml; administer as continuous infusion	

Table continued on following page

Guidelines for Administration of Intravenous Medications in Pediatric Patients (17 Years and Under) *Continued*

Generic Name	Initial Dilution	Maximum Dose	IV Push Administered by Critical Care RN		Intermittent or Continuous Infusion Recommended Rates/Further Dilution	Cautions and Comments
			IV Push Recommended Rate	Exceptions		
Sodium nitroprusside	50 mg/2 ml	8 μg/kg/min	NR		Dilute 200 μg/ml in D₅W; start with 0.1 μg/kg/min and titrate Further dilute any concentration over 3%	Observe for hypotension and extravasation. Protect solution from light.
Sodium salts	Varies	250 mEq/m²/day	NR		NR	
Succinylcholine chloride	20 mg/ml	200 mg	0.5–2 mg/kg over 10–30 sec	Critical care RN may give only if pt on ventilator or MD present	NR	Observe for bradycardia, hypotension, arrhythmias, and respiratory depression. Pretreat children with atropine.
Thiopental sodium	20–50 mg/ml	NI	3–5 mg/kg	Critical care RN may give only if pt on ventilator or MD present	Dilute to 2–4 mg/ml; infuse at 3–6 mg/kg/hour	Observe for respiratory depression, hemolysis, hypotension, and extravasation.
Ticarcillin disodium	1 g/4–10 ml	75 mg/kg/dose	1 g over 10 min		Minimum dilution 1 g/50 ml over 30–120 min	Observe for vein irritation, thrombophlebitis, and possible hypersensitivity reaction.
Tobramycin sulfate	40 mg/ml	2.5 mg/kg/dose	NR		25–50 ml over 20–60 min; adjust dilution for neonates	Observe for respiratory depression. Adjust dosage based on serum levels.

Tolazoline hydrochloride	25 mg/ml	NI	1–2 mg/kg over 10 min	Critical care RN may give only if MD present	1–2 mg/kg/hour	Monitor blood pressure. Observe for arrhythmias and tachycardia.
Trimethoprim (TMP)–sulfamethoxazole (SMX)	80 mg/5 ml TMP 400 mg/5 ml SMX	20 mg/kg/day TMP 100 mg/kg/day SMX	NR		Minimum dilution 5 ml in 50–60 ml D5W over 60 min	
Tromethamine	0.3 molar solution	33–40 ml/kg/day 500 mg/kg	3–5 ml/kg slowly		3–16 ml/kg/hour, up to 33–40 ml/kg/day	Observe for hypoglycemia, vein irritation, respiratory depression, and thrombophlebitis.
Tubocurarine	3 mg/ml	0.3 mg/kg/dose, up to 27 mg	60–90 sec	Critical care RN may give only if pt on ventilator	NR	Observe for hypotension.
Vancomycin	500 mg/10 ml	22 mg/kg/dose, up to 1 g; 5 mg/kg/dose in neonates	NR		Minimum dilution 2.5–5 mg/ml over 30–60 min	Observe for vein irritation and thrombophlebitis.
Vasopressin	20 units/ml	NI	20 units/100 ml over 10 min		100 units/500 ml; 0.2–0.4 unit/min	Monitor blood pressure. Observe for arrhythmias and abdominal pain.
Vidarabine	200 mg/ml	30 mg/kg/day	NR		Dilute 1 mg/2.2 ml over 12–24 hours (may need to warm to dissolve)	Observe for thrombophlebitis. Doses of 15 mg/kg/day increase chance of toxicity.

APPENDIX 2

A Partial Guide to Drug Compatibility*

This is a partial and simplified guide to common two-drug mixtures only. Physical and chemical incompatibilities such as precipitation or degradation are included. COMPATIBILITY MAY VARY WITH DILUENT, CONCENTRATION, OR TEMPERATURE; FOR THE COMPATIBILITY OF SPECIFIC MIXTURES, CONSULT A PHARMACIST. This information is based upon the data reported in the references listed below.

The key to using the table is as follows:

C = compatible for 6 hours or more

Numeral = number of hours compatible if less than 6 hours

Δ = data are inconsistent; variable compatibility depending on drug concentrations, large volume of parenteral diluent solution, age of admixture, etc.

I = incompatible

If the box is blank, no data available—DO NOT ASSUME COMPATIBILITY

Warning: The mixture of incompatible drugs may cause serious harm to the patient. Consult a pharmacist for specific cases and additional information.

REFERENCES

Bosso JA, Townsend RJ: Stability of clindamycin phosphate and ceftizoxime sodium, cefoxitin sodium, cefamandole nafate, or cefazolin sodium in two intravenous solutions. Am J Hosp Pharm 42:2211–2214, 1985.

Kiel D, et al: Visual compatibility of amrinone lactate with various IV secondary additives. Parenterals 3:1, 5–6, 1985.

Klamerus KJ, Ueda CT, Newton DW: Stability of nitroglycerin in intravenous admixtures. Am J Hosp Pharm 41:303–305, 1984.

Nahata MC, Durrel DE: Stability of tobramycin sulfate in admixtures with calcium gluconate. Am J Hosp Pharm 42:1987–1988, 1985.

Newton DW, Fung EXY, Williams DA: Stability of five catecholamines and terbutaline sulfate in 5% dextrose injection in the absence and presence of aminophylline. Am J Hosp Pharm 38:1314–1319, 1981.

Trisell LA: Handbook on Injectable Drugs, 3rd ed. Washington, DC, American Society of Hospital Pharmacists, 1983.

	Albumin	Amikacin	Amino Acids	Aminophylline	Amphotericin B	Ampicillin	Amrinone	Atropine	Bretylium	Bumetanide	Calcium Chloride	Calcium Gluconate	Carbenicillin	Cefamandole	Cefazolin	Cefotaxime	Cefoxitin	Ceftizoxime	Cephalothin	Chloramphenicol	Cimetidine	Clindamycin	Dexamethasone	Diazepam	Digoxin	Diphenhydramine	Dobutamine	Dopamine	Droperidol	Epinephrine	Erythromycin Lactobionate	Fat Emulsion	Furosemide	Gentamicin	Hetastarch
Albumin			C																																
Amikacin			C	I	I						C	C	C		C		C			I	C	C	C	C		C				C	Δ		Δ		
Amino Acids	C			C	I	Δ		Δ			C	C	C	C		C			C	C	C	C				C		C		C	C	C	C	C	
Aminophylline		C	C		Δ	C	C	C				C								I	C	I	I	I	C	C	C	C	I	C		I	C	C	C
Amphotericin B		I	I								I	I	I							I						Δ		I							I
Ampicillin	I	Δ	Δ				I				I	I	I	C		C					1	4	I						1		I	I	I	C	I
Amrinone			C					C	C		C									C						C	C	C		C				I	
Atropine			C		I	C			C	C									C	C	C					C	C	.25	C						
Bretylium			C			C					C	C												C		Δ	Δ	C							
Bumetanide																									I										
Calcium Chloride	C	Δ		I	I	C	C	C										I		I	C					C	C		I		Δ				
Calcium Gluconate	C	C	C	I	I		C	C						I	I				I	C		I	C		C	I			I		I		I		
Carbenicillin	C	C		I	C									C		I			I	C	C					C			I	I	I	C		I	
Cefamandole		C													I				C		I	C											C	I	
Cefazolin	C	C	C		C						I	I	C				C		C	I	C	C	C											I	
Cefotaxime																							C												
Cefoxitin	C	C											I					C		C	C													C	
Ceftizoxime											C	C		C						C															
Cephalothin	I	C	I			C					I	I								C	C	C				I		C		I	I	C		I	
Chloramphenicol	C	C	C	I		C		C	C	I		C							C				C	C	C		C		I	Δ	C				
Cimetidine	C	C	I	I	I	4	C	C			C	I	I	I		C		C			C	C	4	C	4	C			C	C			C	C	
Clindamycin	C	C	I		I					I	C	C	C	C	C	C	C	C		C														C	
Dexamethasone	C		C								C			C					C	C				I		I									
Diazepam			C															C			4	I			C	I				I			I		
Digoxin			C			C													C	C		C	C			Δ									
Diphenhydramine	C	C	C	Δ		C					C								I	C	4	I						.25		C	C	C	I		
Dobutamine		I			C	C	C	Δ	I	C	I								C			I	Δ			C	C		C				I		
Dopamine		C	C	I	I	C		C		C		C					C	C						C				C					C		
Droperidol						.25															.25														
Epinephrine	C	C	I		I	C	C		I	I	I						I	I	C			I			C				I						
Erythromycin Lactobionate	Δ	C	C		I							I							I	Δ	C				C									I	
Fat Emulsion		C	C		C						Δ	I	C	C					C	C					C						I				
Furosemide	Δ	C	C		I														C			I		I	I								I		
Gentamicin		C	C	I	I						I	I	I		C		I		C	C						C				I			I		
Hetastarch																																			
Heparin	I	C	C	C	C		4			4		C				C	C	C	C	4	I	C	4	Δ	C	4	4	I	C	4	I				
Hydralazine		I	I	I														C	C																
Hydrocortisone Phosphate	C		C	C		C				I							Δ	I								C	C				I	I			
Hydrocortisone Succinate	C	C	C	C	I	C	4		C	C	C				C	4	I	C	I		C	4	4	C		4									
Insulin (Regular)		C	I			C			C							C	C			I				C				C							
Isoproterenol		C	I		C			C	C	I			C			C	C			I			C												
Kanamycin		C	C	I	I	C				I	C		I		C		I	C		C	C			C		C					Δ				
Lidocaine	C	C	C	I	Δ	C		C		C	C	C	Δ	I		C		I	C	C	C	Δ	C	C	C	C		C	C			C			
Magnesium Sulfate	4	C		C					I	I	.25	.25	.25		.25		C	C		Δ			C					.25	I		.25				
Mannitol	C			C			C	I			C		C		C			C				C				C									
Metaraminol	C	C	C	I	I	C	C		C						C	C	C			I	I	C	C				C	I		I					
Methyldopa		C	C	I												C			C																
Methylprednisolone		C	C	Δ		C					C	C					Δ	C	C	C			I		C										
Metoclopramide		C		Δ		.25		Δ			I	I			I	I	C	C	C		C			.25		Δ									
Metronidazole	C	I	C	Δ						C	Δ	Δ		Δ		Δ	C	C	C						I							C			
Mezlocillin	I																																	I	
Morphine Sulfate	.25		I		4	C			.25	.25	.25	.25	.25	.25	.25	.25	4	.25			C	C		.25		.25							.25		
Moxalactam																																			
Multi-Vitamins	C	C	C	I		4		4			C	C	C	.25	.25		C		C	C	C	C	C	I	4	4		4	4	C	.25	C	4	C	
Nafcillin			Δ			C										C	C			C	C			C	I		I							I	
Netilmycin		C				C						I						C	C	C		C											I		
Nitroglycerin		C			C		C																C	C					C				C		
Nitroprusside						C													C																
Norepinephrine	C	C	I		I	C	C		C	C							Δ	C	C			I				C	C						I		
Oxacillin	C	C	I		C		C		C						C				C	C								C							

Heparin	Hydralazine	Hydrocortisone Phosphate	Hydrocortisone Succinate	Insulin (Regular)	Isoproterenol	Kanamycin	Lidocaine	Magnesium Sulfate	Mannitol	Metaraminol	Methyldopa	Methylprednisolone	Metoclopramide	Metronidazole	Mezlocillin	Morphine Sulfate	Moxalactam	Multi-Vitamins	Nafcillin	Netilmycin	Nitroglycerin	Nitroprusside	Norepinephrine	Oxacillin	Oxytocin	Penicillin G Potassium	Phenylephrine	Phenytoin	Phytonadione	Piperacillin	Potassium Chloride	Procainamide	Propranolol	Quinidine Gluconate	Ranitidine	Sodium Bicarbonate	Tetracycline	Thiamine	Ticarcillin	Tobramycin	Trimethaphan	Vancomycin	Vasopressin	Verapamil
																		C													C													I
I		C	C				C	4	C	C				C	I	.25		C					C	C	4	C		I	C	I	C					C	C	C		I			C		C
C			C	C	C	C	C	C		C	C	C		I				C		C			C	C	C	C	C		C		C					C	Δ	C	C		C				
C	I	C	C	I	I	C	C			C	C	C	C	C		I		I	Δ		C		I	I	C	I	C	I	I	C	C	C		I		C	I	I			I	I		C
C		C	C			I	I		C	I	I	Δ														I					I			I		I								I
C	I		I			I	Δ	C		I			Δ	Δ		4		4					I	C	4	C			I		C				C	I	I			I		C		C
			C		C		C			C		C									C	C	C				C				C	C				I								C
4		C	4			C				C			.25			C		4	C	C			C	C		C			C		4					I								C
				C			C		C												C							I			C	C		C		C								C
			C		C		C	I	I									C					C	C		C										Δ	I			I				C
4		I	C	C	C	I	C	I		C		C	Δ					C					C			C	C	C	C		C	C				I	I			C		C		C
			C		I	C	C	.25				C		C		.25		C		I					.25						C				C	C	I			I				C
							Δ	.25	C				I	Δ		.25		.25							.25						C				C					I				C
C						I	I	.25					I	Δ		.25		.25						C	C	C					C				C		I			I				C
																.25									.25																			C
						C	C	.25	C					Δ		.25		C							.25										4	C				C				C
																.25																				C	I							
C		Δ	C	C	C	I	I	C		C		Δ	I	Δ		.25		C					Δ	C	.25	C		I	I		C				4	C	I			I				
C		I	C			C	C	C		C	C	C	I	C		.25		C	C				C	C	C	C	C	I	C		C	C				C	I					I		C
C				C	C		C		C	C		C	C	C		4		C	C			C	C			C		I	C		C			C		C	C					C		C
C			C			C		Δ				C	C	C		.25		C		C					.25	C		I			C				C	C				C				C
4			4			C	C			I			C					C	C	C						C			C		4				C		C					I		C
I			I		I		Δ			I								I	C	C			I		Δ						I			I		I		I						C
C	C		C				C											4													C				C									C
4			I			C	C			C	C	I	C			C		4	C	C						C	C	I	C		4	C					C					C		
Δ	C			I	C		C	C		C						C			I		C		C				C	I			Δ	C	C			I								C
C			C			C	C		C			C		I				4			C		C	C		4					C					I	C							C
4			4										.25			.25		4	I												4												
4			4				C			C								C								I					4				C	I	I							C
I			C				C	.25		I			Δ			.25		.25							.25	C					C				C	C	I							C
C		C		C				I										C								C		I			Δ					C	I							
4			4			Δ				I								4		I	C		I								4			I	C		I	I		Δ				C
I		I					C	.25						C	I	.25		C	I						.25	C				I					C				I					C
	4	C	C	4	C	I	C	4		I	C	C	C	C		4		C	C				C	4	4	Δ	C	I	4	C	C	4	4	I		4	Δ			I	4	I		C
4			.25					Δ		C								4			C										4													Δ
C						I				C			C					I								C			I								I					I		C
C	.25			C	4	I	C	C		I	I			C		4		C	I	C			4	4	4	C		C	4	C	C	4	4			C	I				4	C		C
4			C				C	C					C					C								I		I	C		C				C	I								C
C			4				C	C										C		C											C				C	I	C							C
I		I	I					.25		C						.25		4							.25	C	C	I	C	I	C	C				I	C	I	I					
C			C	C	C					C			C				C	C			C		.25			C	C	I		C	C	C			C	Δ	C						C	C
4	Δ		C	C	C	.25					C		C	.25			.25	4	.25				C	.25	C	C			I	.25	4					I	.25		.25	I		.25		C
											I		C				C			C						C					I								C	C				C
I	C	C	I			C	C					I						C						I	C	I	C	I	C		C	C			I	C	C					C		C
C			I					C	I									C		C											C					C	Δ							C
C										I			C					I	I				C			C					C				C	C	I							C
C		C		C			C	C	C			C				C		C								I					C					I	Δ							C
C			C					.25								.25		C							.25	C																	
																				I																				I				
4			4			.25							C	.25			.25	4	.25					.25		.25		I		.25	4					I	I		.25	.25		.25		C
							C	.25	C							.25									.25						C													C
C	4	I	C	C	C	4	C	4		C	C	I	C	C		4			Δ	C			C	4	4	C	C	I	4	4	C	4	4		C	4	C	C	4		4	C		C
C			I					.25				I				.25		Δ					C		.25						C					C	I			Δ				Δ
			C		C				C		C				I			C					C		C				C	I	C	C				C			I					
	C						C																					I																C
																																			C									Δ
C			4				.25	C				C						C	C	C				I	I		C	I			C				C	I	C							C
4			4					.25		I						.25		4					I		.25	Δ					4						I			Δ				C

	Albumin	Amikacin	Amino Acids	Aminophylline	Amphotericin B	Ampicillin	Atropine	Bretylium	Bumetanide	Calcium Chloride	Calcium Gluconate	Carbenicillin	Cefamandole	Cefazolin	Cefotaxime	Ceftizoxime	Cephalothin	Chloramphenicol	Cimetidine	Clindamycin	Dexamethasone	Diazepam	Digoxin	Diphenhydramine	Dobutamine	Dopamine	Droperidol	Epinephrine	Erythromycin Lactobionate	Fat Emulsion	Furosemide	Gentamicin	Hetastarch
Oxytocin	4	C	C		4					.25	.25	C	.25	.25		.25	C			.25			Δ					.25			.25		
Penicillin G Potassium	C	C	I	I	C		C		C	C		C					C	C	C	C	C			C		4		I	C	C		C	
Phenylephrine		C	C		C				C										C							C	C						
Phenytoin	I		I				I		C								I	I	I	I				I	I					I			
Phytonadione	C	C	I		I		C		C								I	C	C		C			C									
Piperacillin	I		C																													I	
Potassium Chloride	C	C	C	C	I	C	C	4	C		C	C	C	C			C	C	C	C	4	I	C	4	Δ	C	4	4	C	Δ	4		
Procainamide			C			C	C		C								C									C	C						
Propanolol																											C						
Quinidine Gluconate			I					C										C				I									I		
Ranitidine	C	C		I	C					C	C	C			4		4	C	C		C							C	C		C	C	
Sodium Bicarbonate	C	Δ	C		I	I	I	I	C	Δ	I	C			C	C	C	C	C	C		I			I	I		I	C	C			
Tetracycline	C	C	I	I	I		I		I	I	I			I			I	I	I	C		C			C		C	I	I	I	I		
Thiamine		C	I																		I										I		
Ticarcillin	I																															I	
Tobramycin		C		I					I	C	I	I	I			C			I		C											Δ	
Trimethaphan			I																														
Vancomycin	C		I		C				C										I	C		I				C							
Vasopressin																																	
Verapamil	I	C		C	I	C	C	C	C	C	C	C	C	C	C	C		C	C	C	C	C	C		C	C		C	C		C	C	

Heparin	Hydralazine	Hydrocortisone Phosphate	Hydrocortisone Succinate	Insulin (Regular)	Isoproterenol	Kanamycin	Lidocaine	Magnesium Sulfate	Mannitol	Metaraminol	Methyldopa	Methylprednisolone	Metoclopramide	Metronidazole	Mezlocillin	Morphine Sulfate	Moxalactam	Multi-Vitamins	Nafcillin	Netilmycin	Nitroglycerin	Nitroprusside	Norepinephrine	Oxacillin	Oxytocin	Penicillin G Potassium	Phenylephrine	Phenytoin	Phytonadione	Piperacillin	Potassium Chloride	Procainamide	Propranolol	Quinidine Gluconate	Ranitidine	Sodium Bicarbonate	Tetracycline	Thiamine	Ticarcillin	Tobramycin	Trimethaphan	Vancomycin	Vasopressin	Verapamil
4			4		.25		C		C					.25		.25	4	.25	C			I	.25		C			C			C	.25	4					C		.25	.25		.25	C
Δ		C	C	I		C	C	C	C	I		C	I	C		.25		C					Δ	C		C	I	C		C	C			C	I	I			I		I		C
C						C	C			C						C					C			C			I	C		C					C	C					C			
I			C	I		I	I			I				I				I		I		I		I			I			I					I	I							I	Δ
4		I	4	C		C			I			C				4		C					C	C	C	I		C			C		C			C		C			I			
C			C			I	C	.25						.25		4		I					.25			C					C			C			I							
C	4		C	C	C	C	C	4	I	C	C	C	C		4	C	C	C	C		C	4	4	C	C	I	C	C		4	4		C	4	C	C		4	C			C	C
4			4			C	C			C						4		C						C		I		4								C					C		C	C
4			4													4												4									C	I						C
I																C																		C	I									C
		C	C		C			C			I		C					C			C	C				C			C			C	C						C					
4			C	I	I		I	Δ	I			C	C	C	I			I			4	C	C		I				I	C	I		C	4			I			I	I		I	Δ
Δ		I	I		C	C	C	.25		C	Δ	I	Δ			I		C	I			C	I		C	I	C	I	C		C	C			I				I				C	
						I										C										C							C					I						C
				I		.25	C									.25	4		I					.25								C							I					C
I							I	C								I	.25		Δ					Δ	.25	I			I				C						I					C
4			4													4												4								4			I					
I		I	C				.25		C							.25	C							.25	I	C	I	I		C	C			C	I	C							C
								C																																				C
C	Δ	C	C	C	C		C	C	C	C	C	C			C	C	C	Δ		C	Δ	C	C	C	C		Δ			C	C	C	C		Δ			C	C		C	C		

Subject Index

Note: Bold face page numbers refer to primary drug discussions. Page numbers in *italics* refer to illustrations. Page numbers followed by b refer to boxed material; page numbers followed by t refer to tables.